THE BEST
DOCTORS
IN
AMERICA

THE BEST DOCTORS IN AMERICA

STEVEN NAIFEH

AND

GREGORY WHITE SMITH

———

Lucienne Potterfield Stec

Senior Editor

———

1992-1993

WOODWARD / WHITE

Aiken, South Carolina

Copyright © 1992 by Woodward/White, Inc.
129 First Avenue, SW, Aiken, SC 29801
All rights reserved. This book, or parts thereof, must not be reproduced in any form without permission.

Designed by JOEL AVIROM

Library of Congress Cataloging-in-Publication Data

Naifeh, Steven W., 1952–
    The best doctors in America / Steven Naifeh and Gregory White
Smith ; Lucienne Potterfield Stec, senior editor.
        p.   cm.
    Includes index.
    ISBN 0-913391-05-0 : $60.00
    1. Physicians—North America—Directories.   I. Smith, Gregory
White.   II. Stec, Lucienne Potterfield.   III. Title.
        [DNLM: 1. Physicians—Canada—directories.   2. Physicians—United
States—directories.   W 22 AA1 N112b]
    R712.A1N25   1992
    610'.25'73—dc20
    DNLM/DLC
    for Library of Congress   92-223
                                                                                CIP

PRINTED IN THE UNITED STATES OF AMERICA

We would like to acknowledge our debt to the thousands of doctors who gave of their time and expertise in the process of compiling these lists.

INTRODUCTION

A fter two years of work and thousands of letters and telephone calls, Woodward/White, Inc., is proud to present the first edition of *The Best Doctors in America*. As difficult as the gestation has been, we have no doubt that it would have been longer, harder, and less fruitful, had it not been for the lessons learned from ten years of publishing our other, more familiar reference work, *The Best Lawyers in America*, now in its fourth edition and widely regarded as the premier referral list to the legal profession.

HOW THIS BOOK WAS COMPILED

The Best Doctors in America was compiled using the same rigorous, peer-review methodology that was developed for *Best Lawyers*. We began by contacting staff doctors at major medical facilities such as Johns Hopkins and the Mayo Clinic and asking them to name the best clinicians at their respective institutions. We then called the recommended doctors and asked them to nominate their most outstanding colleagues. We did not attempt to articulate the criteria for judging professional excellence; we left that to the individual physician. We did, however, routinely couch our inquiry in the following terms: "If you had a friend or loved one who needed a neurological surgeon (for example), and you couldn't perform the operation yourself, for whatever reason, to whom would you refer them?"

The rate of response was remarkable. Out of more than 11,000 telephone calls, only nine of the doctors we contacted refused to cooperate. Many of the respondents called back and shared their views at great length. Many asked if they could take some time to consider the question and get back to us. Others called back later with additional nominations. Although we did not seek official sanction from any national, local, general, or specialized medical associations, individual association officials were among our most cooperative respondents.

As with *Best Lawyers*, we were surprised, and pleased, by the candor of those we interviewed when asked to evaluate their professional colleagues. (Of course, we assured them that their comments would remain confidential.) Often the most difficult problem was to distinguish between doctors who engage primarly or almost exclusively in research and doctors who devote significant time and energy to clinical care. Many outstanding doctors are on the cutting edge of their fields because of their groundbreaking research, but because *Best Doctors* is intended primarily as a referral guide, we asked our respondents to avoid nominating doctors who rarely, if ever, see patients in a clinical setting.

From a few seed names, each list developed gradually into the form in which it appears here. We continued to call doctors on the lists, adding and removing names, until a clear consensus emerged. Many names received unanimous praise. Others earned mixed assessments. In those instances, decisions were made on a case-by-case basis. No name was ever removed from the list on the basis of a single negative vote, nor was any name added on the basis of a single nomination.

While we originally intended to restrict the listings to doctors who practice in the United States, it soon became clear that American doctors think of their Canadian colleagues as members of the same professional community. In the end, we decided to include any doctor to whom American doctors said they would readily recommend their patients. As a result, a substantial number of Canadian doctors are listed.

HOW THIS BOOK IS ORGANIZED

The book is organized alphabetically by field of expertise (see the table of contents for a complete list of fields). General fields of expertise are then subdivided into more specific areas of expertise. Within each field, the entries are arranged alphabetically by last name. Each entry includes the doctor's name; areas of further specialization (if any); academic title(s) and affiliation(s), if any; hospital title(s) and affiliation(s), if any; principal address; and telephone number.

It should be noted that the doctors in this book have been categorized according to the field of expertise in which they were nominated. The doctors themselves may or may not think of themselves as principally engaged in the area of medicine under which they are listed. Similarly, while many of the doctors are board certified in their listed areas of specialization (where such certification is available), some are not. Anyone interested in the certification status of a particular doctor should check with that doctor or the appropriate certifying body.

PREVIOUS DOCTOR REFERRAL GUIDES

In the last decade, several doctor referral guides have been published in the United States. *The Best Doctors in America* should not be confused with any of these previous publications.

THE EDITORS

The Best Doctors in America was edited by Steven Naifeh and Gregory White Smith, both graduates of the Harvard Law School and, between them, authors of fifteen books, including four national bestsellers. The most recent, *Jackson Pollock: An American Saga,* was a nonfiction finalist for the 1990 National Book Award and winner of the 1990 Pulitzer Prize for biography.

The Senior Editor on *The Best Doctors in America* was Lucienne Potterfield Stec. Ms. Stec was assisted by Kathryn White and Suzanne Arnold.

WOODWARD/WHITE REFERRAL SERVICE

In addition to publishing the referral guides, *The Best Doctors in America, The Best Lawyers in America,* and *The Best Lawyers in America: Directory of Experts,* Woodward/White, Inc., now offers to undertake specialized searches for doctors and lawyers using our unique access to sources of information on the best professionals in medicine and law. Prospective patients or clients who require a doctor or lawyer in a particular area of expertise or locale not represented in our books, or who wish assistance in refining the list of candidates, are welcome to write us at Woodard/White, Inc., 129 First Avenue, SW, Aiken, SC 29801, or call 803-648-0300.

PLEASE NOTE

If you are a patient using this book to find a specialist, we recommend that you ask your personal physician to make the initial contact. The specialists in this book are extremely busy and may have questions about your case that only your doctor can answer.

CONTENTS

ADDICTION MEDICINE

ALLERGY & IMMUNOLOGY

ANESTHESIOLOGY

CARDIOVASCULAR DISEASE

CLINICAL PHARMACOLOGY 46

COLON & RECTAL SURGERY

DERMATOLOGY

EATING DISORDERS

ENDOCRINOLOGY & METABOLISM

GASTROENTEROLOGY

GENERAL SURGERY

GERIATRIC MEDICINE

HAND SURGERY

INFECTIOUS DISEASE

MEDICAL ONCOLOGY

MEDICAL ONCOLOGY & HEMATOLOGY

NEPHROLOGY

NEUROLOGICAL SURGERY

NEUROLOGY, ADULT

NEUROLOGY, CHILD

NUCLEAR MEDICINE

OBSTETRICS & GYNECOLOGY

OPHTHALMOLOGY

ORTHOPAEDIC SURGERY

OTOLARYNGOLOGY

PATHOLOGY

PEDIATRICS

PHYSICAL MEDICINE & REHABILITATION

PLASTIC SURGERY

PSYCHIATRY

PULMONARY AND CRITICAL CARE MEDICINE

RADIATION ONCOLOGY

RADIOLOGY

RHEUMATOLOGY

SURGICAL ONCOLOGY

THORACIC SURGERY

UROLOGY

ADDICTION MEDICINE

ADDICTED PREGNANT WOMEN
(See also Pediatrics, Neonatal-Perinatal Medicine)

Elizabeth Ruth Brown · Associate Professor of Pediatrics, Boston University School of Medicine · Director of Neonatology, Boston City Hospital · 818 Harrison Avenue, Maternity 2, Boston, MA 02118 · 617-534-5461

Ira J. Chasnoff · President, National Association for Perinatal Addiction Research & Education, and Associate Professor of Pediatrics & Psychiatry, Northwestern University Medical School · Children's Memorial Hospital · 11 East Hubbard Street, Suite 200, Chicago, IL 60611 · 312-329-2512

Loretta P. Finnegan · (Addicted Pregnant Women & Their Children) · Professor of Pediatrics, Psychiatry and Human Behavior, Jefferson Medical College of Thomas Jefferson University · Senior Advisor on Women's Issues, National Institute on Drug Abuse · 5600 Fishers Lane, Rockwell 2, Suite 615, Rockville, MD 20857 · 301-443-2158

Sidney H. Schnoll · Professor of Internal Medicine and Psychiatry, Virginia Commonwealth University, Medical College of Virginia · Chairman, Division of Substance Abuse Medicine, Medical College of Virginia Hospitals · 1200 East Broad Street, Box 109, Richmond, VA 23298-0109 · 804-786-9914

Robert J. Sokol · (Fetal-Alcohol Syndrome) · Dean, School of Medicine, and Professor of Obstetrics & Gynecology, Wayne State University Medical Center · Chairman of the Medical Board, Detroit Medical Center · 540 East Canfield, Detroit, MI 48201 · 313-577-1335

James R. Woods · (High-Risk Pregnancies) · Professor of Obstetrics & Gynecology, University of Rochester School of Medicine & Dentistry · Associate Chair, Department of Obstetrics & Gynecology, and Director of Obstetrics & Maternal & Fetal Medicine, Strong Memorial Hospital, University of Rochester Medical Center · 601 Elmwood Avenue, Box 668, Rochester, NY 14642 · 716-275-7824

Margaret Lynn Yonekura · Associate Professor of Obstetrics & Gynecology, University of California at Los Angeles School of Medicine · Harbor-UCLA Medical Center · 1000 West Carson Street, Box 3, Torrance, CA 90509 · 213-533-3565

GENERAL ADDICTION MEDICINE

LeClair Bissell · 1932 Woodring Road, Sanibel, FL 33957 · 813-472-5484

Jess W. Bromley · Physicians Community Hospital · 433 Estudillo Avenue, Suite 308, San Leandro, CA 94577 · 510-357-1150

Anne Geller · Chief, Smithers Alcoholism Treatment & Training Center, St. Luke's-Roosevelt Hospital Center · 428 West 59th Street, New York, NY 10019 212-523-6914

Stanley Gitlow · Clinical Professor of Medicine, Mt. Sinai School of Medicine · Attending Physician, Mt. Sinai Hospital · 1136 Fifth Avenue, New York, NY 10128 · 212-722-5731

Mark S. Gold · Professor of Psychiatry, University of Florida College of Medicine P.O. Box 100244, Gainesville, FL 32610 · 904-392-3383

David C. Lewis · Professor of Medicine and Community Health, and Director, Center for Alcohol & Addiction Studies, Brown University School of Medicine · Roger Williams General Hospital · Box G, Providence, RI 02912 · 401-863-1109

Alfonso J. Mooney III · Director, Willingway Hospital · 311 Jones Mill Road, Statesboro, GA 30458 · 912-764-6236

Anthony B. Radcliffe · Physician-in-Charge, Kaiser Permanente Chemical Dependency Recovery Program · 17046 Marygold Avenue, Fontana, CA 92335 · 714-427-5128

Max A. Schneider · Clinical Associate Professor of Psychiatry, University of California at Irvine School of Medicine · Medical Director of Family Recovery Services, St. Joseph Hospital of Orange · 3311 East Kirkwood Avenue, Orange, CA 92669 · 714-771-8080

David E. Smith · (Clinical Toxicology) · Associate Clinical Professor of Occupational Health and Clinical Toxicology, University of California at San Francisco School of Medicine; Honorary Lecturer, Addiction Research Foundation, Clinical Institute, Toronto, Canada; Visiting Clinical Professor of Behavioral Pharmacology, University of Nevada Medical School; Lecturer on Substance Abuse, University of California at Berkeley-University of California at San Francisco Joint Medical School Program · Founder and Medical Director, Haight-Ashbury Free

Clinic; Research Director, Merritt-Peralta Chemical Dependence Recovery Hospital · 409 Clayton Street, San Francisco, CA 94117 · 415-565-1900

Barry Stimmel · Professor of Medicine & Medical Education, and Dean, Academic Affairs, Admissions & Student Affairs, Mt. Sinai School of Medicine · Professor of Medicine & Medical Education, Mt. Sinai Medical Center · One Gustave L. Levy Place, Box 1255, New York, NY 10029 · 212-241-6694

Douglas G. Talbott · Corporate Medical Director, Georgia Alcohol & Drug Associates · 1669 Phoenix Parkway, Stuie 102, Atlanta, GA 30349 · 404-994-0185

MEDICAL TREATMENT FOR DRUG ABUSERS

Frank H. Gawin · Associate Clinical Professor of Psychiatry, University of California at Los Angeles School of Medicine · Director, Substance Abuse Research, Medications Development Unit, Veterans Administration Hospital, Brentwood Division · 760 Westwood Plaza, Los Angeles, CA 90024 · 213-478-3711 x2861

Donald R. Jasinski · Associate Professor, Department of Medicine, Johns Hopkins University School of Medicine · Chief, Center for Chemical Dependence, Francis Scott Key Medical Center · 4940 Eastern Avenue, OPD Room 101, Baltimore, MD 21224 · 301-550-1906

Jack H. Mendelson · Professor of Psychiatry (Neuroscience), Harvard Medical School · Director, Substance Abuse Program, and Co-Director, Alcohol & Drug Abuse Research Center, McLean Hospital · 115 Mill Street, Belmont, MA 02178 617-855-2716

Edward M. Sellers · Professor of Pharmacology and Medicine and Psychiatry, University of Toronto School of Medicine · Director, Clinical Research & Treatment Institute, Addiction Research Foundation · 33 Russell Street, Toronto, Ontario M5S 2S1 · 416-595-6119

Donald Wesson · 8447 Wilshire Boulevard, Beverly Hills, CA 90211 · 213-655-3258

ALLERGY & IMMUNOLOGY

ADULT ALLERGY & IMMUNOLOGY

N. Franklin Adkinson, Jr. · (Drug Allergy) · Professor of Medicine, Johns Hopkins University School of Medicine · Co-Director, Division of Allergy & Clinical Immunology, The Johns Hopkins Medical Institutions; Good Samaritan Hospital Johns Hopkins Asthma and Allergy Center, 5501 Hopkins Bayview Circle, Baltimore, MD 21224-6801 · 410-550-2051

Emil J. Bardana, Jr. · (Occupational and Environmental Hypersensitivity Diseases) · Professor of Medicine and Vice Chairman, Department of Medicine, Oregon Health Sciences University · Head, Division of Allergy & Clinical Immunology, Oregon Health Sciences University · 3181 Southwest Sam Jackson Park Road; L-329, Portland, OR 97201-3098 · 503-494-8531

I. Leonard Bernstein · (Asthma) · Clinical Professor of Medicine, and Co-Director, The Allergy Training & Research Program, University of Cincinnati College of Medicine · Director, Asthma & Allergy Treatment Center, Deaconess Hospital; Jewish Hospital; University of Cincinnati Hospital · 8464 Winton Road, Cincinnati, OH 45231 · 513-931-0775

Malcolm N. Blumenthal · (Genetics of Allergy) · Clinical Professor of Medicine, University of Minnesota School of Medicine · Director, Section of Allergy, University of Minnesota Hospital & Clinics · 420 Delaware Street, SE, Box 434 UMHC, Minneapolis, MN 55455 · 612-624-5456

Robert K. Bush · Professor of Medicine, Section of Allergy & Clinical Immunology, University of Wisconsin-Madison School of Medicine · Chief of Allergy, William S. Middleton Memorial Veterans Hospital; University of Wisconsin Hospital & Clinics · 600 Highland Avenue, Room H6-367, Madison, WI 53792 · 608-263-6174

William W. Busse · (Asthma) · Professor of Medicine, University of Wisconsin-Madison School of Medicine · Head, Allergy/Clinical Immunology, University of Wisconsin Hospital & Clinics · 600 Highland Avenue, Room H6/360, Madison, WI 53792 · 608-263-6183

John J. Condemi · (Allergy) · Clinical Professor of Medicine, University of Rochester School of Medicine & Dentistry · Strong Memorial Hospital; University of Rochester Medical Center; Genesee Valley Medical Center · 919 West Fall Road, Rochester, NY 14618 · 716-442-0150

Max D. Cooper · (Immunodeficiency) · Professor of Medicine, Pediatrics and Microbiology, The University of Alabama School of Medicine · Director, Division of Developmental & Clinical Immunology, The University of Alabama at Birmingham Hospital; The Children's Hospital of Birmingham · 1824 Sixth Avenue South, Tumor Institute, Room 263, Birmingham, AL 35294 · 205-934-3370

Peter S. Creticos · (Pharmacotherapy, Immunotherapy) · Medical Director, Asthma & Allergic Diseases, and Associate Professor of Medicine, Johns Hopkins University School of Medicine · The Johns Hopkins Medical Institutions · Johns Hopkins Asthma & Allergy Center, 301 Bayview Boulevard, Suite 2B.57B, Baltimore, MD 21224 · 410-550-2112

Charlotte Cunningham-Rundles · (Immunodeficiency) · Associate Professor of Medicine/Pediatrics, Mt. Sinai School of Medicine · Mt. Sinai Medical Center · One Gustave L. Levy Place, Annenberg 20332, New York, NY 10029 · 212-241-4014

Murray Dworetzky · (Allergy) · Clinical Professor of Medicine, Cornell University Medical College · The New York Hospital-Cornell Medical Center · 115 East 61st Street, New York, NY 10021 · 212-838-3421

Jordan N. Fink · Professor of Medicine, and Chief, Allergy & Immunology Division, Medical College of Wisconsin · Medical College of Wisconsin Affiliated Hospitals · 8700 West Wisconsin Avenue, Room 253, Milwaukee, WI 53226 · 414-257-6095

Edward J. Goetzl · (Allergy) · Robert L. Kroc Professor of Medicine and Microbiology, University of California at San Francisco School of Medicine · Director, Allergy & Immunology, University of California at San Francisco Medical Center 533 Parnassus Avenue, Box 0724, San Francisco, CA 94143-0724 · 415-476-6725

David Bryant K. Golden · (Insect Hypersensitivity) · Assistant Professor of Medicine, Johns Hopkins University School of Medicine · Sinai Hospital; The Johns Hopkins Medical Institutions; Franklin Square Hospital · 7939 Honeygo Boulevard, Suite 228, Baltimore, MD 21236 · 410-931-0404

Robert A. Good · (Immunodeficiency) · Professor and Chairman, Department of Pediatrics/St. Petersburg, University South Florida College of Medicine · Physician-in-Chief, All Children's Hospital · 801 Sixth Street South, St. Petersburg, FL 33701 · 813-892-4470

J. Andrew Grant · Professor of Medicine and Microbiology, The University of Texas Medical Branch at Galveston · Director of Adult Allergy, and Vice-Chairman for Research, The University of Texas Medical Branch at Galveston · Clinical Sciences Building 409, Ninth And Market Streets, Route G-62, Galveston, TX 77550 · 409-772-3411

Paul Allen Greenberger · Professor of Medicine, Northwestern University Medical School · Northwestern Memorial Hospital · 303 East Chicago Avenue—Tarry 3-705, Chicago, IL 60611 · 312-908-8171

Michael Henry Grieco · (Infectious Diseases, Immunodeficiency, AIDS) · Professor of Clinical Medicine, College of Physicians & Surgeons of Columbia University · Chief, Division of Allergy, Clinical Immunology and Infectious Diseases, St. Luke's-Roosevelt Hospital Center · 25 Central Park West, New York, NY 10023 · 212-974-0766

Michael Aron Kaliner · (Asthma) · Head, Allergic Diseases, National Institute of Allergy & Infectious Disease, National Institutes of Health · 9000 Rockville Pike, Building 10, Room 11C205, Washington, DC 20892 · 301-496-9314

Allen Phillip Kaplan · Professor and Chairman, Department of Medicine, State University of New York Health Science Center at Stony Brook · SUNY at Stony Brook Hospital · Health Sciences Center, T-16, Room 020, Stony Brook, NY 11794-8160 · 516-444-2066

Phillip L. Lieberman · Clinical Professor of Medicine and Pediatrics, Department of Medicine, Division of Allergy & Immunology, The University of Tennessee at Memphis, College of Medicine · Chief of Allergy-Immunology, Baptist Memorial Hospital · 920 Madison Avenue, Suite 909N, Memphis, TN 38103 · 901-527-3954

Richard F. Lockey · (Insect Hypersensitivity, Fire Ant Allergy) · Professor of Medicine, Pediatrics and Public Health, University South Florida College of Medicine · Director, Division of Allergy & Immunology, James A. Haley Veterans Hospital; Tampa General Hospital; Moffitt Cancer Research Hospital; University Community Hospital · 13000 Bruce B. Downs Boulevard, Tampa, FL 33612 · 813-972-7631

Samuel R. Marney · (Asthma, Urticaria) · Associate Professor of Medicine, Department of Internal Medicine, Vanderbilt University School of Medicine · Director of Allergy & Immunology, Vanderbilt University Medical Center · Vanderbilt Allergy Center, The Village at Vanderbilt, 1500 Twenty-First Avenue South, Suite 3500, Nashville, TN 37212 · 615-322-7424

David A. Mathison · (Asthma) · Senior Consultant, Allergy & Immunology, Scripps Clinic & Research Foundation · 10666 North Torrey Pines Road, La Jolla, CA 92037 · 619-554-8616

Harold S. Nelson · (Asthma) · Professor of Medicine, University of Colorado School of Medicine · Senior Staff Physician, National Jewish Center for Immunology & Respiratory Medicine · 1400 Jackson Street, Denver, CO 80206 · 303-398-1562

Philip S. Norman · Professor of Medicine, Johns Hopkins University School of Medicine · Johns Hopkins Asthma & Allergy Center at Francis Scott Key Medical Center · 301 Bayview Boulevard, 2B-71, Baltimore, MD 21212 · 301-550-2101

John L. Ohman, Jr. · Associate Clinical Professor of Medicine, Tufts University School of Medicine · Director, Allergy Unit, New England Medical Center · Five Longfellow Place, Suite 211, Boston, MA 02114-2837 · 617-742-3440

Roy Patterson · Chairman, Department of Allergy & Immunology, Northwestern University Medical School · Northwestern Memorial Hospital · 303 East Chicago Avenue, Chicago, IL 60611 · 312-908-8171

Charles E. Reed · (Asthma) · Professor of Medicine, Mayo Medical School · Mayo Clinic · Division of Allergy & Immunology, 200 First Street, SW, Rochester, MN 55902 · 507-284-2511

Robert E. Reisman · Clinical Professor of Medicine and Pediatrics, State University of New York Health Science Center at Buffalo · Physician, Buffalo General Hospital; Attending Allergist, Buffalo Children's Hospital · 50 High Street, Buffalo, NY 14203 · 716-884-0100

Hal B. Richerson · Professor of Medicine, The University of Iowa College of Medicine · Head, Division of Allergy & Immunology, The University of Iowa Hospitals & Clinics · 200 Hawkins Drive, Iowa City, IA 52242 · 319-356-2117

Stephen I. Rosenfeld · (Rheumatology) · Clinical Professor, Department of Medicine, University of Rochester School of Medicine & Dentistry · Strong Memorial Hospital, University of Rochester Medical Center · 919 Westfall Road, Rochester, NY 14618 · 716-442-0150

Lanny J. Rosenwasser · Professor of Medicine, University of Colorado School of Medicine · Head, Division of Allergy & Clinical Immunology, National Jewish Center for Immunology & Respiratory Medicine · 1400 Jackson Street, Denver, CO 80206 · 303-398-1656

John E. Salvaggio · (Asthma) · Henderson Professor of Medicine, and Vice Chancellor for Research, Tulane University School of Medicine · Tulane University Medical Center · 1700 Perdido Street, Room 305, New Orleans, LA 70112 · 504-588-5228

Andrew Saxon · (Immunodeficiency) · Professor of Medicine, and Chief of Division of Allergy & Immunology, University of California at Los Angeles School of Medicine · University of California at Los Angeles Medical Center · 10833 Le Conte Avenue, Room 52-175CHS, Los Angeles, CA 90024-1680 · 310-825-3718

Michael Schatz · (Asthma, Pregnancy and Asthma) · Associate Clinical Professor of Medicine and Pediatrics, University of California at San Diego School of Medicine · Staff Allergist, Kaiser Permanente · 7060 Claremont-Mesa Boulevard, San Diego, CA 92111 · 619-268-5484

Howard J. Schwartz · Clinical Professor of Medicine, Case Western Reserve University School of Medicine · Associate Physician, and Chief, Adult Allergy Clinic, University Hospitals of Cleveland · University Suburban Health Center, 1611 South Green Road, Cleveland, OH 44121 · 216-381-3333

John C. Selner · Clinical Professor of Pediatrics, University of Colorado School of Medicine · The Children's Hospital · 5800 East Evans Avenue, Denver, CO 80222 · 303-756-3614, 757-4507

Albert L. Sheffer · (Asthma) · Clinical Professor, Harvard Medical School · Brigham & Women's Hospital · 110 Francis Street, Suite 6C, Boston, MA 02115 617-731-3440

Raymond G. Slavin · Professor of Internal Medicine and Microbiology, St. Louis University School of Medicine · Director, Divison of Allergy & Immunology, St. Louis University Medical Center · 1402 South Grand Boulevard, Suite R209, St. Louis, MO 63104-1028 · 314-577-8456

William R. Solomon · Professor of Internal Medicine, The University of Michigan Medical School · Chief, Division of Allergy, The University of Michigan Medical Center · 1500 East Medical Center Drive, Box 0380, Ann Arbor, MI 48109-0380 · 313-936-5634

Sheldon L. Spector · (Asthma) · Clinical Professor of Medicine, University of California at Los Angeles School of Medicine · University of California at Los Angeles Medical Center · 11645 Wilshire Boulevard, Suite 600, Los Angeles, CA 90025 · 213-312-5050

Daniel J. Stechschulte · Professor of Medicine, University of Kansas School of Medicine · University of Kansas Medical Center · Rainbow Boulevard & 39th Street, Kansas City, KS 66103 · 913-588-6008

Donald D. Stevenson · (Asthma, Aspirin Sensitivity) · Senior Consultant, Division of Allergy & Immunology, and Chairman, Department of Medicine, Scripps Clinic & Research Foundation · Ida & Cecil Green Hospital of Scripps Clinic · 10666 North Torrey Pines Road, La Jolla, CA 92037 · 619-455-9100, 554-8614

Timothy J. Sullivan · Chief, Allergy & Immunology Division, The University of Texas Southwestern Medical Center at Dallas · Head, Formulary Committee, Parkland Memorial Hospital · 5323 Harry Hines Boulevard, Dallas, TX 75235-8859 · 214-688-3004

Abba I. Terr · (Allergy) · Professor of Medicine, Stanford University School of Medicine · Director, Allergy Clinic, Stanford University Hospital · 450 Sutter Street, Number 2534, San Francisco, CA 94108 · 415-433-7800

Robert Gordon Townley · (Asthma) · Professor of Medicine & Microbiology, Creighton University School of Medicine · St. Joseph's Hospital · 601 North 30th Street, Omaha, NE 68131-2197 · 402-280-4180

Thomas A. Waldmann · (Immunodeficiency) · Chief, Metabolism Branch, National Cancer Institute, National Institutes of Health · 9000 Rockville Pike, Building 10, Room 4N115, Bethesda, MD 20892 · 301-496-6653

Stephen I. Wasserman · Professor and Chair, Department of Medicine, University of California at San Diego School of Medicine · Chief, Division of Allergy, University of California at San Diego Medical Center · 402 Dickinson Street, Suite 380, San Diego, CA 92103 · 619-543-6170

Betty B. Wray · Professor and Vice-Chairman, Department of Pediatrics, and Professor of Medicine, and Chief, Section of Allergy & Immunology, Medical College of Georgia · 1120 Fifteenth Street, Room CJ141, Augusta, GA 30912 · 404-721-3531

John W. Yunginger · Professor of Pediatrics, Mayo Medical School · Mayo Clinic 200 First Street, SW, Rochester, MN 55905 · 507-284-3454

Chester Raymound Zeiss, Jr. · Professor of Medicine, Northwestern University Medical School · Associate Chief of Staff, Veterans Affairs Lakeside Medical Center · 400 East Ontario, Chicago, IL 60611 · 312-943-6600 x511

Burton Zweiman · Professor of Medicine and Neurology, University of Pennsylvania School of Medicine · Chief, Allergy & Immunology, Hospital of the University of Pennsylvania · 512 Johnson Pavilion, University of Pennsylvania School of Medicine, Philadelphia, PA 19104 · 215-662-2425

PEDIATRIC ALLERGY & IMMUNOLOGY

John Albert Anderson · (Allergy) · Clinical Professor of Pediatrics, The University of Michigan Medical School · Head, Division of Allergy & Immunology, Department of Medicine, Henry Ford Medical Center · 2799 West Grand Boulevard, Detroit, MI 48202 · 313-876-2662

Bernard A. Berman · (Asthma) · Associate Clinical Professor of Pediatrics, Tufts University School of Medicine · St. Elizabeth Hospital · 1714 Beacon Street, Brookline, MA 02146 · 617-738-1700

C. Warren Bierman · (Allergy, Asthma) · Clinical Professor of Pediatrics, University of Washington School of Medicine · Director, Division of Allergy, Children's Hospital & Medical Center · 4540 Sand Point Way NE, Suite 200, Seattle, WA 98105 · 206-527-1200

Robert Michael Blaese · (Immunodeficiency) · Chief, Cellular Immunology Section, and Deputy Chief, Metabolism Branch, National Cancer Institute, National Institutes of Health · Senior Attending Physician, Warren Grant Magnuson Clinical Center, National Institutes of Health · 9000 Rockville Pike, Building 10, Room 6B05, Bethesda, MD 20892 · 301-496-5396

Jerome M. Buckley · (Allergy) · Clinical Associate Professor, Department of Pediatrics, University of Colorado School of Medicine · Colorado Allergy & Asthma Clinic · 1450 S. Havana Street, Suite 500, Aurora, CO 80012 · 303-755-5070

Rebecca Buckley · (Immunodeficiency) · J. Buren Siddury Professor of Pediatrics, and Professor of Immunology, and Chief, Division of Pediatric Allergy & Immunology, Duke University School of Medicine · Duke University Medical Center · Box 2898, DUMC, Durham, NC 27710 · 919-684-5194

Joseph A. Church · (Pediatric AIDS) · Professor of Clinical Pediatrics, University of Southern California School of Medicine · Clinical Director, Children's Aids Center, Children's Hospital Los Angeles · 4650 Sunset Boulevard, Los Angeles, CA 90027 · 213-669-2501

Max D. Cooper · (Immunodeficiency) · Professor of Medicine, Pediatrics and Microbiology, The University of Alabama School of Medicine · Director, Division of Developmental & Clinical Immunology, The University of Alabama at Birmingham Hospital; The Children's Hospital of Birmingham · 1824 Sixth Avenue South, Tumor Institute, Room 263, Birmingham, AL 35294 · 205-934-3370

William J. Davis · (Allergy) · College of Physicians & Surgeons of Columbia University · Director, Division of Allergy, Columbia-Presbyterian Medical Center, Babies Hospital · 3959 Broadway, Suite 107 North, New York, NY 10032 · 212-305-2300

Peyton Eggleston · (Asthma) · Associate Professor of Pediatrics, Johns Hopkins University School of Medicine · The Johns Hopkins Medical Institutions · Childrens Medical and Surgical Center, 600 North Wolfe Street, Room 1103, Baltimore, MD 21205 · 410-955-5883

Elliot F. Ellis · (Allergy) · Chief, Allergy & Immunology Division, Nemours Children's Clinic · 807 Nira Street, Jacksonville, FL 32207 · 904-390-3788

Richard Evans III · Professor of Clinical Pediatrics & Clinical Medicine, Northwestern University Medical School · The Children's Memorial Hospital · Department of Allergy, 2300 North Children's Plaza, Chicago, IL 60614 · 312-880-4920

Philip Fireman · (Allergy, Asthma) · Professor of Pediatrics, University of Pittsburgh School of Medicine · Director, Allergy, Immunology & Rheumatology, Children's Hospital of Pittsburgh · 3705 Fifth Avenue, Pittsburgh, PA 15213 · 412-692-5080

Thomas Joseph Fischer · University of Cincinnati College of Medicine · Acting Director, Division of Allergy/Immunology, Children's Hospital Medical Center Group Health Associates, 8245 Northcreek Drive, Cincinnati, OH 45236 · 513-745-4792

Oscar L. Frick · (Allergy) · Professor of Pediatrics, University of California at San Francisco School of Medicine · Director, Allergy & Immunology Research & Training, University of California at San Francisco Medical Center · 505 Parnassus Avenue, Box 0546, San Francisco, CA 94143-0546 · 415-476-3148

Clifton T. Furakawa · Clinical Professor of Pediatrics, University of Washington School of Medicine · Children's Hospital & Medical Center · 4540 Sand Point Way NE, Seattle, WA 98105 · 206-527-1200

Raif S. Geha · (Immunodeficiency) · The Prince Turki bin Abdul Aziz Al-Saud Professor of Pediatrics, Harvard Medical School · Chief, Division of Immunology, Children's Hospital · The Enders Building, Room 809, 300 Longwood Avenue, Boston, MA 02115 · 617-735-7602

Erwin W. Gelfand · (Immunodeficiency) · Vice-Chairman and Professor of Pediatrics and Microbiology/Immunology, University of Colorado Health Services Center · Chairman of Pediatrics, National Jewish Center for Immunology & Respiratory Medicine · 1400 Jackson Street, Denver, CO 80206 · 303-398-1196

John W. Georgitis · (Allergy) · Associate Professor of Pediatrics, and Director, Allergy, Immunology & Pediatric Pulmonology, The Bowman Gray School of Medicine of Wake Forest University · North Carolina Baptist Hospital · Medical Center Boulevard, Winston-Salem, NC 27157-1081 · 919-748-4431

Robert A. Good · (Immunodeficiency) · Professor and Chairman, Department of Pediatrics/St. Petersburg, University South Florida College of Medicine · Physician-in-Chief, All Children's Hospital · 801 Sixth Street South, St. Petersburg, FL 33701 · 813-892-4470

David F. Graft · University of Minnesota School of Medicine · Rochester Methodist Hospital · 5000 West 39th Street, Minneapolis, MN 55416 · 612-927-3090

Harry R. Hill · (Immunodeficiency, Neutrophil Deficiencies) · Professor of Pathology and Pediatrics, University of Utah School of Medicine · Head, Divison of Clinical Immunology & Allergy, University of Utah Health Sciences Center · 5B114, Department of Pathology, 50 North Medical Drive, Salt Lake City, UT 84132 · 801-581-5873

Bettina C. Hilman · (Cystic Fibrosis, Allergy) · Professor of Pediatrics, Louisiana State University School of Medicine · Louisiana State University Medical Center; Schumpert Medical Center · 1501 Kings Highway, 33932, Shreveport, LA 71130-3932 · 318-674-6094

Richard Hong · (Immunodeficiency, General) · Professor of pediatrics, University of Wisconsin-Madison School of Medicine · University of Wisconsin Children's Hospital · 600 Highland Avenue, Madison, WI 53792-4678 · 608-263-6201

Roger M. Katz · (Allergy) · Clinical Professor, Department of Pediatrics, University of California at Los Angeles School of Medicine · Attending Physician, UCLA Medical Center, Santa Monica Medical Center, Cedar-Sinai Medical Center · 11620 Wilshire Boulevard, Suite 200, Los Angeles, CA 90025 · 310-312-5050

James P. Kemp · Clinical Professor of Pediatrics/Allergy, University of California at San Diego School of Medicine · Allergy & Asthma Medical Group & Research Center · 3444 Kearny Villa Road, Suite 100, San Diego, CA 92123 · 619-292-1144

Allen Lapey · (Cystic Fibrosis, Allergy) · Clinical Assistant Professor of Pediatrics, Harvard Medical School · Associate Pediatrician, and Center Director, Center for Cystic Fibrosis Care & Research, and Director, Pediatric Allergy & Respiratory Disease, Massachusetts General Hospital · 15 Parkman Street, ACC Building, 709, Boston, MA 02114 · 617-726-8707

Robert F. Lemanske · (Asthma, Allergic Diseases) · Associate Professor of Medicine and Pediatrics, University of Wisconsin School of Medicine · University of Wisconsin Hospital & Clinics · 600 Highland Avenue, Room H6362, Madison, WI 53792 · 608-263-6184

Donald Y. M. Leung · (Allergy, Kawasaki Disease) · Professor of Medicine, Head, Division of Pediatric Allergy & Immunology, National Jewish Center for Immunology & Respiratory Medicine · 1400 Jackson Street, Room K-926, Denver, CO 80206-1997 · 303-398-1379

Eli Owen Meltzer · (Allergy, Asthma) · Adjunct Professor, School of Health & Human Services, San Diego State University; Clinical Professor of Pediatrics, Division of Allergy & Immunology, University of California at San Diego School of Medicine · Chief, Division of Allergy & Immunology, Children's Hospital & Health Center · 3444 Kearny Villa Road, Suite 100, San Diego, CA 92123 · 619-292-1144

Harold S. Nelson · (Asthma) · Professor of Medicine, University of Colorado School of Medicine · Senior Staff Physician, National Jewish Center for Immunology & Respiratory Medicine · 1400 Jackson Street, Denver, CO 80206 · 303-398-1562

Hans D. Ochs · (Immunodeficiency) · Professor, Department of Pediatrics, University of Washington School of Medicine · Department of Pediatrics, Mail Stop RD-20, Seattle, WA 98195 · 206-543-3207

Dennis Randall Ownby · Clinical Associate Professor of Pediatrics & Communicable Diseases, The University of Michigan Medical School · Director, Allergy Research Laboratory, Henry Ford Medical Center · 2799 West Grand Boulevard, Detroit, MI 48202-2689 · 313-876-2659

Henry F. Pabst · (Immunodeficiency) · Professor of Pediatrics, University of Alberta · Walter C. Mackenzie Health Sciences Center · 8440 One Hundred Twelfth Street, Room 2C361, Edmonton, Alberta T6G 2R7 · 403-492-4023

Savita G. Pahwa · (Immunodeficiency) · Professor of Pediatrics, Cornell University Medical College · Chief, Division of Allergy/Immunology, Department of Pediatrics, North Shore University Hospital · Research Building, 350 Community Drive, Third Floor, Manhasset, NY 11030 · 516-562-4641

David S. Pearlman · (Allergy) · Clinical Professor of Pediatrics, University of Colorado School of Medicine · Colorado Allergy & Asthma Clinic · 1450 S. Havana Street, Suite 500, Aurora, CO 80012 · 303-755-5070

William E. Pierson · (Allergy, Asthma) · University of Washington School of Medicine · Northwest Asthma & Allergy Center · 4540 Sand Point Way NE, Seattle, WA 29105-3914 · 206-527-1200

Stephen H. Polmar · (Immunodeficiency) · Visiting Professor of Pediatrics, Harvard Medical School · Associate Chief, Division of Immunology of the Department of Medicine, Children's Hospital · 300 Longwood Avenue, Boston, MA 02115 · 617-735-6117

Gary S. Rachelefsky · (Allergy, Asthma) · Clinical Professor, Department of Pediatrics, University of California at Los Angeles School of Medicine · University of California at Los Angeles Medical Center · 11645 Wilshire Boulevard, Suite 600, Los Angeles, CA 90025 · 310-312-5050

Fred Rosen · (Pediatric Immunology, Immunodeficiency) · James L. Gamble Professor of Pediatrics, and President, Center for Blood Research, Harvard Medical School · Senior Associate, Allergy & Immunology, Children's Hospital · Center for Blood Research, 800 Hungtington Avenue, Boston, MA 02115 · 617-731-6470

Arye Rubinstein · (Immunodeficiency, AIDS) · Professor of Pediatrics, Microbiology & Immunology, Albert Einstein College of Medicine · Director, Division of Allergy & Immunology, Albert Einstein University Hospital · 25 Astor Place, Monsey, NY 10952 · 212-430-4227

Hugh A. Sampson · (Food Allergy, Atopic Dermatitis) · Associate Professor of Pediatrics, Johns Hopkins University School of Medicine · The Johns Hopkins Medical Institutions · 600 North Wolfe Street, CMSC 1103, Baltimore, MD 21205 410-955-5883

Robert H. Schwartz · (Asthma, Cow's Milk Allergy) · Professor of Pediatrics and Medicine, University of Rochester School of Medicine & Dentistry · Director of Pediatric Allergy, Strong Memorial Hospital, University of Rochester Medical Center · 919 Westfall Road, Rochester, NY 14618 · 716-442-0150

Jay E. Selcow · (Asthma) · Associate Clinical Professor, Department of Pediatrics, University of Connecticut School of Medicine · Senior Staff, Department of Pediatrics, Hartford Hospital · 836 Farmington Avenue, Suite 207, West Hartford, CT 06119 · 203-232-9911

Gail Greenberg Shapiro · (Allergy, Asthma) · Clinical Professor of Pediatrics, University of Washington School of Medicine · Children's Hospital & Medical Center · Northwest Asthma & Allergy, 4540 Sand Point Way NE, Suite 200, Seattle, WA 98105 · 206-527-1200

William Thomas Shearer · (Immunodeficiency, AIDS) · Professor of Pediatrics & Microbiology & Immunology, Baylor College of Medicine · Chief, Allergy & Immunology Section, Texas Children's Hospital · One Baylor Plaza, Houston, TX 77030 · 713-770-1319

Sheldon C. Siegel · (Allergy) · Clinical Professor of Pediatrics, University of California at Los Angeles School of Medicine · University of California at Los Angeles · 11645 Wilshire Boulevard, Suite 600, Los Angeles, CA 90025 · 213-312-5050

R. Michael Sly · (Allergy) · Professor of Pediatrics, The George Washington University School of Medicine · Chairman, Allergy & Immunology, Children's National Medical Center · 111 Michigan Avenue NW, Washington, DC 20010 · 202-745-2071

E. Richard Stiehm · (Immunodeficiency, AIDS) · Professor of Pediatrics, University of California, Los Angeles School of Medicine · Head, Division of Allergy & Immunology, University of California, Los Angeles Center for Health Sciences Marion Davies Childrens Center, 10833 LeConte Avenue, Room 22-387, Los Angeles, CA 90024-1752 · 310-825-6481

Robert C. Strunk · (Asthma) · Professor of Pediatrics, Washington University School of Medicine · Director, Division of Allergy & Pulmonary Medicine, St. Louis Children's Hospital · Spoehrer Tower, 400 South Kingshighway Boulevard, Room 801, St. Louis, MO 63110 · 314-454-2284

Richard J. Sveum · Clinical Assistant Professor of Allergy & Immunology, University of Minnesota School of Medicine · Park Nicollet Medical Center · 5000 West 39th Street, Minneapolis, MN 55416 · 612-927-3090

Stanley J. Szefler · (Clinical Pharmacology) · Professor of Pediatrics and Pharmacology, University of Colorado School of Medicine · Director, Clinical Pharmacology, National Jewish Center for Immunology & Respiratory Medicine · 1400 Jackson Street, Room K926, Denver, CO 80206 · 303-398-1379

Martin Douglas Valentine · (Insect Hypersensitivity) · Professor of Medicine, Johns Hopkins University School of Medicine · Physician, Francis Scott Key Medical Center; The Johns Hopkins Medical Institutions · Johns Hopkins Asthma and Allergy Center, 301 Bayview Boulevard, Baltimore, MD 21224 · 410-550-2303

Diane Wara · (Immunodeficiency, AIDS) · Professor of Pediatrics, University of California at San Francisco School of Medicine · Director of Pediatric Immunology/Rheumatology, University of California at San Francisco Medical Center · Department of Pediatric Immunology, Parnassus Avenue, Room M601, San Francisco, CA 94143 · 415-476-2865

John W. Yunginger · Professor of Pediatrics, Mayo Medical School · Mayo Clinic 200 First Street, SW, Rochester, MN 55905 · 507-284-3454

Robert S. Zeiger · (Allergy) · Clinical Associate Professor of Pediatrics, University of California at San Diego School of Medicine · Chief of Allergy, Kaiser-Permanente Medical Center · 7060 Clairemont Mesa Boulevard, San Diego, CA 92111 619-268-5408

ANESTHESIOLOGY

ADULT CARDIOVASCULAR

Martin Abel · (Critical Care) · Assistant Professor of Anesthesiology, Mayo Medical School · Consultant, Mayo Clinic · 200 First Street, SW, Rochester, MN 55905 · 507-255-4234

Paul G. Barash · Professor and Chairman of Anesthesiology, Yale University School of Medicine · Chief, Department of Anesthesiology, Yale-New Haven Hospital · 333 Cedar Street, T3, New Haven, CT 06510 · 203-785-4304, 785-2802

Michael K. Cahalan · Associate Professor of Anesthesiology, University of California at San Francisco School of Medicine · University of California at San Francisco Medical Center · 521 Parnassus Avenue, Room C-455, San Francisco, CA 94143-0648 · 415-476-9037

Edward Lowenstein · Professor of Anaesthesia, Harvard Medical School · Anesthetist-in-Chief, Department of Anesthesia & Critical Care, Beth Israel Hospital 330 Brookline Avenue, Boston, MA 02215 · 617-735-2902

Dennis T. Mangano · (Ischemic Heart Disease) · Professor and Vice-Chairman, Department of Anesthesia, University of California at San Francisco, School of Medicine · Anesthesiology Service, Veterans Affairs Medical Center · 4150 Clement Street (129), San Francisco, CA 94121 · 415-750-2069

Edward D. Miller, Jr. · (Hypertension) · E. M. Papper Professor of Anesthesiology, and Chairman, Department of Anesthesiology, College of Physicians & Surgeons of Columbia University · Director, Anesthesiology Service, Columbia-Presbyterian Medical Center · 630 West 168th Street, New York, NY 10032 · 212-305-3117

Joseph Gerald Reves · Professor and Chairman, Department of Anesthesiology, Duke University School of Medicine · Duke University Medical Center · P.O. Box 3094, Durham, NC 27710 · 919-681-6646

Michael F. Roizen · Professor and Chairman, Department of Anesthesiology & Critical Care, University of Chicago, Pritzker School of Medicine · University of Chicago Medical Center · 5841 South Maryland Avenue, Box 428, Chicago, IL 60637-1470 · 312-702-6700

Stephen Slogoff · Professor of Anesthesiology, The University of Texas Health Science Center at Houston · Assistant Chief of Cardiovascular Anesthesiology, Texas Heart Institute · Cardiovascular Anesthesia, 6720 Burtner Street, 1-226, P. O. Box 20345, Houston, TX 77225-0345 · 713-791-2666

Daniel Thys · Professor of Anesthesiology, College of Physicians & Surgeons of Columbia University · Director, Department of Anesthesiology, St. Luke's-Roosevelt Hospital Center · Travers Building Seven, 114th Street and Amsterdam Avenue, New York, NY 10025 · 212-523-2500

John L. Waller · Professor and Chairman, Department of Anesthesiology, Emory University School of Medicine · Chief of Anesthesiology, Emory University Affiliated Hospitals · 1364 Clifton Road NE, Atlanta, GA 30322 · 404-248-3911

Roger D. White · Professor of Anesthesiology, Mayo Medical School · Mayo Clinic · 200 First Street, SW, Rochester, MN 55905 · 507-255-4235

AMBULATORY ANESTHESIA

Burton S. Epstein · Professor of Anesthesiology, The George Washington University School of Medicine · George Washington University Medical Center · 901 Northwest 23rd Street, Washington, DC 20037 · 202-676-5618

Surinder K. Kallar · Professor and Vice Chairman, Department of Anesthesiology, Virginia Commonwealth University, Medical College of Virginia · Director, Ambulatory Anesthesia, Medical College of Virginia Hospital · Box 103, MCV Station, Richmond, VA 23298-0645 · 804-786-8678

Bernard V. Wetchler · Clinical Professor of Anesthesiology, University of Illinois College of Medicine at Peoria · Director, Department of Anesthesiology, and Medical Director, Ambulatory SurgiCare, Methodist Medical Center · 221 Northeast Glen Oak, Peoria, IL 61636 · 309-672-5562

Harry C. Wong · University of Utah School of Medicine · University of Utah Health Sciences Center · Department of Anesthesiology, 50 North Medical Drive, Salt Lake City, UT 84132 · 801-581-6393

CARDIOTHORACIC ANESTHESIOLOGY

Jonathan L. Benumof · (Thoracic Anesthesiology) · Professor of Anesthesia, University of California at San Diego School of Medicine · University of California at San Diego Medical Center · 402 Dickinson Street, Mail Code 8770, San Diego, CA 92103 · 619-543-5562

H. Barrie Fairley · (Pulmonary) · Professor and Chairman, Department of Anesthesiology, Stanford University School of Medicine · Stanford, CA 94305 · 415-723-5024

Thomas F. Hornbein · (Pulmonary, Respiratory Physiology, Respiratory Care) · Professor and Chairman, Department of Anesthesiology, and Professor, Department of Physiology & Biophysics, University of Washington School of Medicine · Department of Anesthesia, Mail Stop RN-10, Seattle, WA 98195 · 206-543-2672

COMPLICATIONS OF ANESTHESIA

David L. Brown · (Regional Anesthesia Pain Management) · Associate Professor of Anesthesiology, Mayo Medical School · Consultant, Department of Anesthesiology, Mayo Clinic · 200 First Street, SW, Rochester, MN 55905 · 507-284-9700

Robert A. Caplan · Associate Clinical Professor of Anesthesiology, University of Washington, Seattle · Staff Anesthesiologist, Virginia Mason Medical Center · 1100 Ninth Avenue (B2-AN), P.O. Box 900, Seattle, WA 98111 · 206-223-6980

Frederick W. Cheney · Professor of Anesthesiology, University of Washington School of Medicine · Director, Respiratory Care Services, University of Washington Medical Center; Seattle Veterans Affairs Medical Center · Department of Anesthesiology, Mail Stop RN-10, Seattle, WA 98195 · 206-543-2672

John H. Eichhorn · Professor and Chairman, Anesthesiology, University of Mississippi · University of Mississippi Medical Center · 2500 North State Street, Room S108A, Jackson, MS 39216-4505 · 601-984-5900

Arthur S. Keats · Associate Professor of Anesthesiology, The University of Texas Health Science Center at Houston · Chief of Cardiovascular Anesthesiology, Texas Heart Institute · Cardiovascular Anesthesia, 6720 Burtner Street, 1-226, P. O. Box 20345, Houston, TX 77225-0345 · 713-791-2666

Richard L. Keenan · Professor and Chairman, Department of Anesthesiology, Virginia Commonwealth University, Medical College of Virginia · Medical College of Virginia Hospital · 1200 East Broad Street, Room 7-102, Richmond, VA 23298 · 804-786-9160

Frederick K. Orkin · Associate Professor of Anesthesiology, University of California at San Francisco School of Medicine · University of California at San Francisco Medical Center · 400 Parnassus Avenue, Room A-3 Plaza Level, Box 0368, San Francisco, CA 94143 · 415-476-8384

CRITICAL CARE MEDICINE

Thomas William Feeley · Professor of Anesthesia, Stanford University School of Medicine · Associate Medical Director of Intensive Care Units, Stanford University Hospital · 300 Pasteur Drive, Stanford, CA 94305 · 415-723-6415

T. James Gallagher · Professor of Anesthesiology and Surgery, University of Florida College of Medicine · Chief, Division of Critical Care Medicine, Shands Hospital at the University of Florida · 1600 Southwest Archer Road, Room 2507 PSB, P.O. Box J-254, Gainesville, FL 32610 · 904-395-0463

John William Hoyt · Clinical Professor of Anesthesiology & Critical Care Medicine, University of Pittsburgh School of Medicine · Chairman, Department of Critical Care, St. Francis Medical Center · 45th Street off Penn Avenue, Pittsburgh, PA 15201 · 412-622-4210

Philip D. Lumb · Professor and Chairman, Department of Anesthesiology, Albany Medical College · 43 New Scotland Avenue, A131, Albany, NY 12208 · 518-445-4305

Donald S. Prough · Professor of Anesthesia & Neurology, and Head, Section on Critical Care, The Bowman Gray School of Medicine of Wake Forest University Associate Chief of Professional Services, North Carolina Baptist Hospital · Medical Center Boulevard, Winston-Salem, NC 27157-1009 · 919-748-4684

Myer H. Rosenthal · Professor of Anesthesia, Medicine and Surgery, Stanford University School of Medicine · Medical Director, Intensive Care Units, Stanford University Hospital · Stanford, CA 94305 · 415-723-7662

Barry A. Shapiro · Professor and Vice-Chairman, Department of Anesthesiology, Northwestern University Medical School · Chief, Section of Respiratory & Critical Care, Department of Anesthesia, Northwestern Memorial Hospital · 250 East Superior Street, Suite 678, Chicago, IL 60611 · 312-908-2280

Robert N. Sladen · Associate Professor of Anesthesiology and Surgery, Duke University School of Medicine · Co-Director, Surgical Intensive Care Unit, Duke University Medical Center; Chief of Anesthesiology, and Co-Director, Surgical Intensive Care Unit, Durham Veterans Affairs Medical Center · 508 Fulton Street, Mail Stop 112-C, Durham, NC 27705 · 919-286-6938

Richard Teplick · Associate Professor of Anesthesia, Harvard Medical School · Director, Division of Critical Care Medicine, Department of Anesthesia, Massachusetts General Hospital · 32 Fruit Street, Boston, MA 02114 · 617-726-5322

Alan S. Tonnesen · Professor of Anesthesiology, The University of Texas Medical School at Houston · Medical Director for Shock Trauma Intensive Care Unit, Hermann Hospital · 6431 Fannin Street, Room 5020, Houston, TX 77030 · 713-797-4011, 792-5566

Roger S. Wilson · Chairman, Department of Anesthesiology & Critical Care Medicine, Memorial Sloan-Kettering Cancer Center · 1275 York Avenue, New York, NY 10021 · 212-639-6848

GENERAL ANESTHESIOLOGY

Allen I. Hyman · Professor of Anesthesiology, College of Physicians & Surgeons of Columbia University · Attending Physician, Columbia-Presbyterian Medical Center · 622 West 168th Street, New York, NY 10032 · 212-305-2068

Ronald D. Miller · Professor and Chairman, Department of Anesthesia, University of California, San Francisco School of Medicine · Anesthesiologist-in-Charge, University of California, San Francisco Medical Center · 521 Parnassus Avenue, Box 0648, San Francisco, CA 94143-0648 · 415-476-1000

Lawrence J. Saidman · Professor, Department of Anesthesiology; and Editor-in-Chief, Journal of Anesthesiology, University of California at San Diego School of Medicine · 9500 Gilman Drive, La Jolla, CA 92093-0815 · 619-543-5710

Robert Stoelting · Chairman, Department of Anesthesiology, Indiana University School of Medicine · 1120 South Drive, Indianapolis IN 46202-5115 · 317-274-0269

John Tinker · (Cardiovascular Anesthesia) · Professor and Head, Department of Anesthesiology, The University of Iowa College of Medicine · Chief of Anesthesiology, The University of Iowa Hospitals & Clinics · Iowa City, IA 52242 · 319-356-2633

Mark A. Warner · (Abdominal, Prostate) · Associate Professor of Anesthesiology, Mayo Medical School · Mayo Clinic · 200 First Street, SW, Rochester, MN 55905 507-255-4236

HEPATIC DISEASE

Burnell R. Brown, Jr. · Professor of Anesthesiology and Pharmacology, The University of Arizona College of Medicine · Head, Department of Anesthesiology, The University of Arizona Health Sciences Center · 1501 North Campbell Avenue, Room 5405, Tucson, AZ 85724 · 602-626-7196

Simon Gelman · Professor and Chairman, Department of Anesthesiology, and Professor of Physiology and Biophysics, The University of Alabama School of Medicine · Chairman, Department of Anesthesiology, The University of Alabama Hospital · 619 Nineteenth Street South, Birmingham, AL 35233 · 205-934-4696

Yoogoo Kang · Associate Professor of Anesthesiology/Critical Care Medicine, University of Pittsburgh School of Medicine · Director, Hepatic Transplantation Anesthesiology Program, Presbyterian University Hospital · DeSoto at O'Hara Streets, Room 2405, Pittsburgh, PA 15213 · 412-647-6969

NEUROANESTHESIA

David P. Archer · Assistant Professor of Anesthesiology, University of Calgary · Director, Anesthesia Residency Program, Foothills Hospital · 1403 Twenty-Ninth Street NW, Calgary, Alberta T2N 2T9 · 403-670-1110

James E. Cottrel · Professor and Chairman, Department of Anesthesiology, State University of New York Health Science Center at Brooklyn · 450 Clarkson Avenue, Brooklyn, NY 11203 · 718-270-1934

Gregory Crosby · Assistant Professor of Anesthesia, Harvard Medical School · Assistant Anesthetist and Director of Neuroanesthesia, Massachusetts General Hospital · 32 Fruit Street, Boston, MA 02114-2696 · 617-726-8812

Roy F. Cucchiara · Professor of Anesthesiology, Mayo Medical School · Consultant, Mayo Clinic · 200 First Street, SW, Rochester, MN 55905 · 507-255-4235

John C. Drummond · Associate Professor of Anesthesiology, University of California at San Diego School of Medicine · Staff Anesthesiologist, San Diego Veterans Administration Medical Center · 9500 Gilman Drive, Mail Code 0629, La Jolla, CA 92093-0629 · 619-534-4496

Adrian Gelb · Professor and Chairman, Department of Anaesthesia, The University of Western Ontario · Chief, Department of Anaesthesia, University Hospital 339 Windermere Road, P.O. Box 5339, London, Ontario N6A 5A5 · 519-663-3000

Arthur M. Lam · Professor, Department of Anesthesiology, University of Washington School of Medicine · Harborview Medical Center · 325 Ninth Avenue, Seattle, WA 98104 · 206-223-3059

William L. Lanier · Associate Professor of Anesthesiology, Mayo Medical School Consultant in Anesthesiology, Mayo Clinic · 200 First Street, SW, Rochester, MN 55905 · 507-255-4235

C. Philip Larson, Jr. · Professor of Anesthesia and Surgery (Neurosurgery), Stanford University School of Medicine · Stanford University Hospital · 300 Pasteur Drive, H3584, Stanford, CA 94305 · 415-723-5439

Pirjo H. Manninen · University of Western Ontario Hospital · 339 Windermere Road, P.O. Box 5339, London, Ontario N6A 5A5 · 519-663-3000

Mary Jane Matjasko · University of Maryland Medical Center · 22 South Greene Street, Baltimore, MD 21201 · 301-328-6122

Robert W. McPherson · Associate Professor of Anesthesiology, Johns Hopkins University School of Medicine · Chief of Neurosurgical Anesthesia, The Johns Hopkins Medical Institutions · 600 North Wolfe Street, Meyer Eight, Baltimore, MD 21205 · 410-955-2611

Joseph M. Messick, Jr. · Professor of Anesthesiology, Mayo Medical School · Mayo Clinic · 200 First Street SW, Rochester, MN 55905 · 507-285-5601

John D. Michenfelder · Professor of Anesthesiology, Mayo Medical School · Mayo Clinic · 200 First Street, SW, Rochester, MN 55905 · 507-255-4235

Leslie N. Milde · Associate Professor of Anesthesiology, Mayo Medical School · Consultant in Anesthesiology, Mayo Clinic · 200 First Street, SW, Rochester, MN 55905 · 507-255-4235

Patricia H. Petrozza · Assistant Professor of Anesthesia, and Director of Neuroanesthesia, Department of Anesthesia, The Bowman Gray School of Medicine of Wake Forest University · North Carolina Baptist Hospital · Medical Center Boulevard, Winston-Salem, NC 27157-1009 · 919-748-2591

Peter A. Raudzens · Senior Clinical Lecturer in Anesthesiology, The University of Arizona Health Sciences Center · Head, Neuroanesthesiology Department, The Barrow Neurological Institute at St. Joseph's Hospital & Medical Center · 7101 North 40th Street, Paradise Valley, AZ 85253 · 602-955-7801, 285-3541

Michael M. Todd · Professor of Anesthesiology, The University of Iowa College of Medicine · The University of Iowa Hospitals & Clinics · Iowa City, IA 52242 319-335-8540

David S. Warner · Associate Professor of Anesthesiology, The University of Iowa College of Medicine · The University of Iowa Hospitals & Clinics · 200 Hawkins Drive, Iowa City, IA 52242 · 319-356-2886

William L. Young · Assistant Professor of Anesthesiology, College of Physicians & Surgeons of Columbia University · Assistant Attending Anesthesiologist, Columbia-Presbyterian Medical Center · 161 Fort Washington Avenue, Room 901, New York, NY 10032 · 212-305-2575

OBSTETRIC ANESTHESIA

David H. Chestnut · Professor of Anesthesiology, Obstetrics & Gynecology, The University of Iowa College of Medicine · Director of Obstetric Anesthesiology, The University of Iowa Hospitals & Clinics · Iowa City, IA 52242 · 319-356-2633, 335-8756

Sheila Evelyn Cohen · Professor of Anesthesiology, Stanford University School of Medicine · Director of Obstetric Anesthesia, Stanford University Hospital · Department of Anesthesia, Stanford University Medical Center, Stanford, CA 94305 415-725-5871

Sanjay Datta · Associate Professor of Anesthesia, Harvard Medical School · Director of Obstetric Anesthesia, Brigham & Women's Hospital · 75 Francis Street, Boston, MA 02115 · 617-732-7346

James C. Eisenach · (Pain Control) · Associate Professor of Anesthesiology, The Bowman Gray School of Medicine of Wake Forest University · Forsyth Memorial Hospital · Winston-Salem, NC 27103 · 919-748-4498

Mieczyslaw Finster · Professor of Anesthesiology, Obstetrics & Gynecology, College of Physicians & Surgeons of Columbia University · Columbia-Presbyterian Medical Center · 622 West 168th Street, Harkness Eight, New York, NY 10032 · 212-305-2564

Brett B. Gutsche · Professor of Anesthesia, and Professor of Obstetrics & Gynecology, University of Pennsylvania School of Medicine · Co-Director, Obstetrics Anesthesia, Hospital of the University of Pennsylvania · Department of Anesthesia, 3400 Spruce Street, Philadelphia, PA 19104 · 215-662-3235

Barbara L. Leighton · Associate Professor of Anesthesiology, Jefferson Medical College of Thomas Jefferson University · Thomas Jefferson University Hospital · 525 Main Building, 132 South 10th Street, Philadelphia, PA 19107-5244 · 215-955-7107

J. Stephen Naulty · Professor of Anesthesiology, The George Washington University School of Medicine · Director of Obstetric Anesthesia, George Washington University Medical Center · 901 Twenty-Third Street, NW, Washington, DC 20037 · 202-994-3864

Mark C. Norris · Associate Professor of Anesthesia, Jefferson Medical College of Thomas Jefferson University · Co-Director of Obstetric Anesthesia, Thomas Jefferson University Hospital · 132 South 10th Street, 524 Main Building, Philadelphia, PA 19107-5244 · 215-955-6161

Gerard W. Ostheimer · Professor of Anesthesia, Harvard Medical School · Interim Chairman, Department of Anesthesia, Brigham & Women's Hospital · 75 Francis Street, Boston, MA 02115 · 617-732-7312

Sol M. Shnider · Professor and Vice-Chairman, Department of Anesthesia, and Professor of Obstetrics, Gynecology & Reproductive Sciences, University of California at San Francisco School of Medicine · Director of Obstetrical Anesthesia, University of California at San Francisco Medical Center · 521 Parnassus Avenue, Box 0648, San Francisco, CA 94143-0648 · 415-476-2274

ORTHOPAEDIC PROCEDURES

David L. Brown · (Regional Anesthesia Pain Management) · Associate Professor of Anesthesiology, Mayo Medical School · Consultant, Department of Anesthesiology, Mayo Clinic · 200 First Street, SW, Rochester, MN 55905 · 507-284-9700

Nigel E. Sharrock · Director of Anesthesiology, The Hospital for Special Surgery 535 East 70th Street, Room 549, New York, NY 10021 · 212-606-1206

PAIN

Stephen E. Abram · (Chronic Pain Management) · Professor and Vice-Chairman, Department of Anesthesiology, Medical College of Wisconsin · Director, Pain Management Center, Milwaukee County Medical Complex · 8700 West Wisconsin Avenue, Milwaukee, WI 53226 · 414-257-6259

F. Michael Ferrante · (Acute Pain Management, Chronic Pain Management) · Assistant Professor of Anesthesiology, Harvard Medical School · Chief of Pain Treatment Service, Brigham & Women's Hospital · 75 Francis Street, Boston, MA 02115 · 617-732-6708

Gabor B. Racz · (Chronic Pain Management) · Professor and Chairman, Department of Anesthesiology, Texas Tech University Health Science Center · Chief of Service and Pain Clinic Director, University Medical Center · 3601 Fourth Street, Lubbock, TX 79430 · 806-743-3112

P. Prithvi Raj · (Chronic Pain Management, Acute Pain Management) · Executive Medical Director, Georgia Baptist Medical Center · 340 Boulevard Northeast, Suite 210, Atlanta, GA 30312 · 404-653-3579

Richard L. Rauck · (Acute Pain Management) · Associate Professor of Anesthesiology, The Bowman Gray School of Medicine of Wake Forest University · Director, Pain Control Center, North Carolina Baptist Hospital · Medical Center Boulevard, Winston-Salem, NC 27157-1077 · 919-748-5530

L. Brian Ready · (Acute Pain Management) · Professor of Anesthesiology, University of Washington School of Medicine · Director of the Acute Pain Service, University of Washington Medical Center · 1959 Northeast Pacific Street, RN-10, Seattle, WA 98195 · 206-548-4260

Steven D. Waldman · (Chronic Pain Management) · Professor of Anesthesiology, University of Missouri at Kansas City School of Medicine · Medical Director, Headache & Pain Center · Pain Consortium of Greater Kansas City, 11111 Nall Avenue, Suite 202, Leawood, KS 66211 · 913-491-3999

Alon P. Winnie · (Chronic Pain Management, Acute Pain Management) · Professor of Anesthesiology, The University of Illinois College of Medicine at Chicago · Director, Pain Control Center, The University of Illinois Hospital · 840 South Wood Street, MC845, Chicago, IL 60612 · 312-996-1127

PEDIATRIC ANESTHESIOLOGY

D. Ryan Cook · Professor of Anesthesiology/Critical Care Medicine and Pharmacology, University of Pittsburgh School of Medicine · Chief Anesthesiologist, Children's Hospital of Pittsburgh · 3705 Fifth Avenue at DeSoto Street, Pittsburgh, PA 15213-2583 · 412-692-5260

Robert K. Crone · Professor of Anesthesiology and Pediatrics, University of Washington School of Medicine · Director of Anesthesiology, Children's Hospital & Medical Center · 4800 Sand Point Way NE, Seattle, WA 98105 · 206-526-2052

John J. Downes · Professor of Anesthesia & Pediatrics, University of Pennsylvania School of Medicine · Anesthesiologist-in-Chief, and Director, Department of Anesthesiology & Critical Care Medicine, The Children's Hospital of Philadelphia · 34th and Civic Center Boulevard, Suite 4330, Philadelphia PA 19104 · 215-590-1863

George Gregory · Professor, Department of Pediatrics & Anesthesia, University of California at San Francisco School of Medicine · University of California at San Francisco Medical Center · 521 Parnassus Avenue, San Francisco, CA 94143-0648 415-476-4887

Raafat S. Hannallah · (Pediatric Ambulatory Anesthesia) · Professor of Anesthesiology, The George Washington University School of Medicine · Children's National Medical Center · 111 Michigan Avenue NW, Washington, DC 20010 · 202-745-2025

Philippa Newfield · (Pediatric Neuroanesthesiology) · Assistant Clinical Professor of Anesthesia and Neurosurgery, University of California San Francisco School of Medicine · Attending Anesthesiologist, California Pacific Medical Center · 3700 California Street, San Francisco, CA 94118 · 415-750-6059

Russell C. Raphaely · Professor of Anesthesia & Pediatrics, University of Pennsylvania School of Medicine · Chief, Division of Critical Care Medicine, and Medical Director, Pediatric Intensive Care Unit, The Children's Hospital of Philadelphia · 34th Street and Civic Center Boulevard, Philadelphia, PA 19104 · 215-590-1872

Mark A. Rockoff · (Pediatric Neuroanesthesia) · Associate Professor of Anesthesia (Pediatrics), Harvard Medical School · Acting Anesthesiologist -in-Chief, and Director of Clinical Services, Children's Hospital · 300 Longwood Avenue, Boston, MA 02115 · 617-735-6457

Mark C. Rogers · Distinguished Faculty Professor and Chairman, Department of Anesthesiology & Critical Care Medicine, and Dean for Clinical Practice, Johns Hopkins University School of Medicine · The Johns Hopkins Medical Institutions 600 North Wolfe Street, Blalock 1415, Baltimore, MD 21205 · 410-955-8408

David J. Steward · Professor of Anesthesiology, University of Southern California School of Medicine · Director, Department of Anesthesiology, Children's Hospital of Los Angeles · 4650 Sunset Boulevard, Suite 866, Los Angeles, CA 90027 · 213-669-2262

Theodore W. Striker · Professor, Anesthesia & Pediatrics, and Director, Pediatric Anesthesia, University of Cincinnati College of Medicine · Director, Department of Anesthesiology, Children's Hospital Medical Center · Elland and Bethesda Avenues, ASB-3, Cincinnati, OH 45229-2899 · 513-559-4408

Jen-Tien Wung · (Neonatal) · Professor of Clinical Anesthesiology (in Pediatrics), College of Physicians & Surgeons of Columbia University · Columbia-Presbyterian Medical Center · Box 115, New York, NY 10032 · 212-305-2575

PEDIATRIC CARDIOVASCULAR

Froukje M. K. Beynen · Assistant Professor of Anesthesiology, Mayo Medical School · Consultant in Anesthesiology, Mayo Clinic · 200 First Street, SW, Rochester, MN 55905 · 507-284-2511

William J. Greeley · Associate Professor of Anesthesiology and Pediatrics, Duke University School of Medicine · Chief, Division of Pediatric Critical Care & Cardiovascular Anesthesia, Duke University Medical Center · P.O. Box 3046, Durham, NC 27710 · 919-681-3543

Dolly D. Hansen · Assistant Professor of Anesthesia, Harvard Medical School · Associate Director, Cardiac Anesthesia Service, Children's Hospital · 300 Longwood Avenue, Pavilion 342, Boston, MA 02115 · 617-735-6225

Paul R. Hickey · Associate Professor of Anesthesia, Harvard Medical School · Senior Associate in Anesthesia, Children's Hospital · 300 Longwood Avenue, Boston, MA 02115 · 617-735-6225

David R. Jobes · Associate Professor of Anesthesia, University of Pennsylvania School of Medicine · Hospital of the University of Pennsylvania; The Children's Hospital of Philadelphia · 3400 Spruce Street, Philadelphia, PA 19104-4283 · 215-662-3778

Susan C. Nicolson · Associate Professor of Anesthesia, University of Pennsylvania School of Medicine · Director of Cardiac Anesthesiology, The Children's Hospital of Philadelphia · Department of Anesthesiology, Thirty-fourth and Civic Center Boulevard, Philadelphia, PA 19104 · 215-590-1874

Hugo S. Raimundo · Assistant Professor of Anesthesiology, Mayo Medical School
Mayo Clinic · 200 First Street, SW, Rochester, MN 55905 · 507-255-4234

David J. Steward · Professor of Anesthesiology, University of Southern California
School of Medicine · Director, Department of Anesthesiology, Children's Hospital of Los Angeles · 4650 Sunset Boulevard, Suite 866, Los Angeles, CA 90027 ·
213-669-2262

Maureen A. Strafford · Assistant Professor of Anesthesiology (Pediatrics), Harvard Medical School · Children's Hospital · 300 Longwood Avenue, Boston, MA
02115 · 617-735-6995

PHARMACOLOGY

Ronald D. Miller · Professor and Chairman, Department of Anesthesia, Univer-
sity of California, San Francisco School of Medicine · Anesthesiologist-in-Charge,
University of California, San Francisco Medical Center · 521 Parnassus Avenue,
Box 0648, San Francisco, CA 94143-0648 · 415-476-1000

CARDIOVASCULAR DISEASE

CARDIAC CATHETERIZATION

John Ambrose · Professor of Medicine, and Director, Catheterization Laboratory, Mt. Sinai Medical Center · One Gustave L. Levy Place, Box 1030, New York, NY 10029 · 212-241-5849

Donald S. Baim · Associate Professor of Medicine, Harvard Medical School · Director, Invasive Cardiology, Beth Israel Hospital · 330 Brookline Avenue, Boston, MA 02215 · 617-735-3015

Peter C. Block · Associate Director, Heart Institute; St. Vincent's Hospital · 9155 Southwest Barnes Road, Suite 230, Portland, OR 97225 · 503-291-2089

Jeffrey A. Brinker · (Interventional Cardiology) · Associate Professor of Medicine and Radiology, Johns Hopkins University School of Medicine · Director, Interventional Cardiology & Pacemaking, The Johns Hopkins Medical Institutions · 600 North Wolfe Street, CMSC 501, Baltimore, MD 21205 · 410-955-6086

Michael Joseph Cowley · Professor of Medicine, Virginia Commonwealth University, Medical College of Virginia · Medical College of Virginia Hospital · MCV Station Box 36, Richmond, VA 23298 · 804-786-9205

John Michael Criley · Professor of Medicine & Radiological Sciences, University of California at Los Angeles School of Medicine · Medical Director of St. John's Heart Institute, Harbor-UCLA Medical Center · Saint John's Heart Institute, 1328 22nd Street, Santa Monica, CA 90404 · 310-533-2532, 829-8755

Gerald Dorros · Assistant Clinical Professor of Medicine, Medical College of Wisconsin · Interventional Cardiologist, St. Luke's Hospital · 2901 West Kinnickinnic River Parkway, Suite 512, Milwaukee, WI 53215 · 414-649-3599

John S. Douglas, Jr. · (Coronary Angioplasty, [PTCA]) · Associate Professor of Medicine (Cardiology), and Assistant Professor of Radiology (Cardiac Radiology), Emory University School of Medicine · Co-director, Cardiac Catheterization Laboratory, Emory University Affiliated Hospitals · 1364 Clifton Road, NE, Room C-430, Atlanta, GA 30322 · 404-727-7034

Stephen G. Ellis · Director, Sones Cardiac Catheterization Laboratories, The Cleveland Clinic Foundation · One Clinic Center, 9500 Euclid Avenue, Cleveland, OH 44195-5066 · 216-445-6712

David Parker Faxon · Professor of Medicine, Boston University School of Medicine · Director, Interventional Cardiology, The University Hospital · 88 East Newton Street, Section D-8, Boston, MA 02118 · 617-638-8700

James S. Forrester · Professor of Medicine, University of California at Los Angeles School of Medicine · Director of Cardiology, Cedars-Sinai Medical Center · 8700 Beverly Boulevard, Room 5347, Los Angeles, CA 90048 · 213-855-3884

William Grossman · Dana Professor of Medicine, Harvard Medical School · Chief, Cardiovascular Division, Beth Israel Hospital · 330 Brookline Avenue, RW453, Boston, MA 02215 · 617-735-2191

Geoffrey O. Hartzler · Clinical Professor of Medicine, University of Missouri at Kansas City School of Medicine · Consulting Cardiologist, Mid America Heart Institute · 4330 Wornall Road, Suite 2000, Kansas City, MO 64111 · 816-931-1883

L. David Hillis · Professor of Internal Medicine, The University of Texas Southwestern Medical Center at Dallas · Parkland Memorial Hospital; Zale-Lipshy University Hospital · 5323 Harry Hines Boulevard, Dallas, TX 75235-9047 · 214-590-8879

David R. Holmes, Jr. · Professor of Medicine, Mayo Medical School · Director of Adult Catheterization Laboratory, Mayo Clinic · 200 First Street, SW, Rochester, MN 55905 · 507-284-3580

Kenneth M. Kent · Washington Cardiology Center · 110 Irving Street, Suite 4B18, Washington, DC 20010 · 202-877-5975

Morton J. Kern · Professor of Medicine, St. Louis University School of Medicine Director, J. Gerard Mudd Cardiac Catheterization Laboratory, St. Louis University Medical Center · 3635 Vista Avenue at Grand Boulevard, P. O. Box 15250, St. Louis, MO 63110-0250 · 314-577-8860

Spencer B. King III · (Angioplasty) · Professor of Medicine (Cardiology), Emory University School of Medicine · Director, Division of Interventional Cardiology, Emory University Affiliated Hospitals · 1364 Clifton Road, NE, Suite F-606, Atlanta, GA 30322 · 404-727-4677

Martin B. Leon · (PTCA) · Director, Investigational Angioplasty Program, Washington Hospital Center · 110 Irving Street, Suite 4B18, Washington, DC 20010 · 202-877-5975

Philip A. Ludbrook · Professor of Medicine, Washington University School of Medicine · Barnes Hospital · Washington University Medical Center Cardiac Unit, Box 8986, 660 South Euclid Avenue, St. Louis, MO 63110 · 314-362-3794

Richard K. Myler · (Interventional Cardiology) · Clinical Professor of Medicine, University of California at San Francisco School of Medicine · Executive Director, San Francisco Heart Institute, Seton Medical Center · 1900 Sullivan Avenue, Daly City, CA 94015 · 415-991-6713

William W. O'Neill · Director, Divison of Cardiology, William Beaumont Hospital 3601 West Thirteen Mile Road, Royal Oak, MI 48073-6769 · 313-551-4163

Carl J. Pepine · Professor of Medicine and Associate Director, Division of Cardiology, University of Florida College of Medicine · Chief, Cardiology Section, Gainesville Veterans Affairs Medical Center; Shands Hospital at the University of Florida · 1600 Southwest Archer Road, P.O. Box 100277, Gainesville, FL 32610 904-374-6103

Cass A. Pinkerton · (Coronary Angioplasty, [PTCA]) · Clinical Professor of Medicine, Indiana University School of Medicine · Director, Interventional Cardiology, St. Vincent Hospital & Health Care Center · Nasser, Smith & Pinkerton Cardiology, 8402 Harcourt Road, Indianapolis, IN 46260 · 317-871-6666

Gary S. Roubin · Director of Cardiac Catheterization & Interventional Laboratories and Associate Professor of Medicine, The University of Alabama School of Medicine · The University of Alabama Hospital · 1919 Seventh Avenue South, 310 LHRB, Birmingham, AL 35294 · 205-934-7898

Patrick J. Scanlon · Professor of Medicine, Loyola Stritch School of Medicine · Chief, Section of Cardiology, Loyola University Medical Center · 2160 South First Avenue, Building 54, Room 131A, Maywood, IL 60153 · 708-216-3308

John B. Simpson · Sequoia Hospital · 2940 Whipple Avenue, Suite 10, Redwood City, CA 94062 · 415-306-2300

Richard S. Stack · Associate Professor, Department of Medicine, Division of Cardiology, Duke University School of Medicine · Director, Interventional Cardiovascular Program, Duke University Medical Center · P.O. Box 3111, Durham, NC 27710 · 919-681-5089

Eric Jeffrey Topol · (Interventional Cardiology) · Chairman, Department of Cardiology, and Director, Center for Thombosis & Arterial Biology, The Cleveland Clinic Foundation · One Clinic Center, 9500 Euclid Avenue, Desk F25, Cleveland, OH 44195 · 216-445-9490

George W. Vetrovec · Professor of Medicine and Associate Chairman for Clinical Affairs, Virginia Commonwealth University, Medical College of Virginia · Director, Adult Catheterization Laboratory, Medical College of Virginia Hospital · 1200 East Broad Street, Box 36, MCV Station, Richmond. VA 23298 · 804-786-9000

Patrick L. Whitlow · Director, Interventional Cardiology, Department of Cardiology, The Cleveland Clinic Foundation · One Clinic Center, 9500 Euclid Avenue, Cleveland, OH 44195-5066 · 216-444-1746

David O. Williams · Professor of Medicine, Brown University School of Medicine Physician-in-Charge, Division of Cardiology, and Director, Cardiac Catheterization Laboratory, Rhode Island Hospital · 593 Eddy Street, APC Building, Fourth Floor, Providence, RI 02903 · 401-277-4581

CARDIAC POSITRON EMISSION TOMOGRAPHY (PET)

Robert Ogden Bonow · Chief, Nuclear Cardiology, National Heart Institute, National Institutes of Health · 9000 Rockville Pike, Building 10, Room 7B 15, Bethesda, MD 20892 · 301-496-9895

Edward M. Geltman · Associate Professor of Medicine, Washington University School of Medicine · Medical Director of the Cardiac Diagnostic Lab, Barnes Hospital · Washington University School of Medicine, 660 South Euclid Avenue, Box 8086, St. Louis, MO 63110 · 314-362-5317

Richard A. Goldstein · Associate Professor of Medicine and Radiology, The University of Texas Medical School at Houston · Director, Nuclear Cardiology, Hermann Hospital · 6341 Fannin Street, Suite MSB 1.246, Houston, TX 77030 · 713-794-4120

CLINICAL EXERCISE TESTING

Bernard R. Chaitman · Professor of Medicine, St. Louis University School of Medicine · Chief of Cardiology, St. Louis University Medical Center · 3635 Vista Avenue at Grand Boulevard, 13th Floor, P.O. Box 15250, St. Louis, MO 63110-0250 · 314-577-8890

Myrvin H. Ellestad · Clinical Professor of Medicine, University of California at Irvine School of Medicine · Medical Director of Memorial Heart Institute, Long Beach Memorial Medical Center · 2801 Atlantic Avenue, Long Beach, CA 90801-1428 · 213-595-2119

Victor F. Froelicher · Professor of Medicine, University of California at Irvine School of Medicine · Chief, Cardiology Section, Long Beach Veterans Affairs Hospital · 5901 East Seventh Street, E119, Long Beach, CA 90822 · 213-494-5486

Paul David Kligfield · Associate Professor of Medicine, Cornell University Medical College · The New York Hospital-Cornell Medical Center · 525 East 68th Street, New York, NY 10021 · 212-746-4686

Daniel B. Mark · Assistant Professor of Medicine, Duke University School of Medicine · Duke University Medical Center · P.O. Box 3485-DUMC, Durham, NC 27710 · 919-681-3519

Paul L. McHenry · Professor and Associate Chairman for Clinical Affairs, Department of Medicine, Indiana University School of Medicine · Director of Clinical Cardiology, Indiana University Medical Center; Senior Research Associate, Krannert Institute of Cardiology · 1111 West 10th Street, Indianapolis, IN 46202 · 317-274-7853

Donald Weiner · Professor of Medicine, Boston University School of Medicine · Director of Exercise Laboratory, The University Hospital · Section of Cardiology, 88 East Newton Street, Boston, MA 02118 · 617-638-8968

ECHOCARDIOGRAPHY

William Armstrong · Professor of Medicine, The University of Michigan Medical School · Interim Division Chief, and Director, Echocardiology Laboratory, The University of Michigan Medical Center · 1500 East Medical Center Drive, UHB1F245 Box 0022, Ann Arbor, MI 48109 · 313-936-9678

Michael H. Crawford · Robert S. Flinn Professor of Cardiology, The University of New Mexico School of Medicine · Chief, Division of Cardiology, The University Hospital · 2211 Lomas Boulevard NE, Albuquerque, NM 87131-5271 · 505-272-6020

Harvey Feigenbaum · Distinguished Professor of Medicine, Indiana University School of Medicine · Director of the Hemodynamic Lab, Indiana University Medical Center · 926 West Michigan Street, Room N562, Indianapolis, IN 46202-5250 · 317-274-1693

Richard E. Kerber · Professor of Medicine, The University of Iowa College of Medicine · Associate Director, Cardiovascular Division, and Program Director of Cardiovascular Fellowship Program, and Chairman, CPR Committee, The University of Iowa Hospitals & Clinics · 200 Hawkins Drive, Room 4207 RCP, Iowa City, IA 52242 · 319-356-2739

Joseph Kisslo · Professor of Medicine, Duke University School of Medicine · Director, Echocardiography Laboratories, Duke University Medical Center · P.O. Box 3818, Durham, NC 27710 · 919-684-6398

Natesa G. Pandian · Associate Professor of Medicine, Tufts University School of Medicine · Director, Noninvasive Cardiac Laboratory, New England Medical Center · 750 Washington Street, Box 32, Boston, MA 02111 · 617-956-6151

Alfred F. Parisi · Professor of Medicine, and Chief, Division of Cardiology, Brown University Program in Medicine · Chief, Cardiology Division, The Miriam Hospital; Rogers Williams General Hospital · 164 Summit Avenue, Room 353, Providence, RI 02906 · 401-331-8500 x4101

Alan S. Pearlman · Professor of Medicine, University of Washington School of Medicine · Director, Echocardiography Laboratory, University of Washington Medical Center · 1959 Northeast Pacific Street, RG-22, Seattle, WA 98195 · 206-685-1397

Richard L. Popp · Professor of Medicine, Stanford University School of Medicine · Stanford University Hospital · 300 Pasteur Drive, Stanford, CA 94305 · 415-723-7493

Miguel A. Quinones · Professor of Medicine, Baylor College of Medicine · The Methodist Hospital · 6535 Fannin Street, MSF-1001, Houston, TX 77030 · 713-790-2783

Nathaniel Reichek · Professor of Medicine, University of Pennsylvania School of Medicine · Director, Noninvasive Laboratories, Hospital of the University of Pennsylvania · 3400 Spruce Street, 942 West Gates Pavilion, Philadelphia, PA 19104 · 215-662-2284

Kent L. Richards · Professor of Medicine, The University of New Mexico School of Medicine · Chief, Cardiology Section, Veterans Affairs Medical Center · 2100 Ridgecrest Drive SE, 111B, Albuquerque, NM 87108 · 505-265-1711 x4495

Nelson B. Schiller · Professor of Medicine, University of California at San Francisco School of Medicine · Director, Adult Echocardiography Laboratory, University of California at San Francisco Medical Center · 505 Parnassus Avenue, Room M-314a, San Francisco, CA 94143-0214 · 415-476-2562

James Bernard Seward · (Invasive Echocardiography, Pediatric Cardiology) · Professor of Medicine and Pediatrics, Mayo Medical School · Mayo Clinic; St. Mary's Hospital · 200 First Street, SW, Rochester, MN 55905 · 507-284-2511

David J. Skorton · Professor of Medicine, and Professor of Electrical and Computer Engineering, The University of Iowa College of Medicine; University of Iowa College of Engineering · The University of Iowa Hospitals & Clinics · 200 Hawkins Drive, Iowa City, IA 52242 · 319-356-4031

William J. Stewart · (Valvular Heart Disease) · Staff, Department of Cardiology, The Cleveland Clinic Foundation · Department of Cardiology, One Clinic Center, 9500 Euclid Avenue, Cleveland, OH 44195 · 216-444-5923

A. Jamil Tajik · Professor of Medicine & Pediatrics, Mayo Medical School · Director of Cardiovascular Ultrasound, Imaging, & Hemodynamic Laboratory, Mayo Clinic · 200 First Street, SW, Rochester, MN 55905 · 507-284-9032

Arthur E. Weyman · Associate Professor of Medicine, Harvard Medical School · Director, Cardiac Ultrasound Laboratories, Massachusetts General Hospital · Zero Emerson Place, Suite 2F, Boston, MA 02114 · 617-726-1840

ELECTROPHYSIOLOGY

Masood Akhtar · Professor of Medicine, University of Wisconsin-Madison School of Medicine · Associate Chief, Cardiovascular Disease Section, and Director of Arrhythmia Service, Sinai Samaritan Medical Center, Mount Sinai Campus · 950 North 12th Street, Milwaukee, WI 53233 · 414-283-7686

Alfred E. Buxton · Associate Professor of Medicine, University of Pennsylvania School of Medicine · Director, Electrophysiologic Laboratory, Hospital of the University of Pennsylvania · 3400 Spruce Street, Nine Founders Pavilion, Philadelphia, PA 19104 · 215-662-6800

Debra S. Echt · Associate Professor of Medicine, Vanderbilt University School of Medicine · Division of Cardiology, CC2218, Medical Center North, Nashville, TN 37232-2170 · 615-322-2318

Andrew E. Epstein · Professor of Medicine, The University of Alabama School of Medicine · The University of Alabama Hospital · Division of Cardiovascular Disease, Tinsley Harrison Tower, Suite 321, Birmingham, AL 35294 · 205-934-7114

John D. Fisher · Professor of Medicine, Albert Einstein College of Medicine · Director, Division of Cardiology, and Director, Arrhythmia Service, Montefiore Medical Center · 111 East 210th Street, Bronx, NY 10467 · 212-920-4291

Richard N. Fogoros · Associate Professor of Medicine, Medical College of Pennsylvania-Allegheny Campus · Director, Electrophysiology Department, Allegheny General Hospital · 320 East North Avenue, Pittsburgh, PA 15212 · 412-359-6444

John J. Gallagher · Director of Electrophysiology, Carolinas Medical Center · The Sanger Clinic, 1001 Blythe Boulevard, Suite 300, Charlotte, NC 28203 · 704-373-1500

J. Anthony Gomes · Professor of Medicine, Mt. Sinai School of Medicine · Director, Electrocardiography & Electrophysiology Section, Division of Cardiology, Mt. Sinai Medical Center · One Gustave L. Levy Place, Box 1030, New York, NY 10029 · 212-241-7272

Warren M. Jackman · Associate Professor of Medicine, The University of Oklahoma Health Sciences Center · Staff Physician and Director, Clinical Electrophysiology, Oklahoma Memorial Hospital · 920 Stanton L. Young Boulevard, Room 5SP300, P.O. Box 26901, Oklahoma City, OK 73190 · 405-270-0501 x3268

Mark E. Josephson · Professor of Medicine, and Robinette Professor of Medicine, University of Pennsylvania School of Medicine · Director, Electrophysiology Program & Arrhythmia Service, Hospital of the University of Pennsylvania · 3400 Spruce Street, Nine Gates Building, Philadelphia, PA 19104 · 215-662-2185

Michael G. Kienzle · Associate Professor of Medicine, The University of Iowa College of Medicine · Assistant Director, Cardiovascular Division, and Director, EKG and EP Laboratories, The University of Iowa Hospitals & Clinics · 200 Hawkins Drive, Iowa City, IA 52242 · 319-356-3641

George J. Klein · Professor of Medicine, The University of Western Ontario · Director, Arrhythmia Service, University Hospital · Station A, P.O. Box 5339, London, Ontario N6A 5A5 · 519-663-3264

Michael H. Lehmann · Associate Professor of Internal Medicine, Wayne State University School of Medicine · Director, Electrophysiology Laboratory & Arrhythmia Service, Harper Hospital · 3990 John R Street, Detroit, MI 48201 · 313-745-2626

Francis E. Marchlinski · Associate Professor of Medicine, University of Pennsylvania School of Medicine · Director, The Arrhythmia Evaluation Center, and Co-Director, Electrophysiologic Laboratory, Hospital of the University of Pennsylvania · 3400 Spruce Street, Nine Founders Pavilion, Philadelphia, PA 19104 · 215-662-2188

John Haynes McNulty · Professor of Medicine, Division of Cardiology, Oregon Health Sciences University · 3181 Southwest Sam Jackson Park Road, Portland, OR 97201 · 503-494-8750

Fred Morady · Professor of Internal Medicine, The University of Michigan Medical School · Director, Clinical Electrophysiology Laboratory, The University of Michigan Medical Center · 1500 East Medical Center Drive, Floor B-1, Room F-245, Box 0022, Ann Arbor, MI 48109-0022 · 313-936-4025

Gerald V. Naccarelli · Professor of Medicine, The University of Texas Medical School at Houston · Director, Clinical Electrophysiology, Hermann Hospital · P.O. Box 20708, Houston, TX 77025 · 713-792-5178

Eric Neal Prystowsky · Consulting Professor of Medicine, Duke University School of Medicine · Director, Clinical Electrophysiology Laboratory, St. Vincent Hospital & Health Care Center · 8402 Harcourt Road, Suite 300, Indianapolis, IN 46260 · 317-872-5050, 871-6024

Jeremy N. Ruskin · Associate Professor of Medicine, Harvard Medical School · Director, Cardiac Arrhythmia Service, & Clinical Electrophysiology Laboratory, Massachusetts General Hospital · 32 Fruit Street, Boston, MA 02114 · 617-726-8514

Melvin M. Scheiman · Professor of Medicine, University of California at San Francisco School of Medicine · Chief of the Electrocardiography & Clinical Cardiac Electrophysiology Section, Moffitt-Long Hospital; University of California at San Francisco Medical Center · 505 Parnassus Avenue, Room M-312, San Francisco, CA 94143 · 415-476-5706

Patrick J. Tchou · Associate Professor of Medicine, University of Pittsburgh School of Medicine · Director of Cardiac Electrophysiology, Presbyterian University Hospital · 552 Scaife Hall, Pittsburgh, PA 152113 · 412-647-5019

David James Wilber · Associate Professor of Medicine, Loyola Stritch School of Medicine · Director, Electrophysiology Laboratory, Loyola University Medical Center · 2160 South First Avenue, Maywood, IL 60153 · 708-216-9449

Roger A. Winkle · Clinical Associate Professor of Medicine, Stanford University School of Medicine · Director, Cardiac Surveillance Unit & Electrophysiology Laboratory, Sequoia Hospital · 770 Welch Road, Suite 100, Palo Alto, CA 94304 415-617-8100

GENERAL CARDIOVASCULAR DISEASE

Stephen C. Achuff · (Cardiac Transplantation) · David J. Carver Professor of Medicine, Johns Hopkins University School of Medicine · Director, Clinical Cardiology, The Johns Hopkins Medical Institutions · 600 North Wolfe Street, Carnegie 568, Baltimore, MD 21205 · 410-955-7670

George A. Beller · Professor of Medicine and Head, Division of Cardiology, University of Virginia Health Sciences Center · University of Virginia Health Sciences Center · Private Clinics Building, Hospital Drive, Room 3591-E, Box 158, Charlottesville, VA 22908 · 804-924-2134

Mark J. Callahan · Assistant Professor, Mayo Medical School · Mayo Clinic · 200 First Street, SW, Rochester, MN 55905 · 507-284-3583

Kanu Chatterjee · Professor of Medicine and Lucie Stern Professor of Cardiology, University of California at San Francisco School of Medicine · Director of the Coronary Care Unit and Associate Chief, Division of Cardiology, University of California at San Francisco Medical Center · 505 Parnassus Avenue, Room M-1186, San Francisco, CA 94143 · 415-476-1326

Lawrence S. Cohen · The Ebenezer K. Hunt Professor of Medicine, Yale University School of Medicine · Yale-New Haven Hospital · 789 Howard Avenue, New Haven, CT 06510 · 203-785-4128

C. Richard Conti · Eminent Scholar and Professor of Medicine, University of Florida College of Medicine · Chief, Division of Cardiology, Shands Hospital at the University of Florida · 1600 Southwest Archer Road, Room M401, P.O. Box 100277, Gainesville, FL 32610 · 904-392-3481

Anthony Nicholas De Maria · Professor of Medicine, University of Kentucky College of Medicine · Chief, Cardiology Division, University of Kentucky Medical Center · 800 Rose Street, Room MN670, Lexington, KY 40536 · 606-233-5843

Roman W. DeSanctis · Physician and Director of Clinical Cardiology, Massachusetts General Hospital · 15 Parkman Street, Suite 467, Boston MA 02114 · 617-726-2889

John P. DiMarco · Professor of Medicine, University of Virginia School of Medicine · Director, Clinical Electrophysiology Laboratory, University of Virginia Health Sciences Center · Private Clinics Building, Hospital Drive, Third Floor, Room 3610, Box 158, Charlottesville, VA 22908 · 804-924-2031

Leonard S. Dreifus · Professor of Medicine, Hahnemann University · Hahnemann University Hospital · Broad and Vine Streets, Philadelphia, PA 19102 · 215-448-3221

Gottlieb C. Friesinger · Professor of Medicine, Division of Cardiology, Vanderbilt University School of Medicine · Vanderbilt University Medical Center · Division of Cardiology, Vanderbilt Medical Center, Nashville, TN 37232-2170 · 615-322-2318

Robert Frye · Chairman, Department of Medicine, Mayo Clinic · 200 First Street, SW, Rochester, MN 55902 · 507-284-3681

Valentine Fuster · Mallinckrodt Professor of Medicine, Harvard Medical School · Chief, Cardiac Unit, Massachusetts General Hospital · Bullfinch Building, 32 Fruit Street, Room 105, Boston, MA 02114 · 617-726-2887

William Grossman · Dana Professor of Medicine, Harvard Medical School · Chief, Cardiovascular Division, Beth Israel Hospital · 330 Brookline Avenue, RW453, Boston, MA 02215 · 617-735-2191

Adolph M. Hutter, Jr. · Associate Professor of Medicine, Harvard Medical School; President-Elect, American College of Cardiology · Chairman, Medical Intensive Care Coordinating Committee, Massachusetts General Hospital · 15 Parkman Street, Boston, MA 02114 · 617-726-2884

Lynne L. Johnson · Associate Professor of Clinical Medicine, and Director, Nuclear Cardiology Laboratory, College of Physicians & Surgeons of Columbia University · Columbia-Presbyterian Medical Center · 630 West 168th Street, PH11 Center, Room 1143, New York, NY 10032 · 212-305-9933

J. Ward Kennedy · Director, Division of Cardiology and Professor of Medicine, University of Washington School of Medicine · Chief of Cardiology, University

Hospital; University of Washington Medical Center · 1959 Northeast Pacific Street, RG22, Seattle, WA 98195 · 206-543-8584

Fletcher A. Miller, Jr. · Associate Professor of Medicine, Mayo Medical School · Mayo Clinic · 200 First Street, SW, Rochester, MN 55905 · 507-284-3682

Rick A. Nishimura · Associate Professor of Medicine, Mayo Medical School · Consultant in Cardiovascular Diseases and Internal Medicine, Mayo Clinic · 200 First Street, SW, Rochester, MN 55905 · 507-284-3265

Robert Anthony O'Rourke · Professor of Medicine, and Director of Cardiology, The University of Texas Health Science Center at San Antonio · 7703 Floyd Curl Drive, San Antonio, TX 78284-7872 · 512-617-5300 x5100

William W. Parmley · Professor of Medicine, University of California at San Francisco School of Medicine · Chief, Division of Cardiology, University of California at San Francisco Medical Center · 505 Parnassus Avenue, Room M-1186, San Francisco, CA 94143 · 415-476-1326

Thomas F. Ryan · Assistant Professor of Medicine, Indiana University School of Medicine · Director, Coronary Care, Wishard Memorial Hospital; Indiana University Medical Center · 1001 West 10th Street, Indianapolis, IN 46202 · 317-630-7462

John S. Schroeder · Professor of Medicine, Stanford University School of Medicine · Stanford University Hospital · Falk Cardiovascular Research Center, CVRC, 300 Pasteur Drive, Stanford, CA 94305-5246 · 415-723-5561

Hugh Smith · Chairman, Division of Cardiovascular Disease, Mayo Clinic · 200 First Street, SW, Rochester, MN 55902 · 507-284-2511

Myron L. Weisfeldt · Chairman and Professor of Medicine, College of Physicians & Surgeons of Columbia University · Columbia-Presbyterian Medical Center · 630 West 168 th Street, New York, NY 10032 · 212-305-5838

James T. Willerson · Professor and Chairman, Department of Internal Medicine, The University of Texas Medical School at Houston · Chief of Medical Services, Hermann Hospital, and Lyndon B. Johnson General Hospital; Director, Cardiology Research, St. Luke's Episcopal Hospital/Texas Heart Institute · 6431 Fannin Street, Room 1.150, Houston, TX 77030 · 713-792-5075

HEART FAILURE

Eugene Braunwald · Hersey Professor of Medicine, Harvard Medical School · Chairman, Department of Medicine, Brigham & Women's Hospital · 75 Francis Street, Boston, MA 02115 · 617-732-6340

Kanu Chatterjee · Professor of Medicine and Lucie Stern Professor of Cardiology, University of California at San Francisco School of Medicine · Director of the Coronary Care Unit and Associate Chief, Division of Cardiology, University of California at San Francisco Medical Center · 505 Parnassus Avenue, Room M-1186, San Francisco, CA 94143 · 415-476-1326

Jay N. Cohn · Professor of Medicine and Head, Cardiovascular Division, Department of Medicine, University of Minnesota School of Medicine · University of Minnesota Hospital & Clinics · 420 Delaware Street SE, Box 488 UMHC, Minneapolis, MN 55455 · 612-625-5646

Barry H. Greenberg · Professor of Medicine, Oregon Health Sciences University Director of Coronary Care, Oregon Health Sciences University · 3181 Southwest Sam Jackson Park Road, Portland, OR 97201-3098 · 503-494-8750

Thierry H. Le Jentel · Professor of Medicine, Albert Einstein College of Medicine Attending, Montefiore Medical Center · Albert Einstein College of Medicine, 1300 Morris Park Avenue, Bronx, NY 10461 · 212-904-2193

Carl V. Leier · James W. Overstreet Professor of Medicine & Pharmacology, and Director, Division of Cardiology, Ohio State University College of Medicine · The Ohio State University Hospitals · 1654 Upham Drive, 669 Means Hall, Columbus, OH 43210 · 614-293-8963

John Nicklas · Associate Professor of Internal Medicine, The University of Michigan Medical School · Director, Congestive Heart Failure Program, and Director, Coronary Care Unit, The University of Michigan Medical Center · 3910 Taubman Center, 1500 East Medical Center Drive, Box 0366, Ann Arbor, MI 48109-0366 · 313-936-5260

John B. O'Connell · (Pre and Post Heart Transplantation Care, Heart Muscle Disease) · Professor and Chairman, Department of Medicine, University of Mississippi · University of Mississippi Medical Center · 2500 North State Street, Jackson, MS 39216 · 601-984-5600

Milton Packer · Professor of Medicine, Mt. Sinai School of Medicine · Mt. Sinai Medical Center · Division of Cardiology, 100th Street & Fifth Avenue, Box 1030, New York, NY 10029 · 212-241-4029

William W. Parmley · Professor of Medicine, University of California at San Francisco School of Medicine · Chief, Division of Cardiology, University of California at San Francisco Medical Center · 505 Parnassus Avenue, Room M-1186, San Francisco, CA 94143 · 415-476-1326

Robert C. Schlant · Professor of Medicine (Cardiology), Emory University School of Medicine · Chief of Cardiology, Grady Memorial Hospital; Attending Cardiologist, Emory University Hospital; Crawford W. Long Hospital · 69 Butler Street, SE, Atlanta, GA 30303 · 404-248-3467

Edmond H. Sonnenblick · Assistant Professor of Medicine, Albert Einstein College of Medicine · Weiler Hospital of the Albert Einstein College of Medicine · 1300 Morris Park Avenue, Bronx, NY 10461 · 212-430-2000

Barry F. Uretsky · (Interventional Cardiology) · Associate Professor of Medicine, University of Pittsburgh School of Medicine · Co-Director of the Cardiac Catheterization Laboratories, and Director of the Heart Failure Unit, Presbyterian University Hospital · 3494 P.U.H., DeSoto at O'Hara Streets, PIttsburgh, PA 152113 412-647-3431

John R. Wilson · Associate Professor of Medicine, University of Pennsylvania School of Medicine · Acting Chief, Cardiology Division, and Director, Heart Failure Program, Hospital of the University of Pennsylvania · 3400 Spruce Street, Third Floor, White Building, Philadelphia, PA 19104 · 215-662-6809

HEART TRANSPLANTATION
(See also General Surgery, Transplantation; Infectious Disease, Transplantation Infections; Thoracic Surgery, Transplantation)

Sharon A. Hunt · (Post Heart Transplantation Care) · Clinical Associate Professor of Medicine, Stanford University School of Medicine, Division of Cardiovascular Medicine · Director, Post-Transplant Program, Stanford University Hospital · 300 Pasteur Drive, Stanford, CA 94305 · 415-723-5771

John B. O'Connell · (Pre and Post Heart Transplantation Care, Heart Muscle Disease) · Professor and Chairman, Department of Medicine, University of Mississippi · University of Mississippi Medical Center · 2500 North State Street, Jackson, MS 39216 · 601-984-5600

Dale Renlund · (Pre and Post Heart Transplantation Care) · University of Utah School of Medicine · Medical Director, University of Utah Health Sciences Center 50 North Medical Drive, Suite 4A100, Salt Lake City, UT 84132 · 801-581-7715

MAGNETIC RESONANCE IMAGING
(See also Adult Neurology, Magnetic Resonance Imaging; Radiology, Magnetic Resonance Imaging)

Justin D. Pearlman · Assistant Professor of Medicine, with joint appointment at MIT, Harvard Medical School · Director of NMR Computing & Technology,

Massachusetts General Hospital · Cardiac Group, Bulfinch Four, MSH, Boston, MA 02114 · 617-726-1707

Ronald Michael Peshock · Associate Professor of Radiology & Cardiology, and Director of Clinical MRI, The University of Texas Southwestern Medical Center at Dallas · 5801 Forest Park Road, Dallas, TX 75235 · 214-688-8112

Gerald M. Pohost · Professor of Medicine and Radiology, and Director, Division of Cardiovascular Disease, The University of Alabama School of Medicine · 1900 University Boulevard, THT 311, Birmingham, AL 35294 · 205-934-3624

Nathaniel Reichek · Professor of Medicine, University of Pennsylvania School of Medicine · Director, Noninvasive Laboratories, Hospital of the University of Pennsylvania · 3400 Spruce Street, 942 West Gates Pavilion, Philadelphia, PA 19104 · 215-662-2284

Gerald Wisenberg · Professor of Medicine, The University of Western Ontario · Chief, Division of Cardiology, St. Joseph's Health Centre · 268 Grosvenor Street, London, Ontario N6A 4V2 · 519-439-2506

NUCLEAR CARDIOLOGY
(See also Nuclear Medicine, Nuclear Cardiology)

George A. Beller · Professor of Medicine and Head, Division of Cardiology, University of Virginia Health Sciences Center · University of Virginia Health Sciences Center · Private Clinics Building, Hospital Drive, Room 3591-E, Box 158, Charlottesville, VA 22908 · 804-924-2134

Daniel S. Berman · Professor of Medicine, University of California at Los Angeles School of Medicine · Director, Nuclear Cardiology, Cedars-Sinai Medical Center 8700 Beverly Boulevard, Room A-042, Los Angeles, CA 90048 · 213-855-4223

Robert Ogden Bonow · Chief, Nuclear Cardiology, National Heart Institute, National Institutes of Health · 9000 Rockville Pike, Building 10, Room 7B 15, Bethesda, MD 20892 · 301-496-9895

Elias H. Botvinick · Professor of Medicine and Radiology, University of California at San Francisco School of Medicine · University of California at San Francisco Medical Center · 505 Parnassus Avenue, Room L-340, San Francisco, CA 94143 415-476-1521

Charles A. Boucher · Associate Professor of Medicine, Harvard Medical School · Massachusetts General Hospital · Cardiac Unit, MGH, Boston, MA 02114 · 617-726-8511

Raymond J. Gibbons · Associate Professor of Medicine, Mayo Medical School · Mayo Clinic · 200 First Street, SW, Rochester, MN 55905 · 507-284-2541

Ami S. Iskandrian · Clinical Professor of Medicine, University of Pennsylvania School of Medicine · Co-Director, Philadelphia Heart Institute; Director, Non Invasive Cardiac Imaging, Presbyterian Medical Center of Philadelphia · 51 North 39th Street, Philadelphia, PA 19104 · 215-662-9068

Lynne L. Johnson · Associate Professor of Clinical Medicine, and Director, Nuclear Cardiology Laboratory, College of Physicians & Surgeons of Columbia University · Columbia-Presbyterian Medical Center · 630 West 168th Street, PH11 Center, Room 1143, New York, NY 10032 · 212-305-9933

Jeffrey A. Leppo · Professor and Clinical Director, Nuclear Cardiology, University of Massachusetts Medical School · University of Massachusetts Medical Center · Department of Nuclear Medicine, 55 Lake Avenue North, H2569, Worcester, MA 01655 · 508-856-3711

Jamshid Maddahi · (Positron Emission Tomography [PET]) · Professor of Radiological Sciences, University of California at Los Angeles School of Medicine · Director, Clinical Positron Emission Tomography (PET) Center, University of California at Los Angeles Medical Center · 10833 LeConte Avenue, AR175, Los Angeles, CA 90024-1721 · 213-206-9896

James L. Ritchie · Professor of Medicine, University of Washington School of Medicine · Seattle Veterans Affairs Medical Center · 1660 South Columbian Way, 111C, Seattle, WA 98108 · 206-764-2008

Alan Rozanski · (Preventive Cardiology) · Associate Professor of Medicine, College of Physicians & Surgeons of Columbia University · Director of Nuclear Cardiology & Cardiac Stress Testing, St. Luke's-Roosevelt Hospital Center · 114th Street and Amsterdam Avenue, New York, NY 10025 · 212-523-4011

Mario S. Verani · Professor of Medicine, Baylor College of Medicine · Director, Nuclear Cardiology Laboratory, The Methodist Hospital · 6535 Fannin Street, F905, Houston, TX 77030 · 713-790-3385

Frans Wackers · Professor of Diagnostic Radiology and Medicine, Yale University School of Medicine · Attending, Diagnostic Imaging (Nuclear Cardiology) and Internal Medicine (Cardiology), and Director, Cardiovascular Nuclear Imaging and Stress Laboratories, Yale-New Haven Hospital · 333 Cedar Street, Thompkins East 2, New Haven, CT 06510 · 203-785-4915

Barry L. Zaret · Robert W. Berliner Professor of Medicine and Chief, Section of Cardiology, Yale University School of Medicine · Chief of Cardiology, Attending Physician, Yale-New Haven Hospital · 333 Cedar Street, New Haven, CT 06510 203-785-4127

PACEMAKERS

Jerry C. Griffin · (Clinical Cardiac Electrophysiology) · Professor of Medicine, University of California at San Francisco School of Medicine · Director of Cardiology Laboratories, University of California at San Francisco Medical Center · 505 Parnassus Avenue, Room M-312, Box 0214, San Francisco, CA 94143 · 415-476-5706

J. Warren Harthorne · Associate Professor of Medicine, Harvard Medical School Director, Pacemaker Laboratory, Massachusetts General Hospital · Wang Ambulatory Care Center, Fourth Floor, Suite 478, 15 Parkman Street, Boston, MA 02114 · 617-726-2876

Victor Parsonnet · Clinical Professor of Surgery, University of Medicine & Dentistry of New Jersey · Director of Surgery, and Director of the Pacemaker Center, Newark Beth Israel Medical Center · 201 Lyons Avenue, Newark, NJ 07112 · 201-926-8038

VASO-SPASTIC DISEASES

Jay D. Coffman · (Raynaud's Disease) · Professor of Medicine, and Chief, Peripheral Vascular Section, Boston University School of Medicine · The University Hospital · 88 East Newton Street, Evans Building, #411, Boston, MA 02116 · 617-638-7260

Mark A. Creager · (Raynaud's Disease) · Associate Professor of Medicine, Harvard Medical School · Director of Noninvasive Vascular Laboratory, Brigham & Women's Hospital · 75 Francis Street, Boston, MA 02115 · 617-732-6631

CLINICAL PHARMACOLOGY

Darrell Abernethy · Professor of Medicine, and Director, Program in Clinical Pharmacology, Brown University School of Medicine · Roger Williams General Hospital · 825 Chalkstone Avenue, Providence, RI 02908 · 401-456-2312

Arthur J. Atkinson, Jr. · (Drug Metabolism) · Professor, Department of Clinical Pharmacology, Northwestern University Medical School · Medical Director, Clinical Pharmacology, Northwestern Memorial Hospital · 707 North Fairbanks Court, 209 Jennings, Chicago, IL 60611 · 312-908-3235

Neal L. Benowitz · (Substance Abuse, Nicotine) · Professor of Medicine, University of California at San Francisco School of Medicine · Chief, Division of Clinical Pharmacology and Experimental Therapeutics, San Francisco General Hospital · 1001 Potrero Avenue, Building 30, Fifth Floor, San Francisco, CA 94110 · 415-821-3125

Thorir D. Bjornsson · Professor, Division of Clinical Pharmacology, Jefferson Medical College of Thomas Jefferson University · Director, Division of Clinical Pharmacology, Thomas Jefferson University Hospital · 1100 Walnut Street (MOB-601), Philadelphia, PA 19107 · 215-955-6086

Terrence F. Blaschke · (Drug Metabolism) · Professor of Medicine and Pharmacology, Stanford University School of Medicine · Stanford University Hospital · 300 Pasteur Drive, Stanford, CA 94305 · 415-723-7801

D. Craig Brater · (Drug Induced Kidney Disease) · Professor and Chairman, Department of Medicine, Professor of Pharmacology, and Chief, Division of Clinical Pharmacology, Indiana University School of Medicine · Indiana University Medical Center · 545 Barnhill Drive, Room EM317, Indianapolis, IN 46202 · 317-630-8796

Garret A. FitzGerald · (Thrombosis, Hypertension) · Professor of Medicine and Pharmacology, and Chief, Division of Clinical Pharmacology, Vanderbilt University School of Medicine · Division of Clinicial Pharmacology, Room 532, Medical Research Building, Nashville, TN 37232-6002 · 615-322-2274

Perry V. Halushka · (Prostaglandins, Platelet Function, Hypertension) · Professor of Pharmacology and Medicine, Medical University of South Carolina · Director,

Division of Clinical Pharmacology, Medical University of South Carolina Hospital Department of Cell and Molecular Pharmacology and Experimental Therapeutics, Division of Clinical Pharmacology, 171 Ashley Avenue, Charleston, SC 29425 · 803-792-2501

Paul S. Lietman · Professor of Medicine, Johns Hopkins University School of Medicine · Chief, Division of Clinical Pharmacology, The Johns Hopkins Medical Institutions · 600 North Wolfe Street, Osler 527, Baltimore, MD 21205 · 410-955-3100

Bernard L. Mirkin · (Pediatric, Cancer Research) · Professor of Pediatrics and Pharmacology, Northwestern University Medical School · Head and Director of Research, and William G. Swartchild, Jr. Distinguished Chair in Research, Children's Memorial Institute for Education & Research · 2300 Children's Plaza, Box 17, Chicago, IL 60614 · 312-880-4590

David Nierenberg · Associate Professor of Medicine and Pharmacology, Dartmouth Medical School · Chief, Division of Clinical Pharmacology, Dartmouth-Hitchcock Medical Center · Lebanon, NH 03756 · 603-650-7679

Alan S. Nies · (Prostaglandins, Hypertension) · Professor of Medicine and Pharmacology, and Head of the Division of Clinical Pharmacology, University of Colorado School of Medicine · University of Colorado Health Sciences Center · 4200 East Ninth Avenue, Box C237, Denver, CO 80262 · 303-270-8455

John A. Oates · (Hypertension, Drug Interactions, Prostaglandins (Eicosasnoid Pharmacology)) · The Thomas F. Frist, Sr. Professor and Chairman, Department of Medicine, Vanderbilt University School of Medicine · Physician-in-Chief, Vanderbilt University Medical Center · Department of Medicine, D3100,Medical Center North, Nashville, TN 37232-2358 · 615-322-3146

Marcus M. Reidenberg · Professor of Medicine & Pharmacology, Cornell University Medical College · Attending Physician, The New York Hospital-Cornell Medical Center · 1300 York Avenue, Box 70, New York, NY 10021 · 212-746-6227

COLON & RECTAL SURGERY

COLON & RECTAL CANCER
(See also Surgical Oncology, Colon & Rectal Cancer)

Herand Abcarian · Professor and Chairman, Department of Surgery, The University of Illinois College of Medicine at Chicago · The University of Illinois Hospital · 840 South Wood Street, Chicago, IL 60612 · 312-782-4828

Victor W. Fazio · Chairman, Department of Colorectal Surgery, The Cleveland Clinic Foundation · One Clinic Center, 9500 Euclid Avenue, Desk A-111, Cleveland, OH 44195 · 216-444-6672

Lee E. Smith · The George Washington University School of Medicine · Director, Division of Colon & Rectal Surgery, George Washington University Medical Center · Department of Surgery, 2150 Pennsylvania Avenue, NW, Washington, DC 20037 · 202-994-4840

Malcolm C. Veidenheimer · (Inflammatory Bowel Disease) · Staff Surgeon, Lahey Clinic Medical Center · 41 Mall Road, Burlington, MA 01805 · 617-273-8571

GENERAL COLON & RECTAL SURGERY

Harold Randolph Bailey · Clinical Professor of Surgery, The University of Texas Medical School at Houston · Hermann Hospital · 6550 Fannin Street, Suite 2307, Houston, TX 77030 · 713-790-9250

Zane Cohen · (Inflammatory Bowel Disease) · Professor of Surgery, University of Toronto School of Medicine · Surgeon-in-Chief, Department of Surgery, Mt. Sinai Hospital · 600 University Avenue, Suite 451, Toronto, Ontario M5G 1X5 · 416-586-8346

Thomas Dailey · St. Luke's-Roosevelt Hospital Center · 53 East 67th Street, New York, NY 10021 · 212-988-7410

Roger R. Dozois · Professor of Surgery, Mayo Medical School · Head, Section of Colon & Rectal Surgery, Mayo Clinic · 200 First Street, SW, Rochester, MN 55905 · 507-284-2218

Victor W. Fazio · Chairman, Department of Colorectal Surgery, The Cleveland Clinic Foundation · One Clinic Center, 9500 Euclid Avenue, Desk A-111, Cleveland, OH 44195 · 216-444-6672

J. Byron Gathright, Jr. · Associate Medical Director, and Chairman, Department of Colon & Rectal Surgery, Ochsner Clinic · 1514 Jefferson Highway, New Orleans, LA 70121 · 504-838-4001

Philip H. Gordon · Professor of Surgery, McGill University · Director, Colon & Rectal Surgery, Sir Mortimer B. Davis Jewish General Hospital · 3755 Cote St. Catherine Road, Pavilion G310, Montreal, Quebec H3T 1E2 · 514-342-1772

David G. Jagelman · (Familial Polyposis) · Chairman, Department of Colorectal Surgery, and Chief, Department of Surgery, The Cleveland Clinic Florida · 3000 Cyprus Creek Road West, Fort Lauderdale, FL 33309 · 305-978-5234

John M. MacKeigan · (Anal, Rectal Surgery) · Associate Professor of Surgery, Michigan State University College of Human Medicine · Chief of Staff, Ferguson Hospital and Ferguson Clinic · 75 Sheldon Boulevard SE, Grand Rapids, MI 49503 · 616-456-0290

W. Patrick Mazier · Clinical Professor of Surgery, Michigan State University College of Human Medicine · Director of Residency Training, and President, Ferguson Clinic · 75 Sheldon Boulevard SE, Grand Rapids, MI 49503 · 800-456-0290

David A. Rothenberger · Clinical Professor of Surgery, University of Minnesota School of Medicine · University of Minnesota Hospital & Clinics · 420 Delaware Street, SE, Box 450 UMHC, Minneapolis, MN 55455 · 612-625-3288, 291-1151

David J. Schoetz, Jr. · Chairman, Department of Colon & Rectal Surgery, Lahey Clinic Medical Center · 41 Mall Road, Department Six West, Burlington, MA 01805 · 617-273-8889

Theodore R. Schrock · (Inflammatory Bowel Disease) · Professor of Surgery, University of California at San Francisco School of Medicine · University of California at San Francisco Medical Center · 505 Parnassus Avenue, Room 887M, San Francisco, CA 94143-0144 · 415-476-2592

Lee E. Smith · (Pelvic Floor Disorders) · The George Washington University School of Medicine · Director, Division of Colon & Rectal Surgery, George Washington University Medical Center · Department of Surgery, 2150 Pennsylvania Avenue, NW, Washington, DC 20037 · 202-994-4840

Malcolm C. Veidenheimer · (Inflammatory Bowel Disease) · Staff Surgeon, Lahey Clinic Medical Center · 41 Mall Road, Burlington, MA 01805 · 617-273-8571

Peter A. Volpe · Clinical Assistant Professor, University of California, San Francisco · Active Staff, St. Mary's Hospital & Medical Center; California Pacific Medical Center · 3838 California Street, Suite 616, San Francisco, CA 94118 · 415-668-0411

Bruce G. Wolff · Associate Professor of Surgery, Mayo Medical School · Rochester Methodist Hospital; St. Marys Hospital · 200 First Street SW, Rochester, MN 55905 · 507-284-2472

DERMATOLOGY

ACNE

James J. Leyden · (Cutaneous Infections, Cosmetics) · Professor of Dermatology, University of Pennsylvania School of Medicine · Hospital of the University of Pennsylvania · Maloney Building, 3400 Spruce Street, Second Floor, Philadelphia, PA 19104 · 215-662-7339

Donald Paul Lookingbill · Professor of Medicine, Pennsylvania State University Chief, Division of Dermatology, The Milton S. Hershey Medical Center · 500 University Drive, P.O. Box 850, Hershey, PA 17033 · 717-531-8307

Alan R. Shalita · Professor and Chairman of Dermatology, and Clinical Associate Dean, State University of New York Health Science Center at Brooklyn · Chief of Dermatology, University Hospital of Brooklyn; Chief of Dermatology, Kings County Hospital Center; Consultant in Dermatology, Brooklyn Veterans Administration Medical Center; Consultant in Dermatology, Brookdale Hospital Medical Center · 450 Clarkson Avenue, Brooklyn, NY 11203 · 718-270-1229

John S. Strauss · Professor and Head, Department of Dermatology, The University of Iowa College of Medicine · Head, Department of Dermatology, The University of Iowa Hospitals & Clinics · 200 Hawkins Drive, Room 2045BT, Iowa City, IA 52242 · 319-356-2274

AGING SKIN

Barbara A. Gilchrest · (Photoaging) · Professor & Chairman, Department of Dermatology, and Director of the Laser Center, Boston University School of Medicine; Senior Scientist, USDA Human Nutrition Research Center on Aging, Tufts University · Dermatologist-in-Chief, The University Hospital; Boston City Hospital · 80 East Concord Street, Boston, MA 02118 · 617-638-5500

James J. Leyden · (Cosmetics) · Professor of Dermatology, University of Pennsylvania School of Medicine · Hospital of the University of Pennsylvania · Maloney Building, 3400 Spruce Street, Second Floor, Philadelphia, PA 19104 · 215-662-7339

ALLERGIC REACTIONS OF THE SKIN

Robert Stern · Associate Professor of Dermatology, Harvard Medical School · Beth Israel Hospital · Libby Building, 330 Brookline Avenue, Room 134, Boston, MA 02215 · 617-735-4592

Bruce U. Wintroub · Professor and Chairman, Department of Dermatology, University of California at San Francisco School of Medicine · University of California at San Francisco Medical Center · 515 Spruce Street, Box 1214, San Francisco, CA 94143-1214 · 415-476-2545

ATOPIC DERMATITIS

Kevin D. Cooper · Associate Professor of Dermatology, The University of Michigan Medical School · Director, Immunodermatology Unit, The University of Michigan Medical Center · 1910 Taubman Center, 1500 East Medical Center Drive, Box 0314, Ann Arbor, MI 48109-0314 · 313-747-0091

Jon M. Hanifin · Professor of Dermatology, Oregon Health Sciences University · 3181 Southwest Sam Jackson Park Road, Portland, OR 97201-3098 · 503-494-5603

CLINICAL DERMATOLOGY

Elizabeth A. Abel · Clinical Associate Professor of Dermatology, Stanford University School of Medicine · Stanford University Hospital; El Camino Hospital · 525 South Drive, Suite 115, Mountain View, CA 94040 · 415-969-5600

Kenneth A. Arndt · (Vascular Birthmarks) · Professor of Dermatology, Harvard Medical School · Dermatologist-in-Chief, Beth Israel Hospital · 330 Brookline Avenue, Boston, MA 02215 · 617-735-4591

Philip L. Bailin · Chairman, Department of Dermatology, and Vice-Chairman, Division of Medicine, Head, Section of Micrographic Surgery (Mohs) & Oncology, The Cleveland Clinic Foundation · One Clinic Center, 9500 Euclid Avenue, Desk A-61, Cleveland, OH 44195-5032 · 216-444-3345

David Rinsey Bickers · Associate Dean, and Professor & Chairman, Department of Dermatology, Case Western Reserve University School of Medicine · Chief of Staff and Senior Vice-President for Medical Affairs, and Director, Department of Dermatology, University Hospitals of Cleveland · Department of Dermatology, 2074 Abington Road, Cleveland, OH 44106 · 216-844-3177

Irwin M. Braverman · Vice-Chairman, Department of Dermatology, Yale University School of Medicine · Yale-New Haven Hospital · 333 Cedar Street, Room LCI5004092, New Haven, CT 06510 · 203-785-4092

Jeffrey P. Callen · (Collagen Vascular Diseases) · Professor and Chief, Division of Dermatology, University of Louisville School of Medicine · University Associates in Dermatology, 310 East Broadway, Louisville, KY 40202 · 502-588-7287

Mark V. Dahl · (Dermatologic Immunology) · Professor of Dermatology, University of Minnesota Medical School · University of Minnesota Hospital a&d Clinics 420 Delaware Street, SE, Box 98, Minneapolis, MN 55455 · 612-625-8625

Vincent A. DeLeo · George Fox Assistant Professor of Dermatology, College of Physicians & Surgeons of Columbia University · Director, Environmental Dermatology, Columbia-Presbyterian Medical Center · 630 West 168th Street, VC15-230A, New York, NY 10032 · 212-305-8484, 305-5293

Richard L. Dobson · Professor of Dermatology, Medical University of South Carolina · Medical University of South Carolina Hospital · 171 Ashley Avenue, Charleston, SC 29425-2215 · 803-792-5858

John Howard Epstein · Clinical Professor of Dermatology, University of California at San Francisco School of Medicine · Mt. Zion Hospital & Medical Center · 450 Sutter Street, Suite 1306, San Francisco, CA 94108 · 415-781-4083

Nancy B. Esterly · (Pediatric) · Professor of Dermatology and Pediatrics, Medical College of Wisconsin · Children's Hospital of Wisconsin · MACC Fund Research Center, 8701 Watertown Plank Road, Milwaukee, WI 53226 · 414-266-4608

Mark Allen Everett · Regents' Professor and Head, Department of Dermatology, The University of Oklahoma College of Medicine · Service Chief, Children's Hospital; Oklahoma Memorial Hospital · 619 Northeast 13th Street, Oklahoma City, OK 73104 · 405-271-6112

Robert M. Fine · Professor of Dermatology, and Clinical Associate Professor of Pathology, Emory University School of Medicine · DeKalb Medical Center · 2675 North Decatur Road, Suite 601, Decatur, GA 30033 · 404-294-0121

Irwin M. Freedberg · Professor and Chairman, Department of Dermatology, New York University School of Medicine · Dermatologist-in-Chief, Tisch Hospital; Bellevue Hospital · Dermatologic Associates, 566 First Avenue, New York, NY 10016 · 212-263-5889

Lowell A. Goldsmith · (Congenital Skin Disorders) · The James H. Sterner Professor and Chairman, Department of Dermatology, University of Rochester School of Medicine & Dentistry · Strong Memorial Hospital, University of Rochester Medical Center · 601 Elmwood Avenue, Box 697, Rochester, NY 14642 · 716-275-3871

Robert W. Goltz · Adjunct Professor, University of California at San Diego School of Medicine · University of California at San Diego Medical Center · 225 Dickinson Street, Mail Code 8420, San Diego, CA 92103-8420 · 619-534-7350

G. Thomas Jansen · Clinical Professor of Dermatology, University of Arkansas for Medical Sciences · St. Vincent's Infirmary · 500 South University Avenue, Suite 501, Little Rock, AR 72205 · 501-664-4161

Brian V. Jegasothy · Professor and Chairman, Department of Dermatology, University of Pittsburgh School of Medicine · Chief, Dermatology Service, Presbyterian University Hospital; University of Pittsburgh Medical Center · 190 Lothrop Street, Suite 145, Pittsburgh, PA 15213 · 412-648-3250

Joseph L. Jorizzo · Professor and Chairman, Department of Dermatology, The Bowman Gray School of Medicine of Wake Forest University · North Carolina Baptist Hospital · Medical Center Boulevard, Winston-Salem, NC 27157-1071 · 919-748-3926

Stephen I. Katz · (Blistering Disorders) · Chief, Dermatology Branch, National Cancer Institute, National Institutes of Health · Building 10, Room 12N238, Bethesda, MD 20892 · 301-496-2481

A. Paul Kelly · Professor and Chief, Division of Dermatology, King Drew Medical Center · Martin Luther King Jr. General Hospital · 12021 South Wilmington Avenue, Room 4016, Los Angeles, CA 90059 · 213-603-4571

John Andrew Kenney, Jr. · Professor of Dermatology, Howard University College of Medicine · Attending Physician, Children's Hospital National Medical Center, Howard University Hospital · 8830 Cameron Street, Suite 201, Silver Spring, MD 20910 · 301-588-8313

Lloyd E. King, Jr. · (Dermatology Research) · Professor of Medicine and Chief, Division of Dermatology, Vanderbilt University School of Medicine · Chief, Dermatology, Vanderbilt University Medical Center; Director, Photophoresis Unit, Veterans Administration Medical Center · 608 Medical Arts Building, 1211 Twenty-First Avenue South, Nashville, TN 37212 · 615-343-9530, 327-5342

Nicholas J. Lowe · Clinical Professor of Dermatology, University of California at Los Angeles School of Medicine · 2001 Santa Monica Boulevard, Santa Monica, CA 90404 · 213-828-2282

Peter John Lynch · Professor and Head, Department of Dermatology, University of Minnesota School of Medicine · University of Minnesota Hospital & Clinics · Dermatology, 420 Delaware Street, SE, Box 98 UMHC, Minneapolis MN 55455 612-625-8625

Frederick D. Malkinson · Professor and Chairman, Department of Dermatology, Rush Medical College · Senior Attending Physician, Rush-Presbyterian-St. Luke's Medical Center · 1653 West Congress Parkway, Chicago, IL 60612-3864 · 312-942-6096

Charles J. McDonald · Professor and Head of Dermatology, Brown University School of Medicine · Physician-in-Charge of Dermatology, Roger Williams Medical Center, The Rhode Island Hospital · 825 Chalkstone Avenue, Providence, RI 09208 · 401-456-2590

Laurence Herbert Miller · Assistant Professor of Dermatology, The George Washington University School of Medicine · Special Advisor for Skin Diseases, National Institutes of Health · 5454 Wisconsin Avenue, Suite 747, Chevy Chase, MD 20815 · 301-652-2882

Larry E. Millikan · Professor and Chairman, Department of Dermatology, Tulane University School of Medicine · Tulane University Medical Center · 1430 Tulane Avenue, New Orleans, LA 70112 · 504-588-5114

Samuel Leonard Moschella · Clinical Professor of Dermatology, Emeritus, Harvard Medical School · Senior Consultant, Department of Dermatology, Lahey Clinic Medical Center · 41 Mall Road, Burlington, MA 01805 · 617-273-8443

Richard B. Odom · Clinical Professor and Associate Chairman, Department of Dermatology, University of California, San Francisco School of Medicine · University of California, San Francisco Medical Center · 400 Parnassus Avenue, San Francisco, CA 94143 · 415-476-2066

Neal S. Penneys · Professor and Director of Dermatology, Saint Louis University School of Medicine · Saint Louis University Affiliated Hospitals · 1402 South Grand Boulevard, St. Louis, MO 63104 · 314-577-8762

Harold Otto Perry · Professor Emeritus, Mayo Medical School · Mayo Clinic · 200 First Street, SW, Rochester, MN 55905 · 507-284-2522

Colin A. Ramsay · Professor of Dermatology, University of Toronto School of Medicine · Head, Division of Dermatology, The Toronto Hospital; Women's College Hospital · 123 Edward Street, Suite 725, Toronto, Ontario M5G 1E2 · 416-599-0403

Daniel N. Sauder · Professor and Chief of Dermatology, University of Toronto School of Medicine · Sunnybrook Health Science Center · 2075 Bayview Avenue, Toronto, Ontario M4N 3M5 · 416-480-4767

Walter B. Shelley · Professor of Dermatology, Medical College of Ohio · Medical College of Ohio Hospital · Division of Dermatology, P.O. Box 10008, Toledo, OH 43699-0008 · 419-381-3720

Nicholas Arthur Soter · Professor of Dermatology, New York University School of Medicine · New York University Medical Center · 550 First Avenue, New York, NY 10016 · 212-263-5253

Frances J. Storrs · Professor, Physician and Surgeon,Department of Dermatology, Oregon Health Sciences University · 3181 Southwest Sam Jackson Park Road, Portland, OR 97201-3098 · 503-494-5604

Denny L. Tuffanelli · (Collagen Vascular Diseases) · Clinical Professor of Dermatology, University of California at San Francisco School of Medicine · California Pacific Hospital · 450 Sutter Street Suite 1306, San Francisco, CA 94108 · 415-781-4083

Dennis Allen Weigand · Professor of Dermatology, The University of Oklahoma College of Medicine · Veterans Affairs Medical Center · 619 Northeast 13th Street, Oklahoma City, OK 73104 · 405-271-6112

CONTACT DERMATITIS

Robert M. Adams · (Occupational Dermatology) · Clinical Professor of Dermatology, Stanford University School of Medicine · Stanford University Hospital · 1300 University Drive, Suite Six, Menlo Park, CA 94025 · 415-323-0276

Donald Vincent Belsito · Associate Professor of Dermatology, New York University School of Medicine · New York University Medical Center · 550 First Avenue, New York, NY 10016 · 212-263-5889

Vincent A. DeLeo · George Fox Assistant Professor of Dermatology, College of Physicians & Surgeons of Columbia University · Director, Environmental Dermatology, Columbia-Presbyterian Medical Center · 630 West 168th Street, VC15-230A, New York, NY 10032 · 212-305-8484, 305-5293

Howard I. Maibach · Professor and Vice-Chairman, Department of Dermatology, University of California at San Francisco School of Medicine · Professor of Dermatology, University of California at San Francisco Medical Center · University of California Medical Center, 400 Parnassus, San Francisco, CA 94122 · 415-476-2468; 476-4256

James Garfield Marks, Jr. · Professor of Medicine, Pennsylvania State University The Milton S. Hershey Medical Center · 500 University Drive, P.O. Box 850, Hershey, PA 17033 · 717-531-8307

Robert L. Rietschel · Clinical Associate Professor of Dermatology, Tulane University School of Medicine; Louisiana State University School of Medicine · Chairman, Department of Dermatology, Ochsner Clinic · 1514 Jefferson Highway, 11th Floor North, New Orleans, LA 70123 · 504-838-3940

William F. Schorr · Clinical Professor of Dermatology, University of Wisconsin-Madison School of Medicine · St. Joseph's Hospital; Marshfield Clinic · 1000 North Oak Avenue, Marshfield, WI 54449-5777 · 715-387-5311

Frances J. Storrs · Professor, Physician and Surgeon,Department of Dermatology, Oregon Health Sciences University · 3181 Southwest Sam Jackson Park Road, Portland, OR 97201-3098 · 503-494-5604

James S. Taylor · Head, Section of Industrial Dermatology, The Cleveland Clinic Foundation · One Clinic Center, 9500 Euclid Avenue, A-61, Cleveland, OH 44195-5032 · 216-444-5723

CUTANEOUS IMMUNOLOGY

Grant J. Anhalt · (Blistering Disorders) · Associate Professor of Dermatology, Johns Hopkins University School of Medicine · Director, Dermato-Immunology Labs, The Johns Hopkins Medical Institutions · Richard Starr Ross Research Building, Room 771, 720 Rutland Avenue, Baltimore, MD 21205-2196 · 410-955-2992

Eugene A. Bauer · (Blistering Disorders, Epidermolysis Bullosa) · Professor and Chairman, Department of Dermatology, Stanford University School of Medicine Chief of the Dermatology Service, Stanford University Hospital · 300 Pasteur Drive, Room R-150, Stanford, CA 94305 · 415-723-6105

Paul R. Bergstresser · Chairman, Department of Dermatology, The University of Texas Southwestern Medical Center at Dallas · Chief, Dermatology Service, Parkland Memorial Hospital · 5323 Harrry Hines Boulevard, Dallas, TX 75235-9069 · 214-688-2969

Robert Alan Briggaman · (Blistering Disorders) · Professor and Chairman, Department of Dermatology, University of North Carolina School of Medicine · University of North Carolina Hospitals · 137 UNC Hospitals, Campus Box 7600, Chapel Hill, NC 27514 · 919-966-3322

Jean-Claude Bystryn · (Blistering Disorders) · Professor of Dermatology, New York University School of Medicine · New York University Medical Center, Tisch Hospital · 530 First Avenue, New York, NY 10016 · 212-889-3846

Luis A. Diaz · (Blistering Disorders) · Professor and Chairman, Department of Dermatology, Medical College of Wisconsin · Veterans Affairs Medical Center, Froedtert Memorial Lutheran Hospital, Children's Hospital of Wisconsin, Milwaukee County Medical Complex · 8701 Watertown Plank Road, Milwaukee, WI 53226 · 414-266-4087

Jo-David Fine · (Blistering Disorders) · Associate Professor of Dermatology, University of North Carolina School of Medicine · Principal Investigator, National Epidermolysis Bullosa Registry, University of North Carolina Hospitals · Campus Box 7600, Chapel Hill, NC 27514 · 919-966-3321

W. Ray Gammon · (Blistering Disorders) · Professor of Dermatology, University of North Carolina School of Medicine · University of North Carolina Hospitals · Manning Drive, Campus Box 7600, Chapel Hill, NC 27514 · 919-966-3321

Russell P. Hall · (Blistering Disorders) · Assistant Professor of Medicine, Duke University School of Medicine · Duke University Medical Center · Box 3135, DUMC, Durham, NC 27710 · 919-684-5337

J. Clark Huff · (Blistering Disorders) · Professor of Dermatology, University of Colorado School of Medicine · University of Colorado Health Sciences Center · 4200 East Ninth Avenue, Box E-153, Denver, CO 80262 · 303-372-1132

Robert E. Jordon · (Blistering Disorders) · Professor and Chairman, Department of Dermatology, The University of Texas Medical School at Houston · Chief of Dermatology, Hermann Hospital · 6431 Fannin Street, Room 1204, Houston, TX 77030 · 713-792-5115

Stephen I. Katz · (Blistering Disorders) · Chief, Dermatology Branch, National Cancer Institute, National Institutes of Health · Building 10, Room 12N238, Bethesda, MD 20892 · 301-496-2481

Thomas J. Lawley · (Vasculitis, Immune-Complex Vasculitis, Blistering Disorders) · Professor and Chairman, Department of Dermatology, Emory University School of Medicine · Department of Dermatology, 5001 Woodruff Memorial Building, Atlanta, GA 30322 · 404-727-5872

Lela A. Lee · (Collagen Vascular Diseases) · Assistant Professor of Dermatology, University of Colorado School of Medicine · 4200 East Ninth Avenue, Box E-153, Denver, CO 80262 · 303-372-1132

David A. Norris · (Collagen Vascular Disease) · Professor of Dermatology, University of Colorado School of Medicine · University of Colorado Health Sciences Center · 4200 East Ninth Avenue, Box E-153, Denver, CO 80262 · 303-372-1132

Thomas T. Provost · (Blistering Disorders, Collagen Vascular Diseases, Lupus) · Noxell Professor and Chairman of Dermatology, Johns Hopkins University School of Medicine · The Johns Hopkins Medical Institutions · 600 North Wolfe Street, Blalock 920, Baltimore, MD 21205 · 410-955-3397

W. Mitchell Sams, Jr. · (Vasculitis) · Professor and Chairman, Department of Dermatology, The University of Alabama School of Medicine · Kracke Building, 1922 Seventh Avenue South, Room 101, Birmingham, AL 35233 · 205-934-4141

Richard D. Sontheimer · (Collagen Vascular Disease, Lupus, Erythematosus) · Vice Chairman, Department of Dermatology, The University of Texas Southwestern Medical Center at Dallas · Parkland Memorial Hospital; Children's Medical Center; Zale-Lipshy University Hospital; St. Paul Medical Center · 5323 Harry Hines Boulevard, Dallas, TX 75235 -9069 · 214-688-3436

John Roger Stanley · (Blistering Disorders) · Medical Officer, Dermatology Branch, National Cancer Institute, National Institutes of Health · Building 10, Room 12N238, Bethesda, MD 20892 · 301-496-2481

Michael D. Tharp · (Urticaria) · Professor and Vice-Chairman, Department of Dermatology, and Director of Clinical & Basic Science Research, University of Pittsburgh School of Medicine · Presbyterian University Hospital · 190 Lothrop Street, Suite 145, Pittsburgh, PA 15213 · 412-648-3252

Denny L. Tuffanelli · (Collagen Vascular Diseases) · Clinical Professor of Dermatology, University of California at San Francisco School of Medicine · California Pacific Hospital · 450 Sutter Street Suite 1306, San Francisco, CA 94108 · 415-781-4083

Kim B. Yancey · Associate Professor of Dermatology, Uniformed Services University of Health Sciences · 4301 Jones Bridge Road, Building B, Room B4082, Bethesda, MD 20814-4799 · 301-295-3699

John Zone · (Blistering Disorders) · Chief Professor of Dermatology, University of Utah School of Medicine · University of Utah Health Sciences Center · 50 North Medical Drive, Salt Lake City, UT 84132 · 801-581-7837

CUTANEOUS LYMPHOMAS

Richard L. Edelson · (Immunologic Diseases of the Skin) · Professor and Chairman, Department of Dermatology, Yale University School of Medicine · Professor and Chairman, Department of Dermatology, Yale-New Haven Hospital · 333 Cedar Street, LCI500, New Haven, CT 06510 · 203-785-4632

Robert E. Tigelaar · Professor of Dermatology and Immunobiology, Yale University School of Medicine · Attending Physician, Yale-New Haven Hospital · 333 Cedar Street, P.O. Box 3333, New Haven, CT 06510 · 203-785-4093

DEPIGMENTING DISEASES

John Andrew Kenney, Jr. · Professor of Dermatology, Howard University College of Medicine · Attending Physician, Children's Hospital National Medical Center, Howard University Hospital · 8830 Cameron Street, Suite 201, Silver Spring, MD 20910 · 301-588-8313

David A. Norris · (Vitiligo, Autoimmune Depigmenting Diseases) · Professor of Dermatology, University of Colorado School of Medicine · University of Colorado Health Sciences Center · 4200 East Ninth Avenue, Box E-153, Denver, CO 80262 303-372-1132

DERMATOPATHOLOGY
(See also Pathology, Dermatopathology)

A. Bernard Ackerman · Professor, Department of Dermatology & Pathology; and Director of Dermatopathology, New York University School of Medicine · New York University Medical Center · 530 First Avenue, Suite 7J, New York, NY 10016 · 212-263-7250

John C. Maize · Professor & Chairman of Dermatology, and Professor of Pathology, Medical University of South Carolina · Medical University of South Carolina Hospital · 171 Ashley Avenue, Charleston, SC 29425-2215 · 803-792-5858

ECZEMA

Kevin D. Cooper · Associate Professor of Dermatology, The University of Michigan Medical School · Director, Immunodermatology Unit, The University of Michigan Medical Center · 1910 Taubman Center, 1500 East Medical Center Drive, Box 0314, Ann Arbor, MI 48109-0314 · 313-747-0091

Irwin M. Freedberg · Professor and Chairman, Department of Dermatology, New York University School of Medicine · Dermatologist-in-Chief, Tisch Hospital; Bellevue Hospital · Dermatologic Associates, 566 First Avenue, New York, NY 10016 · 212-263-5889

Jon M. Hanifin · Professor of Dermatology, Oregon Health Sciences University · 3181 Southwest Sam Jackson Park Road, Portland, OR 97201-3098 · 503-494-5603

GENITAL DERMATOLOGICAL DISEASE
(See also Obstetrics & Gynecology, Genital Dermatological Disease)

Libby I. E. Edwards · Clinical Associate Professor, University of North Carolina · Chief of Dermatology, Carolinas Medical Center · Department of Internal Medicine, 1000 Blythe Avenue, Charlotte, NC 28203 · 704-355-3165

Peter John Lynch · Professor and Head, Department of Dermatology, University of Minnesota School of Medicine · University of Minnesota Hospital & Clinics · Dermatology, 420 Delaware Street, SE, Box 98 UMHC, Minneapolis MN 55455 612-625-8625

Marilynne McKay · (Vulvar Diseases) · Associate Professor of Dermatology, Emory University School of Medicine · Chief of Dermatology Service, Grady Memorial Hospital · Dermatology-The Emory Clinic,1365 Clifton Road NE, Atlanta, GA 30322 · 404-248-3681

Stephanie Hoyer Pincus · (Vulvar Diseases) · Professor & Chairman, Department of Dermatology, and Professor, Department of Medicine, State University of New York at Buffalo, School of Medicine & Biomedical Sciences · Buffalo General Hospital · 100 High Street, Suite C319, Buffalo, NY 14203 · 716-845-1566

Maria L. Turner · (Vulvar Diseases) · Medical Officer, Dermatology Branch, National Institutes of Health · 9000 Rockville Pike, Building 10, Room 13C306, Bethesda, MD 20982 · 301-496-6421

HAIR

Wilma F. Bergfeld · (Hair Disorders) · Head, Clinical Research, Department of Dermatology, and Head, Dermatopathology, Department of Pathology, Cleveland Clinic Foundation; Professor, Department of Dermatology, Cleveland Clinic Foundation, Education · The Cleveland Clinic Foundation · One Clinic Center, 9500 Euclid Avenue, Desk A-61, Cleveland, OH 44195-5032 · 216-444-5722

Arthur P. Bertolino · (Hair Disorders) · Assistant Clinical Professor of Dermatology, New York University Medical Center · Director, Hair Consultation Unit, New York University Medical Center · Three East 76th Street, New York, NY 10021; 190 Dayton Street, Ridgewood, NJ 07450 · 212-861-9393, 201-444-7888

Rebecca Jo Ann Caserio · (Hair Disorders) · Clinical Assistant Professor of Dermatology, University of Pittsburgh School of Medicine · St. Margaret's Hospital · 241 Freeport Road, Pittsburgh, PA 15215 · 412-784-1606

Richard L. DeVillez · (Hair Disorders) · Chief, Division of Dermatology, The University of Texas at San Antonio · 7703 Floyd Curl Drive, San Antonio, TX 78284 · 512-567-4887

Virginia C. Fiedler · (Hair Disorders) · Professor and Director, Department of Dermatology, Northwestern University Medical School · 303 East Chicago Avenue, Ward Building 3-179, Chicago, IL 60611 · 312-908-8173

Lowell A. Goldsmith · (Hair Disorders) · The James H. Sterner Professor and Chairman, Department of Dermatology, University of Rochester School of Medicine & Dentistry · Strong Memorial Hospital, University of Rochester Medical Center · 601 Elmwood Avenue, Box 697, Rochester, NY 14642 · 716-275-3871

John T. Headington · (Hair Disorders) · Professor of Pathology and Dermatology, The University of Michigan Medical School · The University of Michigan Medical Center · Medical Science I, 1301 Catherine, M5242/0602, Box 0602, Ann Arbor, MI 48109-0602 · 313-936-1874

Maria K. Hordinsky · (Hair Disorders) · Associate Professor of Dermatology, University of Minnesota School of Medicine · University of Minnesota Hospital & Clinics · 4-240 Phillips Wagensteen Building, 420 Delaware Street SE, Box 98, Minneapolis, MN 55455 · 615-625-8625

Elise A. Olsen · (Hair Disorders) · Associate Professor of Medicine, Duke University School of Medicine · Director of the Dermatopharmacology Study Center, Duke University Medical Center · P.O. Box 3294, Durham, NC 27710 · 919-684-6844

Norman Orentreich · (Hair Transplantation, Hair Disorders) · Clinical Professor, Department of Dermatology, New York University School of Medicine · Associate Attending Physican, Department of Dermatology, New York University Medical Center · 909 Fifth Avenue, New York, NY 10021 · 212-606-0828

Vera H. Price · (Hair Disorders) · Professor of Clinical Dermatology, University of California at San Francisco School of Medicine · 350 Parnassus Avenue, Suite 404, San Francisco, CA 94117 · 415-476-9350

Robert L. Rietschel · (Hair Disorders) · Clinical Associate Professor of Dermatology, Tulane University School of Medicine; Louisiana State University School of Medicine · Chairman, Department of Dermatology, Ochsner Clinic · 1514 Jefferson Highway, 11th Floor North, New Orleans, LA 70123 · 504-838-3940

Ronald C. Savin · (Hair Disorders) · Clinical Professor of Dermatology, Yale University School of Medicine · Yale-New Haven Hospital · 134 Park Street, New Haven, CT 06513 · 203-865-6143

Nia Terezakis · (Hair Disorders) · 2633 Napoleon Avenue, Suite 905, New Orleans, LA 70115 · 504-897-6267

David A. Whiting · (Hair Disorders) · Clinical Professor of Dermatology & Pediatrics, The University of Texas Southwestern Medical Center at Dallas · Children's Medical Center of Dallas · 3600 Gaston Avenue, Suite 1051, Dallas, TX 75246 · 214-824-2087

HANSEN'S DISEASE

Thomas H. Rea · Professor of Dermatology, University of Southern California School of Medicine · Chief of Dermatology, The Los Angeles County + University of Southern California Medical Center · 1200 North State Street, Romm 8440, Los Angeles, CA 90033 · 213-226-3373

HERPES VIRUS INFECTIONS
(See also Infectious Disease, Herpes Virus Infections)

J. Clark Huff · Professor of Dermatology, University of Colorado School of Medicine · University of Colorado Health Sciences Center · 4200 East Ninth Avenue, Box E-153, Denver, CO 80262 · 303-372-1132

LASER SURGERY
(See also Plastic Surgery, Laser Surgery)

Kenneth A. Arndt · (Vascular Birthmarks) · Professor of Dermatology, Harvard Medical School · Dermatologist-in-Chief, Beth Israel Hospital · 330 Brookline Avenue, Boston, MA 02215 · 617-735-4591

Philip L. Bailin · Chairman, Department of Dermatology, and Vice-Chairman, Division of Medicine, Head, Section of Micrographic Surgery (Mohs) & Oncology, The Cleveland Clinic Foundation · One Clinic Center, 9500 Euclid Avenue, Desk A-61, Cleveland, OH 44195-5032 · 216-444-3345

Jeffrey S. Dover · (Vascular Birthmarks) · Assistant Professor of Dermatology, Harvard Medical School · Chief, Division of Dermatology, New England Deaconess Hospital · 110 Francis Street, Suite 7H, Boston, MA 02215 · 617-732-9681

Jerome M. Garden · (Vascular Birthmarks) · Associate Professor, Department of Dermatology, Northwestern University Medical School · Northwestern Memorial Hospital; Children's Memorial Hospital · 150 East Huron Street, Suite 910, Chicago, IL 60611 · 312-280-0890

Roy G. Geronemus · (Vascular Birthmarks) · Chief, Surgery & Laser Section, Skin & Cancer Unit, Mohs Micrographic Surgeon Skin Cancer, Department of Dermatology, New York University School of Medicine · New York University Medical Center · 566 First Avenue, New York, NY 10016 · 212-263-7306

Nicholas J. Lowe · Clinical Professor of Dermatology, University of California at Los Angeles School of Medicine · 2001 Santa Monica Boulevard, Santa Monica, CA 90404 · 213-828-2282

Ronald G. Wheeland · (Vascular Birthmarks) · Professor and Chairman, Department of Dermatology, University of California at Davis School of Medicine · Chief, Mohs & Laser Surgery, University of California at Davis Medical Center · 1700 Alhambra Boulevard, Sacramento, CA 95816 · 916-734-6191

MUCOUS MEMBRANE DISEASES

Edward Alexander Krull · (Mouth Diseases) · Chairman, Department of Dermatology, Henry Ford Medical Center · Detroit, MI 48202 · 313-876-2170

Roy S. Rogers III · (Mouth Diseases) · Professor of Dermatology, Mayo Medical School · Dean, Mayo School of Health-Related Sciences, Mayo Clinic; St. Mary's Hospital; Rochester Methodist Hospital · 200 First Street, SW, Rochester, MN 55905-0001 · 507-284-3837

PEDIATRIC DERMATOLOGY
(See also Pediatrics, Pediatric Dermatology)

Bernard Alan Cohen · Associate Professor of Pediatrics & Dermatology, Johns Hopkins University School of Medicine · Director, Pediatric Dermatology, The Johns Hopkins Medical Institutions · 600 North Wolfe Street, Baltimore, MD 21205 · 410-955-2049

Ilona Frieden · Assistant Clinical Professor of Pediatrics in Dermatology, University of California at San Francisco School of Medicine · University of California at San Francisco Medical Center · Department of Dermatology, 400 Parnassus, Third Floor, Box 0316, San Francisco, CA 94143-0316 · 415-476-4239

Ronald C. Hansen · Professor, The University of Arizona College of Medicine · The University of Arizona Health Sciences Center · Section of Dermatology, 1501 North Campbell, Tucson, AZ 85724 · 602-626-7783

Adelaide A. Hebert · Assistant Professor of Dermatology and Pediatrics, The University of Texas Health Science Center at Houston · Attending Staff, The University of Texas MD Anderson Cancer Center; Hermann Hospital · 6431 Fannin Street, Suite 1.204, Houston, TX 77030 · 713-794-5230

Paul Joseph Honig · Professor of Pediatrics & Dermatology, University of Pennsylvania School of Medicine · Director, Pediatric Dermatology, The Children's Hospital of Philadelphia · Department of Dermatology, 34th and Civic Center Boulevard, Philadelphia, PA 19104 · 215-590-2169

Sidney Hurwitz · Clinical Professor of Pediatrics & Dermatology, Yale University School of Medicine · Yale-New Haven Hospital, Hospital of St. Raphael · 2 Church Street South, New Haven, CT 06519 · 203-776-0600

Alvin H. Jacobs · Professor Emeritus of Dermatology, Stanford University School of Medicine · Lucile Salter Packard Children's Hospital at Stanford · Edwards Building, R-144, 300 Pasteur Drive, Stanford, CA 94305 · 415-723-6101

Alfred T. Lane · Associate Professor of Dermatology and Pediatrics, Stanford University School of Medicine · Director of Pediatric Dermatology, Stanford University Hospital; Lucile Salter Packard Children's Hospital at Stanford · 300 Pasteur Drive, Edwards Building R-144, Stanford CA 94305-5334 · 415-725-7022

Moise L. Levy · Assistant Professor of Dermatology and Pediatrics, Baylor College of Medicine · Chief, Pediatric Dermatology, Texas Children's Hospital · 6621 Fannin Street, Houston, TX 77030 · 713-770-3720

Anne Lucky · (Acne) · Children's Hospital Medical Center · 7691 Five Mile Road, Cincinnati, OH 45230 · 513-559-4215, 232-3332, 791-6161

Susan B. Mallory · Associate Professor of Dermatology and Pediatrics, Washington University School of Medicine · Director of Pediatric Dermatology, St. Louis Children's Hospital · 400 South Kingshighway Boulevard, Room 8E6, St. Louis, MO 63110 · 314-454-2714

Joseph McGuire · (Psoriasis) · Carl Herzog Professor of Dermatology and Pediatrics, Stanford University School of Medicine · Stanford University Hospital; Lucile Salter Packard Children's Hospital at Stanford · 300 Pasteur Drive, Edwards Building, R114, Stanford, CA 94305 · 415-725-5272

Joseph G. Morelli · (Birthmarks, Laser Surgery) · Assistant Professor of Dermatology and Pediatrics, University of Colorado School of Medicine · University Hospital · 4200 East Ninth Avenue, Room B153, Denver, CO 80262 · 303-372-1111

Arthur L. Norins · Professor and Chairman, Department of Dermatology, Indiana University School of Medicine · Indiana University Medical Center · 1100 West Michigan Street, Room RG524, Indianapolis, IN 46202 · 317-630-6691

Amy S. Paller · Associate Professor of Pediatrics and Dermatology, Northwestern University Medical School · Head, Division of Dermatology, The Children's Memorial Hospital · 2300 Children's Plaza, Box 107, Chicago, IL 60614 · 312-880-4698

Neil S. Prose · (AIDS, General) · Duke University School of Medicine · Duke University Medical Center · Box 3252, DUMC, Durham, NC 27710 · 919-684-5146

Lawrence Schachner · Professor of Dermatology and Pediatrics, University of Miami School of Medicine · Director, Division of Pediatric Dermatology, University of Miami-Jackson Memorial Medical Center · P.O. Box 016250 (R-250), Miami, FL 33101 · 305-547-6742

Lawrence M. Solomon · Professor of Dermatology, The University of Illinois College of Medicine at Chicago · The University of Illinois Hospital · Box 6998, Chicago, IL 60680 · 312-996-6966

Mary K. Spraker · Associate Professor of Dermatology and Pediatrics, Emory University School of Medicine · Chief of Dermatology, Henrietta Egleston Hospital for Children; Emory University Affiliated Hospitals · 1365 Clifton Road, NE, Atlanta, GA 30322 · 404-248-3336

Oon Tian Tan · (Pediatric Laser Surgery) · Associate Professor of Pathology, Boston University School of Medicine · Director, Laser Research Laboratory, Boston City Hospital · 29 Commonwealth Avenue, Suite 101, Boston, MA 02116 617-424-8335

Samuel Weinberg · Clinical Professor of Dermatology, New York University School of Medicine · Attending Staff, Dermatology, New York University Medical Center · 2035 Lakeville Road, New Hyde Park, NY 11040 · 516-352-6151

William L. Weston · Professor and Chairman, Department of Dermatology; and Professor of Pediatrics, University of Colorado School of Medicine · University of Colorado Health Sciences Center · 4200 East Ninth Avenue, Box E-153, Denver, CO 80262 · 303-372-1111

Mary L. Williams · (Keratinizing Disorders) · Associate Professor of Dermatology and Pediatrics, University of California at San Francisco School of Medicine · University of California at San Francisco Medical Center; San Francisco Veterans Administration Medical Center · 400 Parnassus Avenue, San Francisco, CA 94143-0316 · 415-476-4239

PHOTOBIOLOGY

Elizabeth A. Abel · Clinical Associate Professor of Dermatology, Stanford University School of Medicine · Stanford University Hospital; El Camino Hospital · 525 South Drive, Suite 115, Mountain View, CA 94040 · 415-969-5600

Paul R. Bergstresser · Chairman, Department of Dermatology, The University of Texas Southwestern Medical Center at Dallas · Chief, Dermatology Service, Parkland Memorial Hospital · 5323 Harrry Hines Boulevard, Dallas, TX 75235-9069 · 214-688-2969

David Rinsey Bickers · Associate Dean, and Professor & Chairman, Department of Dermatology, Case Western Reserve University School of Medicine · Chief of Staff and Senior Vice-President for Medical Affairs, and Director, Department of Dermatology, University Hospitals of Cleveland · Department of Dermatology, 2074 Abington Road, Cleveland, OH 44106 · 216-844-3177

Vincent A. DeLeo · George Fox Assistant Professor of Dermatology, College of Physicians & Surgeons of Columbia University · Director, Environmental Dermatology, Columbia-Presbyterian Medical Center · 630 West 168th Street, VC15-230A, New York, NY 10032 · 212-305-8484, 305-5293

John Howard Epstein · Clinical Professor of Dermatology, University of California at San Francisco School of Medicine · Mt. Zion Hospital & Medical Center · 450 Sutter Street, Suite 1306, San Francisco, CA 94108 · 415-781-4083

Nicholas J. Lowe · (Phototherapy, Sun Screen Research) · Clinical Professor of Dermatology, University of California at Los Angeles School of Medicine · 2001 Santa Monica Boulevard, Santa Monica, CA 90404 · 213-828-2282

Warwick L. Morison · (Phototherapy) · Associate Professor of Dermatology, Johns Hopkins University School of Medicine · The Johns Hopkins Medical Institutions 8422 Bellona Lane, Suite 205, Towson, MD 21204 · 301-296-5400

Colin A. Ramsay · Professor of Dermatology, University of Toronto School of Medicine · Head, Division of Dermatology, The Toronto Hospital; Women's College Hospital · 123 Edward Street, Suite 725, Toronto, Ontario M5G 1E2 · 416-599-0403

Nicholas Arthur Soter · Professor of Dermatology, New York University School of Medicine · New York University Medical Center · 550 First Avenue, New York, NY 10016 · 212-263-5253

PSORIASIS

Elizabeth A. Abel · Clinical Associate Professor of Dermatology, Stanford University School of Medicine · Stanford University Hospital; El Camino Hospital · 525 South Drive, Suite 115, Mountain View, CA 94040 · 415-969-5600

Robert Auerbach · Clinical Associate Professor of Dermatology, New York University School of Medicine · Attending Staff, Tisch Hospital, and New York University Medical Center · 440 East 57th Street, New York, NY 10022 · 212-935-9610

Howard P. Baden · Professor of Dermatology, Harvard Medical School · Dermatologist, Massachusetts General Hospital · Department of Dermatology, CBRC, Building 149, 13th Street, Charlestown, MA 02129 · 617-726-3993

David Rinsey Bickers · Associate Dean, and Professor & Chairman, Department of Dermatology, Case Western Reserve University School of Medicine · Chief of Staff and Senior Vice-President for Medical Affairs, and Director, Department of Dermatology, University Hospitals of Cleveland · Department of Dermatology, 2074 Abington Road, Cleveland, OH 44106 · 216-844-3177

William E. Clendenning · Professor of Clinical Medicine, Department of Dermatology, Dartmouth Medical School · Dartmouth-Hitchcock Medical Center · One Medical Center Drive, Lebanon, NH 03756 · 603-650-5175

Irwin M. Freedberg · Professor and Chairman, Department of Dermatology, New York University School of Medicine · Dermatologist-in-Chief, Tisch Hospital; Bellevue Hospital · Dermatologic Associates, 566 First Avenue, New York, NY 10016 · 212-263-5889

Gerald G. Krueger · Professor of Dermatology, University of Utah School of Medicine · University of Utah Health Sciences Center · 50 North Medical Drive, Salt Lake City, UT 84132 · 801-581-7837

Gerald S. Lazarus · Professor and Chairman, Department of Dermatology, University of Pennsylvania School of Medicine · Hospital of the University of Pennsylvania · 3400 Spruce Street, Philadelphia, PA 19104 · 215-662-6536

Nicholas J. Lowe · Clinical Professor of Dermatology, University of California at Los Angeles School of Medicine · 2001 Santa Monica Boulevard, Santa Monica, CA 90404 · 213-828-2282

Howard I. Maibach · Professor and Vice-Chairman, Department of Dermatology, University of California at San Francisco School of Medicine · Professor of Dermatology, University of California at San Francisco Medical Center · University of California Medical Center, 400 Parnassus, San Francisco, CA 94122 · 415-476-2468; 476-4256

M. Alan Menter · Associate Clinical Professor of Dermatology, The University of Texas Southwestern Medical Center at Dallas · Director, Baylor Psoriasis Center-Dallas · 3409 Worth Street, Suite 500, Dallas, TX 75246 · 214-826-8390

Warwick L. Morison · (Phototherapy) · Associate Professor of Dermatology, Johns Hopkins University School of Medicine · The Johns Hopkins Medical Institutions 8422 Bellona Lane, Suite 205, Towson, MD 21204 · 301-296-5400

Sheldon R. Pinnell · J. Lamar Callaway Professor of Dermatology, Duke University School of Medicine · Chief, Division of Dermatology, Duke University Medical Center · Box 3135, DUMC, Durham, NC 27710 · 919-684-5337

John J. Voorhees · Professor and Chairman, Department of Dermatology, The University of Michigan Medical School · The University of Michigan Medical Center · 1500 East Medical Center Drive, Box 0314, Ann Arbor, MI 48109-0314 313-936-4078

Gerald D. Weinstein · Professor and Chairman, Department of Dermatology, University of California at Irvine School of Medicine · University of California at Irvine Medical Center · Irvine, CA 92717 · 714-856-5515

SKIN CANCER SURGERY & RECONSTRUCTION

Michael J. Albom · (Mohs Micrographic Surgery & Reconstruction) · Associate Clinical Professor, Department of Dermatology, New York University School of Medicine · New York University Medical Center, Skin & Cancer Unit · 33 East 70th Street, New York, NY 10021 · 212-517-2121

Rex A. Amonette · Clinical Professor of Dermatology, The University of Tennessee, The Health Science Center · Baptist Memorial Hospital · 1455 Union Avenue, Memphis, TN 38104 · 901-726-6655

Philip L. Bailin · Chairman, Department of Dermatology, and Vice-Chairman, Division of Medicine, Head, Section of Micrographic Surgery (Mohs) & Oncology, The Cleveland Clinic Foundation · One Clinic Center, 9500 Euclid Avenue, Desk A-61, Cleveland, OH 44195-5032 · 216-444-3345

Richard G. Bennett · Assistant Clinical Professor of Dermatology, University of Southern California School of Medicine · The Los Angeles County + University of Southern California Medical Center · 1301 Twentieth Street, Suite 570, Santa Monica, CA 90404 · 310-315-0171

Martin Braun III · Associate Professor of Medicine & Dermatology, The George Washington University School of Medicine · George Washington University Medical Center · 2112 F Street, NW, Suite 701, Washington, DC 20037 · 202-293-7618

Roger I. Ceilley · (Mohs Micrographic Surgery and Reconstruction) · Assistant Clinical Professor of Dermatology, The University of Iowa College of Medicine Director, Mohs Micrographic Surgery & Cutaneous Oncology Fellowship Program, Iowa Methodist Medical Center; The University of Iowa Hospitals & Clinics · 1212 Pleasant Street, Suite 402, Des Moines, IA 50309 · 515-244-0136

Roy G. Geronemus · (Vascular Birthmarks) · Chief, Surgery & Laser Section, Skin & Cancer Unit, Mohs Micrographic Surgeon Skin Cancer, Department of Dermatology, New York University School of Medicine · New York University Medical Center · 566 First Avenue, New York, NY 10016 · 212-263-7306

Arthur H. Gladstein · Professor of Clinical Dermatology, New York University School of Medicine · New York University Medical Center, Skin & Cancer · 566 First Avenue, New York, NY 10016 · 212-263-5247

Hubert T. Greenway · (Mohs Skin Cancer Surgery & Reconstruction) · Head, Mohs Surgery & Cutaneous Laser Unit, Scripps Clinic & Research Foundation · 10666 North Torrey Pines Road, La Jolla, CA 92037 · 619-554-8646

Roy C. Grekin · Associate Clinical Professor, Department of Dermatology, University of California at San Francisco School of Medicine · Chief of Dermatologic Surgery, University of California at San Francisco Medical Center · 400 Parnassus Avenue, Third Floor, Box 0316, San Francisco, CA 94143-0316 · 415-476-4239

Alfred Walter Kopf · (Medical Diagnosis, Pigmented Lesions, Melanoma) · Clinical Professor of Dermatology, New York University School of Medicine · New York University Medical Center · Skin & Cancer Unit, 550 First Avenue, New York, NY 10116 · 212-263-5260

Edward Alexander Krull · Chairman, Department of Dermatology, Henry Ford Medical Center · Detroit, MI 48202 · 313-876-2170

June Robinson · Professor of Dermatology and Surgery, Northwestern University Medical School · Northwestern Memorial Hospital · 222 East Superior, Sixth Floor, Chicago, IL 60611 · 312-908-8106

Stuart J. Salasche · Assistant Professor of Dermatology, Harvard Medical School Co-Director of Dermatology Surgery, Massachusetts General Hospital · 15 Parkman Street, Boston, MA 02114 · 617-726-1869

Neil A. Swanson · Professor of Dermatology and Otolaryngology, Head & Neck Surgery, Oregon Health Sciences University · University Hospital; St. Vincent's Hospital; Portland Veterans Administration Hospital · 3181 Southwest Sam Jackson Park Road, 1468, Portland, OR 97201 · 503-494-4713

Duane C. Whitaker · Associate Professor of Dermatology, The University of Iowa College of Medicine · Director, Dermatologic Surgery, The University of Iowa Hospitals & Clinics · 200 Hawkins Drive, Room 2045BT, Iowa City, IA 52242 · 319-356-2274

John A. Zitelli · Montefiore University Hospital; Shadyside Hospital; St. Francis Hospital · 3471 Fifth Avenue, Suite 1011, Pittsburgh, PA 15213 · 412-681-9400

WOUND HEALING
(See also General Surgery, Wound Healing; Plastic Surgery, Wound Healing)

Claude S. Burton · Assistant Professor of Medicine, Duke University School of Medicine · Duke University Medical Center · P.O. Box 3511, Durham, NC 27710 919-684-5037

William H. Eaglstein · (Leg Ulcers) · Chairman and Harvey Blank Professor, Department of Dermatology & Cutaneous Surgery, University of Miami School of Medicine · Chief of Dermatology, Jackson Memorial Hospital; Mt. Sinai Medical Center; University of Miami Hospital & Clinics; Cedars Medical Center · 1444 Northwest Ninth Avenue, Miami, FL 33136 · 305-547-6704

Vincent Falanga · Associate Professor of Dermatology, University of Miami School of Medicine · University of Miami Affiliated Hospitals · 15600 Northwest 10th Avenue, Room RMSB 2023A (R-250), Miami, FL 33101 · 305-547-5958

John A. Zitelli · Montefiore University Hospital; Shadyside Hospital; St. Francis Hospital · 3471 Fifth Avenue, Suite 1011, Pittsburgh, PA 15213 · 412-681-9400

EATING DISORDERS
(See also Psychiatry, Eating Disorders)

George A. Bray · (Obesity, Nutrition) · Professor of Medicine and Executive Director, Louisiana State University, Pennington Biomedical Research Center · Physician, Pennington Biomedical Research Center · 6400 Perkins Road, Baton Rouge, LA 70808-4124 · 504-765-2513

ENDOCRINOLOGY & METABOLISM

DIABETES

Lloyd Axelrod · Associate Professor of Medicine, Harvard Medical School · Physician and Chief of the James Howard Means Firm, Massachusetts General Hospital · Bulfinch Building, Fourth Floor, 32 Fruit Street, Boston, MA 02114 · 617-726-2874

Richard Bergenstal · Associate Clinical Professor of Medicine, University of Minnesota School of Medicine · Senior Vice-President, International Diabetes Center, Chairman, Department of Endocrinology & Metabolism, Park Nicollet Medical Center · 5000 West 39th Street, Minneapolis, MN 55416 · 612-927-3393

Aubrey E. Boyd III · Professor of Medicine, Tufts University School of Medicine Chief, Division of Endocrinology, Diabetes, Metabolism & Molecular Medicine, New England Medical Center · 750 Washington Street, Box 268, Boston, MA 02111 · 617-956-5689

Oscar B. Crofford · Professor of Medicine, and Director, Diabetes Research & Training Center, Vanderbilt University School of Medicine · Chief, Vanderbilt Diabetes Clinics, Vanderbilt University Hospital · B3307 Medical Center North, 21st Avenue South at Garland, Nashville, TN 37232-2230 · 615-322-2197

Philip E. Cryer · Professor of Medicine, Washington University School of Medicine · Director of the Division of Endocrinology, Diabetes & Metabolism, and Director of General Clinical Research Center, Barnes Hospital · 660 South Euclid Avenue, St. Louis, MO 63110 · 314-362-7617

Mayer B. Davidson · Professor of Medicine, University of California at Los Angeles School of Medicine · Director of the Diabetes Program, Cedars-Sinai Medical Center · Division of Endocrinology, Becker 131, 8700 Beverly Boulevard, Los Angeles, CA 90048 · 310-855-4618

Saul Genuth · Professor of Medicine, Case Western Reserve University School of Medicine · Director, Saltzman Institute for Clinical Investigation, The Mt. Sinai Medical Center · One Mt. Sinai Drive, Cleveland, OH 44106 · 216-421-4013

John E. Godine · Assistant Professor of Medicine, Harvard Medical School · Assistant Physician, Massachusetts General Hospital · Bulfinch Building, 32 Fruit Street, Boston, MA 02114 · 617-726-2874

John H. Karam · Professor of Medicine, University of California at San Francisco School of Medicine · Chief, Clinical Endocrinology, Metabolic Research Unit, University of California at San Francisco Medical Center · Health Science West Building, Third and Parnassus Avenue, Room 1141, San Francisco, CA 94143 · 415-476-1364

Orville G. Kolterman · Professor of Medicine, University of California, San Diego School of Medicine · Director of General Clinical Research Center, and Medical Director, University of California, San Diego Diabetes Program, University of California, San Diego Medical Center · 225 Dickinson Street, 8203, San Diego, CA 92103 · 619-543-3968

Robert S. Mecklenburg · Associate Clinical Professor of Medicine, University of Washington Medical School · Virginia Mason Medical Center · 1100 Ninth Avenue, Seattle, WA 98101 · 206-223-6625

David M. Nathan · Associate Professor of Medicine, Harvard Medical School · Associate Physician and Director, Diabetes Research Center, and Director of the Mallinckrodt General Clinical Research Center, and Director, Diabetes Clinic, Massachusetts General Hospital · Bulfinch Building, 32 Fruit Street, Boston, MA 02114 · 617-726-2874

Jerry P. Palmer · Professor of Medicine, University of Washington School of Medicine · Chief of Endocrinology & Metabolism, Seattle Veterans Administration Medical Center · 1660 South Columbian Way, Seattle, WA 98108 · 206-764-2495

P. J. Palumbo · (Clinical Nutrition, Lipid Abnormalities) · Professor of Medicine, Mayo Medical School · Consultant, Internal Medicine and Endocrinology & Metabolism, and Director, Clinical Nutrition, Mayo Clinic; St. Mary's Hospital; Rochester Methodist Hospital · 200 First Street, SW, Rochester, MN 55905 · 507-284-2784

Kenneth Polansky · Professor of Medicine, University of Chicago, Pritzker School of Medicine · Chief, Section of Endocrinology, University of Chicago Medical Center · 5841 South Maryland Avenue, Chicago, IL 60637 · 312-702-6217

Philip Raskin · Professor of Medicine, The University of Texas Southwestern Medical Center at Dallas · Director, Diabetes Clinic, and University Diabetes Treatment Center/Parkland Memorial Hospital; Dallas VA Medical Center; Zale-Lipshy University Medical Center; Presbyterian Hospital; Medical City · 5323 Harry Hines Boulevard, Dallas, TX 75235-8858 · 214-688-2017

Matthew C. Riddle · Associate Professor of Medicine, Oregon Health Sciences University · Head, Section of Diabetes, Oregon Health Sciences University · 3181 Southwest Sam Jackson Park Road, L-345, Portland, OR 97201 · 503-494-8488

Harold Rifkin · Clinical Professor of Medicine, Albert Einstein College of Medicine; Professor of Clinical Medicine, New York University School of Medicine · Principal Consultant, Diabetes Research & Training Center, Montefiore Medical Center · 35 East 75th Street, New York, NY 10021 · 212-288-1538

Robert A. Rizza · Professor of Medicine, Mayo Medical School · Director of Endocrine Research, and Vice Chairman of Medicine (Research), Mayo Clinic · 200 First Street, SW, Rochester, MN 55905 · 507-284-2784

R. Paul Robertson · Professor of Medicine and Cell Biology, and Pennock Chair for Diabetes Research, and Director, Diabetes Center, and Director, Clinical Research Center, University of Minnesota School of Medicine · University of Minnesota Hospital & Clinics · 516 Delaware Street SE, Box 101 UMHC, Minneapolis, MN 55455 · 612-626-1960

Arthur H. Rubenstein · Chairman, Department of Medicine, and Lowell T. Coggershall Distinguished Service Professor of Medical Sciences, University of Chicago, Pritzker School of Medicine · Attending Staff, Bernard Mitchell Hospital 5841 South Maryland Avenue, Chicago, IL 60637 · 312-702-1051

David S. Schade · Professor of Medicine, The University of New Mexico School of Medicine · The University Hospital · 2211 Lomas Boulevard NE, Albuquerque, NM 87131 · 505-272-4657

F. John Service · Professor of Medicine, Mayo Medical School · Mayo Clinic · 200 First Street, SW, Rochester, MN 55905 · 507-284-4738

Harry Shamoon · Professor of Medicine, Albert Einstein College of Medicine · 1300 Morris Park Avenue, Bronx, NY 10461 · 212-430-2908

Robert S. Sherwin · Professor of Medicine, Yale University School of Medicine · Yale-New Haven Hospital · P.O. Box 3333, Fitkin 1, New Haven, CT 06510 · 203-785-4183

Jay S. Skyler · Professor of Medicine, Pediatrics, and Psychology, University of Miami School of Medicine · University of Miami Affiliated Hospitals · 1500 Northwest 12th Avenue, 14th Floor, Miami, FL 33136 · 305-547-6146

Karl E. Sussman · Professor of Medicine, University of Colorado School of Medicine · Associate Chief of Staff, Research & Development, Denver Department of Veterans Affairs Medical Center · 1055 Clermont Street, 151, Denver, CO 80220 303-393-4619

Bruce R. Zimmerman · Associate Professor of Medicine, Mayo Medical School · Mayo Clinic · 200 First Street, SW, Rochester, MN 55905 · 507-284-2776

Bernard Zinman · Professor of Medicine, University of Toronto School of Medicine · Director, Division of Endocrinology & Metabolism, and Director, Diabetes Clinical Research Unit, Mt. Sinai Hospital/Toronto Hospital · 600 University Avenue, Suite 782, Toronto, Ontario M5G 1X5 · 416-586-8747

NEUROENDOCRINOLOGY

George Panagiotis Chrousos · (Pediatric Neuroendocrinology) · Professor of Pediatrics, Georgetown University School of Medicine · Chief, Pediatric Endocrinology Section, National Institute on Child Development, National Institutes of Health · 9000 Rockville Pike, Building 10, Room 10N262, Bethesda, MD 20892 301-496-4686

Lawrence A. Frohman · Professor of Medicine, and Director, Division of Endocrinology & Metabolism, University of Cincinnati College of Medicine · University of Cincinnati Hospital · 231 Bethesda Avenue, ML 547, Cincinnati, OH 45267 513-558-4444

David Lewis Kleinberg · Professor of Medicine, New York University School of Medicine · Chief, Endocrinology, and Attending Physician, Veterans Affairs Medical Center, New York University Medical Center, Bellevue Hospital · 530 First Avenue, New York, NY 10016 · 212-263-6772

Anne Klibanski · Associate Professor of Medicine, Harvard Medical School · Chief, Neuroendocrine Unit, and Associate Physician, Massachusetts General Hospital · Massachusetts General Neuroendocrine Unit, Jackson 1021, Boston, MA 02114 · 617-726-3870

D. Lynn Loriaux · Professor of Medicine, Oregon Health Sciences University · 3181 Southwest Sam Jackson Park Road, Portland, OR 97201-3098 · 503-494-8459

Shlomo Melmed · Professor of Medicine, University of California at Los Angeles School of Medicine · Director of Endocrinology, Cedars-Sinai Medical Center · 8700 Beverly Boulevard, Room B-131, Los Angeles, CA 90048 · 310-855-4691

Mark E. Molitch · Professor of Medicine, Northwestern University Medical School · Attending, Northwestern Memorial Hospital · 222 E. Superior Street, Chicago, IL 60611 · 312-908-7970

David N. Orth · (Cushing's Disease) · Professor of Medicine, and Professor of Molecular Physiology and Biophysics, Vanderbilt University School of Medicine · Room AA-4206, Medical Center North, Division of Endocrinology, Nashville, TN 37232 · 615-322-6199

Seymour Reichlin · Professor of Medicine, Tufts University School of Medicine New England Medical Center · Tupper Building, Ninth Floor, 750 Washington Street, Box 268, Boston, MA 02111 · 617-956-5689

E. C. Ridgway · Professor of Medicine, Head, Division of Endocrinology and Director, General Clinical Research Center, University of Colorado School of Medicine · University of Colorado Health Science Center · 4200 East Ninth Avenue, Box B-151, Denver, CO 80262 · 303-270-8443

Alan G. Robinson · Professor and Vice-Chairman, Department of Medicine, University of Pittsburgh School of Medicine · Chief, Division of Endocrinology & Metabolism, University of Pittsburgh Medical Center · East 1140 Biomedical Science Tower, Pittsburgh, PA 15261 · 412-648-9770

Peter Joseph Snyder · (Male Reproductive Endocrinology) · Professor of Medicine, University of Pennsylvania School of Medicine · Hospital of the University of Pennsylvania · University of Pennsylvania Medical Group, 36th and Spruce Streets, Philadelphia, PA 19104 · 215-662-2300

Michael O. Thorner · Kenneth R. Crispell Professor of Medicine, University of Virginia School of Medicine · Chief Division of Endocrinology & Metabolism, and Director, General Clinical Research Center, University of Virginia Health Sciences Center · Box 511-66, Charlottesville, VA 22908 · 804-982-3297

J. Blake Tyrrell · (Pituitary Tumors, Cushing's Syndrome, Adrenal Disorders) · Clinical Professor of Medicine, University of California, San Francisco · Chief, Clinical Endocrinology, University of California, San Francisco · 350 Parnassus Avenue, San Francisco, CA 94117 · 415-664-8344

Mary Lee Vance · Associate Professor of Medicine, University of Virginia School of Medicine · University of Virginia Health Sciences Center · Department of Internal Medicine, Box 511, Charlottesville, VA 22908 · 804-924-5629

PAGET'S DISEASE
(See also Rheumatology, Paget's Disease)

Frederick R. Singer · Professor of Medicine, University of California at Los Angeles School of Medicine · Director, Cedars-Sinai Medical Center Bone Center 444 South San Vicente Boulevard, Suite 1004, Los Angeles, CA 90048 · 213-855-2434

Ethel Silverman Siris · Professor of Clinical Medicine, College of Physicians & Surgeons of Columbia University · Attending Physician, Columbia-Presbyterian Medical Center · 622 West 168th Street, PH4-124, New York, NY 10032 · 212-305-2663

Stanley Wallach · Professor and Associate Chairman, Department of Internal Medicine, University South Florida College of Medicine · Attending Physician and Consultant, Tampa General Hospital; H. Lee Moffitt Cancer Center & Research Institute; James A. Haley Veterans Hospital · 1200 80th Street South, St. Petersburg, FL 33707 · 813-343-0048

REPRODUCTIVE ENDOCRINOLOGY

William J. Bremner · Professor of Medicine, University of Washington School of Medicine · Chief of Medical Service, Seattle Veterans Affairs Medical Center · 1660 South Columbian Way (111), Seattle, WA 98108 · 206-764-2345

William F. Crowley, Jr. · Associate Professor of Medicine, Harvard Medical School · Chief, Reproductive Endocrine Unit, Massachusetts General Hospital · Bartlett Extension, 32 Fruit Street, Boston, MA 02114 · 617-726-5390

John C. Marshall · (Hypothalmic-Pituitary Disorders) · Arthur & Margaret Ebbert Professor of Medical Science, and Professor and Chairman, Department of Medicine, University of Virginia School of Medicine · Physician-in-Chief, Internal Medicine, University of Virginia Health Sciences Center · Box 466, Charlottesville, VA 22908 · 804-924-2105

Ronald S. Swerdloff · Professor of Medicine, University of California at Los Angeles School of Medicine · Chief, Division of Endocrinology, Harbor-UCLA Medical Center · 1124 West Carson Street, RB1, Torrance, CA 90502 · 213-212-1867

Jean D. Wilson · Professor of Internal Medicine, The University of Texas Southwestern Medical Center at Dallas · Charles Cameron Sprague Distinguished Chair in Biomedical Science, Parkland Memorial Hospital; Zale Lipshy University Hospital · 5323 Harry Hines Boulevard, Dallas, TX 75235-8857 · 214-688-3494

THYROID
(See also Nuclear Medicine, Thyroid)

Lewis E. Braverman · Director and Professor of Medicine & Physiology, University of Massachusetts Medical School · University of Massachusetts Medical Center · 55 Lake Avenue North, Worcester, MA 01655 · 508-856-3115

Ralph R. Cavalieri · Professor of Medicine & Radiology, University of California at San Francisco School of Medicine · Chief of Nuclear Medicine, Department of Veterans Affairs Medical Center · 4150 Clement Street, San Francisco, CA 94121 415-750-2070

Gilbert H. Daniels · Massachusetts General Hospital · Thyroid Unit, ACC-730, Boston, MA 02114 · 617-726-8430

Leslie J. DeGroot · Professor of Medicine, University of Chicago, Pritzker School of Medicine · University of Chicago Medical Center · 5841 South Maryland Avenue, Box 138, Chicago, IL 60637-1470 · 312-702-1470

Colum A. Gorman · Professor of Medicine, Mayo Medical School · Mayo Clinic 200 First Street, SW, Rochester, MN 55905 · 507-284-4738

Francis S. Greenspan · Clinical Professor of Medicine and Radiology, and Chief, Thyroid Clinic, University of California, San Francisco School of Medicine · University of California, San Francisco Medical Center · 350 Parnassus Avenue, Suite 609, San Francisco, CA 94117 · 415-476-1121

Ian D. Hay · Professor of Medicine, Mayo Medical School · Consultant in Endocrinology and Internal Medicine, Mayo Clinic · 200 First Street, SW, Rochester, MN 55905 · 507-284-3915

Jerome M. Hershman · Professor of Medicine, University of California, Los Angeles School of Medicine · Chief, Division of Endocrinology & Metabolism, Veterans Affairs Medical Center West Los Angeles · Wilshire & Sawtelle Boulevard, W111D, Los Angeles, CA 90073 · 213-824-4442

James R. Hurley · Associate Professor of Radiology & Medicine, Cornell University Medical College · Associate Director, Division of Nuclear Medicine, The New York Hospital-Cornell Medical Center · 525 East 68th Street, Room Starr 221, New York, NY 10021 · 212-746-4584

Paul W. Ladenson · John Eager Howard Professor of Medicine, Johns Hopkins University School of Medicine · Director, Division of Endocrinology & Metabolism, The Johns Hopkins Medical Institutions · 600 North Wolfe Street, Blalock 904, Baltimore, MD 21205 · 410-955-3663

P. Reed Larsen · Professor of Medicine, Harvard Medical School · Senior Physician, and Director, Thyroid Division, Brigham & Women's Hospital · 75 Francis Street, Boston, MA 02115 · 617-732-5666

J. Maxwell McKenzie · The Kathleen & Stanley Glaser Professor and Chairman, Department of Medicine, University of Miami School of Medicine · Chief of the Medical Service, Jackson Memorial Medical Center; University of Miami Hospital & Clinics · 1611 Northwest 12th Avenue, South Wing 630, Miami, FL 33136 · 305-585-7023

John T. Nicoloff · Professor of Medicine, University of Southern California School of Medicine · The Los Angeles County + University of Southern California Medical Center · 2025 Zonal Avenue, Room 18415, Los Angeles, CA 90033 · 213-226-4632

E. C. Ridgway · Professor of Medicine, Head, Division of Endocrinology and Director, General Clinical Research Center, University of Colorado School of Medicine · University of Colorado Health Science Center · 4200 East Ninth Avenue, Box B-151, Denver, CO 80262 · 303-270-8443

Douglas S. Ross · Assistant Professor of Medicine, Harvard Medical School · Assistant Physician and Co-Director of Thyroid Associates, Massachusetts General Hospital · 15 Parkman Street, ACC 730, Boston, MA 02114 · 617-726-3872

Peter A. Singer · Clinical Professor of Medicine, University of Southern California School of Medicine · Chief, Clinical Endocrinology, Hospital of the Good Samaritan; University of Southern California University Hospital · 1510 San Pablo Street, Suite 451, Los Angeles, CA 90033 · 213-342-5724

Robert Volpé · Professor of Medicine, and Director, Division of Endocrinology & Matabolism, University of Toronto School of Medicine · Wellesley Hospital · 160 Wellesley Street East, Toronto, Ontario M4Y 1J3 · 416-926-7777

Leonard Wartofsky · Professor of Medicine, Uniformed Services University of Health Sciences · Chief, Department of Medicine, Walter Reed Army Medical Center · Building 2, Washington, DC 20307-5001 · 202-576-1205

GASTROENTEROLOGY

ENDOSCOPY

Jamie S. Barkin · Professor of Medicine, University of Miami · Chief of Gastroenterology, Mt. Sinai Medical Center · Division of Gastroenterology, 4300 Alton Road, Miami Beach, FL 33140 · 305-674-2240

H. Worth Boyce, Jr. · Professor of Medicine, University South Florida College of Medicine · Director, Center for Swallowing Disorders, University of South Florida Medical Center · 12901 Bruce B. Downs Boulevard, MDC19, Tampa, FL 33612-4733 · 813-974-3374

Peter Cotton · Professor of Medicine and Chief of Endoscopy, Duke University School of Medicine · Duke University Medical Center · Box 3341, DUMC, Durham, NC 27710 · 919-684-3341

David E. Fleischer · Professor of Medicine, Georgetown University School of Medicine · Chief of Endoscopy, Georgetown University Medical Center · Main Hospital, Second Floor, 3800 Reservoir Road, NW, Washington, DC 20007 · 202-687-8741

Joseph E. Geenen · (Biliary Endoscopy) · Clinical Professor of Medicine, Medical College of Wisconsin · Director, Digestive Disease Center, St. Luke's Hospital · 1333 College Avenue, Racine, WI 53403 · 414-636-8100

Walter J. Hogan · (Biliary Tract) · Professor of Medicine and Co-Chief, Division of Gastroenterology, Medical College of Wisconsin · Medical College of Wisconsin Affiliated Hospitals · 9200 West Wisconsin Avenue, Milwaukee, WI 53226 · 414-259-2730

Richard H. Hunt · Professor of Medicine and Head, Division of Gastroenterology, McMaster University · Chief of Gastrointestinal Endoscopy, Chedoke-McMaster Hospital · 1200 Main Street West, Hamilton, Ontario L8N 3Z5 · 416-521-9800 x6404

Dennis Jensen · Professor of Medicine, University of California at Los Angeles School of Medicine · University of California at Los Angeles Medical Center · 10833 LeConte Avenue, CHF-44138, Los Angeles, CA 90024 · 310-825-7025

Ronald Melvin Katon · Professor of Medicine, and Director of Endoscopy, Oregon Health Sciences University · 3181 Southwest Sam Jackson Park Road, Portland, OR 97201-3098 · 503-494-8577

Richard A. Kozarek · (Biliary Tract) · Clinical Professor of Medicine, University of Washington School of Medicine · Chief, Department of Gastroenterology, Virginia Mason Medical Center · 1100 Ninth Avenue, Seattle, WA 98111 · 206-223-6934

Loren A. Laine · Associate Professor of Medicine, University of Southern California School of Medicine · The Los Angeles County + University of Southern California Medical Center; Kenneth Morris, Jr., Cancer Hospital; University of Southern California University Hospital; Gastrointestinal Division, Department of Medicine, University of Southern California School of Medicine · 2025 Zonal Avenue, Los Angeles, CA 90033 · 213-226-7995

Glen A. Lehman · (Pancreatobiliary Diseases) · Professor of Medicine, Indiana University School of Medicine · Director of Clinical Gastroenterology/Hepatology, Indiana University Medical Center · 926 West Michigan Street, Suite 2300, Indianapolis, IN 46202-5250 · 317-274-4821

Robert H. Schapiro · (Biliary Endoscopy) · Harvard Medical School · Chief of Medical Endoscopy, Massachusetts General Hospital · Zero Emerson Place, Boston, MA 02114 · 617-523-1466

Fred E. Silverstein · Professor of Medicine, University of Washington School of Medicine · University of Washington Medical Center · 1959 Northeast Pacific Street, BB1361, Seattle, WA 98195 · 206-543-3183

Michael V. Sivak, Jr. · Chairman, Department of Gastroenterology, The Cleveland Clinic Foundation · One Clinic Center, 9500 Euclid Avenue, Cleveland, OH 44195-5001 · 216-444-6528

Jerome D. Waye · (Colon Cancer, Colon Polyps, Colonoscopy) · Clinical Professor of Medicine, Mt. Sinai School of Medicine · Chief, Gastointestinal Endoscopy Unit, Mt. Sinai Medical Center; Lenox Hill Hospital · 650 Park Avenue, New York, NY 10021 · 212-439-7779

Wilfred M. Weinstein · Professor of Medicine, Division of Gastroenterology, University of California at Los Angeles School of Medicine · Director, Gastroenterology Procedures Unit, Division of Gastroenterology, University of California at Los Angeles Center for Health Sciences · 10833 LeConte Avenue, Los Angeles, CA 90024 · 310-825-3659

ESOPHAGEAL DISEASE

H. Worth Boyce, Jr. · Professor of Medicine, University South Florida College of Medicine · Director, Center for Swallowing Disorders, University of South Florida Medical Center · 12901 Bruce B. Downs Boulevard, MDC19, Tampa, FL 33612-4733 · 813-974-3374

Donald O. Castell · (Esophageal Motility) · Rorer Professor of Medicine, Jefferson Medical College of Thomas Jefferson University · Director, Gastroenterology & Hepatology, Thomas Jefferson University Hospital · 1025 Walntut Street, 901 College, Philadelphia, PA 19107 · 215-955-6944

FUNCTIONAL GASTROINTESTINAL DISORDERS

Douglas A. Drossman · Professor of Medicine and Psychiatry, University of North Carolina School of Medicine · University of North Carolina Hospitals · 420 Burnett-Womack Building, Manning Drive, Campus Box 7080, Chapel Hill, NC 27599-7080 · 919-966-2511

Robert S. Fisher · Professor of Medicine, Temple University School of Medicine Chairman, Gastroenterology Section, Temple University Hospital · 3401 North Broad Street, Philadelphia, PA 19140 · 215-221-3496

GASTROENTEROLOGIC CANCER

Jerome D. Waye · (Colon Cancer, Colon Polyps, Colonoscopy) · Clinical Professor of Medicine, Mt. Sinai School of Medicine · Chief, Gastrointestinal Endoscopy Unit, Mt. Sinai Medical Center; Lenox Hill Hospital · 650 Park Avenue, New York, NY 10021 · 212-439-7779

Sidney J. Winawer · (Colon Cancer, Colon Polyps) · Chief, Gastroenterology Service, Memorial Sloan-Kettering Cancer Center · 1275 York Avenue, Room C278, New York, NY 10021 · 212-639-7675

GASTROINTESTINAL BLEEDING

Dennis Jensen · Professor of Medicine, University of California at Los Angeles School of Medicine · University of California at Los Angeles Medical Center · 10833 LeConte Avenue, CHF-44138, Los Angeles, CA 90024 · 310-825-7025

Loren A. Laine · Associate Professor of Medicine, University of Southern California School of Medicine · The Los Angeles County + University of Southern California Medical Center; Kenneth Morris, Jr., Cancer Hospital; University of Southern California University Hospital; Gastrointestinal Division, Department of Medicine, University of Southern California School of Medicine · 2025 Zonal Avenue, Los Angeles, CA 90033 · 213-226-7995

GASTROINTESTINAL MOTILITY

Sidney Cohen · (Colon Motility) · Richard Laylord Evans Professor of Medicine, Temple University School of Medicine · Chairman & Program Director, Department of Medicine, Temple University Hospital · 3401 North Broad Street, Parkinson Pavillon, Eighth Floor, Philadelphia, PA 19140 · 215-221-4947

Robert S. Fisher · Professor of Medicine, Temple University School of Medicine Chairman, Gastroenterology Section, Temple University Hospital · 3401 North Broad Street, Philadelphia, PA 19140 · 215-221-3496

John R. Mathias · (Small Intestinal Motility) · Professor of Medicine, The University of Texas Medical Branch at Galveston · Associate Director of Gastroenterology, The University of Texas Medical Branch at Galveston · 4.106 McCullough Building, Route G-64, Galveston, TX 77550 · 409-772-1501

James C. Reynolds · (Colon Motility) · Associate Professor of Medicine, University of Pittsburgh School of Medicine · Chief, Division of Gastroenterology, University of Pittsburgh Medical Center · M2, DeSoto at O'Hara Streets, Pittsburgh, PA 15213-2582 · 412-648-9115

Lawrence Schiller · (Diarrheal Disease, Colon Motility, Colon Motility Disorder) Baylor University · Baylor University Medical Center · Department of Internal Medicine, 3500 Gaston Avenue, Dallas, TX 75246 · 214-820-2671

Marvin M. Schuster · (Colon Motility) · Professor of Medicine with Joint Appointments in Psychiatry, Johns Hopkins University School of Medicine · Chief, Division of Digestive Diseases, Francis Scott Key Medical Center · 4940 Eastern Avenue, Baltimore, MD 21224 · 410-550-0790

William J. Snape, Jr. · (Colon Motility) · Clinical Professor of Medicine, University of California at Los Angeles School of Medicine · Director, Bowel Disease and Motility Center, Long Beach Memorial Medical Center · 2650 Elm Avenue, Suite 201, Long Beach, CA 90806 · 213-424-7010, 595-5421

GENERAL GASTROENTEROLOGY

James L. Achord · Professor of Medicine, University of Mississippi · Director, Division of Digestive Diseases, University of Mississippi Medical Center · 2500 North State Street, Room N136, Jackson, MS 39216-4505 · 601-984-4540

Eugene M. Bozymski · Professor of Medicine and Chief of Endoscopy, and Co-Chief, Division of Gastroenterology, University of North Carolina School of Medicine · Chief of Endoscopy, and Co-Chief, Division of Gastroenterology, U.N.C. Hospitals & Medical Center · 324 Burnett-Womack Building, Manning Drive, Campus Box 7080, Chapel Hill, NC 27599-7080 · 919-966-2511

Sarkis John Chobanian · (Diagnostic & Therapeutic Endoscopy of the Pancreaticobiliary Tract) · Assistant Professor of Medicine, Uniformed Services University of Health Sciences; Trustee, American College of Gastroenterology · Director, Digestive Disease Institute, St. Mary's Medical Center · 801 Weisgarber Road, Knoxville, TN 37909 · 615-588-5121

Harris Reynold Clearfield · Professor of Medicine, Hahnemann University · Director, Division of Gastroenterology, and Director, Krancer Center for Inflammatory Bowel Disease Research, Hahnemann Hospital · Broad & Vine Streets, MS 131, Philadelphia, PA 19102 · 215-246-5064,448-8101

Franz Goldstein · Professor of Medicine, Jefferson Medical College of Thomas Jefferson University · Past Chief, Division of Gastroenterology, Lankenau Hospital · 252 Lankenau Medical Building, East, 100 Lancaster Avenue and City Line, Wynnewood, PA 19096 · 215-896-7360

Walter J. Hogan · (Biliary Tract) · Professor of Medicine and Co-Chief, Division of Gastroenterology, Medical College of Wisconsin · Medical College of Wisconsin Affiliated Hospitals · 9200 West Wisconsin Avenue, Milwaukee, WI 53226 · 414-259-2730

Myron Lewis · Associate Professor of Medicine, The University of Tennessee at Memphis, College of Medicine · Baptist Memorial Hospital · 930 Madison Avenue, Suite 870, Memphis, TN 38103 · 901-526-4222

William H. Lipshutz · Clinical Professor of Medicine, Hospital of the University of Pennsylvania · Head, Gastroenterology Section, Pennsylvania Hospital · Eighth and Spruce Streets, Philadelphia, PA 19107 · 215-829-3561

Christina M. Surawicz · Associate Professor of Medicine, University of Washington School of Medicine · Harborview Medical Center · 325 Ninth Avenue, Seattle, WA 98104 · 206-223-3650

HEPATOLOGY

Joseph R. Bloomer · Professor of Medicine, University of Minnesota School of Medicine · Director, Division of Gastroenterology, Hepatology, & Nutrition, University of Minnesota Hospital & Clinics · 516 Delaware Street SE, Box 36 UMHC, Minneapolis, MN 55455 · 612-625-8999

James L. Boyer · Professor of Medicine, Yale University School of Medicine · Yale-New Haven Hospital · 333 Cedar Street, Room 1080LMP, New Haven, CT 06510 · 203-785-4138

Gary Gitnick · Professor of Medicine, and Professor and Director, Department of Gastroenterology, University of California at Los Angeles School of Medicine · Chief of Staff and Medical Director, University of California at Los Angeles Health Care Programs, University of California at Los Angeles Medical Center · 10833 LeConte Avenue, 924 Westwood Boulevard, Suite 515, Los Angeles, CA 90024-7018 · 310-825-6671

Marshall M. Kaplan · Professor of Medicine, Tufts University School of Medicine Chief of Gastroenterology Division, New England Medical Center · 750 Washington Street, Boston, MA 02111 · 617-956-5877

Emmet B. Keeffe · Professor of Medicine, and Chief, Hepatology Section, Oregon Health Sciences University · Division of Gastroenterology, L461, 3181 Southwest Sam Jackson Park Road, Portland, OR 97201-3098 · 503-494-8578

Willis C. Maddrey · Vice-President for Clinical Affairs, and Professor of Internal Medicine, The University of Texas Southwestern Medical Center at Dallas · 5323 Harry Hines Boulevard, Dallas, TX 75235-8570 · 214-688-2024

Telfer B. Reynolds · Professor of Medicine, University of Southern California School of Medicine · The Los Angeles County + University of Southern California Medical Center · 2025 Zonal Avenue, Los Angeles, CA 90033 · 213-226-4641

Eugene R. Schiff · Professor of Medicine and Chief, Division of Hepatology, and Director, Center for Liver Diseases, University of Miami School of Medicine · Chief, Hepatology Section, Miami Veterans Affairs Medical Center; University of Miami Hospital; Jackson Memorial Hospital; Cedars Medical Center · The Jackson Medical Towers, 1500 Northwest 12th Avenue, Suite 1101, Miami, FL 33136 305-547-5821

Michael F. Sorrell · Professor of Internal Medicine, University of Nebraska College of Medicine · University of Nebraska Medical Center · 600 South 42nd Street, Omaha, NE 68198-3332 · 402-559-7912

INFLAMMATORY BOWEL DISEASE

Theodore M. Bayless · Professor of Medicine, Johns Hopkins University School of Medicine · Medical Director of the Meyerhoff Digestive Disease-Inflammatory Bowel Disease Center, The Johns Hopkins Medical Institutions · 600 North Wolfe Street, Blalock Room 461, Baltimore, MD 21205 · 410-955-4916

Lawrence J. Brandt · Professor of Medicine, Albert Einstein College of Medicine Director, Division Gastroenterology, Moses Division of Montefiore Medical Center, and North Central Bronx Hospital · 111 East 210th Street, Bronx, NY 10467 212-920-4476

Harris Reynold Clearfield · Professor of Medicine, Hahnemann University · Director, Division of Gastroenterology, and Director, Krancer Center for Inflammatory Bowel Disease Research, Hahnemann Hospital · Broad & Vine Streets, MS 131, Philadelphia, PA 19102 · 215-246-5064,448-8101

Richard G. Farmer · Consultant, Department of Colorectal Surgery, The Cleveland Clinic Foundation · One Clinic Center, 9500 Euclid Avenue, Cleveland, OH 44195-5001 · 216-444-6515

John S. Fordtran · (Chronic Diarrheal Disease) · Chief, Department of Internal Medicine, Baylor University · Baylor University Medical Center · 3500 Gaston Avenue, Dallas, TX 75246 · 214-820-2671

Stephen B. Hanauer · Associate Professor of Medicine, University of Chicago, Pritzker School of Medicine · University of Chicago Medical Center · 5841 South Maryland Avenue, Box 400, Chicago, IL 60637-1470 · 312-702-1466

Joseph Barnett Kirsner · Professor of Medicine, University of Chicago, Pritzker School of Medicine · University of Chicago Medical Center · 5841 South Maryland Avenue, Box 319, Chicago, IL 60637 · 312-702-6101

Burton I. Korelitz · Clinical Professor of Medicine, Cornell University Medical College · Chief of Gastroenterology, Lenox Hill Hospital · 45 East 95th Street, New York, NY 10028 · 212-988-3800

Daniel H. Present · Clinical Professor of Medicine, Mt. Sinai School of Medicine Mt. Sinai Medical Center · 12 East 86th Street, New York, NY 10028 · 212-861-2000

Arvey I. Rogers · (Disorders of Gastrointestinal Function) · Professor of Medicine, University of Miami School of Medicine · President of the Medical Staff, University of Miami Hospital & Clinics; Jackson Memorial Hospital; Miami Veterans Affairs Medical Center · Veterans Affairs Medical Center, 1201 Northwest 16th Street, Suite 111B, Miami, FL 33125 · 305-324-3162

David B. Sachar · Professor of Medicine, Mt. Sinai School of Medicine · Chief, Division of Gastroenterology, Mt. Sinai Medical Center · One Gustave L. Levy Place, Box 1069, New York, NY 10029 · 212-241-6749

PANCREATIC DISEASE

Jamie S. Barkin · Professor of Medicine, University of Miami · Chief of Gastroenterology, Mt. Sinai Medical Center · Division of Gastroenterology, 4300 Alton Road, Miami Beach, FL 33140 · 305-674-2240

Joseph E. Geenen · (Biliary Endoscopy) · Clinical Professor of Medicine, Medical College of Wisconsin · Director, Digestive Disease Center, St. Luke's Hospital · 1333 College Avenue, Racine, WI 53403 · 414-636-8100

PEPTIC DISORDERS

Harris Reynold Clearfield · Professor of Medicine, Hahnemann University · Director, Division of Gastroenterology, and Director, Krancer Center for Inflammatory Bowel Disease Research, Hahnemann Hospital · Broad & Vine Streets, MS 131, Philadelphia, PA 19102 · 215-246-5064,448-8101

Robert S. Fisher · (Acid-Peptic Disorders) · Professor of Medicine, Temple University School of Medicine · Chairman, Gastroenterology Section, Temple University Hospital · 3401 North Broad Street, Philadelphia, PA 19140 · 215-221-3496

John S. Fordtran · (Chronic Diarrheal Disease) · Chief, Department of Internal Medicine, Baylor University · Baylor University Medical Center · 3500 Gaston Avenue, Dallas, TX 75246 · 214-820-2671

Richard H. Hunt · Professor of Medicine and Head, Division of Gastroenterology, McMaster University · Chief of Gastrointestinal Endoscopy, Chedoke-McMaster Hospital · 1200 Main Street West, Hamilton, Ontario L8N 3Z5 · 416-521-9800 x6404

Jon I. Isenberg · Professor of Medicine and Head, Division of Gastroenterology, University of California at San Diego School of Medicine · University of California at San Diego Medical Center · 225 Dickinson Street, Mail Code 8413, San Diego, CA 92103-8413 · 619-543-3542

GENERAL SURGERY

BREAST SURGERY
(See also Plastic Surgery, Breast Surgery)

David W. Kinne · Memorial Sloan-Kettering Cancer Center · 1275 York Avenue, New York, NY 10021 · 212-639-7962

William C. Wood · Joseph B. Whitehead Professor & Chairman, Department of Surgery, Emory University School of Medicine · Emory University Affiliated Hospitals · 1364 Clifton Road, NE, Atlanta, GA 30322 · 404-727-5800

ENDOCRINE SURGERY

Maria D. Allo · (Surgical Critical Care) · Clinical Associate Professor in Surgery, Stanford University School of Medicine · Chairman, Department of Surgery, and Chief, Division of General Surgery, Santa Clara Valley Medical Center · 751 South Bascom Avenue, San Jose, CA 95128 · 408-299-6789

Dana K. Anderson · Professor of Medicine, University of Chicago, Pritzker School of Medicine · Chief, Section of General Surgery, University of Chicago Medical Center · 5841 South Maryland Avenue, Box 168, Chicago, IL 60637-1470 312-702-6214

Joseph N. Attie · Associate Professor of Surgery at New York University School of Medicine; Professor of Surgery, Albert Einstein College of Medicine · Director, Division of Head & Neck Surgery, Long Island Jewish Medical Center · 200 Middle Neck Road, Great Neck, NY 11021 · 516-487-2212

Edward L. Bradley III · (Pancreatic Surgery) · William G. Whittaker, Jr. Professor of Surgery, Emory University School of Medicine · Piedmont Hospital · Department of Surgery, 1968 Peachtree Road, NW, Atlanta, GA 30309 · 404-605-3228

Murray Frederick Brennan · (Pancreatic Cancer, Adrenal Parathyroid, Islet Carcinoma) · Chairman, Department of Surgery, Memorial Sloan-Kettering Cancer Center · 1275 York Avenue, New York, NY 10021 · 212-639-6586

Blake Cady · Professor of Surgery, Harvard Medical School · Chief, Surgical Oncology, New England Deaconess Hospital · 110 Francis Street, Suite 2H, Boston, MA 02215 · 617-732-8990

Orlo H. Clark · (Endocrine-Thyroid, Parathyroid, Adrenal and Pancreatic Tumors) · Professor and Vice-Chairman, Department of Surgery, University of California at San Francisco School of Medicine · Chief of Surgery, Mt. Zion Medical Center of the University of California at San Francisco · 1600 Divisadero Street, P.O. Box 7921, San Francisco, CA 94120 · 415-476-1070, 885-7616

Caldwell B. Esselstyn, Jr. · Head, Section of Thyroid & Parathyroid Surgery, The Cleveland Clinic Foundation · One Clinic Center Drive, 9500 Euclid Avenue, Cleveland, OH 44195 · 216-444-6662

Randall David Gaz · Assistant Professor of Surgery, Harvard Medical School · Massachusetts General Hospital · Department of Surgery, Boston, MA 02114 · 617-726-3510

Armando E. Giuliano · Clinical Professor of Surgery, University of California, Los Angeles Medical Center · Chief of Surgical Oncology, St. John's Hospital & Health Center · 1328 Twenty-Second Street, Three West, Santa Monica, CA 90404 · 213-829-8089

Clive S. Grant · Associate Professor of Surgery, Mayo Medical School · Head, General and Gastrointestinal Surgery, Mayo Clinic · 200 First Street, SW, Rochester, MN 55905 · 507-284-2511

George L. Irvin · Professor of Surgery, University of Miami School of Medicine · Chief of Surgical Service, Miami Veterans Affairs Medical Center; Jackson Memorial/University of Miami Medical Center · 1201 Northwest 16th Street, Mail Code 112, Miami, FL 33125 · 305-324-3244

Edwin L. Kaplan · Professor of Surgery, University of Chicago, Pritzker School of Medicine · University of Chicago Medical Center · 5841 South Maryland Avenue, Box 402, Chicago, IL 60637-1470 · 312-702-6155

Barbara Kinder · Professor of Surgery, Yale University School of Medicine · Yale-New Haven Hospital · 333 Cedar Street, New Haven, CT 06510 · 203-785-2562

Paul Lo Gerfo · Professor of Surgery, College of Physicians & Surgeons of Columbia University · Director, General Surgical Service, Columbia-Presbyterian Medical Center · 161 Fort Washington Avenue, New York, NY 10032 · 212-305-8501

Eberhard Mack · Professor of Surgery, University of Wisconsin-Madison School of Medicine · University of Wisconsin Hospital & Clinics · 600 Highland Avenue, H4/744A CSC, Madison, WI 53792 · 608-263-1387

Jack M. Monchik · Associate Clinical Professor of Surgery, Brown University School of Medicine · Director, Division of Endocrine Surgery, Rhode Island Hospital · 154 Waterman Street, Providence, RI 02906 · 401-273-2450

H. H. Newsome, Jr. · Professor of Surgery, and Associate Dean of Clinical Activities, Virginia Commonwealth University, Medical College of Virginia · Medical College of Virginia Hospital · 1200 East Broad Street, Richmond, VA 23298 · 804-786-9661

Jeffrey A. Norton · Head, Surgical Metabolism Section, Surgery Branch, National Cancer Institute, National Institutes of Health · 9000 Rockville Pike, Building 10, Room 2B07, Bethesda, MD 20892 · 301-496-2195

Patricia J. Numann · Professor of Surgery, and Director, Comprehensive Breast Care Program, State University of New York Health Science Center at Syracuse · University Hospital · Department of Surgery, 750 East Adams Street, Syracuse, NY 13210 · 315-464-4603

Edward Paloyan · Professor of Surgery, Loyola University Stritch School of Medicine · Associate Chief of Staff for Research, Department of Veterans Affairs, Edward Hines, Jr., Hospital; Chief, Endocrine Surgery, Loyola University Medical Center, Foster G. McGaw Hospital; Staff Surgeon, Hinsdale Hospital · P.O. Box 5, Hines, IL 60141 · 708-216-4430

Richard A. Prinz · (Pancreatic and Biliary Surgery, Laparoscopic Surgery) · Professor of Surgery, Loyola Stritch School of Medicine · Foster G. McGaw Hospital 2160 South First Avenue, Room 2668, Maywood, IL 60153 · 708-216-4596

Irving B. Rosen · Associate Professor of Surgery, University of Toronto School of Medicine · Mt. Sinai Hospital · 600 University Avenue, Suite 478, Toronto, Ontario M5G 1X5 · 416-586-4656

Gary B. Talpos · Clinical Assistant Professor of Surgery, The University of Michigan Medical School · Staff Surgeon, Henry Ford Medical Center · 2799 West Grand Boulevard, Detroit, MI 48202 · 313-876-3042

Colin G. Thomas, Jr. · Byah Thomason Doxey-Sanford Doxey Professor of Surgery, University of North Carolina School of Medicine · Attending Surgeon, University of North Carolina Hospitals · 3010 Old Clinic Building, Manning Drive, Campus Box 7210, Chapel Hill, NC 27599-7210 · 919-966-4597

Norman W. Thompson · Professor of Surgery, The University of Michigan Medical School · Chief, Division of Endocrine Surgery, The University of Michigan Medical Center · 2920 Taubman Center, 1500 East Medical Center Drive, Box 0331, Ann Arbor, MI 48109-0331 · 313-936-5818

Jon van Heerden · (Endocrine-Thyroid Tumors, Pancreatic Islet-Cell Tumors) · Professor of Surgery, Mayo Medical School · Mayo Clinic · 200 First Street, SW, Rochester, MN 55905 · 507-284-3364

Charles G. Watson · (Thyroid Surgery, Parathyroid and Adrenal Surgery) · Professor of Surgery, University of Pittsburgh School of Medicine · Montefiore University Hospital; Presbyterian University Hospital · 497 Scaife Hall, Pittsburgh, PA 15261 · 412-648-3173

Samuel A. Wells · Professor and Chairman of Surgery, Washington University School of Medicine · Surgeon-in-Chief, Barnes Hospital · 4960 Audubon Avenue, Box 8109, St. Louis, MO 63110 · 314-362-8020

Stuart D. Wilson · Professor of Surgery, Medical College of Wisconsin · Senior Attending Surgeon, Milwaukee County Medical Complex; Medical College of Wisconsin Clinics at Froedtert Memorial Luther Hospital · 9200 West Wisconsin Avenue, Milwaukee, WI 53226 · 414-454-5723

GASTROENTEROLOGIC SURGERY

Arthur H. Aufses, Jr. · (Inflammatory Bowel Disease) · Franz W. Sichel Professor of Surgery, Mt. Sinai School of Medicine · Chairman, Department of Surgery, Mt. Sinai Medical Center · Five East 98th Street, Box 1259, New York, NY 10029 · 212-241-7646

James Becker · (Inflammatory Bowel Disease) · Associate Professor of Surgery, Harvard Medical School · Chief, Division of General & Gastrointestinal Surgery, Brigham & Women's Hospital · 75 Francis Street, Boston, MA 02115 · 617-732-6944

George Edward Bloch · Thomas D. Jones Professor of Surgery, University of Chicago, Pritzker School of Medicine · Acting Chairman, Department of Surgery, University of Chicago Medical Center · 5841 South Maryland Avenue, Box 168, Chicago, IL 60637 · 312-702-6142

John W. Braasch · Senior Consultant, Department of General Surgery, Lahey Clinic Medical Center · 41 Mall Road, Burlington, MA 01805 · 617-273-8585

John L. Cameron · (Pancreatic Cancer, Biliary Cancer) · Professor and Chairman, Department of Surgery, Johns Hopkins University School of Medicine · Chief of Surgery, The Johns Hopkins Hospital · 720 Rutland Avenue, Ross Building 759, Baltimore, MD 21205 · 410-955-5166

Larry C. Carey · Professor and Chairman, Department of Surgery, University South Florida College of Medicine · Chief of Surgery, Tampa General Hospital · 4 Columbia Drive, Suite 430, Tampa, FL 33606 · 813-253-6901

Laurence Y. Cheung · Professor and Chairman of Surgery, University of Kansas School of Medicine · Chief of Surgery, University of Kansas Medical Center · 39th and Rainbow Boulevard, Kansas City, KS 66103 · 913-588-6101

Haile T. Debas · Professor of Surgery, University of California at San Francisco School of Medicine · Chairman, Department of Surgery, University of California at San Francisco Medical Center · 513 Parnassus Avenue, Room S-320, San Francisco, CA 94143-0104 · 415-476-1236

Tom R. DeMeester · (Esophageal, Gastric and Pulmonary Diseases) · Professor and Chairman, Department of Surgery, University of Southern California School of Medicine · Chief of Surgery, University of Southern California University Hospital, and Kenneth Norris, Jr. Cancer Hospital, and The Los Angeles County + University of Southern California Medical Center · 1510 San Pablo Street, Suite 514, Los Angeles, CA 90033-4612 · 213-342-5925

Frederic E. Eckhauser · Professor of Surgery, The University of Michigan Medical School · Chief, Division of Gastrointestinal Surgery, The University of Michigan Medical Center · 1500 East Medical Center Drive, Box 0331, Ann Arbor, MI 48109-0331 · 313-936-4866

E. Christopher Ellison · Assistant Clinical Professor, Department of Surgery, Ohio State University College of Medicine · Director, Ohio Digestive Disease

Institute, Grant Medical Center · 423 East Town Street, Second Floor, Columbus, OH 43215 · 614-224-8422

Peter Jeffrey Fabri · (Critical Care) · Professor and Vice-Chairman, Department of Surgery, University of South Florida College of Medicine · Chief, Surgical Service, James A. Haley Veterans Hospital; Tampa General Hospital; H. Lee Moffitt Cancer Center & Research Institute · 13000 Bruce B. Downs Boulevard, Surgical Service, Tampa, FL 33612 · 813-972-2000 x6513

Josef E. Fischer · Christian R. Holmes Professor and Chairman, Department of Surgery, University of Cincinnati College of Medicine · Surgeon-in-Chief, University of Cincinnati Hospital · 231 Bethesda Avenue, ML 558, Cincinnati, OH 45267-0558 · 513-558-4202

Robert E. Hermann · Chairman, Department of General Surgery, The Cleveland Clinic Foundation · One Clinic Center, 9500 Euclid Avenue, Desk A-110, Cleveland, OH 44195 · 216-444-6663

Bernard M. Jaffe · Professor and Chairman, Department of Surgery, State University of New York Health Science Center at Brooklyn · University Hospital of Brooklyn; Kings County Hospital Center; Brooklyn Veterans Affairs Medical Center · 450 Clarkson Avenue, Box 40, Brooklyn, NY 11203 · 718-270-1973

R. Scott Jones · (Hepatic Surgery, Biliary Surgery, Pancreatic Surgery) · Professor and Chairman, Department of Surgery, University of Virginia School of Medicine University of Virginia Health Sciences Center · Private Clinics Building, Hospital Drive, Second Floor, Room 2537, Charlottesville, VA 22908 · 804-924-2000

Gordon Lee Kauffman · Professor of General Surgery, Pennsylvania State University · Chief of General Surgery, The Milton S. Hershey Medical Center · 500 University Drive, P.O. Box 850, Hershey, PA 17033 · 717-531-8521

Keith A. Kelly · (Inflammatory Bowel Disease) · Professor of Surgery, Mayo Medical School · Chairman, Department of Surgery, Mayo Clinic · 200 First Street, SW, Rochester, MN 55905 · 507-284-2511

William C. Meyers · Professor of Surgery, Duke University School of Medicine · Chief of Gastrointestinal Surgery, and Director of Liver Transplantation, Duke University Medical Center · P.O. Box 3041, Durham, NC 27710 · 919-684-6437

Thomas A. Miller · Professor of Surgery, The University of Texas Medical School at Houston · Attending Physician, Hermann Hospital · 6431 Fannin Street, MSMB 4.266, Houston, TX 77030 · 713-792-5463

Ashby Moncure · Massachusetts General Hospital · 32 Fruit Street, Boston, MA 02114 · 617-726-2819

Frank G. Moody · Professor and Chairman, Department of Surgery, The University of Texas Medical School at Houston · Chief of Surgery, Hermann Hospital 6431 Fannin Street, Suite 4020, Houston, TX 77030 · 713-792-5400

A. R. Moossa · (Oncologic Surgery) · Professor and Chairman, Department of Surgery, University of California at San Diego School of Medicine · Surgeon-in-Chief, University of California at San Diego Medical Center · 225 Dickinson Street, San Diego, CA 92103-8400 · 619-543-5860

Michael W. Mulholland · Associate Professor of Surgery, The University of Michigan Medical School · The University of Michigan Medical Center · 2922 Taubman Center, 1500 East Medical Center Drive, Box 0331, Ann Arbor, MI 48109-0331 · 313-936-3236

David M. Nagorney · (Hepatic Surgery) · Associate Professor of Surgery, Mayo Medical School · Mayo Clinic; Rochester Methodist Hospital; St. Mary's Hospital 200 First Street, SW, Rochester, MN 55905 · 507-284-2644

David L. Nahrwold · Loyal and Edith Davis Professor & Chairman, Department of Surgery, Northwestern University Medical School · Surgeon-in-Chief, Northwestern Memorial Hospital · 250 East Superior Street, Suite 201, Chicago, IL 60611 · 312-908-8060

Leslie W. Ottinger · Associate Professor of Surgery, Harvard Medical School · Visiting Surgeon, Massachusetts General Hospital · 15 Parkman Street, Room 465, Boston, MA 02114 · 617-726-3414

Theodore N. Pappas · Assistant Professor of Surgery, Duke University School of Medicine · Duke University Medical Center · Box 3479, DUMC, Durham, NC 27710 · 919-681-3442

Edward Passaro, Jr. · (Acid-Peptic Disease, Gastrinoma (Zollinger-Ellison Syndrome)) · Professor of Surgery, University of California at Los Angeles School of Medicine · Chief, Surgical Service, Wadsworth Veterans Hospital · Wilshire & Sawtelle Boulevards, Los Angeles, CA 90073 · 213-824-3236

Carlos Pellegrini · University of California at San Francisco School of Medicine University of California at San Francisco Medical Center · 533 Parnassus Avenue, Room U-122, San Francisco, CA 94143-0788 · 415-476-0974

Henry A. Pitt · (Hepatic Surgery, Biliary Surgery, Pancreatic Surgery) · Professor of Surgery, Johns Hopkins University School of Medicine · Vice Chairman, Department of Surgery, The Johns Hopkins Medical Institutions · 600 North Wolfe Street, Blalock 688, Baltimore, MD 21205 · 410-955-7794

Hiram C. Polk, Jr. · Ben A. Reid, Sr. Professor and Chairman, Department of Surgery, University of Louisville School of Medicine · Humana Hospital University of Louisville, Norton Hospital, Jewish Hospital · Department of Surgery, University of Louisville, Louisville, KY 40292 · 502-588-5442

Jeffrey L. Ponsky · (Endoscopy) · Professor of Surgery, Case Western Reserve University School of Medicine · Director, Department of Surgery, The Mt. Sinai Medical Center · One Mt. Sinai Drive, Cleveland, OH 44106 · 216-421-3945

John Hugh C. Ranson · (Pancreatic Surgery) · Professor of Surgery, New York University School of Medicine · New York University Medical Center · 530 First Avenue, Suite 6B, New York, NY 10016 · 212-263-7301

Howard A. Reber · (Pancreatic Surgery) · Professor and Vice-Chairman, Department of Surgery, University of California at Los Angeles School of Medicine · University of California at Los Angeles Medical Center · 10833 LeConte Avenue, Los Angeles, CA 90026 · 310-825-4976

Layton F. Rikkers · (General, Hepatic Surgery, Biliary Surgery) · Professor and Chairperson, Department of Surgery, University of Nebraska College of Medicine University of Nebraska Medical Center · 600 South 42nd Street, Omaha, NE 68198-3280 · 402-559-6719

Wallace P. Ritchie, Jr. · (Acid-Peptic Disease) · Professor & Chairman, Department of Surgery, Temple University School of Medicine · Temple University Hospital · Broad and Ontario Streets, Philadelphia, PA 19140 · 215-221-3626

Ernest F. Rosato · Professor of Surgery, University of Pennsylvania School of Medicine · Chief, Division of Gastrointestinal Surgery, Hospital of the University of Pennsylvania · 3400 Spruce Street, Philadelphia, PA 19104 · 215-662-2013

Joel Roslyn · (General) · Associate Professor, Division of General Surgery, University of California at Los Angeles School of Medicine · University of California at Los Angeles Center for the Health Sciences · Department of Surgery, Division of General Surgery, 10833 LeConte Avenue, Los Angeles, CA 90024-1749 · 310-825-6156

Michael G. Sarr · (Pancreatic Surgery, Bariatric Surgery, Gastrointestinal Motility Disorders) · Associate Professor of Surgery, Mayo Medical School · Consultant in Gastroenterologic, General Surgery and Surgical Research, Mayo Clinic · 200 First Street, SW, Rochester, MN 55905 · 507-284-2644

William Silen · Johnson & Johnson Professor of Surgery, Harvard Medical School Surgeon-In-Chief, Beth Israel Hospital · 330 Brookline Avenue, Boston, MA 02215 · 617-735-3788

Nathaniel J. Soper · (Laparoscopic Surgery) · Assistant Professor of Surgery, Washington University School of Medicine · Barnes Hospital · One Barnes Hospital Plaza, Suite 6108, St. Louis, MO 63110 · 314-362-6900

James R. Starling · Professor of Surgery, University of Wisconsin-Madison School of Medicine · Chief of Surgical Services, William S. Middleton Memorial Veterans Hospital; University of Wisconsin Hospital & Clinics · University of Wisconsin Clinical Science Center, Room H4-750, 600 Highland Avenue, Madison, WI 53792 · 608-263-2521

James C. Thompson · John Woods Harris Professor & Chairman, Department of Surgery, The University of Texas Medical Branch at Galveston · Chief of Surgery, The John Sealy Hospital · Department of Surgery, University of Texas Medical Branch at Galveston, Galveston, TX 77550 · 409-772-1285

Ronald K. Tompkins · (Biliary Surgery) · Professor of Surgery, University of California, Los Angeles School of Medicine · Chief, Section of Gastrointestinal Surgery, University of California, Los Angeles Center for the Health Sciences · 10833 LeConte Avenue, Room 74-125, Los Angeles, CA 90024 · 310-825-6846

Andrew L. Warshaw · Harold and Ellen Danser Professor of Surgery, Harvard Medical School · Associate Chief of Surgery, Massachusetts General Hospital · The Ambulatory Care Center, Suite 336, 15 Parkman Street, Boston, MA 02114 617-726-8254

Lawrence W. Way · (Hepatic Surgery, Biliary Surgery, Pancreatic Surgery, Laparoscopic Surgery) · Professor of Surgery, University of California at San Francisco School of Medicine · University of California at San Francisco Medical Center · 400 Parnassus Avenue, Suite 680, San Francisco, CA 94143 · 415-476-1161

Michael J. Zinner · (Inflammatory Bowel Disease) · Professor and Chairman, Department of Surgery, and The William P. Longmire, Jr. Chair in Surgery, University of California at Los Angeles School of Medicine · Chief, Division of General Surgery, and Chairman, Department of Surgery, University of California at Los Angeles Medical Center · Room 72-131 CHS, Los Angeles, CA 90024 · 310-825-7017

GENERAL VASCULAR SURGERY

William Henry Baker · (Carotid Surgery) · Professor & Chief, Section of Peripheral Vascular Surgery, Loyola Stritch School of Medicine · Foster G. McGaw Hospital · 2160 South First Avenue, Maywood, IL 60153 · 708-216-9187

Dennis F. Bandyk · (Graft Infections, Infrainguinal Bypass Surgery) · Professor of Surgery, University South Florida College of Medicine · Chief, Vascular Surgery Section, Tampa General Hospital; James A. Haley Veterans Hospital · Harbourside Medical Towers, Four Columbia Drive, Suite 730, Tampa, FL 33606 · 813-974-2201, 253-6001

Robert W. Barnes · (Noninvasive Study) · Professor and Chairman, General Surgery, University of Arkansas for Medical Sciences · Chief of Staff, The University Hospital of Arkansas · Slot #520, 4301 West Markham, Little Rock, AR 72205 · 501-686-5610

John J. Bergen · (Venous Disease) · Clinical Professor of Surgery, University of California at San Diego School of Medicine · Scripps Memorial Hospital; Veterans Administration Medical Center · Northcoast Surgeons, 9900 Genesee Avenue, Suite D, La Jolla, CA 92037 · 619-452-0306

Ramon Berguer · (Carotid Surgery, Vertebral Surgery, Brachiocephalic Surgery) · Professor and Chief, Division of Vascular Surgery, Wayne State University School of Medicine · Chief, Section of Vascular Surgery, Director, Acute Stroke Unit, Harper Hospital · 3990 John R Street, Detroit, MI 48201 · 313-745-8637

Henry D. Berkowitz · (Infrainguinal Bypass Surgery) · Associate Professor of Surgery, University of Pennsylvania School of Medicine · Chief, Division of Vascular Surgery, Presbyterian Medical Center of Philadelphia · 39th and Market Streets, Medical Arts Building, Suite 101, Philadelphia, PA 19104 · 215-662-0800

Victor Bernhard · (Infrainguinal Bypass Surgery, Graft Infection) · Professor and Chief, Section of Vascular Surgery, The University of Arizona College of Medicine The University of Arizona Health Sciences Center · Department of Surgery, 1501 North Campbell Avenue, Tucson, AZ 85724 · 602-626-6670

Eugene F. Bernstein · (Carotid Surgery, Noninvasive Testing) · Clinical Professor of Surgery, University of California at San Diego School of Medicine · Member, Division of Vascular and Thoracic Surgery, and Adjunct Member, Research Institute of Scripps Clinic, Scripps Clinic & Research Foundation · 10666 North Torrey Pines Road, La Jolla, CA 92037 · 619-554-8147

William F. Blaisdell · (Arterial Trauma, Bleeding Disorders) · Professor and Chairman, Department of Surgery, University of California at Davis School of Medicine · Chief of Surgery, University of California at Davis Medical Center · 4301 X Street, Suite 2310, Sacramento, CA 95817 · 916-734-2207

David C. Brewster · (Infrainguinal Bypass Surgery, Aortic Surgery) · Harvard Medical School · Massachusetts General Hospital · One Hawthorne Place, Boston, MA 02114 · 617-726-3567

Herbert Dardik · (Infrainguinal Bypass Surgery) · Chief of Surgery, Englewood Hospital · 375 Engle Street, Englewood, NJ 07631 · 201-894-0400

Richard H. Dean · (Renal Vascular Surgery, Aortic Surgery) · Director of Surgical Sciences, Division of Surgical Sciences, The Bowman Gray School of Medicine of Wake Forest University · North Carolina Baptist Hospital · Medical Center Boulevard, Winston-Salem, NC 27157-1095 · 919-748-4443

Ralph G. DePalma · (Impotence, Venous Disease) · Professor and Chairman, Department of Surgery, The George Washington University School of Medicine · George Washington University Medical Center · 2150 Pennsylvania Avenue, NW, Suite 6B415, Washington, DC 20037 · 202-994-4011

Allan R. Downs · (Aortic Surgery) · Professor of Surgery, University of Manitoba School of Medicine · Head, Vascular Surgery Service, The Health Sciences Centre 820 Sherbrook Street, Room GC405, Winnipeg, Manitoba R3A 1R9 · 204-787-2857

William K. Ehrenfeld · (Thoracic Outlet Disorders, Carotid Surgery) · Professor of Surgery, University of California at San Francisco School of Medicine · University of California at San Francisco Medical Center · 505 Parnassus Avenue, Room M488, San Francisco, CA 94143 · 415-476-2381

Calvin Ernst · (Graft Infections) · Clinical Professor of Surgery, The University of Michigan Medical School · Head, Division of Vascular Surgery, Henry Ford Medical Center · 2799 West Grand Boulevard, Detroit, MI 48202 · 313-876-1777

Joseph Martin Giordano · Professor of Surgery, The George Washington University School of Medicine · Chief, Division of Vascular Surgery, and Director, Vascular Laboratory, George Washington University Medical Center · 2150 Pennsylvania Avenue NW, Washington, DC 20037 · 202-994-4429

Peter Gloviczki · (Venous Disease, Vascular Malformations & Lymphoedema) · Associate Professor of Surgery, Mayo Medical School · Mayo Clinic · 200 First Street, SW, Rochester, MN 55905 · 507-284-2644

Jerry Goldstone · (Carotid Disease, Graft Infection) · Professor and Vice-Chairman, Department of Surgery, University of California at San Francisco School of Medicine · Chief, Vascular Surgery, University of California at San Francisco Medical Center · 505 Parnassus Avenue, Room M-488, San Francisco, CA 94143 · 415-476-2381

Richard M. Green · (Carotid Surgery, Aneurysms) · Associate Professor of Surgery, University of Rochester School of Medicine & Dentistry · Chief, Vascular Surgery, Strong Memorial Hospital, University of Rochester Medical Center · 125 Lattimore Road, Rochester, NY 14620 · 716-473-1112

Lazar J. Greenfield · (Thromboembolism, Venous Disease) · Professor and Chairman, Department of Surgery, The University of Michigan Medical School · The University of Michigan Medical Center · 2101 Taubman Center, 1500 East Medical Center Drive, Box 0346, Ann Arbor, MI 48109-0346 · 313-936-6398

Norman R. Hertzer · (Carotid Disease, Aortic Disease) · Chairman, Department of Vascular Surgery, The Cleveland Clinic Foundation · One Clinic Center, 9500 Euclid Avenue, Cleveland, OH 44195-5272 · 216-444-5705

Robert W. Hobson II · (Carotid Surgery) · Professor of Surgery, and Chief, Section of Vascular Surgery, University of Medicine & Dentistry of New Jersey · University Hospital, St. Michael's Medical Center, Newark, NJ; St. Clare's Medical Center, Danville, NJ; Department of Veterans Affairs Medical Center, E. Orange, NJ · 185 South Orange Avenue, G-532, Newark, NJ 07103 · 201-456-6633

Larry H. Hollier · (Thoraco-Abdominal Aneurysms, Aortic Surgery) · Chairman, Department of Surgery, Ochsner Clinic; Clinical Professor of Surgery, Louisiana State University School of Medicine, and Tulane University School of Medicine · Chief of Surgery, Ochsner Clinic · 1514 Jefferson Highway, New Orleans, LA 70121 · 504-838-4072

Michael Hume · (Venous Disease) · Professor of Surgery, Tufts University School of Medicine · New England Baptist Hospital · 125 Parker Hill Avenue, Boston, MA 02120 · 617-277-0020

George Johnson · (Arterial Trauma, Venous Disease, Aneurysms) · Professor of Surgery, University of North Carolina School of Medicine · University of North Carolina Hospitals · 210 Burnett Womack Building, Campus Box 7210, Chapel Hill, NC 27599-7210 · 919-966-3391

K. Wayne Johnson · (Aortic Surgery) · Professor of Surgery, University of Toronto School of Medicine · Head, Division of Vascular Surgery, The Toronto Hospital 200 Elizabeth Street, Ninth Floor, Eaton Wing, Room 217, Toronto, Ontario M5G 2C4 · 416-340-3552

David R. Knighton · Associate Professor of Surgery, University of Minnesota School of Medicine · University of Minnesota Hospital & Clinics · 420 Delaware Street SE, Box 120 UMHC, Minneapolis, MN 55455-0415 · 612-626-5464

Robert P. Leather · (Infrainguinal Bypass Surgery) · Professor of Surgery, Albany Medical College · Albany Medical Center · 47 New Scotland Avenue, Suite ME622, Albany, NY 12208 · 518-445-5158

Herbert I. Machleder · (Thoracic Outlet Disorders) · Professor of Surgery, University of California, Los Angeles School of Medicine · University of California,

Los Angeles Center for the Health Sciences · 10833 LeConte Avenue, Room 72-170, Los Angeles, CA 90024-6904 · 310-825-7433

John A. Mannick · (Infrainguinal Bypass Surgery, Aneurysms) · Moseley Professor of Surgery, Harvard Medical School · Surgeon-in-Chief, Brigham & Women's Hospital · 75 Francis Street, Boston, MA 02115 · 617-732-6820

Kenneth L. Mattox · (Arterial Trauma) · Professor of Surgery, Baylor College of Medicine · Chief of Staff, Ben Taub General Hospital · One Baylor Plaza, Houston, TX 77030 · 713-798-4557

Wesley S. Moore · (Carotid Disease, Carotid Surgery, Graft Infection) · Professor of Surgery, University of California, Los Angeles School of Medicine · Chief, Section of Vascular Surgery, University of California, Los Angeles Center for the Health Sciences · 10833 LeConte Avenue, Los Angeles, CA 90024-6904 · 310-825-9641

Thomas F. O'Donnell · (Carotid Disease, Venous Disease) · Professor of Surgery, Tufts University School of Medicine · Chief of Vascular Surgery, New England Medical Center · 750 Washington Street, Boston, MA 02111 · 617-956-5660

Victor Parsonnet · (Cardio-Vascular Surgery) · Clinical Professor of Surgery, University of Medicine & Dentistry of New Jersey · Director of Surgery, and Director of the Pacemaker Center, Newark Beth Israel Medical Center · 201 Lyons Avenue, Newark, NJ 07112 · 201-926-8038

Malcolm O. Perry · (Arterial Trauma, Aortic Surgery) · Professor and Chief of Vascular Surgery, Texas Tech University Health Sciences Center · University Surgical Associates, 3502 Ninth Street, Suite 210, Lubbock, TX 79415 · 806-743-1613

John M. Porter · (Vaso-Spastic Diseases, Raynaud's Disease, Infrainguinal Bypass Surgery) · Professor of Surgery, Division of Vascular Surgery, Oregon Health Sciences University · 3181 Southwest Sam Jackson Park Road, OP11, Portland, OR 97201-3098 · 503-494-7593

Thomas S. Riles · (Carotid Disease) · Professor of Surgery, New York University School of Medicine · New York University Medical Center, Tisch Hospital · 530 First Avenue, 6F, New York, NY 10016 · 212-263-7311

David B. Roos · (Thoracic Outlet Disorders) · Clinical Professor of Surgery, University of Colorado School of Medicine · Presbyterian-St. Luke's Medical Center · 1721 East 19th Avenue, Suite 138, Denver, CO 80218-1239 · 303-863-7667

Robert B. Rutherford · (Aortic Surgery, Infrainguinal Bypass Surgery, Peripheral Artery Surgery, Extraanatomic Surgery) · Professor of Surgery, and Chief of Vascular Surgery, Department of Surgery, University of Colorado School of Medicine University of Colorado Health Sciences Center · 4200 East Ninth Avenue, Box C-312, Denver CO 80262 · 303-270-8552

Richard J. Sanders · (Thoracic Outlet Disorders) · Clinical Professor of Surgery, University of Colorado School of Medicine · Rose Medical Center · 4545 East Ninth Avenue, Suite 240, Denver, CO 80220 · 303-388-6461

Gregorio A. Sicard · (Aortic Surgery) · Professor of Surgery, Washington University School of Medicine · Director of Vascular Service, Barnes Hospital · One Barnes Hospital Plaza, Suite 5103, St. Louis, MO 63110 · 314-362-7841

James C. Stanley · (Renal Vascular Surgery) · Professor and Associate Chairman, Department of Surgery, The University of Michigan Medical School · Head, Section of Vascular Surgery, The University of Michigan Medical Center · 2210 Taubman Center, 1500 East Medical Center Drive, Box 0329, Ann Arbor, MI 48109-0329 · 313-936-5786

Ronald J. Stoney · (Infections, Thoracic Outlet Disorders, Graft Infections, Aneurysms, Aortic Surgery) · Professor of Surgery, University of California at San Francisco Medical Center · Vascular Surgery, M488, Box 0222, 505 Parnassus Avenue, San Francisco, CA 94143-0222 · 415-476-2381

D. Eugene Strandness, Jr. · (Noninvasive) · Professor of Surgery and Head, Division of Vascular Surgery, University of Washington School of Medicine · Attending Vascular Surgeon, University of Washington Medical Center · Department of Surgery, Mail Stop: RF-25, 1959 N.E. Pacific Street, Seattle, WA 98195 206-543-3653

David Spurgeon Sumner · (Noninvasive Diagnosis) · Distinguished Professor of Surgery, Southern Illinois University School of Medicine · Memorial Medical Center; St. John's Hospital · 301 North Eighth Street, St. John's Pavilion, Third Floor, Springfield, IL 62701 · 217-782-7804

Brian L. Thiele · (Noninvasive Diagnosis) · Professor of Surgery, Pennsylvania State University · Chief of Vascular Surgery, The Milton S. Hershey Medical Center · 500 University Drive, Hershey, PA 17033 · 717-531-8866

Jonathan B. Towne · (Infrainguinal Bypass Surgery, Coagulation Problems, Graft Infections) · Professor of Surgery and Chairman, Department of Vascular Surgery, Medical College of Wisconsin · Milwaukee County Medical Complex · 8700 West Wisconsin Avenue, Milwaukee, WI 53226 · 414-257-5516

Frank J. Veith · (Infrainguinal Bypass Surgery, Redo Vascular Surgery) · Professor of Surgery, Albert Einstein College of Medicine · Interim Chairman, Department of Surgery, and Chief of Vascular Surgery, Montefiore Medical Center · 111 East 210th Street, Bronx, NY 10467 · 212-920-4108

J. Leonel Villavicencio · (Venous Disease) · Professor of Surgery, Uniformed Services University of Health Sciences · Senior Consultant and Staff, Department of Surgery and Vascular Surgery, Walter Reed Army Medical Center · 4301 Jones Bridge Road, Bethesda, MD 20814-4799 · 301-295-3155

Marshall W. Webster · Professor of Surgery, University of Pittsburgh School of Medicine · Chief, Section of Vascular Surgery & Wound Healing, Presbyterian University Hospital · 1084 Scaife Hall, Pittsburgh, PA 15261 · 412-648-9867

Anthony D. Whittemore · (Infrainguinal Bypass Surgery) · Associate Professor of Surgery, Harvard Medical School · Chief, Division of Vascular Surgery, Brigham & Women's Hospital · 75 Francis Street, Boston, MA 02115 · 617-732-6816

G. Melville Williams · (Aneurysms) · Bertram M. Bernheim Professor and Surgeon-in-Charge, Johns Hopkins University School of Medicine · Chairman, Division of Transplantation & Vascular Surgery Service, The Johns Hopkins Medical Institutions · Blalock Building, 600 North Wolfe Street, Room 606, Baltimore, MD 21205 · 410-955-5165

James See-Tao Yao · (Aneurysms, Infrainguinal Bypass Surgery, Noninvasive Testing) · Professor of Surgery, Northwestern University Medical School · Attending Surgeon, Northwestern Memorial Hospital · 251 East Chicago, Chicago, IL 60611 · 312-908-2714

PEDIATRIC SURGERY

R. Peter Altman · (Liver, Biliary Tract) · Professor of Surgery and Pediatrics, College of Physicians & Surgeons of Columbia University · Director of Pediatric Surgery, Columbia Presbyterian Medical Center; Surgeon-in-Chief, Columbia-Presbyterian Medical Center, Babies Hospital · 3959 Broadway, Rom 203 North, New York, NY 10032 · 212-305-5870

Kathryn Duncan Anderson · Professor of Surgery, The George Washington University School of Medicine · Acting Chairman, Department of Surgery, Children's National Medical Center · 111 Michigan Avenue NW, Washington, DC 20010 · 202-745-2153

Arnold G. Coran · (Pediatric Thoracic Surgery, Pediatric Surgical Critical Care) · Professor of Surgery, The University of Michigan Medical School · Head, Section of Pediatric Surgery, and Surgeon-in-Chief, C.S. Mott Children's Hospital, The University of Michigan Medical Center · L2110 Maternal Child Health Care

Center, 1500 East Medical Center Drive, Room 2G332, Box 0245, Ann Arbor, MI 48109-0245 · 313-764-4151

Patricia Donahoe · Professor of Surgery, Harvard Medical School · Chief, Department of Pediatric Surgical Services, Massachusetts General Hospital · 32 Fruit Street, Boston, MA 02114 · 617-726-8839

Philip R. Exelby · (Pediatric Surgical Oncology) · Chief, Pediatric Surgical Service, Memorial Sloan-Kettering Cancer Center · 1275 York Avenue, New York, NY 10021 · 212-639-7966

Robert M. Filler · Professor of Surgery and Pediatrics, University of Toronto School of Medicine · Surgeon-in-Chief, The Hospital for Sick Children · 555 University Avenue, Room 1526, Toronto, Ontario M5G 1X8 · 416-598-6400

Howard Church Filston · Professor of Pediatric Surgery & Pediatrics, Duke University School of Medicine · Duke University Medical Center · Box 3815, Knoxville, TN 27710 · 615-544-9240

Jay L. Grosfeld · Professor and Chairman, Department of Surgery, Indiana University School of Medicine · Surgeon-in-Chief, James Whitcomb Riley Hospital for Children; Indiana University Medical Center · 545 Barnhill Drive, Emerson Hall 244, Indianapolis IN 46202-5124 · 317-274-4681

Michael R. Harrison · (Fetal Surgery) · Professor of Surgery, University of California at San Francisco School of Medicine · Chief of Pediatric Surgery, University of California at San Francisco Medical Center · 505 Parnassus Avenue, Room U112, San Francisco, CA 94143 · 415-476-2538

W. Hardy Hendren · (Pediatric Urology) · Robert E. Gross Professor of Surgery, Harvard Medical School · Chief of Surgery, Children's Hospital · 300 Longwood Avenue, Boston, MA 02115 · 617-735-8001

John Lilly · (Biliary Atresia) · Professor of Surgery, University of Colorado School of Medicine · Surgeon-in-Chief, The Children's Hospital · 1950 Ogden Street, B-323, Denver, CO 80218 · 303-861-6526

James A. O'Neill · Koop Professor of Pediatric Surgery, University of Pennsylvania School of Medicine · Surgeon-in-Chief, The Children's Hospital of Philadelphia · General Surgery, 34th and Civic Center Boulevard, Philadelphia, PA 19104 215-590-2727

Alberto Pena · (Colorectal Problems in Children) · Professor of Surgery, Albert Einstein College of Medicine · Chief, Pediatric Surgery, Schneiders Children's Hospital; Long Island Jewish Medical Center · 269-01 Seventy-Sixth Avenue, Room 158, New Hyde Park, NY 11042 · 718-470-3637

Bradley Moreland Rodgers · Professor and Chief, Division of Pediatric Surgery, University of Virginia School of Medicine · University of Virginia Health Sciences Center · Jefferson Park Avenue, Box 181, Charlottesville, VA 22908 · 804-924-2673

Marc I. Rowe · Professor of Pediatric Surgery, University of Pittsburgh School of Medicine · Chief, Surgical Services, Children's Hospital of Pittsburgh · 3705 Fifth Avenue at DeSoto Street, Pittsburgh, PA 15213 · 412-692-5043

Moritz M. Ziegler · Professor of Surgery and Pediatrics, University of Cincinnati College of Medicine · Director, Pediatric Surgery, and Surgeon-in-Chief, Children's Hospital Medical Center · 240 Bethesda Avenue, Cincinnati, OH 45229-2899 · 513-559-4371

TRANSPLANTATION
(See also Adult Nephrology, Kidney Transplantation; Cardiovascular Disease, Heart Transplantation; Infectious Disease, Transplantation Infections; Thoracic Surgery, Transplantation; Urology, Kidney Transplantation)

Nancy L. Ascher · (Liver and Kidney Transplantation) · Professor of Surgery, University of California at San Francisco School of Medicine · Chief, Liver & Kidney Transplant Service, University of California at San Francisco Medical Center · 505 Parnassus Avenue, M-896, San Francisco, CA 94143 · 415-476-8028

Clyde F. Barker · (Kidney Transplantation) · Chairman, Department of Surgery, University of Pennsylvania School of Medicine · Chief of Surgery, Chief of Vascular Surgery & Transplant Surgery, Hospital of the University of Pennsylvania · 3400 Spruce Street, Philadelphia, PA 19104 · 215-662-2027

Folkert O. Belzer · (Organ Preservation) · Professor and Chairman, Department of Surgery, University of Wisconsin-Madison School of Medicine · University of Wisconsin Hospital & Clinics · 600 Highland Avenue, Room H4-710, Madison, WI 53792 · 608-263-1377

R. Randal Bollinger · (Kidney Transplantation) · Professor of Surgery, and Associate Professor of Immunology, Duke University School of Medicine · Chief of Surgical Transplantation, Duke University Medical Center · P.O. Box 2910, Durham, NC 27710 · 919-684-5209

Ronald W. Busuttil · (Liver Transplantation) · Professor of Surgery, University of California, Los Angeles School of Medicine · Director, University of California, Los Angeles Liver Transplant Program, University of California, Los Angeles Center for Health Sciences · 10833 LeConte Avenue, Los Angeles, CA 90024 · 310-825-5318

Robert J. Corry · (Pancreas and Kidney Transplantation) · Professor and Head, Department of Surgery, The University of Iowa College of Medicine · Chief of Surgery, The University of Iowa Hospitals & Clinics · Iowa City, IA 52242 · 319-356-2545

Arnold G. Diethelm · (Kidney Transplantation) · Professor and Chairman, Department of Surgery, The University of Alabama School of Medicine · Chief of Surgery, The University of Alabama Hospital · 701 South 19th Street, Birmingham, AL 35294 · 205-934-5200

Jean C. Emond · (Liver Transplantation) · Assistant Professor, Department of Surgery, University of Chicago, Pritzker School of Medicine · University of Chicago Medical Center · 5841 South Maryland Avenue, Box 259, Chicago, IL 60637-1470 · 312-702-6319

Carlos O. Esquivel · (Liver Transplantation) · Assistant Clinical Professor of Surgery, University of California at Davis School of Medicine · Director, Liver Transplantation, California Pacific Medical Center · 2340 Clay Street, Suite 425, San Francisco, CA 94115 · 415-923-3450

John Fung · (Liver Transplantation, Transplantation Immunology) · Associate Professor of Surgery, and Chief, Division of Transplantation Surgery, University of Pittsburgh School of Medicine · 3601 Fifth Avenue, Department of Surgery, Pittsburgh, PA 15213 · 412-648-3200

Mark A. Hardy · (Kidney Transplantation) · Auchincloss Professor of Surgery, College of Physicians & Surgeons of Columbia University · Attending in Surgery, Columbia-Presbyterian Medical Center · 630 West 168th Street, New York, NY 10032 · 212-305-5502

Roger L. Jenkins · (Liver Transplantation) · Associate Professor of Surgery, Harvard Medical School · Chief, Division of Hepatobiliary Surgery & Liver Transplantation, New England Deaconess Hospital · 110 Francis Street, Suite 8C, Boston, MA 02215 · 617-732-9779

Barry Donald Kahan · (Kidney Transplantation) · Professor of Surgery, The University of Texas Health Science Center at Houston · Director, Division of Immunology & Organ Transplantation, Hermann Hospital · 6431 Fannin Street, Suite 6240, Houston, TX 77030 · 713-792-5670

Munci Kalayoğlu · (Liver Transplantation) · Professor of Surgery and Pediatrics, University of Wisconsin-Madison School of Medicine · Director, Liver Transplant Program, University of Wisconsin Hospital & Clinics · 600 Highland Avenue, Room H4-780, Madison, WI 53792 · 608-263-9903

Goran B. Klintmalm · (Liver Transplantation) · Director, Transplantation Services, Baylor University · Baylor University Medical Center · Transplantation Services, 3500 Gaston Avenue, Dallas, TX 75246 · 214-820-2050

Ruud A.F. Krom · (Liver Transplantation) · Professor of Surgery, Mayo Medical School · Head of Liver Transplant,Mayo Clinic · 200 First Street, SW, Rochester, MN 55905 · 507-284-5115

Anthony Monaco · (Kidney and Pancreas Transplantation) · Professor of Surgery, Harvard Medical School · Chief, Division of Organ Transplantation, New England Deaconess Hospital · 185 Pilgrim Road, Boston, MA 02215 · 617-732-8549

John S. Najarian · (Pediatric Liver & Kidney Transplantation) · Regents' Professor, and Jay Phillips Chair in Surgery, University of Minnesota School of Medicine · Chairman, Department of Surgery, University of Minnesota Hospital & Clinics · 516 Delaware Street, SE, Minneapolis, MN 55455 · 612-625-8444

Byers W. Shaw Jr. · (Liver Transplantation) · Professor of Surgery, University of Nebraska College of Medicine · Chief of Transplantation Service, University of Nebraska Medical Center · 600 South 42nd Street, Omaha, NE 68198-3280 · 402-559-4076

Richard L. Simmons · (Kidney Transplantation) · Professor and Chairman, Department of Surgery, University of Pittsburgh School of Medicine · University of Pittsburgh Medical Center · 497 Scaife Hall, Pittsburgh, PA 15261 · 412-648-1823

Hans W. Sollinger · (Pancreas and Kidney Transplantation) · Professor of Surgery, University of Wisconsin-Madison School of Medicine · Director, Pancreas Transplant Program, University of Wisconsin Hospital & Clinics · 600 Highland Avenue, Room H4-780, Madison, WI 53792 · 608-263-9903

Thomas E. Starzl · (Liver & Kidney Transplantation) · Professor of Surgery, University of Pittsburgh School of Medicine · Director of the Transplantation Institute, Presbyterian University Hospital; Children's Hospital of Pittsburgh; VA Medical Center · 3601 Fifth Avenue, 5C Falk Clinic, Pittsburgh, PA 15213 · 412-624-0112

Sylvester Sterioff · (Kidney Transplantation) · Professor of Surgery, Mayo Medical School · Director of Transplantation, Mayo Clinic · 200 First Street, SW, Rochester, MN 55905 · 507-284-8392

David E. Sutherland · (Kidney and Pancreas Transplantation) · Professor of Surgery, University of Minnesota School of Medicine · University of Minnesota Hospital & Clinics · 420 Delaware Street, SE, Box 280 UMHC, Minneapolis, MN 55455 · 612-625-7600

J. Richard Thistlethwaite, Jr. · (Kidney, Liver and Pancreas Transplantation) · Associate Professor of Surgery, University of Chicago, Pritzker School of Medicine Chief, Transplant Surgery Section, University of Chicago Medical Center · 5841 South Maryland Avenue, Box 77, Chicago, IL 60637-1470 · 312-702-6104

G. Melville Williams · (Kidney Transplantation) · Bertram M. Bernheim Professor and Surgeon-in-Charge, Johns Hopkins University School of Medicine · Chairman, Division of Transplantation & Vascular Surgery Service, The Johns Hopkins Medical Institutions · Blalock Building, 600 North Wolfe Street, Room 606, Baltimore, MD 21205 · 410-955-5165

WOUND HEALING
(See also Dermatology, Wound Healing; Plastic Surgery, Wound Healing)

Adrian Barbul · Associate Professor of Surgery, Johns Hopkins University School of Medicine · Sinai Hospital of Baltimore · 123 West Lanvale Street, Baltimore, MD 21217 · 301-578-5843

Thomas K. Hunt · Professor of Surgery and Vice-Chairman for Research, Department of Surgery, University of California at San Francisco School of Medicine · University of California at San Francisco Medical Center · 513 Parnassus Avenue, Room HSE-839, San Francisco, CA 94143 · 415-476-0410

David R. Knighton · Associate Professor of Surgery, University of Minnesota School of Medicine · University of Minnesota Hospital & Clinics · 420 Delaware Street SE, Box 120 UMHC, Minneapolis, MN 55455-0415 · 612-626-5464

GERIATRIC MEDICINE

GENERAL GERIATRIC MEDICINE

Edwin J. Olsen · (Geriatric Psychiatry) · University of Miami School of Medicine; Mount Sinai Medical Center, Miami Beach, FL · Vice Chairman, Department of Psychiatry, University of Miami School of Medicine; Chairman, Mount Sinai Medical Center, Miami Beach, FL; University of Miami-Jackson Memorial Medical Center · 4300 Alton Road, Main #204, Miami Beach, FL 33140 · 305-647-2194

Itamar B. Abrass · (Endocrinology, Diabetes) · Professor of Medicine, Division of Gerontology and Geriatric Medicine, University of Washington School of Medicine · Head, Division of Gerontology & Geriatric Medicine, Harborview Medical Center · 325 Ninth Avenue (ZA-87), Seattle, WA 98104 · 206-223-3089

Richard M. Allman · Associate Professor of Medicine and Director, Division of Gerontology and Geriatric Medicine, The University of Alabama School of Medicine · Chief, Geriatrics Section, Birmingham Veterans Affairs Medical Center; The University of Alabama Hospital · 1717 Eleventh Avenue South, Room 731, Birmingham, AL 35294 · 205-934-9261

William B. Applegate · (Cardiovascular, Hypertension) · Professor of Preventive Medicine and Medicine, The University of Tennessee at Memphis, College of Medicine · University of Tennessee Bowld Hospital · 66 North Pauline Street, Suite 232, Memphis, TN 38163 · 901-528-5903

Patricia P. Barry · Associate Professor of Medicine, University of Miami School of Medicine · Associate Chief of Staff for Geriatrics & Extended Care, Miami Veterans Affairs Medical Center · 1201 Northwest 16th Street, Room C1209, Miami, FL 33125 · 305-324-3204

Richard W. Besdine · Director, Travelers Center on Aging, University of Connecticut School of Medicine · University of Connecticut Health Center, MC5215, 263 Farmington Avenue, Farmington, CT 06030 · 203-679-3956

Marlene Bluestein · Assistant Professor of Medicine, Arizona Health Sciences Center, and Professor of Medicine, The University of Arizona College of Medicine · Chief, Geriatrics Section, Tucson Veterans Affairs Medical Center · 3601 South Sixth Street, Tucson, AZ 85723 · 602-792-1450 x6447

Kenneth V. Brummel-Smith · (Rehabilitation) · Associate Professor of Medicine and Family Medicine, Oregon Health Sciences University · Portland Veterans Affairs Medical Center · Division of Geriatrics (111), 3710 SW U.S.Veterans Hospital Road, P.O. Box 1034, Portland, OR 97207 · 503-273-5015

George J. Caranasos · Professor of Internal Medicine, University of Florida College of Medicine · Ruth S. Jewett Professor of Medicine in Geriatrics, Shands Hospital at the University of Florida · 1600 Southwest Archer Road, Room M405, P.O. Box 100277, Gainesville, FL 32610 · 904-392-3197

Christine K. Cassel · Professor of Medicine and Professor of Public Policy, University of Chicago, Pritzker School of Medicine · Chief, Section of General Internal Medicine, University of Chicago Medical Center · 5841 South Maryland Avenue, Box 12, Chicago, IL 60637-1470 · 312-702-3045

A. Mark Clarfield · Professor and Assistant Dean, Faculty of Medicine, McGill University · Sir Mortimer B. Davis Jewish General Hospital · Division of Geriatrics, 3755 Cote St. Catherine Road, Suite E0018, Montreal, Quebec H3T 1E2 · 514-340-7501

Harvey Jay Cohen · Professor of Medicine, Duke University School of Medicine Chief, Division of Geriatric Medicine, Department of Medicine, Duke University Medical Center; Director of Geriatric Research, Education & Clinical Center, GRECC, Durham Veterans Affairs Medical Center · P.O. Box 3003, Duke University Medical Center, Durham, NC 27710 · 919-684-3176

Patrick P. Coll · (Family Medicine) · Assistant Professor, Department of Family Medicine, University of Connecticut School of Medicine · John Dempsey Hospital; St. Francis Hospital & Medical Center · 123 Sigourney Street, Hartford, CT 06105-2756 · 203-566-8994

Leo M. Cooney · Professor of Medicine, Yale University School of Medicine · Director, Continuing Care Unit, and Director, Utilization Review, Yale-New Haven Hospital · 20 York Street, New Haven, CT 06504 · 203-785-6361

Edmund H. Duthie · Professor of Medicine and Chief, Division of Geriatrics, Medical College of Wisconsin · Chief, Section of Geriatrics, Veterans Affairs Medical Center; Froedtert Memorial Lutheran Hospital; Milwaukee County Medical Complex · 9200 West Wisconsin Avenue, Milwaukee, WI 53226 · 414-384-2000 x2775, 259-2000

Maria A. Fiatarone · Assistant Professor of Medicine, Harvard Medical School; Scientist II, U.S.D.A. Human Nutrition Research Center on Aging at Tufts University · Consultant Staff, Brigham & Women's Hospital; Associate in Medicine, Beth Israel Hospital · 711 Washington Street, Boston, MA 02111 · 617-556-3075

Suzanne L. Fields · Assistant Professor of Medicine, New York Medical College Chief of Geriatric Medicine, St. Vincent's Hospital & Medical Center of New York · 153 West 11th Street, New York, NY 10011 · 212-790-8904

Cornelius James Foley · Assistant Professor of Medicine, State University of New York Health Science Center at Stony Brook · Long Island Jewish Medical Center 271-11 Seventhy-Sixth Street, New Hyde Park, NY 11042 · 718-343-2100

Michael L. Freedman · Professor of Medicine, and The Diane and Arthur Belfer Professor of Geriatric Medicine, New York University School of Medicine · Director, Division of Geriatrics, New York University Medical Center, Bellevue Hospital · 550 First Avenue, Suite 4C, New York, NY 10016 · 212-561-6380

Marsha D. Fretwell · Clinical Associate Professor of Medicine, Brown University Program in Medicine · Attending Physician, Roger Williams Medical Center · 12 Madden Lane, Little Compton, RI 02837 · 401-635-4562

Meghan B. Gerety · Assistant Professor of Medicine, The University of Texas Health Science Center at San Antonio · Acting Clinical Director—GRECC and Medical Director—Geriatric Evaluation Unit, Audie L. Murphy Memorial Veterans Hospital · 7400 Merton Minter Boulevard, GEU 18(C), San Antonio, TX 78284 · 512-617-5197

Mary Kane Goldstein · (Family Practice) · Fellow in Health Services Research, Stanford University School of Medicine · Director of Graduate Medical Education for Geriatrics, Palo Alto Veterans Affairs Medical Center; Stanford University Hospital · Division of General Internal Medicine, MSOB X215, Stanford, CA 94305-5479 · 415-723-3288

Susan L. Greenspan · Assistant Professor of Medicine, Harvard Medical School · Associate in Medicine, Beth Israel Hospital · Division of Gerontology, 330 Brookline Avenue, Boston, MA 02215 · 617-735-4580

Richard T. Ham · State University of New York Distinguished Chair in Geriatric Medicine, State University of New York Health Science Center at Syracuse · University Hospital · 750 East Adams Street, Syracuse, NY 13210 · 315-464-5167

William R. Hazzard · (Lipid Disorders) · Professor and Chairman, Department of Internal Medicine, The Bowman Gray School of Medicine of Wake Forest University · North Carolina Baptist Hospital · Medical Center Boulevard, Winston-Salem, NC 27157-1052 · 919-748-2020

Patrick W. Irvine · Assistant Professor of Medicine, University of Minnesota School of Medicine · Hennepin County Medical Center · 701 Park Avenue, 834, Minneapolis, MN 55415 · 612-337-7490

Dennis W. Jahnigen · Head, Department of Geriatric Medicine, The Cleveland Clinic Foundation · One Clinic Center, 9500 Euclid Avenue, Cleveland, OH 44195 · 216-444-8091

Jerry C. Johnson · Associate Professor of Medicine, and Director, Geriatric Medicine Fellowship, University of Pennsylvania School of Medicine · Chief, Geriatric Section of the Philadelphia VAMC, Hospital of the University of Pennsylvania; Philadelphia VA Medical Center · The Ralston-Penn Center, The Geriatrics Program, 3615 Chestnut Street, Philadelphia, PA 19104-2676 · 215-898-1548

Joseph M. Keenan · (Home Care) · Assistant Professor of Family Medicine, University of Minnesota School of Medicine · Director of Geriatrics, Department of Family Practice, University of Minnesota Hospital & Clinics · 825 Washington Avenue SE, Box 25 UMHC, Minneapolis, MN 55414 · 612-627-4943

Robert D. Kennedy · Clinical Professor of Medicine, Albert Einstein College of Medicine · Interim Chairman, Division of Geriatrics, Montefiore Medical Center 111 East 210th Street, Bronx, NY 10467 · 212-920-6721

Steven Levenson · Director, Medical Office, Levindale Hebrew Geriatric Center & Hospital · 2434 West Belvedere Avenue, Baltimore, MD 21215 · 301-466-8700

Elaine Annette Leventhal · Associate Professor of Medicine, Robert Wood Johnson Medical School-University of Medicine & Dentistry of New Jersey · Head of Geriatrics, Robert Wood Johnson University Hospital · The Professional Building, 97 Patterson Street, New Brunswick, NJ 08903 · 908-418-8145

Leslie S. Libow · Anna A. Greenwall Professor of Geriatrics & Adult Development, Mt. Sinai School of Medicine · Chief, Medical Services, The Jewish Home & Hospital for the Aged · 120 West 106th Street, New York, NY 10025 · 212-240-5457

David A. Lipschitz · (Hematology) · Professor of Medicine and Head, Division on Aging, University of Arkansas for Medical Sciences · Director, Geriatric Research & Education & Clinical Center, John L. McClellan Veterans Hospital · 4300 West Seventh Street, Little Rock, AR 72205 · 501-660-2031

Lewis A. Lipsitz · (Long-Term Care) · Assistant Professor of Medicine and Director, Harvard Geriatric Fellowship Program, Harvard Medical School · The Irving & Edyth Usen Director of Clinical Research, Hebrew Rehabilitation Center for Aged · 1200 Centre Street, Roslindale, MA 02131 · 617-325-8000

Robert J. Luchi · Professor of Medicine, Baylor College of Medicine · Chief, Geriatrics, The Methodist Hospital; and, Houston Veterans Affairs Medical Center · 6550 Fannin Street, Suite 1035, Houston, TX 77030 · 713-798-3967

Kenneth W. Lyles · (Metabolic Bone Disease) · Associate Professor of Medicine, Duke University School of Medicine · Clinical Director, Geriatric Research, Education & Clinical Center, Durham Veterans Affairs Medical Center · P.O. Box 3881, Duke University Medical Center, Durham, NC 27710 · 919-684-6977

Michael E. Maddens · Director, Division of Geriatric Medicine, William Beaumont Hospital · 3601 West Thirteen Mile Road, Royal Oak, MI 48073 · 313-551-0615

David Charles Martin · Chief, Division of Geriatric Medicine, The Senior Health Center of Western Pennsylvania Hospital · 251 Pearl Street, Pittsburgh, PA 15224 · 412-578-7366

Diane Meier · Associate Professor of Medicine, Mt. Sinai School of Medicine · Mt. Sinai Medical Center · One Gustave L. Levy Place, P.O. Box 1070, New York, NY 10029-6574 · 212-241-5561

Graydon S. Meneilly · Assistant Professor, Department of Medicine, The University of British Columbia · University Hospital, Shaughnessy Site · Jean Matheson Pavilion, 4500 Oak Street, Suite G437, Vancouver, British Columbia V6H 3N1 604-822-7031,875-2003

Kenneth L. Minaker · Associate Professor of Medicine, Harvard Medical School Director, Geriatric Research Education and Clinical Center, Brockton/West Roxbury VAMC; Associate Director, The Clinical Research Center, Beth Israel Hospital · Gerontology Division, 330 Brookline Avenue, Boston, MA 02215 · 617-735-2692

Fitzhugh C. Pannill III · Assistant Professor of Medicine, Yale University School of Medicine · West Haven Veterans Affairs Medical Center · 950 Campbell Avenue, West Haven, CT 06516 · 203-785-6361

Robert A. Pearlman · Associate Professor of Medicine and Health Services, Division of Gerontology and Geriatric Medicine, University of Washington School of Medicine · Seattle Veterans Affairs Medical Center · 1660 South Columbian Way, Seattle, WA 98108 · 206-764-2308

Jane F. Potter · Associate Professor of Internal Medicine, and Chief, Section of Geriatrics and Gerontology, University of Nebraska College of Medicine · University of Nebraska Medical Center · 600 South 42nd Street, Omaha, NE 68198-5620 · 402-559-4427

David B. Reuben · Assistant Professor of Medicine, University of California at Los Angeles School of Medicine · Associate Director, Multicampus Division of Geriatric Medicine & Gerontology, University of California at Los Angeles Center for Health Sciences · 10833 LeConte Avenue, Los Angeles, CA 90024-1687 · 310-825-8255

Laurence J. Robbins · Associate Professor of Medicine, University of Colorado School of Medicine · Associate Chief of Staff for Geriatrics & Extended Care, Denver Department of Veterans Affairs Medical Center · 1055 Clermont Street, Geriatrics (111D), Denver, CO 80220 · 303-399-8020

Bruce Eugene Robinson · Associate Professor and Director, Division of Geriatric Medicine, University South Florida College of Medicine · Chief, Section of Geriatrics, James A. Haley Veterans Hospital; Medical Director, Hospice of Hillsborough; and, Tampa General Hospital · 12901 Bruce B. Downs Boulevard, Box 19, Tampa FL 33612 · 813-974-2201

Laurence Z. Rubenstein · Associate Professor of Medicine, University of California at Los Angeles School of Medicine · Director, Geriatric Research Education & Clinical Center, University of California at Los Angeles Geriatric Psychiatry Service · 16111 Plummer Street, Mail Code 11-E, Sepulveda, CA 91343 · 818-895-9311

Robert S. Schwartz · (Endocrinology, Metabolism, Nutrition) · Associate Professor of Medicine, Division of Gerontology and Geriatric Medicine, University of Washington School of Medicine · Harborview Medical Center · 325 Ninth Avenue (ZA-87), Seattle, WA 98104 · 206-223-3537

Fredrick Todd Sherman · Clinical Associate Professor of Medicine, State University of New York Health Science Center at Stony Brook · Huntington Hospital 158 East Main Street, Huntington, NY 11743 · 516-351-3434

Philip D. Sloane · Associate Professor of Family Medicine and Associate Clinical Professor of Epidemiology, University of North Carolina School of Medicine · University of North Carolina Hospitals · William B. Aycock Building, Manning Drive, Campus Box 7595, Chapel Hill, NC 27599-7595 · 919-966-3711

Stephanie A. Studenski · Assistant Professor of Medicine, Duke University School of Medicine · Fellow, Duke University Center for the Study of Aging in Human Development; Chief of Rehabilitation Medicine Service & Aging Center, Durham Veterans Affairs Medical Center · 508 Fulton Street, Durham, NC 27705 919-286-6874

George Taler · (Family Medicine) · University of Maryland School of Medicine · Family Medicine, 405 West Redwood Street, First Floor, Baltimore, MD 21201 · 301-448-2770

Mary E. Tinetti · Associate Professor, Department of Internal Medicine, Yale University School of Medicine · Yale-New Haven Hospital · 333 Cedar Street, P.O. Box 3333, New Haven, CT 06510-8056 · 203-785-6361

Richard P. Tonino · Associate Professor, Department of Medicine, University of Vermont School of Medicine · Medical Center Hospital of Vermont · Given Health Care, One South Prospect, Burlington, VT 05401 · 802-656-4531

Gregg Warshaw · (Ambulatory Care) · Director, Office of Geriatric Medicine, and The Martha Betty Semmons Associate Professor, Geriatric Medicine, and Associate Professor of Family Medicine, University of Cincinnati College of Medicine University of Cincinnati Hospital · Office of Geriatric Medicine, 231 Bethesda Avenue, Cincinnati, OH 45267-0582 · 513-558-0650

Mark E. Williams · Associate Professor and Director of the Program on Aging, University of North Carolina School of Medicine · University of North Carolina Hospitals · 141 MacNider Building. Campus Box 7550, Chapel Hill, NC 27599-7550 · 919-966-5945

Carol Hutner Winograd · (Family Medicine) · Associate Professor of Medicine, and Assistant Director, Division of Endocrinology, Gerontology & Metabolism, and Chief of Clinical Programs, Geriatric Medicine, Stanford University School of Medicine · Director of Clinical Activities, Geriatric Research, Education & Clinical Center, Palo Alto Veterans Affairs Medical Center · 3801 Miranda Avenue, GRECC 182-B, Palo Alto, CA 94304 · 415-852-3415

Gisele P. Wolf-Klein · Assistant Professor of Medicine, Albert Einstein College of Medicine · Physician-in-Charge of the Geriatric Community Health Care Center, Parker Jewish Geriatric Institute; Chief, Division of Geriatric Medicine, Long Island Jewish Medical Center · 271-11 Seventy-Sixth Avenue, Medical Department, Second Floor, New Hyde Park, NY 11042 · 718-343-2100 x307

URINARY INCONTINENCE
(See also Urology, Neuro-Urology & Voiding Dysfunction)

John Russell Burton · Associate Professor of Medicine, Johns Hopkins University School of Medicine · Director, Geriatric Medicine, Francis Scott Key Medical Center · Johns Hopkins Geriatrics Center, 5505 Hopkins Bayview Circle, Baltimore, MD 21224 · 301-550-0520

Joseph G. Ouslander · Associate Professor of Medicine, University of California at Los Angeles School of Medicine · Medical Director, Jewish Home for the Aging, University of California at Los Angeles Center for Health Sciences · 18855 Victory Boulevard, Reseda, CA 91335 · 818-774-3051

Neil M. Resnick · Assistant Professor of Medicine, Harvard Medical School · Chief of Geriatrics, and Director, Continence Center, Brigham & Women's Hospital · 75 Francis Street, Boston, MA 02115 · 617-732-6844

HAND SURGERY

ELBOW SURGERY

Ralph W. Coonrad · (Elbow Reconstruction) · Associate Clinical Professor of Orthopaedic Surgery, Duke University School of Medicine · Durham General Hospital · 1828 Hillandale Road, Durham, NC 27705 · 919-220-5593

GENERAL HAND SURGERY

Peter C. Amadio · Associate Professor of Orthopaedic Surgery, Mayo Medical School · Mayo Clinic · 200 First Street, SW, Rochester, MN 55905 · 507-284-2806

William Patrick Cooney III · Professor of Orthopaedics, Mayo Medical School · Head, Section of Hand Surgery, Mayo Clinic · 200 First Street, SW, Rochester, MN 55905 · 507-284-2994

David P. Green · Clinical Professor of Orthopaedics, The University of Texas Health Science Center at San Antonio · St. Luke's Lutheran Hospital · 7940 Floyd Curl Drive, Suite 900, San Antonio, TX 78229 · 512-614-7025

Neil F. Jones · Associate Professor of Plastic and Hand Surgery, University of Pittsburgh School of Medicine · Chief of Hand Surgery and Microsurgery, Presbyterian University Hospital; Children's Hospital of Pittsburgh · 660 Scaife Hall, Pittsburgh, PA 15261 · 412-648-9674

William Kleinman · Clinical Associate Professor of Orthopaedic Surgery, Indiana University School of Medicine · The Indiana Hand Center; St. Vincent Hospital & Health Care Center; Riley Children's Hospital at IUMC · 8501 Harcourt Road, Indianapolis, IN 46260 · 317-875-9105

Roy A. Meals · Associate Clinical Professor of Orthopaedic Surgery, University of California at Los Angeles School of Medicine · Chief of Hand Surgery Service, University of California at Los Angeles Medical Center · 100 UCLA Medical Plaza, Suite 305, Los Angeles, CA 90024-6970 · 213-206-6337

Lawrence H. Schneider · Clinical Professor of Orthopaedic Surgery, Jefferson Medical College of Thomas Jefferson University · Director, Division of Hand Surgery, Department of Orthopaedic Surgery, Thomas Jefferson University Hospital · Hand Rehabilitation Center, 901 Walnut Street, Philadelphia, PA 19107 · 215-629-0980

Peter Joseph Stern · Clinical Professor of Orthopaedic Surgery, and Director, Division of Hand Surgery, Department of Orthopaedic Surgery, University of Cincinnati College of Medicine · Bethesda Hospital; Children's Hospital Medical Center; The Christ Hospital; The Deaconess Hospital; Good Samaritan Hospital; The Jewish Hospital of Cincinnati; Jewish Hospital Kenwood; Shriners Burn Institute; University of Cincinnati Medical Center · Cincinnati Hand Surgery Consultants, 2800 Windslow Avenue, Suite 401, Cincinnati, OH 45206 · 513-961-4263

MICROSURGERY
(See also Plastic Surgery, Microsurgery)

Harry J. Buncke · (Microvascular) · Clinical Professor of Surgery, University of California at San Francisco School of Medicine · Director, Neurosurgical Division, Davies Medical Center; Peninsula-Mills Hospitals · Davies Medical Center, M.O.B. Annex Suite 140, 45 Castro Street, San Francisco, CA 94114 · 415-342-8989

Graham D. Lister · (Tendons, Congenital) · Professor and Chairman, Division of Plastic & Reconstructive Surgery, University of Utah School of Medicine · 50 North Medical Drive, Room 3C-127, Salt Lake City, UT 84132 · 801-585-3251

Hani S. Matloub · Associate Professor of Plastic Surgery, Medical College of Wisconsin · Director of Microsurgery and Hand Surgery, Froedtert Memorial Lutheran Hospital · 9200 West Wisconsin Avenue, Milwaukee, WI 53226 · 414-454-5446

James Baptiste Steichen · Clinical Professor of Orthopaedic Surgery, Indiana University Medical Center · Surgeon-in-Chief, St. Vincent Hospital & Health Care Center · 8501 Harcourt Road, P.O. Box 80434, Indianapolis, IN 46280-0434 317-875-9105

James R. Urbaniak · (Microvascular) · Virginia Flowers Baker Professor of Orthopaedic Surgery, and Chief, Division of Orthopaedic Surgery, Duke University School of Medicine · Duke University Medical Center · P.O. Box 2912, Duke University Medical Center, Durham, NC 27710 · 919-684-2476

Andrew J. Weiland · Professor of Surgery, Orthopaedic and Plastic, Cornell University Medical College · Surgeon-in-Chief, The Hospital for Special Surgery · 535 East 70th Street, New York, NY 10021 · 212-606-1575

Michael B. Wood · Professor of Orthopaedic Surgery, Mayo Medical School, and Mayo Graduate School of Medicine · St. Mary's Hospital · 200 First Street, SW, Rochester MN 55902 · 507-284-2511

PARALYTIC DISORDERS

Charles Hamlin · Assistant Clinical Professor of Orthopaedics, University of Colorado School of Medicine · Craig Rehabilitation Hospital · 850 East Harvard, Suite 405, Denver, CO 80210 · 303-744-7078

Vincent R. Hentz · Professor of Surgery, Stanford University School of Medicine Chief, Division of Hand Surgery, Stanford University Hospital · 520 Sand Hill Road, Clinic C, Stanford, CA 94304 · 415-723-5256

James H. House · (Tendon Transfer Reconstruction, Congenital) · Professor of Orthopaedic Surgery, University of Minnesota School of Medicine · University of Minnesota Hospital & Clinics · 420 Delaware Street SE, Box 190 UMHC, Minneapolis, MN 55455 · 612-625-1177

Charles Lindsey McDowell · Clinical Professor of Plastic & Orthopaedic Surgery, Virginia Commonwealth University, Medical College of Virginia · Retreat Hospital; Humana Hospital; St. Mary's Hospital · 2911 Grove Avenue, Richmond, VA 23221 · 804-257-7261

PEDIATRIC ORTHOPAEDIC SURGERY

Harold Michael Dick · (Musculoskeletal Tumor Surgery) · Professor and Chairman, Department of Orthopaedic Surgery, College of Physicians & Surgeons of Columbia University · Director, Orthopaedic Surgery, Columbia-Presbyterian Medical Center · 161 Fort Washington Avenue, New York, NY 10032 · 212-305-5561

PERIPHERAL NERVE SURGERY
(See also Neurological Surgery, Peripheral Nerve Surgery; Orthopaedic Surgery, Peripheral Nerve Surgery; Plastic Surgery, Peripheral Nerve Surgery)

Edward E. Almquist · Clinical Professor, Department of Orthopaedics, University of Washington · Seattle Hand Surgery Group · 600 Broadway, Medical Center, Suite 440, Seattle, WA 98122 · 206-292-6252

Frank William Bora, Jr. · Professor of Orthopaedic Surgery, University of Pennsylvania School of Medicine · Chief, Hand Surgery, Hospital of the University of Pennsylvania · Penn Tower Hotel, 34th Street and Civic Center Boulevard, Eighth Floor, Philadelphia, PA 19104 · 215-662-6106

Richard M. Braun · Board Member, Rehabilitation Committee, Sharp Memorial Hospital; Chairman, Orthopaedic Department, Alvarado Hospital · 6699 Alvarado Road, Suite 2302, San Diego, CA 92120 · 619-287-4477

A. Lee Dellon · Associate Professor of Plastic Surgery, and Associate Professor of Neurosurgery, Johns Hopkins University School of Medicine · The Johns Hopkins Medical Institutions; Children's Hospital & Center for Reconstructive Surgery · 3901 Greenspring Avenue, Suite 104, Baltimore, MD 21211 · 301-225-0300

Richard H. Gelberman · Professor of Orthopaedic Surgery, Harvard Medical School · Chief, Hand Surgery Service, Department of Orthopaedic Surgery, Massachusetts General Hospital · 15 Parkman Street, WACC 527, Boston, MA 02114 617-726-2946

Michael E. Jabaley · Clinical Professor of Plastic & Orthopaedic Surgery, University of Mississippi · University of Mississippi Medical Center; St. Dominic Hospital; River Oaks Hospital · 971 Lakeland Drive, Suite 515, Jackson, MS 39216 · 601-981-2525

Joseph E. Kutz · Clinical Professor of Surgery (Hand), University of Louisville School of Medicine · Jewish Hospital · One Medical Center Plaza, 225 Abraham Flexner Way, Louisville, KY 40202 · 502-561-4263

Robert D. Leffert · (Thoracic Outlet Disorders) · Professor of Orthopaedic Surgery, Harvard Medical School · Chief, Surgical Upper Extremity Rehabilitation Unit, Massachusetts General Hospital · 32 Fruit Street, Boston, MA 02114 · 617-726-2954

George E. Omer · Professor Emeritus, the University of New Mexico School of Medicine · The University Hospital · University of New Mexico Medical Center, Department of Orthopaedics, Albuquerque, NM 87131-5296 · 505-272-4107

Morton Spinner · (Nerve Compression Lesions) · Clinical Professor of Orthopaedic Surgery, Albert Einstein College of Medicine · Consultant in Hand Surgery, Franklin Hospital Medical Center; North Shore University Hospital; Long Island Jewish Medical Center · 557 Central Avenue, Cedarhurst, NY 11516 · 516-569-6323

Jack W. Tupper · Clinical Professor of Orthopaedic Surgery, University of California at San Francisco School of Medicine · Director, Hand Clinic, Children's Hospital of the East Bay, Samuel Merritt Hospital · 2938 Webster Street, Oakland, CA 94609 · 510-893-9589

James R. Urbaniak · Virginia Flowers Baker Professor of Orthopaedic Surgery; and Chief, Division of Orthopaedic Surgery, Duke University School of Medicine Duke University Medical Center · P.O. Box 2912, Duke University Medical Center, Durham, NC 27710 · 919-684-2476

Allen L. Van Beek · Clinical Associate Professor of Surgery, University of Minnesota School of Medicine · North Memorial Medical Center; Fairview South Dale Hospital; Abbott Northwestern Hospital; Minneapolis Children's Medical Center · 7373 France Avenue South, Suite 510, Minneapolis, MN 55435 · 612-588-0593, 830-1028

E. F. Shaw Wilgis · (Vascular Disorders of the Hand) · Associate Professor of Plastic & Orthopaedic Surgery, Johns Hopkins University School of Medicine · Chief, Division of Hand Surgery, and Director, Raymond Curtis Hand Center, Union Memorial Hospital · 1400 Front Avenue, Suite 100, Lutherville, MD 21093 410-296-6232

Virchel E. Wood · Professor of Orthopaedic Surgery, Loma Linda University School of Medicine · Chief of Hand Surgery Service, Loma Linda University Medical Center · 11234 Anderson Street, Room A519, Loma Linda, CA 92350 · 714-824-4413

RECONSTRUCTIVE SURGERY
(See also Orthopaedic Surgery, Reconstructive Surgery; Plastic Surgery, Reconstructive Surgery)

Loui Garrett Bayne · (Congenital) · 960 Johnson Ferry Road NE, Suite 430, Atlanta, GA 30342 · 404-255-0226

Richard Irving Burton · (Thumb Reconstruction, Arthritis) · Professor, Department of Orthopaedics, University of Rochester School of Medicine and Dentistry Chairman, Department of Orthopaedics, Strong Memorial Hospital; University of Rochester Medical Center · 601 Elmwood Avenue, Rochester, NY 14642 · 716-275-5168

Richard G. Eaton · (Fingers & Thumb Reconstruction) · Professor of Clinical Surgery, College of Physicians & Surgeons of Columbia University · Director, Hand Surgery Center, St. Luke's-Roosevelt Hospital Center · 428 West 59th Street, New York, NY 10019 · 212-523-7590

Vincent R. Hentz · (Tendons, Paralytic Disorders) · Professor of Surgery, Stanford University School of Medicine · 520 Sand Hill Road, Clinic C, Palo Alto, CA 94304 · 415-723-5256

James H. House · (Tendon Transfer Reconstruction, Congenital) · Professor of Orthopaedic Surgery, University of Minnesota School of Medicine · University of Minnesota Hospital & Clinics · 420 Delaware Street SE, Box 190 UMHC, Minneapolis, MN 55455 · 612-625-1177

James M. Hunter · (Tendons) · Distinguished Professor of Orthopaedic Surgery, Jefferson Medical College of Thomas Jefferson University · Thomas Jefferson University Hospital · 901 Walnut Street, Philadelphia, PA 19107 · 215-629-0980

Jesse B. Jupiter · (Trauma) · Associate Professor of Orthopaedic Surgery, Harvard Medical School · Associate Orthopaedic Surgeon, Massachusetts General Hospital Five Whittier Place, Suite 102, Boston, MA 02114 · 617-726-5100

Terry Richard Light · (Congenital) · The Dr. William M. Scholl Professor and Chairman, Department of Orthopaedic Surgery, Loyola Stritch School of Medicine · Attending, Loyola University Medical Center · 2160 South First Avenue, Building 54, Room 167, Maywood, IL 60153 · 708-216-3834

Ronald Linscheid · (Wrist Problems) · Mayo Medical School · Mayo Clinic · 200 First Street, SW, Rochester, MN 55905 · 507-284-2511

Graham D. Lister · (Tendons, Congenital) · Professor and Chairman, Division of Plastic & Reconstructive Surgery, University of Utah School of Medicine · 50 North Medical Drive, Room 3C-127, Salt Lake City, UT 84132 · 801-585-3251

Dean S. Louis · Professor of Surgery, The University of Michigan Medical School Head, Orthopaedic Hand Service, The University of Michigan Medical Center · 2914 Taubman Center, 1500 East Medical Center Drive, Box 0328, Ann Arbor, MI 48109-0328 · 313-936-5200

Paul R. Manske · (Tendons, Congenital) · Chairman, Orthopaedic Surgery Department, Washington University School of Medicine · Barnes Hospital · One Barnes Hospital Plaza, Suite 11300, St. Louis, MO 63110 · 314-362-4080

Lewis H. Millender · (Arthritis) · Clinical Professor, Orthopaedic Surgery, Tufts University School of Medicine · Assistant Chief, Hand Surgical Section, New England Baptist Hospital · 125 Parker Hill Avenue, Suite 540, Boston, MA 02120 617-738-0857

Edward A. Nalebuff · (Arthritis) · Clinical Professor of Orthopaedic Surgery, and Chief, Hand Surgical Section, New England Baptist Hospital · 125 Parker Hill Avenue, Suite 540, Boston, MA 02120 · 617-738-0857

Alan E. Seyfer · (Rheumatoid Arthritis) · Professor of Surgery, and Head of Plastic Surgery, Oregon Health Sciences University · 3181 Southwest Sam Jackson Park Road, L352A, Portland, OR 97201-3098 · 503-494-7824

David John Smith, Jr. · (Burn Reconstruction) · Associate Professor of Surgery, and Section Head, Plastic & Reconstructive Surgery, The University of Michigan Medical School · The University of Michigan Medical Center · 1500 East Medical Center Drive, Taubman Center, Room 2130, Ann Arbor, MI 48109-0340 · 313-936-8925

James W. Strickland · (Tendon Work, Rheumatoid Arthritis) · Clinical Professor of Orthopaedic Surgery, Indiana University School of Medicine · Chief, Section of Hand Surgery, St. Vincent Hospital & Health Care Center · 8501 Harcourt Road, P.O. Box 80434, Indianapolis, IN 46280-0434 · 317-875-9105

Julio Taleisnik · (Wrist Problems, Arthritis) · Clinical Professor of Orthopaedic Surgery, University of California at Irvine School of Medicine · Consultant, Hand Surgery Service, University of California at Irvine Medical Center · 1201 West Laveta, Suite 501, Orange, CA 92668 · 714-835-4881

James R. Urbaniak · Virginia Flowers Baker Professor of Orthopaedic Surgery; and Chief, Division of Orthopaedic Surgery, Duke University School of Medicine Duke University Medical Center · P.O. Box 2912, Duke University Medical Center, Durham, NC 27710 · 919-684-2476

H. Kirk Watson · (Wrist Reconstruction) · Associate Clinical Professor, University of Connecticut; Associate Professor of Orthopaedics & Surgery, University of Massachusetts Medical Center; Assistant Clinical Professor of Orthopaedics &

Rehabilitation & Surgery (Plastic), Yale Medical School · Director, Connecticut Combined Hand Surgery Service (Hartford); Chief, Hand Service, Newington Children's Hospital; Senior Staff, Hartford Hospital · 85 Seymour Street, Suite 816, Hartford, CT 06106 · 203-527-7161

Paul M. Weeks · Professor of Surgery (Plastic & Reconstructive), Washington University School of Medicine · Chief, Division of Plastic Surgery, Barnes Hospital; St. Louis Children's Hospital · One Barnes Hospital Plaza, Suite 17424, St. Louis, MO 63110 · 314-362-4593

Andrew J. Weiland · Professor of Surgery, Orthopaedic and Plastic, Cornell University Medical College · Surgeon-in-Chief, The Hospital for Special Surgery · 535 East 70th Street, New York, NY 10021 · 212-606-1575

Michael B. Wood · Professor of Orthopaedic Surgery, Mayo Medical School, and Mayo Graduate School of Medicine · St. Mary's Hospital · 200 First Street, SW, Rochester MN 55902 · 507-284-2511

Virchel E. Wood · (Thoracic Outlet Disorders, Congenital Anomalies) · Professor of Orthopaedic Surgery, Loma Linda University School of Medicine · Chief of Hand Surgery Service, Loma Linda University Medical Center · 11234 Anderson Street, Room A519, Loma Linda, CA 92350 · 714-824-4413

INFECTIOUS DISEASE

AIDS
(See also Child Neurology, AIDS; Medical Oncology & Hematology, AIDS; Pulmonary & Critical Care Medicine, AIDS)

Donald Armstrong · Chief, Infectious Disease Service, Memorial Sloan-Kettering Cancer Center · 1275 York Avenue, New York, NY 10021 · 212-639-7809

John G. Bartlett · Professor of Medicine, Johns Hopkins University School of Medicine · Chief, Division of Infectious Disease, The Johns Hopkins Medical Institutions · Johns Hopkins Hospital, 600 North Wolfe Street, Blalock Building, Room 1111, Baltimore, MD 21205 · 410-955-3150

Deborah J. Cotton · Assistant Professor of Medicine, Harvard Medical School · Infectious Diseases Division, Beth Israel Hospital · 330 Brookline Avenue, Da-617, Boston, MA 02215 · 617-735-3661

Donald Edward Craven · Professor of Medicine & Microbiology, Boston University School of Medicine; Professor of Epidemiology and Biostatistics, Boston University School of Public Health · Boston City Hospital · Boston, MA 02118 · 617-534-4800

Anthony Stephen Fauci · Director, National Institute of Allergy & Infectious Diseases, National Institutes of Health · 9000 Rockville Pike, Building 31,7A-O3, Bethesda, MD 20892 · 301-496-2263

Gerald H. Friedland · Professor of Medicine & Epidemiology & Public Health, and Director, Yale AIDS Program, Yale University School of Medicine · Yale-New Haven Hospital · 20 York Street, 3C Welch Center, New Haven, CT 06504 · 203-737-2450

Michael S. Gottlieb · (Adult AIDS) · Assistant Clinical Professor of Internal Medicine, University of California at Los Angeles School of Medicine · Medical Director of the Immune Suppressed Unit at, Sherman Oaks Community Hospital 4955 Van Nuys Boulevard, Suite 715, Sherman Oaks, CA 91403 · 818-501-2600

Martin S. Hirsch · Professor of Medicine, Harvard Medical School · Physician, Massachusetts General Hospital · Infectious Disease Unit, Gray Five, Fruit Street, Boston, MA 02114 · 617-726-3815

King K. Holmes · Director, University of Washington Center for AIDS & STDs, University of Washington School of Medicine · Harborview Medical Center · 1001 Broadway, Suite 215, Seattle, WA 98122 · 206-720-4239

Benjamin J. Luft · (Toxoplasmic Encephalitis in AIDS Patients) · Associate Professor of Medicine, State University of New York at Stony Brook · SUNY at Stony Brook Hospital · Department of Medicine, Division of Infectious Diseases, HSC, Tower 15, Room 080, Stony Brook, NY 11794-8153 · 516-444-1660

Henry Masur · Chief, Critical Care Medicine Department, National Institutes of Health · 9000 Rockville Pike, Building 10, Room 7D43, Bethesda, MD 20892 · 301-496-9565

John Mills · Professor of Medicine, Microbiology and Laboratory Medicine, University of California at San Francisco School of Medicine · Chief, Infectious Diseases, San Francisco General Hospital · 995 Potrero Avenue, San Francisco, CA 94110 · 415-821-8666

John P. Phair · Section Chief, Infectious Disease, Northwestern University Medical School · Director, Comprehensive AIDS Center, Northwestern Memorial Hospital, HIV Center · 680 North Lakeshore Drive, Suite 1106, Chicago, IL 60611 · 312-908-8196

Thomas C. Quinn · Associate Professor of Medicine and International Health, Johns Hopkins University School of Medicine · Senior Investigator, Laboratory of Immunoregulation, National Institute of Allergy & Infectious Diseases; Head of International AIDS Research, National Institutes of Health · Blalock Building, 600 North Wolfe Street, Room 1111, Baltimore, MD 21205 · 410-955-7635

Jack Remington · (CNS Infections of AIDS, Toxoplasmic Encephalitis in AIDS Patients) · Professor of Medicine, Division of Infectious Disease, Stanford University School of Medicine · Marcus A. Krupp Research Chair, and Chairman, Department of Immunology & Infectious Diseases Research Institute, Palo Alto Medical Foundation · 860 Bryant Street, Palo Alto, CA 94301 · 415-853-4832

Douglas D. Richman · Professor of Pathology and Medicine, University of California, San Diego School of Medicine · Chief, Virology Section, and Director, Research Center for AIDS and HIV Infection, San Diego Veterans Affairs Medical Center · 3350 La Jolla Village Drive, 111F, San Diego, CA 92161 · 619-552-7439

Merle A. Sande · (Upper Respiratory Tract Infections) · Professor and Vice-Chairman of Medicine, University of California at San Francisco School of Medicine · Chief, Medical Service, San Francisco General Hospital · 1001 Potrero Avenue, Room 5H22, San Francisco, CA 94110 · 415-476-4520

Robert Yarchoan · Chief, Retroviral Diseases Section, Medicine Branch, National Cancer Institute, National Institutes of Health · National Institutes of Health Clinical Center · 9000 Rockville Pike, Building 10, 13N248, Bethesda, MD 20892 · 301-496-0328

ANAEROBIC INFECTIONS

John G. Bartlett · Professor of Medicine, Johns Hopkins University School of Medicine · Chief, Division of Infectious Disease, The Johns Hopkins Medical Institutions · Johns Hopkins Hospital, 600 North Wolfe Street, Blalock Building, Room 1111, Baltimore, MD 21205 · 410-955-3150

Sydney M. Finegold · Professor of Medicine, University of California at Los Angeles School of Medicine · Associate Chief of Staff/Research & Development, Wadsworth Veterans Affairs Medical Center · Wilshire and Sawtelle Boulevards, Los Angeles, CA 90073 · 213-824-4328

Ellie J. C. Goldstein · Clinical Professor of Medicine, University of California at Los Angeles School of Medicine · Director, R.M. Alden Research Laboratory, Santa Monica Hospital Medical Center; Chief, Infectious Diseases Section, St. John's Hospital & Health Center of Santa Monica · 2021 Santa Monica Boulevard, Suite 640 East, Santa Monica, CA 90404 · 310-315-1511

Sherwood L. Gorbach · Professor of Community Health and Medicine, Tufts University School of Medicine · New England Medical Center · Arnold 205 Building, 136 Harrison Avenue, Boston, MA 02111 · 617-956-5811

ANTIOBIOTIC PHARMACOLOGY

William A. Craig · Professor of Medicine & Pharmaceutics, University of Wisconsin-Madison School of Medicine · Chief, Infectious Diseases, William S. Middleton Memorial Veterans Hospital · 2500 Overlook Terrace, Madison, WI 53705 608-262-7020

Harold C. Neu · Professor of Medicine & Pharmacology, College of Physicians & Surgeons of Columbia University · Attending Physician and Hospital Epidemiologist, Columbia-Presbyterian Medical Center · 630 West 168th Street, New York, NY 10032 · 212-305-3395

BONE INFECTIONS

Layne O. Gentry · Clinical Professor of Immunology, Baylor College of Medicine St. Luke's Episcopal Hospital · 6720 Bertner Avenue, Box 233, Houston, TX 77030 · 713-794-6198

CANCER & INFECTIONS

Donald Armstrong · Chief, Infectious Disease Service, Memorial Sloan-Kettering Cancer Center · 1275 York Avenue, New York, NY 10021 · 212-639-7809

Gerald P. Bodey · Professor of Medicine, The University of Texas · Chairman, Department of Medical Specialties; Chief, Section of Infectious Diseases, The University of Texas MD Anderson Cancer Center · 1515 Holcombe Boulevard, Department of Medical Specialties/47), Houston, TX 77030 · 713-792-6830

Joel D. Meyers · (Bone Marrow Tranplantations) · Professor of Medicine, University of Washington School of Medicine · Member and Head, Program in Infectious Diseases, Fred Hutchinson Cancer Research Center · 1124 Columbia Street, Seattle, WA 98104 · 206-667-4338

James C. Wade · (Medical Oncology) · Professor of Medicine & Oncology, University of Maryland School of Medicine · Head, Section of Infectious Diseases & Microbiology, University of Maryland Cancer Center · 22 South Greene Street, Baltimore, MD 21201 · 301-328-7823

Thomas John Walsh · Associate Professor of Medicine, University of Maryland School of Medicine · Senior Investigator, Section of Infectious Diseases, Pediatric Branch, National Cancer Institute · 9000 Rockville Pike, Building 10, Room 13N240, Bethesda, MD 20892 · 301-402-0023

DIARRHEA

Herbert L. DuPont · Mary W. Kelsey Professor and Director, Center for Infectious Diseases, The University of Texas Medical School at Houston/School of Public Health · Hermann Hospital; Lyndon B. Johnson General Hospital · John Freeman Building, 6431 Fannin Street, Room 1.729, Houston, TX 77030 · 713-794-4254

Robert Fekety, Jr. · Professor of Internal Medicine, The University of Michigan Medical School · Chief, Division of Infectious Diseases, Department of Internal Medicine, The University of Michigan Hospitals · 3116 Taubman Center, 1500 East Medical Center Drive, Ann Arbor, MI 48109-0378 · 313-936-5205

Sherwood L. Gorbach · Professor of Community Health and Medicine, Tufts University School of Medicine · New England Medical Center · Arnold 205 Building, 136 Harrison Avenue, Boston, MA 02111 · 617-956-5811

ENDOCARDITIS

William Ernest Dismukes · Professor and Vice-Chairman for Educational Programs and Director, Division of Infectious Diseases, The University of Alabama School of Medicine · Director, Medicine House Staff, and Attending Physician, The University of Alabama Hospital · 1900 University Boulevard, Tinsley Harrison Tower, Suite 229, Birmingham, AL 35294 · 205-934-2186

David T. Durack · Professor of Medicine, Microbiology and Immunology, Duke University School of Medicine · Chief, Division of Infectious Disease & International Health, Duke University Medical Center · P.O. Box 3876, Durham, NC 27710 · 919-684-2660

Adolf W. Karchmer · Associate Professor of Medicine, Harvard Medical School · Chief, Division of Infectious Diseases, New England Deaconess Hospital · Kennedy Building, 185 Pilgrim Road, Sixth Floor, Boston, MA 02215 · 617-735-0760

Merle A. Sande · Professor and Vice-Chairman of Medicine, University of California at San Francisco School of Medicine · Chief, Medical Service, San Francisco General Hospital · 1001 Potrero Avenue, Room 5H22, San Francisco, CA 94110 · 415-476-4520

Walter R. Wilson · Professor of Medicine, Mayo Medical School · Mayo Clinic · 200 First Street, SW, Rochester, MN 55905 · 507-284-2916

FUNGAL INFECTIONS

John Eugene Bennett · Professor of Medicine, Uniformed Services University of Health Sciences · Clinical Center, National Institutes of Health · Bethesda, MD 20892 · 301-496-3461

William Ernest Dismukes · Professor and Vice-Chairman for Educational Programs and Director, Division of Infectious Diseases, The University of Alabama School of Medicine · Director, Medicine House Staff, and Attending Physician, The University of Alabama Hospital · 1900 University Boulevard, Tinsley Harrison Tower, Suite 229, Birmingham, AL 35294 · 205-934-2186

John E. Edwards, Jr. · Professor of Medicine, University of California at Los Angeles School of Medicine · Chief of Infectious Diseases, Harbor-UCLA Medical Center · 1000 West Carson Street, Building E-5, Torrance, CA 90509 · 213-533-3813

GENERAL INFECTIOUS DISEASE

Vincent T. Andriole · Professor of Medicine, Yale University School of Medicine Attending Physician, Yale-New Haven Hospital · 333 Cedar Street, 201LCI, New Haven, CT 06510 · 203-785-4141

Gordon L. Archer · Professor of Medicine and Microbiology & Immunology, Virginia Commonwealth University, Medical College of Virginia · Medical College of Virginia Hospital · 1101 East Marshall Street, Room 7076, Richmond, VA 23298 · 804-786-9711

Arnold S. Bayer · Professor of Medicine, University of California at Los Angeles School of Medicine · Associate Chief, Division of Infectious Diseases, Harbor-UCLA Medical Center · 1000 West Carson Street, Building E-5, Los Angeles, CA 90509 · 213-533-3815

C. Glenn Cobbs · Professor of Medicine, The University of Alabama School of Medicine · Chief, Medical Service, The Department of Veterans Affairs Medical Center-Birmingham · 700 South 19th Street (111), Birmingham, AL 35233 · 205-934-9089

Robert Fekety, Jr. · Professor of Internal Medicine, The University of Michigan Medical School · Chief, Division of Infectious Diseases, Department of Internal Medicine, The University of Michigan Hospitals · 3116 Taubman Center, 1500 East Medical Center Drive, Ann Arbor, MI 48109-0378 · 313-936-5205

Dale Nicholas Gerding · Professor of Medicine, Laboratory Medicine, & Pathology, University of Minnesota School of Medicine · Chief, Infectious Disease Section, Minneapolis Veterans Affairs Medical Center · One Veterans Drive, Infectious Disease-111F, Minneapolis, MN 55417 · 612-725-2000 x4185

Richard H. Glew · Chairperson of Department of Medicine, Medical Center of Central Massachusetts, The Medical Center of Central Massachusetts · The Med Center—Memorial, 119 Belmont Street, Worcester, MA 01605-2982 · 508-793-6256

W. Lee Hand · Professor of Medicine and Director, Division of Infectious Diseases, Emory University School of Medicine · Chief, Infectious Diseases, Grady Memorial Hospital; Emory University Affiliated Hospitals · Division of Infectious Diseases, 69 Butler Street, SE, Atlanta, GA 30303 · 404-616-3600

William J. Holloway · Clinical Professor of Medicine, Jefferson Medical College of Thomas Jefferson University · Director, Infectious Disease Research Laboratory, Medical Center of Delaware · 501 West 14th Street, Wilmington, DE 19899 302-428-2744

Donald Kaye · Chairman & Professor of Medicine, Medical College of Pennsylvania · Chief of Medicine, Hospital of the Medical College of Pennsylvania; Consultant, Veterans Affairs Medical Center, Philadelphia · 3300 Henry Avenue, Philadelphia, PA 19129 · 215-842-6950

Gerald L. Mandell · Professor of Medicine, Owen R. Cheatham Professor of the Sciences, and Head, Division of Infectious Diseases, University of Virginia School of Medicine · University of Virginia Health Sciences Center · Box 385 University of Virginia Medical Center, Charlottesville, VA 22908 · 804-924-5942

Robert C. Moellering, Jr. · Shields Warren—Mallinckrodt Professor of Medical Research, Harvard Medical School · Physician-in-Chief, New England Deaconess Hospital · Suite 6A, Department of Medicine, 185 Pilgrim Road, Boston, MA 02215 · 617-732-8586

George A. Pankey · Clinical Professor of Medicine, Louisiana State University School of Medicine; Tulane University School of Medicine · Head, Section of Infectious Diseases, Ochsner Clinic; Ochsner Foundation Hospital · Section on Infectious Diseases, 1514 Jefferson Highway, New Orleans, LA 70121 · 504-842-4005

Charles V. Sanders · Edgar Hull Professor and Chairman, Department of Medicine, Louisiana State University School of Medicine · Charity Hospital at New Orleans; Hotel Dieu Hospital · 1542 Tulane Avenue, New Orleans, LA 70112 · 504-568-5036

W. Michael Scheld · Professor of Medicine and Neurosurgery, University of Virginia School of Medicine · Associate Chair, Residency Programs, University of Virginia Health Sciences Center · University of Virginia Health Sciences Center, Box 385, Charlottesville, VA 22908 · 804-924-5241

H. Grant Stiver · Associate Professor of Medicine, The University of British Columbia · Assistant Head, Divison of Infectious Disease, Vancouver General Hospital · 2733 Heather Street, Heather Pavilion, Room 452 D, Vancouver, British Columbia V5Z 3J5 · 604-875-4588

Morton N. Swartz · Professor of Medicine, Harvard Medical School · Chief of the James Jackson Firm, Massachusetts General Hospital · Infectious Disease Unit, Massachusetts General Hospital, Boston, MA 02114 · 617-726-3811

George F. Thornton · Clinical Professor of Medicine, Yale University School of Medicine, and University of Connecticut School of Medicine · Director, Division of Medicine, Waterbury Hospital · 64 Robbins Street, Waterbury, CT 06721 · 203-573-7228

Marvin Turck · Professor of Medicine, University of Washington School of Medicine · University of Washington Medical Center; Harborview Medical Center · 1910 Fairview Avenue E, Suite 210, Seattle, WA 98102 · 206-543-3660

Robert Van Scoy · Mayo Clinic · 200 First Street, SW, Rochester, MN 55905 · 507-284-3309

HERPES VIRUS INFECTIONS
(See also Dermatology, Herpes Virus Infections)

Lawrence Corey · (Viral Sexually Transmitted Disease, AIDS) · Professor, Laboratory Medicine and Medicine, University of Washington School of Medicine · Pacific Medical Center · 1200 Twelth Avenue South, Ninth Floor, Seattle, WA 98144 · 206-326-4177

Clyde S. Crumpacker · Associate Professor of Medicine, Harvard Medical School Physician, Beth Israel Hospital · 330 Brookline Avenue, Boston, MA 02215 · 617-735-3661

John M. Douglas · Assistant Professor of Medicine, University of Colorado School of Medicine · Assistant Director, Disease Control Services, Denver General Hospital · 605 Bannock Street, Mail Code 2600, Denver, CO 80204 · 303-893-7051

Gregory J. Mertz · Associate Professor, Department of Medicine, The University of New Mexico School of Medicine · The University Hospital · Department of Medicine, HHSB301, Box 608, Albuquerque, NM 87131-5271 · 505-277-8207

Stephen E. Straus · Chief, Laboratory of Clinical Investigation, National Institutes of Health · 9000 Rockville Pike, Building 10, Room 11N-228, Bethesda, MD 20892 · 301-496-5221

HOSPITAL-ACQUIRED INFECTIONS

John P. Burke · Professor, Department of Internal Medicine, University of Utah School of Medicine · Chief, Division of Infectious Diseases, Latter Day Saints Hospital · Eighth Avenue and C Street, Salt Lake City, UT 84143 · 801-321-1006

Donald Edward Craven · Professor of Medicine & Microbiology, Boston University School of Medicine; Professor of Epidemiology and Biostatistics, Boston University School of Public Health · Boston City Hospital · Boston, MA 02118 · 617-534-4800

Richard E. Dixon · Associate Professor of Medicine, Hahnemann University · Medical Director, and Hospital Epidemiologist, Helene Fuld Medical Center · 750 Brunswick Avenue, Trenton, NJ 08638 · 609-394-6208

Richard A. Garibaldi · Professor of Medicine, University of Connecticut School of Medicine · Hospital Epidemiologist, and Vice Chairman, Department of Medicine, John Dempsey Hospital · 263 Farmington Avenue, Room LG004, Farmington, CT 06030 · 203-679-3553

Allen B. Kaiser · Associate Professor of Medicine, Vanderbilt University School of Medicine · D3100 Medical Center North, Nashville, TN 37232-2358 · 615-343-6821

Calvin M. Kunin · Professor of Internal Medicine, Ohio State University College of Medicine · The Ohio State University Hospitals · 320 West 10th, M 110 Starling Loving Hall, Columbus, OH 43210 · 614-293-8976

F. Marc LaForce · Professor of Medicine, University of Rochester School of Medicine & Dentistry · Physician-in-Chief, Department of Medicine, The Genesee Hospital · 224 Alexander Street, Rochester, NY 14607 · 716-263-2236

Dennis G. Maki · (Critical Care Medicine, Nosocomial Infections) · Professor of Medicine, University of Wisconsin-Madison School of Medicine · Head, Section of Infectious Disease, University of Wisconsin Health Center · 600 Highland Avenue, H4-574, Madison WI 53792 · 608-263-1545

C. Glen Mayhall · Professor of Medicine, The University of Tennessee at Memphis, College of Medicine · Hospital Epidemiologist, Regional Medical Center at Memphis; University of Tennessee Bowld Hospital · 956 Court Avenue, Room H-308, Memphis, TN 38163 · 901-528-5770

John E. McGowan, Jr. · (Medical Microbiology) · Professor of Pathology & Medicine, Emory University School of Medicine · Grady Memorial Hospital · 80 Butler Street, SE, Box 26248, Atlanta, GA 30335 · 404-616-3431

Frank S. Rhame · Associate Professor of Medicine, University of Minnesota School of Medicine · University of Minnesota Hospital & Clinics · 420 Delaware Street SE, Box 421, Minneapolis, MN 55455 · 612-626-5036

Louis D. Saravolatz · (Legionnaires' Disease) · Clinical Professor of Medicine, The University of Michigan Medical School · Division Head, Infectious Diseases, Henry Ford Medical Center · 2799 West Grand Boulevard, CFP 104, Detroit, MI 48202 · 313-876-2573

William Schaffner · Professor and Chairman, Department of Preventive Medicine, Vanderbilt University School of Medicine · Vanderbilt University Medical Center · A1124 Medical Center North, Nashville, TN 37232-2637 · 615-322-2037

William E. Scheckler · (Hospital Epidemiology) · Professor of Family Medicine & Practice, and Professor of Medicine, University of Wisconsin-Madison School of Medicine · University of Wisconsin Hospital & Clinics · 777 South Mills Street, Madison, WI 53715 · 608-263-4550

Timothy R. Townsend · Associate Professor of Pediatrics, Johns Hopkins University School of Medicine · Senior Director of Medical Affairs, The Johns Hopkins Medical Institutions · 600 North Wolfe Street, Administration 125B, Baltimore, MD 21205 · 410-955-0620

Richard P. Wenzel · (Assessing Quality Health Care) · Professor and Director, Division of General Medicine, Clinical Epidemiology, and Health Services Research, Department of Internal Medicine, The University of Iowa College of Medicine · The University of Iowa Hospitals & Clinics · General Hospital, Room C-41, Iowa City, IA 52242 · 319-356-1838

LYME DISEASE

Benjamin J. Luft · Associate Professor of Medicine, State University of New York at Stony Brook · SUNY at Stony Brook Hospital · Department of Medicine, Division of Infectious Diseases, HSC, Tower 15, Room 080, Stony Brook, NY 11794-8153 · 516-444-1660

PEDIATRIC INFECTIOUS DISEASE
(See also Pediatrics, Pediatric Infectious Disease)

Marian E. Melish · (Kawasaki Disease) · Professor of Pediatrics, Tropical Medicine and Medical Microbiology, John A. Burns School of Medicine, University of Hawaii · Kapiolani Medical Center · 1319 Punahou Street, Honolulu, HI 96826 · 808-973-8387

RESPIRATORY INFECTIONS
(See also Pulmonary & Critical Care Medicine, Lung Infections)

Thomas R. Cate · Professor of Medicine & Microbiology & Immunology, Baylor College of Medicine · Chief, Infectious Disease Service, and Director, Thomas Street Clinic, Ben Taub General Hospital · Influenza Research Center, One Baylor Plaza, Houston, TX 77030-2397 · 713-798-4469

SEXUALLY TRANSMITTED DISEASE

William R. Bowie · Professor of Medicine, Faculty of Medicine, The University of British Columbia · Vancouver General Hospital · 2733 Heather Street, D Floor, Room 425, Vancouver, British Columbia V5Z 3J5 · 604-875-4147

Robert C. Brunham · Professor and Head, Department of Medical Microbiology, University of Manitoba School of Medicine · Health Sciences Center · 730 William Avenue, Room 543, Winnipeg, Manitoba R3E OW3 · 204-788-6524

Lawrence Corey · (Viral Sexually Transmitted Disease, AIDS) · Professor, Laboratory Medicine and Medicine, University of Washington School of Medicine · Pacific Medical Center · 1200 Twelth Avenue South, Ninth Floor, Seattle, WA 98144 · 206-326-4177

John M. Douglas · Assistant Professor of Medicine, University of Colorado School of Medicine · Assistant Director, Disease Control Services, Denver General Hospital · 605 Bannock Street, Mail Code 2600, Denver, CO 80204 · 303-893-7051

H. Hunter Handsfield · Professor of Medicine, University of Washington School of Medicine; Director, STD Control Program, Seattle-King County Department of Public Health · Harvorview Medical Center · 325 Ninth Avenue (ZA-89), Seattle, WA 98104 · 206-223-5899

King K. Holmes · Director, University of Washington Center for AIDS & STDs, University of Washington School of Medicine · Harborview Medical Center · 1001 Broadway, Suite 215, Seattle, WA 98122 · 206-720-4239

Edward W. Hook III · Associate Professor of Medicine, Johns Hopkins University School of Medicine · Chief, Clinical Sexually Transmitted Disease Services, Baltimore City Health Department, The Johns Hopkins Medical Institutions · 600 North Wolfe Street, Blalock 1111, Baltimore, MD 21205 · 410-955-3150

Franklyn N. Judson · Professor, Department of Medicine & Preventive Medicine, University of Colorado School of Medicine · Chief, Infectious Diseases, Denver General Hospital · 605 Bannock Street, Mail Code 2600, Denver, CO 80204 · 303-893-7051

David H. Martin · Professor of Medicine, Louisiana State University School of Medicine · Charity Hospital of New Orleans · 1542 Tulane Avenue, New Orleans, LA 70112 · 504-568-5031

William M. McCormack · Professor of Medicine and Obstetrics & Gynecology, and Chief, Infectious Diseases Division, State University of New York Health Science Center at Brooklyn · 450 Clarkson Avenue, Brooklyn, NY 11203 · 718-270-1432

Michael F. Rein · Professor of Internal Medicine, Division of Infectious Diseases, University of Virginia School of Medicine · Attending Physician, University of Virginia Health Sciences Center · Jefferson Park Avenue, Box 385, Charlottesville, VA 22908 · 804-924-9668

Allan Ronald · Distinguished Professor of Medicine & Medical Microbiology, University of Manitoba School of Medicine · Head, Microbiology, St. Boniface General Hospital · 409 Tache Avenue, Winnipeg, Manitoba R2H 2A6 · 204-237-2927

Jack D. Sobel · Professor of Medicine, Immunology, Microbiology, and Obstetrics & Gynecology, and Chief, Division of Infectious Diseases, Wayne State University School of Medicine · Chief of Infectious Diseases, Detroit Medical Center-Harper Hospital · Harper Professional Building, Suite 202, 4160 John R Street, Detroit, MI 48201 · 313-745-7104

Walter E. Stamm · Professor of Medicine, University of Washington School of Medicine · Head, Infectious Disease Division, Harborview Medical Center · 325 Ninth Avenue (ZA-89), Seattle, WA 98104 · 206-223-8493

Sumner Edward Thompson III · Professor of Medicine, Emory University School of Medicine · Medical Director, Infectious Disease Clinic, Grady Memorial Hospital · Infectious Disease Clinic, 69 Butler Street SE, Atlanta, GA 30303 · 404-616-2444

Thomas C. Quinn · Associate Professor of Medicine and International Health, Johns Hopkins University School of Medicine · Senior Investigator, Laboratory of Immunoregulation, National Institute of Allergy & Infectious Diseases; Head of International AIDS Research, National Institutes of Health · Blalock Building, 600 North Wolfe Street, Room 1111, Baltimore, MD 21205 · 410-955-7635

TOXOPLASMOSIS

Rima Linnea McLeod · (Congenital Toxoplasmosis) · Professor of Medicine, Immunology & Microbiology, University of Illinois at Chicago College of Medicine; Lecturer in Medicine and The Committee on Immunology, Pritzker School of Medicine, The University of Chicago · Attending Physician, Humana Hospital,

Michael Reese Hospital · 2929 South Ellis, Room 114 Baum, Chicago, IL 60616
312-791-4152

Jack Remington · (Congenital Toxoplasmosis, Toxoplasmic Encephalitis in AIDS Patients) · Professor of Medicine, Division of Infectious Disease, Stanford University School of Medicine · Marcus A. Krupp Research Chair, and Chairman, Department of Immunology & Infectious Diseases Research Institute, Palo Alto Medical Foundation · 860 Bryant Street, Palo Alto, CA 94301 · 415-853-4832

TRANSPLANTATION INFECTIONS

Monto Ho · (Medical Virology) · Professor of Medicine & Chief, Division of Infectious Diseases, University of Pittsburgh School of Medicine; Chairman & Professor, Department of Infectious Diseases & Microbiology, Graduate School of Public Health, University of Pittsburgh · Chief of Infectious Diseases, and Director of Clinical Microbiology, Presbyterian University Hospital · A 427 Crabtree Hall, Pittsburgh, PA 15261 · 412-624-3092

Joel D. Meyers · (Bone Marrow Tranplantations) · Professor of Medicine, University of Washington School of Medicine · Member and Head, Program in Infectious Diseases, Fred Hutchinson Cancer Research Center · 1124 Columbia Street, Seattle, WA 98104 · 206-667-4338

Jack Remington · Professor of Medicine, Division of Infectious Disease, Stanford University School of Medicine · Marcus A. Krupp Research Chair, and Chairman, Department of Immunology & Infectious Diseases Research Institute, Palo Alto Medical Foundation · 860 Bryant Street, Palo Alto, CA 94301 · 415-853-4832

Robert H. Rubin · Harvard Medical School · Chief of Infectious Disease for Transplantation, Massachusetts General Hospital · 55 Fruit Street, Gray-1, Boston, MA 02114 · 617-726-3706

Lowell S. Young · Clinical Professor of Medicine, University of California at San Francisco School of Medicine · Chief, Division of Infectious Diseases, and Director of the Kuzell Institute for Arthritis & Infectious Diseases of the Medical Research Institute of San Francisco, California Pacific Medical Center · 2200 Webster Street, Room 305, San Francisco, CA 94115 · 415-923-3262

TROPICAL DISEASES

Bruce M. Greene · (Travel Medicine) · Professor of Medicine and Director, Division of Geographic Medicine, The University of Alabama School of Medicine Attending Physician and Consultant, University of Alabama Hospital; Birmingham Veterans Affairs Hospital; Cooper-Green Hospital; Kirklin Clinic · Department of Medicine, University of Alabama, Birmingham, AL 35294 · 205-934-1630

Warren D. Johnson · B. H. Kean Professor of Tropical Medicine, and Chief of International Medicine, Cornell University Medical College · The New York Hospital-Cornell Medical Center · 1300 York Avenue, Rom A-431, New York, NY 10021 · 212-746-6306

Adel A. F. Mahmoud · Chairman, Department of Medicine, and The John H. Hord Professor of Medicine, Case Western Reserve University School of Medicine Physician-in-Chief, University Hospitals of Cleveland · 2074 Abington Road, Cleveland, OH 44106 · 216-844-3293

URINARY TRACT INFECTIONS
(See also Urology, Urologic Infections)

Donald Kaye · Chairman & Professor of Medicine, Medical College of Pennsylvania · Chief of Medicine, Hospital of the Medical College of Pennsylvania; Consultant, Veterans Affairs Medical Center, Philadelphia · 3300 Henry Avenue, Philadelphia, PA 19129 · 215-842-6950

Calvin M. Kunin · Professor of Internal Medicine, Ohio State University College of Medicine · The Ohio State University Hospitals · 320 West 10th, M 110 Starling Loving Hall, Columbus, OH 43210 · 614-293-8976

VASCULITIS
(See also Rheumatology, Vasculitis)

Anthony Stephen Fauci · Director, National Institute of Allergy & Infectious Diseases, National Institutes of Health · 9000 Rockville Pike, Building 31,7A-O3, Bethesda, MD 20892 · 301-496-2263

VIROLOGY

Martin S. Hirsch · Professor of Medicine, Harvard Medical School · Physician, Massachusetts General Hospital · Infectious Disease Unit, Gray Five, Fruit Street, Boston, MA 02114 · 617-726-3815

Robert T. Schooley · Professor of Medicine, University of Colorado School of Medicine · Head, Division of Infectious Disease, University of Colorado Health Sciences Center · 4200 East Ninth Avenue, Box B-168, Denver, CO 80262 · 303-270-6753

MEDICAL ONCOLOGY

BONE MARROW TRANSPLANTATION
(See also Medical Oncology & Hematology, Bone Marrow Transplantation)

Richard Champlin · Chief, Section of Bone Marrow Transplantation, The University of Texas MD Anderson Cancer Center · 1515 Holcombe Boulevard, Houston, TX 77030 · 713-792-3611

Stephen J. Forman · Director, Department of Hematology & Bone Marrow Transplantation, City of Hope National Medical Center · 1500 East Duarte Road, Duarte, CA 91010-0269 · 818-359-8111

Geoffrey P. Herzig · Professor of Medicine, State University of New York Health Science Center at Buffalo · Chief, Divisions of Hematologic Oncology and Bone Marrow Transplantation, Roswell Park Cancer Institute · Elm & Carlton Streets, Buffalo, NY 14263 · 716-845-7610

William P. Vaughan · Professor of Medicine and Pharmacology, and Director, Marrow Transplantation Program, and Associate Director of Clinical Research, Comprehensive Cancer Center, The University of Alabama School of Medicine · The University of Alabama Hospital · 1900 University Boulevard, Birmingham, AL 35294 · 205-934-1908

BREAST CANCER
(See also Medical Oncology & Hematology, Breast Cancer; Radiation Oncology, Breast Cancer; Surgical Oncology, Breast Cancer)

John H. Glick · Director of University of Pennsylvania Cancer Center, and Professor of Medicine, University of Pennsylvania School of Medicine · University of Pennsylvania Cancer Center · 3400 Spruce Street, Six Penn Tower, Philadelphia PA 19104 · 215-662-6334

Charles M. Haskell · Professor of Medicine, University of California at Los Angeles School of Medicine · Director, Wadsworth Cancer Center; Chief, Hematology-Oncology Section, Veterans Affairs Medical Center, West Los Angeles · Wilshire and Sawtelle Boulevards, Los Angeles, CA 90073 · 310-824-6661

Gabriel N. Hortobagyi · Professor of Medicine, The University of Texas · Internist, Chief, Breast Medical Oncology, The University of Texas MD Anderson Cancer Center · 1515 Holcombe Boulevard, Houston, TX 77030 · 713-792-2817

James N. Ingle · Professor of Oncology, Mayo Medical School · Mayo Clinic · 200 First Street, SW, Rochester, MN 55905 · 507-284-4849

B. J. Kennedy · (Lymphoma, Cancer & Aging, Chemotherapy) · Regents' Professor of Medicine, Emeritus, and Masonic Professor of Oncology, Emeritus, University of Minnesota School of Medicine · University of Minnesota Hospital & Clinics · Harvard Street at East River Road, Box 286 UMHC, Minneapolis, MN 55455 · 612-624-9611

Kathleen Isabel Pritchard · Associate Professor of Medicine, University of Toronto School of Medicine · Head, Medical Oncology, Toronto Bayview Regional Cancer Center · 2075 Bayview Avenue, Toronto, Ontario M4N 3M5 · 416-480-4616

Sandra M. Swain · Assistant Professor of Medicine, Georgetown University School of Medicine · Director, Comprehensive Breast Center, Vincent T. Lombardi Cancer Research Center, Georgetown University Medical Center · Lombardi Cancer Research Center—Podium Level, 3800 Reservoir Road, NW, Washington, DC 20007 · 202-687-2198

Ian F. Tannock · Professor of Medicine, University of Toronto School of Medicine · Chief of Medicine, Princess Margaret Hospital · 500 Sherbourne Street, Toronto, Ontario M4X 1K9 · 416-924-0671

William P. Vaughan · Professor of Medicine and Pharmacology, and Director, Marrow Transplantation Program, and Associate Director of Clinical Research, Comprehensive Cancer Center, The University of Alabama School of Medicine · The University of Alabama Hospital · 1900 University Boulevard, Birmingham, AL 35294 · 205-934-1908

Charles L. Vogel · Clinical Professor of Oncology, University of Miami School of Medicine · Medical Director, South Florida Comprehensive Cancer Centers · 11750 Bird Road, Miami, FL 33175 · 305-227-5556

CLINICAL PHARMACOLOGY

Stephen B. Howell · Professor of Medicine, University of California at San Diego School of Medicine · Division of Hematology/Oncology, University of California at San Diego Medical Center · 220 West Dickinson Street, Room 339, San Diego, CA 92103 · 619-543-5530

Martin Newman Raber · (Clinical Trials) · Associate Professor of Medicine, The University of Texas MD Anderson Cancer Center · Director, Educational Programs, Division of Medicine; Director, Clinical Trials Administration; Deputy Head, Division of Medicine, The University of Texas MD Anderson Cancer Center · 1515 Holcombe Boulevard, Box 92, Houston, TX 77030 · 713-792-7765

Daniel D. Von Hoff · (New Drug Development) · Professor of Medicine and Head, Section of Drug Development, The University of Texas Health Science Center at San Antonio · Head, Research Department, Cancer Therapy Research Center · 7703 Floyd Curl Drive, San Antonio, TX 78284-7884 · 512-567-4747

GASTROINTESTINAL ONCOLOGY

Jaffer A. Ajani · Associate Professor of Medicine, The University of Texas · The University of Texas MD Anderson Cancer Center · 1515 Holcombe Boulevard, 78, Houston, TX 77030 · 713-792-2828

Daniel G. Haller · Associate Professor of Medicine, University of Pennsylvania School of Medicine · Hospital of the University of Pennsylvania · 3400 Spruce Street, Sixth Floor, Penn Tower, Philadelphia, PA 19104 · 215-662-6318

David P. Kelsen · Associate Professor of Medicine, Cornell University Medical College · Chief, Gastrointestinal Oncology Service, Memorial Sloan-Kettering Cancer Center · 1275 York Avenue, New York, NY 10021 · 212-639-8470

Nancy E. Kemeny · Gastrointestinal Oncology Service, Memorial Sloan-Kettering Cancer Center · 1275 York Avenue, New York, NY 10021 · 212-639-8068

Bernard Levin · Professor of Medicine, The University of Texas · The University of Texas MD Anderson Cancer Center · 1515 Holcombe Boulevard, Houston, TX 77030 · 713-792-2828

John S. Macdonald · Professor of Medicine and Chief, Division of Medical Oncology, Temple University School of Medicine · Medical Director, Temple University Comprehensive Cancer Center · 3322 North Broad Street, P.O. Box 38346, Philadelphia, PA 19140 · 215-221-8030

Robert J. Mayer · Associate Professor of Medicine, Harvard Medical School · Associate Physician, Dana-Farber Cancer Institute · 44 Binney Street, Boston, MA 02115 · 617-732-3474

Charles G. Moertel · (Neuroendocrine Tumors, Colon Cancer) · Professor of Oncology, Mayo Medical School · Mayo Clinic · 200 First Street, SW, Rochester, MN 55905 · 507-284-2511

Michael J. O'Connell · Professor of Oncology, Mayo Medical School · Mayo Clinic · 200 First Street, SW, Rochester, MN 55905 · 507-284-3903

GENERAL MEDICAL ONCOLOGY

Samuel A. Jacobs · Clinical Associate Professor of Medicine, University of Pittsburgh School of Medicine · Co-Medical Director, the Forbes Hospice, Montefiore University Hospital, and Medical Oncology Associates · 3471 Fifth Avenue, Suite 401, Pittsburgh, PA 15213 · 412-621-7778

John Andrew Laurie · Grand Forks Clinic · Grand Forks, ND 58201 · 701-780-6000

Ronald G. Stoller · Clinical Associate Professor of Medicine, University of Pittsburgh School of Medicine · Co-Medical Director, the Forbes Hospice, Montefiore University Hospital · 3471 Fifth Avenue, Suite 401, Pittsburgh, PA 15213 · 412-621-7778

John E. Ultmann · (Hodgkin's Disease, Unknown Primary Cancer) · Professor of Medicine, University of Chicago, Pritzker School of Medicine · Associate Director, Cancer Research Center, and Attending Physician, University of Chicago

Medical Center · 5841 South Maryland Avenue, Box 420, Chicago, IL 60637-1470
312-702-6180

Charles L. Vogel · Clinical Professor of Oncology, University of Miami School of Medicine · Medical Director, South Florida Comprehensive Cancer Centers · 11750 Bird Road, Miami, FL 33175 · 305-227-5556

Daniel D. Von Hoff · (New Drug Development) · Professor of Medicine and Head, Section of Drug Development, The University of Texas Health Science Center at San Antonio · Head, Research Department, Cancer Therapy Research Center · 7703 Floyd Curl Drive, San Antonio, TX 78284-7884 · 512-567-4747

Stanley Winokur · 993 Johnson Ferry Road NE, Suite D, Atlanta GA 30342 · 404-256-4777

LEUKEMIA
(See also Medical Oncology & Hematology, Leukemia)

Zalmen Amos Arlin · Chief Professor of Medicine, New York Medical College · Westchester County Medical Center · Munger Pavilion, Valhalla, NY 10595 · 914-993-4400

Clara D. Bloomfield · Professor of Medicine, and Chief, Division of Oncology, State University of New York at Buffalo · Head, Department of Medicine, Roswell Park Cancer Institute · Elm and Carlton Street, Buffalo, NY 14263 · 716-845-3300

Richard Champlin · Chief, Section of Bone Marrow Transplantation, The University of Texas MD Anderson Cancer Center · 1515 Holcombe Boulevard, Houston, TX 77030 · 713-792-3611

Stephen J. Forman · Director, Department of Hematology & Bone Marrow Transplantation, City of Hope National Medical Center · 1500 East Duarte Road, Duarte, CA 91010-0269 · 818-359-8111

Emil J Freireich · Ainsworth Professor of Medicine, The University of Texas Medical School at Houston · Director, Adult Leukemia Research Program, The University of Texas MD Anderson Cancer Center · 1515 Holcombe Boulevard, Box 55, Houston, TX 77030 · 713-792-2660

Harvey M. Golomb · (Hairy Cell Leukemia) · Professor of Medicine, University of Chicago, Pritzker School of Medicine · Director, Section of Hematology/ Oncology, University of Chicago Medical Center · 5841 South Maryland Avenue, Box 420, Chicago, IL 60637-1470 · 312-702-6115

Geoffrey P. Herzig · Professor of Medicine, State University of New York Health Science Center at Buffalo · Chief, Divisions of Hematologic Oncology and Bone Marrow Transplantation, Roswell Park Cancer Institute · Elm & Carlton Streets, Buffalo, NY 14263 · 716-845-7610

Hagop Kantarjian · Associate Professor of Medicine, and Associate Internist, Department of Hematology/Leukemia Section, The University of Texas Medical School at Houston · The University of Texas MD Anderson Cancer Center · 1515 Holcombe Boulevard, Box 61, Houston, TX 77030 · 713-792-7026

Michael J. Keating · Associate Vice President for Clinical Investigations, The University of Texas · Professor of Medicine and Internist, The University of Texas MD Anderson Cancer Center · 1515 Holcombe Boulevard, Box 38, Houston, TX 77030 · 713-792-2933

Charles Albert Linker · Associate Clinical Professor of Medicine, University of California at San Francisco School of Medicine · University of California at San Francisco Medical Center · 400 Parnassus Avenue, A-502, Box 0324, San Francisco, CA 94143-0324 · 415-476-1421

Robert J. Mayer · Associate Professor of Medicine, Harvard Medical School · Associate Physician, Dana-Farber Cancer Institute · 44 Binney Street, Boston, MA 02115 · 617-732-3474

Harvey D. Preisler · Professor of Medicine, University of Cincinnati College of Medicine · University of Cincinnati Hospital · 231 Bethesda Avenue, Cincinnati, OH 45267 · 513-558-3459

Kanti R. Rai · (Chronic Lymphatic Leukemia) · Professor of Medicine, Albert Einstein College of Medicine · Chief of Hematology/Oncology, Long Island Jewish Medical Center · Institute of Oncology, Second Floor, 269-11 Seventy-Sixth Avenue, New Hyde Park, NY 11042 · 718-470-7135

Charles A. Schiffer · Professor of Medicine and Oncology, University of Maryland School of Medicine · Head, Division of Hematologic Malignancies, University of Maryland Cancer Center · 22 South Greene Street, Baltimore, MD 21201 · 410-328-7394

William P. Vaughan · Professor of Medicine and Pharmacology, and Director, Marrow Transplantation Program, and Associate Director of Clinical Research, Comprehensive Cancer Center, The University of Alabama School of Medicine · The University of Alabama Hospital · 1900 University Boulevard, Birmingham, AL 35294 · 205-934-1908

W. Ralph Vogler · Professor of Medicine, Emory University School of Medicine Emory University Affiliated Hospitals, Emory Clinic · 1365 Clifton Road, Atlanta, GA 30322 · 404-248-3361

LUNG CANCER
(See also Medical Oncology & Hematology, Lung Cancer; Radiation Oncology, Lung Cancer)

Robert L. Comis · Professor of Medicine, Temple University School of Medicine Vice President, Medical Science, and Medical Director, The Fox Chase Cancer Center · 7701 Burholme Avenue, Philadelphia, PA 19111 · 215-728-3060

Robert T. Eagan · Professor of Oncology, Mayo Medical School · Mayo Clinic · 200 First Street, SW, Rochester, MN 55905 · 507-284-4430

John Dorrance Minna · Professor of Internal Medicine and Pharmacology, The University of Texas Southwestern Medical Center at Dallas · Director, Harold C. Simmons Comprehensive Cancer Center · 5323 Harry Hines Boulevard, Dallas, TX 75235-8590 · 214-688-7689

LYMPHOMAS
(See also Medical Oncology & Hematology, Lymphomas)

Clara D. Bloomfield · Professor of Medicine, and Chief, Division of Oncology, State University of New York at Buffalo · Head, Department of Medicine, Roswell Park Cancer Institute · Elm and Carlton Street, Buffalo, NY 14263 · 716-845-3300

John H. Glick · Director of University of Pennsylvania Cancer Center, and Professor of Medicine, University of Pennsylvania School of Medicine · University of Pennsylvania Cancer Center · 3400 Spruce Street, Six Penn Tower, Philadelphia PA 19104 · 215-662-6334

Geoffrey P. Herzig · Professor of Medicine, State University of New York Health Science Center at Buffalo · Chief, Divisions of Hematologic Oncology and Bone Marrow Transplantation, Roswell Park Cancer Institute · Elm & Carlton Streets, Buffalo, NY 14263 · 716-845-7610

John E. Ultmann · (Hodgkin's Disease, Unknown Primary Cancer) · Professor of Medicine, University of Chicago, Pritzker School of Medicine · Associate Director, Cancer Research Center, and Attending Physician, University of Chicago Medical Center · 5841 South Maryland Avenue, Box 420, Chicago, IL 60637-1470 312-702-6180

MEDICAL ONCOLOGY & HEMATOLOGY

AIDS
(See also Child Neurology, AIDS; Infectious Disease, AIDS; Pulmonary &
Critical Care Medicine, AIDS)

Margaret A. Fischl · Professor of Medicine and Director, Comprehensive AIDS
Program, University of Miami School of Medicine · University of Miami-Jackson
Memorial Medical Center · 1800 Northwest 10th Avenue, Miami, FL 33136 ·
305-547-3847

Jerome E. Groopman · (AIDS Related Malignancies) · Chief, Department of
Hematology & Oncology, New England Deaconess Hospital · 785 Pilgrim Road,
Boston, MA 02215 · 617-732-7000

Alexandra M. Levine · (AIDS Lymphomas) · Professor of Medicine, and Chief,
Division of Hematology, University of Southern California School of Medicine ·
The Los Angeles County + University of Southern California Medical Center;
Kenneth Norris, Jr., Cancer Hospital & Research Institute · 1975 Zonal Avenue,
KAM-110, Los Angeles, CA 90033 · 213-224-6668

Paul A. Volberding · Professor of Medicine, University of California at San Francisco School of Medicine · Director, AIDS Program, San Francisco General Hospital · 995 Potrero Avenue, Ward 84, San Francisco, CA 94110 · 415-476-4082
x84232

BONE MARROW TRANSPLANTATION
(See also Medical Oncology, Bone Marrow Transplantation)

Karen Antman · (Sarcomas) · Associate Professor of Medicine, Harvard Medical
School · Director, Solid Tumor Autologous Bone Marrow Program, Dana-Farber
Cancer Institute · 44 Binney Street, Boston, MA 02115 · 617-732-3339

Frederick R. Appelbaum · Professor of Medicine, University of Washington School of Medicine · Fred Hutchinson Cancer Research Center · 1124 Columbia Street, Seattle, WA 98104 · 206-667-4412

James O. Armitage · Professor and Chairman, Department of Internal Medicine, University of Nebraska College of Medicine · University of Nebraska Medical Center · Department of Internal Medicine, 600 South 42nd Street, Omaha, NE 68198-3332 · 402-559-7290

Patrick G. Beatty · Professor of Medicine, and Director of Bone Marrow Transplant Program, Division of Hematology & Oncology, University of Utah School of Medicine · University of Utah Health Sciences Center · 50 North Medical Drive, Salt Lake City, UT 84132 · 801-585-3229

Jacob D. Bitran · Clinical Professor of Medicine, University of Chicago Medical Center · Director of Division of Hematology/Oncology, Lutheran General Hospital · 1875 Dempster Street, Suite 405, Park Ridge, IL 60068 · 708-696-6889

Karl G. Blume · Professor of Medicine (Hematology, Oncology), Stanford University School of Medicine · Director of the Bone Marrow Transplantation Program, Stanford University Hospital · 300 Pasteur Drive, Room H-1353, Palo Alto, CA 94305 · 415-723-0822

Nancy E. Davidson · Assistant Professor of Oncology, Johns Hopkins University School of Medicine · Active Staff, The Johns Hopkins Medical Institutions · 600 North Wolfe Street, Baltimore, MD 21205 · 410-955-8489

Hans A. Messner · Professor, Department of Medicine, University of Toronto School of Medicine · Director, Bone Marrow Transplant Service, Ontario Cancer Institute, Princess Margaret Hospital · 500 Sherbourne Street, Room 673, Toronto, Ontario M4X 1K9 · 416-924-0671

William P. Peters · Associate Professor of Medicine, Duke University School of Medicine · Director, Bone Marrow Transplantation Program, Duke University Medical Center · P.O. Box 3961, Durham, NC 27710 · 919-684-6707

Gordon L. Phillips · Professor of Medicine, and Director, Leukemia/Bone Marrow Transplantation Program of British Columbia, The University of British Columbia · Vancouver General Hospital; Cancer Agency of British Columbia · 910 West 10th Avenue, Department of Medicine, LSP-3, Room 3329, Vancouver, British Columbia V5Z 4E3 · 604-875-4161

Stephanie F. Williams · Assistant Professor of Medicine, Section of Hematology/Oncology, University of Chicago, Pritzker School of Medicine · University of Chicago Medical Center · 5841 South Maryland Avenue, Box 420, Chicago, IL 60637-1470 · 312-702-6956

BREAST CANCER
(See also Medical Oncology, Breast Cancer, Radiation Oncology, Breast Cancer; Surgical Oncology, Breast Cancer)

Martin D. Abeloff · Professor of Medicine and Oncology, Johns Hopkins University School of Medicine · Clinical Director, Oncology Center, The Johns Hopkins Medical Institutions · 600 North Wolfe Street, Johns Hopkins Oncology Center, Room 124, Baltimore, MD 21205 · 410-955-8838

David L. Ahmann · Professor of Oncology, Mayo Medical School · Mayo Clinic · 200 First Street, SW, Rochester, MN 55905 · 507-284-2779

Tom Anderson · Director of Adult Hematology & Oncology, Medical College of Wisconsin · The Milwaukee County Medical Complex, 8700 West Wisconson Avenue,Box 133, Milwaukee, WI 53226 · 414-257-4565

Karen Antman · (Sarcomas) · Associate Professor of Medicine, Harvard Medical School · Director, Solid Tumor Autologous Bone Marrow Program, Dana-Farber Cancer Institute · 44 Binney Street, Boston, MA 02115 · 617-732-3339

John M. Bennett · Professor of Oncology, Medicine, Pathology & Laboratory Medicine, University of Rochester School of Medicine & Dentistry · Associate Director for Clinical Affairs, and Head of Medical Oncology Unit, University of Rochester Cancer Center · 601 Elmwood Avenue, Box 704, Rochester, NY 14642 716-275-4915

Jacob D. Bitran · Clinical Professor of Medicine, University of Chicago Medical Center · Director of Division of Hematology/Oncology, Lutheran General Hospital · 1875 Dempster Street, Suite 405, Park Ridge, IL 60068 · 708-696-6889

George P. Canellos · William Rosenberg Professor of Medicine, Harvard Medical School · Chief, Division of Medical Oncology, Dana-Farber Cancer Institute · 44 Binney Street, Boston, MA 02115 · 617-732-3470

John Topham Carpenter, Jr. · Professor of Medicine and The American Cancer Society Professor of Clinical Oncology, The University of Alabama School of Medicine · The University of Alabama Hospital · University Station, WTI229, Birmingham, AL 35294 · 205-934-2084

Nancy E. Davidson · Assistant Professor of Oncology, Johns Hopkins University School of Medicine · Active Staff, The Johns Hopkins Medical Institutions · 600 North Wolfe Street, Baltimore, MD 21205 · 410-955-8489

I. Craig Henderson · Professor of Medicine, University of California, San Francisco · Chief, Division of Medical Oncology, Moffitt-Long Hospital; Mt. Zion Hospital & Medical Center · Moffitt 1282, University of California, San Francisco, Box 0128, San Francisco, CA 94143 · 415-476-2201

Marc E. Lippman · Professor of Medicine and Pharmacology, Georgetown University School of Medicine · Director, Lombardi Cancer Research Center, Georgetown University Medical Center · 3800 Reservoir Road, NW, Podium Level, Washington, DC 20007 · 202-687-2110

Robert B. Livingston · Professor of Medicine and Head of the Division of Oncology, University of Washington School of Medicine · 1959 Northeast Pacific Street, Seattle, WA 98195 · 206-548-4125

Franco M. Muggia · Professor of Medicine, University of Southern California School of Medicine · Associate Director, Clinical Investigations, The Los Angeles County + University of Southern California Medical Center; Kenneth Norris, Jr. Cancer Hospital & Research Institute · 1441 Eastlake Avenue, Suite 162, Los Angeles, CA 90033 · 213-224-6677

Hyman B. Muss · Professor of Medicine, Section of Hematology/Oncology, and Associate Director of Clinical Research, Comprehensive Cancer Center of Wake Forest University, The Bowman Gray School of Medicine of Wake Forest University · North Carolina Baptist Hospital · Medical Center Boulevard, Winston-Salem, NC 27157-1082 · 919-748-4397

Larry Norton · Chief, Breast & Gynecologic Cancer Medicine Service, Memorial Sloan-Kettering Cancer Center · 1275 York Avenue, New York, NY 10021 · 212-639-6425

C. Kent Osborne · Professor of Medicine; and Head, Section of Clinical Medical Oncology, The University of Texas Health Science Center at San Antonio · Attending Physician, Medical Center Hospital; Cancer Therapy and Research Center · 7703 Floyd Curl Drive, San Antonio, TX 78284 · 512-567-4777

Steven Papish · Clinical Assistant Professor of Medicine, College of Physicians & Surgeons of Columbia University · Morristown Memorial Hospital · 261 James Street, Suite 1B, Morristown, NJ 07960 · 201-538-5210

A. H. Paterson · Director, Department of Medical Oncology, Tom Baker Cancer Center · 1331 Twenty-Ninth Street NW, Calgary, Alberta T2N 4N2 · 403-670-1767

Nichoas J. Robert · Clinical Associate Professor of Medicine, Georgetown University · Associate Physician, Fairfax Hospital · 3301 Woodburn Road, Suite 206, Annandale, VA 22003 · 703-560-7210

Douglass C. Tormey · Professor, Departments of Human Oncology and Medicine, and Chairman, Eastern Cooperative Oncology Group, University of Wisconsin Comprehensive Cancer Center · University of Wisconsin Hospital & Clinics · 600 Highland Avenue, Room K4/666, Madison, WI 53792 · 608-263-9269

Stephanie F. Williams · Assistant Professor of Medicine, Section of Hematology/Oncology, University of Chicago, Pritzker School of Medicine · University of Chicago Medical Center · 5841 South Maryland Avenue, Box 420, Chicago, IL 60637-1470 · 312-702-6956

CLINICAL PHARMACOLOGY

Joseph Bertino · Program Chairman, Department of Molecular Pharmacology & Therapeutics, Memorial Sloan-Kettering Cancer Center · 1275 York Avenue, New York, NY 10021 · 212-639-8230

Bruce A. Chabner · Director, Division of Cancer Treatment, National Cancer Institute, National Institutes of Health · 9000 Rockville Pike, Building 31, Room 3A44, Bethesda, MD 20892 · 301-496-4291

Ross C. Donehower · (New Drug Development) · Associate Professor of Medicine and Oncology, Johns Hopkins University School of Medicine · The Johns Hopkins Medical Institutions · 600 North Wolfe Street, Johns Hopkins Oncology Center, Room 121, Baltimore, MD 21205 · 410-955-8902

James H. Doroshow · Director of Medical Oncology, City of Hope National Medical Center · 1500 East Duarte Road, Duarte, CA 91010 · 818-359-8111

David S. Ettinger · (New Drug Development) · Associate Professor of Medicine and Oncology, Johns Hopkins University School of Medicine · Director, Lung Cancer Program, and Director, Outpatient Department, The Johns Hopkins Medical Institutions · 600 North Wolfe Street, Johns Hopkins Oncology Center, Room 130, Baltimore, MD 21205 · 410-955-8847

Franco M. Muggia · Professor of Medicine, University of Southern California School of Medicine · Associate Director, Clinical Investigations, The Los Angeles County + University of Southern California Medical Center; Kenneth Norris, Jr. Cancer Hospital & Research Institute · 1441 Eastlake Avenue, Suite 162, Los Angeles, CA 90033 · 213-224-6677

Charles E. Myers · Chief, Clinical Pharmacology, National Cancer Institute, National Institutes of Health · 9000 Rockville Pike, Building 10, Room 12C103, Bethesda, MD 20892 · 301-402-1357

Peter James O'Dwyer · Director of Developmental Chemotherapy, The Fox Chase Cancer Center · 7701 Burholme Avenue, Department of Medical Oncology, Philadelphia, PA 19111 · 215-728-2674

Mark Jeffrey Ratain · Associate Professor of Medicine, and Director of Clinical Pharmacology, Section of Hematology/Oncology, University of Chicago, Pritzker School of Medicine · University of Chicago Medical Center · 5841 South Maryland Avenue, Box 420, Chicago, IL 60637-1470 · 312-702-1815

Richard L. Schilsky · (New Drug Development) · Professor of Medicine, and Director of The University of Chicago Cancer Research Center, The University of Chicago, Pritzker School of Medicine · University of Chicago Medical Center · 5841 South Maryland Avenue, Box 420, Chicago, IL 60637-1470 · 301-702-9305

David R. Spriggs · (New Drug Development) · Assistant Professor of Human Oncology, University of Wisconsin-Madison School of Medicine · University of Wisconsin Hospital & Clinics · 600 Highland Avenue, Madison, WI 53792 · 608-263-8600

Donald L. Trump · Professor of Medicine and Director of Experimental Therapeutics, Duke University School of Medicine · Duke University Medical Center Box 3398, DUMC, Durham, NC 27710 · 919-684-3869

David Andrew VanEcho · (New Drug Development) · Professor of Medicine and Oncology, University of Maryland School of Medicine; Affiliate Professor of Clinical Pharmacology, University of Maryland Cancer Center · Chairman, Institutional Review Board, and Director of Clinical Programs, University of Maryland Cancer Center · 22 South Greene Street, Baltimore, MD 21201 · 301-328-2565

GENERAL MEDICAL ONCOLOGY & HEMATOLOGY

William Steven Dalton · Associate Professor of Medicine and Director of Bone Marrow Transplantation, Department of Internal Medicine, Arizona Cancer Center, The University of Arizona College of Medicine · Arizona Cancer Center · Room 3945, Tucson, AZ 85724 · 602-626-4196

Thomas P. Duffy · Professor of Medicine, Yale University School of Medicine · Yale-New Haven Hospital · 333 Cedar Street, WWW4, New Haven, CT 06510 · 203-785-4144

Emil Frei III · Richard & Susan Smith Professor of Medicine, Harvard Medical School · Physician and Chief, Emeritus, and Chief, Division of Cancer Pharmacology, Dana-Farber Cancer Institute · 44 Binney Street, Boston, MA 02115 · 617-732-3555

William N. Hait · Associate Professor of Medicine and Pharmacology and Chief, Section of Medical Oncology, Yale University School of Medicine · Yale-New Haven Hospital · 333 Cedar Street, New Haven, CT 06510 · 203-785- 4191

H. Clark Hoagland · Associate Professor of Medicine, Mayo Medical School · Chairman, Division of Hematology, Mayo Clinic · 200 First Street, SW, Rochester, MN 55905 · 507-284-3151

Howard E. Lessner · Professor Emeritus of Oncology, University of Miami School of Medicine · Baptist Hospital · 8950 North Kendall Drive, Suite 410, Miami, FL 33176 · 305-271-6467

Joseph O. Moore · Associate Professor of Medicine, Duke University School of Medicine · Duke University Medical Center · P.O. Box 3536, Durham, NC 27710 · 919-684-5202

GENITO-URINARY CANCER
(See also Radiation Oncology, Genito-Urinary Cancer)

George Joseph Bosl · Associate Professor of Medicine, Cornell University Medical College · Head, Division of Solid Tumor Oncology, Memorial Sloan-Kettering Cancer Center · 1275 York Avenue, Box 64, New York, NY 10021 · 212-639-8473

Ronald M. Bukowski · Acting Director, Cleveland Clinic Cancer Center, The Cleveland Clinic Foundation · One Clinic Center, 9500 Euclid Avenue, Cleveland, OH 44195 · 216-444-6825

Lawrence Einhorn · Distinguished Professor of Medicine, Indiana University School of Medicine · 926 West Michigan Avenue, Room 1730, Indianapolis, IN 46202 · 317-274-5555

Marc B. Garnick · (Biotechnology) · Associate Clinical Professor of Medicine, Harvard Medical School · Associate Physician, Dana Farber Cancer Institute; Vice-President of Clinical Development, Genetics Institute, Inc. · 87 Cambridge Park Drive, Cambridge, MA 02140 · 617-876-1170

L. Michael Glode · Professor of Medicine, Division of Medical Oncology, University of Colorado School of Medicine · University of Colorado Health Sciences Center · 4200 East Ninth Avenue, Box B-171, Denver, CO 80262 · 303-270-8801

F. Anthony Greco · Professor of Medicine, and Director of Division of Medical Oncology, Vanderbilt University School of Medicine · 1956 The Vandebilt Clinic, Nashville, TN 37232-5536 · 615-322-4967

Philip W. Kantoff · Assistant Professor of Medicine, Harvard Medical School · Program Director, Genitourinary Oncology, Dana-Farber Cancer Institute · 44 Binney Street, Boston, MA 02115 · 617-732-3466

Patrick J. Loehrer · (Testicular Cancer, Bladder Cancer) · Associate Professor of Medicine, Indiana University School of Medicine · Indiana University Medical Center · 926 West Michigan Street, Room 1730, Indianapolis, IN 46202-5265 · 317-274-0920

Robert J. Motzer · Assistant Professor of Medicine, Cornell University Medical College · Assistant Attending Physician-Medical Oncology, Memorial Sloan-Kettering Cancer Center · 1275 York Avenue, New York, NY 10021 · 212-639-6667

Derek Raghavan · Professor of Medicine, State University of New York at Buffalo Chief, Divisions of Investigational Therapeutics and Solid Tumor Oncology, Roswell Park Cancer Institute · Elm & Carlton Streets, Buffalo, NY 14263 · 716-845-7614

Ronald Lee Richardson · (Genito-Urinary Tumors) · Assistant Professor of Medicine, Mayo Medical School · Mayo Clinic · 200 First Street, SW, E-12, Rochester, MN 55905 · 507-284-4430

Howard Isador Scher · Memorial Sloan-Kettering Cancer Center · 1275 York Avenue, New York, NY 10021 · 212-639-7585

Frank M. Torti · Associate Professor of Medicine, Division of Oncology, Stanford University School of Medicine · Chief, Oncology Section, and Clinical Investigator, Palo Alto Veterans Affairs Medical Center · 3801 Miranda Avenue, 154-N, Palo Alto, CA 94304 · 415-852-3249

Donald L. Trump · Professor of Medicine and Director of Experimental Therapeutics, Duke University School of Medicine · Duke University Medical Center Box 3398, DUMC, Durham, NC 27710 · 919-684-3869

George Wilding · (Prostate Cancer) · Assistant Professor of Human Oncology and Medicine, University of Wisconsin-Madison School of Medicine, and University of Wisconsin Comprehensive Cancer Center · University of Wisconsin Hospital & Clinics · 600 Highland Avenue, Room K4-666, CSC, Madison, WI 53792 · 608-263-8600

Stephen D. Williams · (Ovarian Cancer) · Professor of Medicine, Indiana University School of Medicine · Indiana University Medical Center; Veterans Affairs Hospital · 926 West Michigan Street, Room A109, Indianapolis, IN 46202 · 317-274-0920

Alan Yagoda · Professor of Surgery/Urology, Cornell University Medical College The New York Hospital-Cornell Medical Center · 525 East 68th Street, P.O. Box 94, Room K908, New York, NY 10021 · 212-746-5478

GYNECOLOGIC CANCER
(See also Obstetrics & Gynecology, Gynecologic Cancer)

David Alberts · (Ovarian Cancer) · Professor of Medicine and Pharmacology, and Director of Cancer Prevention & Control Program, The University of Arizona College of Medicine · Deputy Director, Arizona Cancer Center, The University of Arizona · 1515 North Campbell Avenue, Tucson, AZ 85724 · 602-626-7685

James Charles Arseneau · (Ovarian Cancer) · Co-Chairman, Medical Oncology Committee, Gynecologic Oncology Group; and Clinical Associate Professor of Medicine, Albany Medical College · Associate Attending Staff, Department of Medicine, St. Peters Hospital · 317 South Manning Boulevard, Suite 330, Albany, NY 12208 · 518-489-2607

Maurie Markman · (Ovarian Cancer) · Vice-Chairman, Department of Medicine, Memorial Sloan-Kettering Cancer Center · 1275 York Avenue, New York, NY 10021 · 212-639-8354

William P. McGuire III · (Ovarian Cancer) · Associate Professor of Medicine and Oncology, Johns Hopkins University School of Medicine · The Johns Hopkins Medical Institutions · Johns Hopkins Oncology Center, 600 North Wolfe Street, Room 128, Baltimore, MD 21205 · 410-955-3300

Franco M. Muggia · (Ovarian Cancer) · Professor of Medicine, University of Southern California School of Medicine · Associate Director, Clinical Investigations, The Los Angeles County + University of Southern California Medical Center; Kenneth Norris, Jr.Cancer Hospital & Research Institute · 1441 Eastlake Avenue, Suite 162, Los Angeles, CA 90033 · 213-224-6677

Hyman B. Muss · Professor of Medicine, Section of Hematology/Oncology, and Associate Director of Clinical Research, Comprehensive Cancer Center of Wake Forest University, The Bowman Gray School of Medicine of Wake Forest University · North Carolina Baptist Hospital · Medical Center Boulevard, Winston-Salem, NC 27157-1082 · 919-748-4397

George A. Omura · (Ovarian Cancer) · Professor of Medicine; and Professor of Gynecology, The University of Alabama School of Medicine · Active Staff, The University of Alabama Hospital · 1824 Sixth Avenue South, Room 223, Birmingham, AL 35294-3300 · 205-934-3204

Robert Ozols · (Ovarian Cancer) · Professor of Medicine, Temple University School of Medicine · Chief of Oncology, The Fox Chase Cancer Center · 7701 Burholme Avenue, Philadelphia, PA 19111 · 215-728-2673

James Tate Thigpen · (Ovarian Cancer) · Professor of Medicine, University of Mississippi · Director, Division of Medical Oncology, University of Mississippi Medical Center · 2500 North State Street, Clinical Sciences Building L504, Jackson, MS 39216 · 601-984-5590

Stephen D. Williams · (Ovarian Cancer) · Professor of Medicine, Indiana University School of Medicine · Indiana University Medical Center; Veterans Affairs Hospital · 926 West Michigan Street, Room A109, Indianapolis, IN 46202 · 317-274-0920

Robert C. Young · (Ovarian Cancer) · President, Fox Chase Cancer Center · 7701 Burholme Avenue, Philadelphia, PA 19111 · 215-728-2781

HEAD & NECK CANCER
(See also Radiation Oncology, Head & Neck Cancer)

Muhyi Al-Sarraf · (Combined Modality Therapy) · Professor of Medicine, Wayne State University School of Medicine · Chief, Head & Neck Cancer Service, Detroit Medical Center; Harper Hospital · 3990 John R Street, Detroit, MI 48201 · 313-745-9184

Thomas J. Ervin · Dana-Farber Cancer Institute; Maine Medical Center · 180 Park Avenue, Portland, ME 04102 · 207-773-1754

Arlene A. Forastiere · (Esophageal Cancer) · Associate Professor of Oncology, Johns Hopkins University School of Medicine · The Johns Hopkins Medical Institutions · Johns Hopkins Oncology Center, 600 North Wolfe Street, Room 128, Baltimore, MD 21205 · 410-955-8847

Waun Ki Hong · Professor of Medicine, The University of Texas · The University of Texas MD Anderson Cancer Center · 1515 Holcombe Boulevard, Box 80, Houston, TX 77030 · 713-792-6363

Charlotte Jacobs · Senior Associate Dean for Education, Stanford University School of Medicine · Stanford University Hospital · 300 Pasteur Drive, Room M-121, Stanford, CA 94305-5302 · 415-725-8738

Everett E. Vokes · Associate Professor of Medicine and Radiation & Cellular Oncology, University of Chicago, Pritzker School of Medicine · Director of Clinical Research, University of Chicago Medical Center · 5841 South Maryland Avenue, Box 420, Chicago, IL 60637-1470 · 312-702-9306

HEMATOLOGICAL MALIGNANCIES

George P. Canellos · William Rosenberg Professor of Medicine, Harvard Medical School · Chief, Division of Medical Oncology, Dana-Farber Cancer Institute · 44 Binney Street, Boston, MA 02115 · 617-732-3470

Morton Coleman · Clinical Professor of Medicine, Cornell University Medical College · Attending Physician, The New York Hospital-Cornell Medical Center · 407 East 70th Street, New York, NY 10021 · 212-517-5900

Robert Owen Dillman · Clinical Professor of Medicine, University of California, Irvine · Director, Hoag Cancer Center of Hoag Memorial Hospital · 301 Newport Boulevard, Box Y, Newport Beach, CA 92658-8912 · 714-645-8600

Richard Fisher · (Hodgkin's Disease) · Professor of Medical Oncology & Hematology, Loyola Stritch School of Medicine · Chief, Section of Hematology Oncology, Loyola University Medical Center · 2160 South First Avenue, Building 54, Suite 067A, Maywood, IL 60153 · 708-216-9000

Paul Klimo · Associate Professor of Medicine, The University of British Columbia Staff Oncologist, Lions Gate Hospital · 126 East 15th Street, Suite 207, North Vancouver, British Columbia V7L 2P9 · 604-988-4899

Richard A. Larson · Associate Professor of Medicine, University of Chicago, Pritzker School of Medicine · Director, Acute Leukemia Program, University of Chicago Medical Center · 5841 South Maryland Avenue, Box 420, Chicago, IL 60637-1470 · 312-702-6783

Alexandra M. Levine · Professor of Medicine, and Chief, Division of Hematology, University of Southern California School of Medicine · The Los Angeles County + University of Southern California Medical Center; Kenneth Norris, Jr., Cancer Hospital & Research Institute · 1975 Zonal Avenue, KAM-110, Los Angeles, CA 90033 · 213-224-6668

Saul A. Rosenberg · (Hodgkin's Disease) · Professor of Medicine and Radiation Oncology, Stanford University School of Medicine · Chief, Division of Oncology, Stanford University Hospital · 300 Pasteur Drive, Stanford, CA 94305 · 415-725-6455

Gregory P. Sarna · Cedars-Sinai Comprehensive Cancer Center · 8700 Beverly Boulevard, Los Angeles, CA 90048-1869 · 213-855-8030

IMMUNOTHERAPY, BIOLOGICAL RESPONSE MODIFIERS ONCOLOGY

(See also Surgical Oncology, Immunotherapy, Biological Response Modifiers Oncology)

Robert C. Bast, Jr. · (Immunodiagnosis) · Professor of Medicine, Duke University School of Medicine · Director, Duke Comprehensive Cancer Center, Duke University Medical Center · P.O. Box 3843, Durham, NC 27710 · 919-684-3377

Ernest C. Borden · Professor of Medicine, Microbiology, and Pediatrics and American Cancer Society Professor, Medical College of Wisconsin · Director, Cancer Center, Medical College of Wisconsin · 8701 Watertown Plank Road, Milwaukee, WI 53226 · 414-257-4559

Robert Owen Dillman · Clinical Professor of Medicine, University of California, Irvine · Director, Hoag Cancer Center of Hoag Memorial Hospital · 301 Newport Boulevard, Box Y, Newport Beach, CA 92658-8912 · 714-645-8600

Jordan U. Gutterman · Professor of Medicine, The University of Texas · Chairman of Clinical Immunology & Biological Therapy, The University of Texas MD Anderson Cancer Center · 1515 Holcombe Boulevard, AC6005, Houston, TX 77030 · 713-792-2676

Alan N. Houghton · (Monoclonal Antibodies) · Associate Professor of Medicine, Cornell University Medical College · Chief of Clinical Immunology, and Head of Melanoma Section for the Division of Medical Oncology, Memorial Sloan-Kettering Cancer Center · 1275 York Avenue, New York, NY 10021 · 212-639-7505

Ronald Levy · Professor of Medicine, Stanford University School of Medicine · Stanford University Hospital · Department of Medicine, Division of Oncology, Room M-207, Stanford, CA 94305-5306 · 415-725-6452

Albert S. Lobuglio · Professor of Medicine, The University of Alabama School of Medicine · Director, Comprehensive Cancer Center, The University of Alabama Hospital · 1824 Sixth Avenue South, Room 237, Birmingham, AL 35294 · 205-934-5077

Malcolm S. Mitchell · (Vaccine Therapy, Cytokines) · Professor of Medicine and Microbiology, University of Southern California School of Medicine · The Los Angeles County + University of Southern California Medical Center, Kenneth Norris, Jr. Cancer Hospital · 2025 Zonal Avenue, Division of Medical Oncology, Los Angeles, CA 90033 · 213-226-6352

Lee M. Nadler · Associate Professor of Medicine, Harvard Medical School · Dana-Farber Cancer Institute · 44 Binney Street, Boston, MA 02115 · 617-732-3332

Robert K. Oldham · (Cancer Biotherapy) · Clinical Professor of Medicine, University of Missouri, Columbia, MO · Williamson Medical Center Biological Therapy Institute · Hospital Drive, P.O. Box 1700, Franklin, TN 37065 · 615-790-7535

David R. Parkinson · (Adoptive Immunotherapy) · Senior Staff, Immunotherapy Service, Surgery Branch, Clinical Oncology Program, and Head, Biologics Evaluation Section, Investigational Drug Branch, Cancer Therapy Evaluation Program, Division of Cancer Treatment, National Cancer Institute, National Institutes of Health · Clinical Center, National Institutes of Health · Executive Plaza North, 6130 Executive Boulevard, Room 715, Rockville, MD 20892 · 301-496-8798

Steven A. Rosenberg · Chief of Surgery, Surgery Branch, National Cancer Institute, National Institutes of Health · 9000 Rockville Pike, Building 10, Room 242, Bethesda, MD 20892 · 301-496-4164

LEUKEMIA
(See also Medical Oncology, Leukemia)

John M. Bennett · Professor of Oncology, Medicine, Pathology & Laboratory Medicine, University of Rochester School of Medicine & Dentistry · Associate Director for Clinical Affairs, and Head of Medical Oncology Unit, University of Rochester Cancer Center · 601 Elmwood Avenue, Box 704, Rochester, NY 14642 716-275-4915

Robert L. Capizzi · Director of the Comprehensive Cancer Center of Wake Forest University; Charles L. Spurr Professor of Medicine, Section Head, Hematology/Oncology, The Bowman Gray School of Medicine of Wake Forest University · North Carolina Baptist Hospital · Medical Center Boulevard, Winston-Salem, NC 27157-1082 · 919-748-4464

Richard A. Larson · Associate Professor of Medicine, University of Chicago, Pritzker School of Medicine · Director, Acute Leukemia Program, University of Chicago Medical Center · 5841 South Maryland Avenue, Box 420, Chicago, IL 60637-1470 · 312-702-6783

Peter Harris Wiernik · (Hodgkin's Disease) · Head of the Division of Medical Oncology, Albert Einstein College of Medicine · Gutman Professor and Chairman, Department of Oncology, Montefiore Medical Center · 111 East 210th Street, Bronx, NY 10467 · 212-920-4826

LUNG CANCER
(See also Medical Oncology, Lung Cancer; Radiation Oncology, Lung Cancer)

Paul A. Bunn, Jr. · Professor of Medicine and Division Head, Division of Medical Oncology, University of Colorado School of Medicine · Director, University of Colorado Cancer Center, University of Colorado Health Sciences Center · 4200 East Ninth Avenue, Box B-171, Denver, CO 80262 · 303-270-8801

Lawrence Einhorn · Distinguished Professor of Medicine, Indiana University School of Medicine · 926 West Michigan Avenue, Room 1730, Indianapolis, IN 46202 · 317-274-5555

David S. Ettinger · (New Drug Development) · Associate Professor of Medicine and Oncology, Johns Hopkins University School of Medicine · Director, Lung Cancer Program, and Director, Outpatient Department, The Johns Hopkins Medical Institutions · 600 North Wolfe Street, Johns Hopkins Oncology Center, Room 130, Baltimore, MD 21205 · 410-955-8847

Richard J. Gralla · Section Head of Hematology-Oncology, and Director, Ochsner Cancer Institute, Ochsner Clinic · 1514 Jefferson Highway, New Orleans, LA 70121 · 504-838-3261

F. Anthony Greco · Professor of Medicine, Division of Medical Oncology, Vanderbilt University School of Medicine · Director, Medical Oncology, Vanderbilt University Medical Center · 1956 The Vanderbilt Clinic, Nashville TN 37232-5536 · 615-322-4967

Mark R. Green · Professor of Medicine, University of California at San Diego School of Medicine · Chief, Division of Hematology/Oncology, University of California at San Diego Medical Center · 225 Dickinson Street, Mail Code 8421, San Diego, CA 92103-8421 · 619-543-6631

Daniel C. Ihde · Professor of Medicine, Uniformed Services University for Health Sciences · Deputy Director, Clinical Center, National Institutes of Health; National Naval Medical Center · 9000 Rockville Pike, Building 31, Room 11A48, Bethesda, MD 20892 · 301-496-1927

David Johnson · Associate Professor of Medicine, Division of Medical Oncology, Vanderbilt University School of Medicine · Vanderbilt University Medical Center 1956 The Vanderbilt Clinic, Nashville, TN 37232-5536 · 615-322-4967

Mark G. Kris · Associate Professor of Medicine, Cornell University Medical College · Associate Attending Physician and Chief, Thoracic Oncology Service, Division of Solid Tumor Oncology, Memorial Sloan-Kettering Cancer Center · 1275 York Avenue, New York, NY 10021 · 212-639-7590

Robert B. Livingston · Professor of Medicine and Head of the Division of Oncology, University of Washington School of Medicine · 1959 Northeast Pacific Street, Seattle, WA 98195 · 206-548-4125

Ronald B. Natale · Professor of Internal Medicine, The University of Michigan Medical School · The University of Michigan Medical Center · 3700 Upjohn Center, 1310 East Catherine Street, Ann Arbor, MI 48109-0504 · 313-747-1417

John C. Ruckdeschel · Professor of Medicine, University South Florida College of Medicine · Director/CEO, H. Lee Moffitt Cancer Center & Research Institute P.O. Box 280179, Tampa, FL 33682-8401 · 813-972-4673

LYMPHOMAS
(See also Medical Oncology, Lymphomas)

Tom Anderson · Director of Adult Hematology & Oncology, Medical College of Wisconsin · The Milwaukee County Medical Complex, 8700 West Wisconson Avenue, Box 133, Milwaukee, WI 53226 · 414-257-4565

James O. Armitage · Professor and Chairman, Department of Internal Medicine, University of Nebraska College of Medicine · University of Nebraska Medical Center · Department of Internal Medicine, 600 South 42nd Street, Omaha, NE 68198-3332 · 402-559-7290

John M. Bennett · Professor of Oncology, Medicine, Pathology & Laboratory Medicine, University of Rochester School of Medicine & Dentistry · Associate Director for Clinical Affairs, and Head of Medical Oncology Unit, University of Rochester Cancer Center · 601 Elmwood Avenue, Box 704, Rochester, NY 14642 716-275-4915

Paul A. Bunn, Jr. · Professor of Medicine and Division Head, Division of Medical Oncology, University of Colorado School of Medicine · Director, University of Colorado Cancer Center, University of Colorado Health Sciences Center · 4200 East Ninth Avenue, Box B-171, Denver, CO 80262 · 303-270-8801

Fernando Cabanillas · Professor of Medicine, The University of Texas MD Anderson Cancer Center · Chief, Section of Lymphoma, The University of Texas MD Anderson Cancer Center · 1515 Holcolmbe Boulevard, Box 68, Houston, TX 77030 · 713-792-2860

George P. Canellos · William Rosenberg Professor of Medicine, Harvard Medical School · Chief, Division of Medical Oncology, Dana-Farber Cancer Institute · 44 Binney Street, Boston, MA 02115 · 617-732-3470

Morton Coleman · Clinical Professor of Medicine, Cornell University Medical College · Attending Physician, The New York Hospital-Cornell Medical Center · 407 East 70th Street, New York, NY 10021 · 212-517-5900

Charles A. Coltman, Jr. · Professor, Department of Medicine, The University of Texas Health Science Center at San Antonio · Medical Director, The Cancer Therapy and Research Center · 4450 Medical Drive, San Antonio, TX 78229 · 512-616-5580

Joseph M. Connors · Clinical Associate Professor of Medicine, Division of Medical Oncology, The University of British Columbia · British Columbia Cancer Agency · 600 West 10th Avenue, Vancouver, British Columbia V5Z 4E6 · 604-877-6000

Richard Fisher · (Hodgkin's Disease) · Professor of Medical Oncology & Hematology, Loyola Stritch School of Medicine · Chief, Section of Hematology Oncology, Loyola University Medical Center · 2160 South First Avenue, Building 54, Suite 067A, Maywood, IL 60153 · 708-216-9000

Sandra J. Horning · Associate Professor of Medicine, Stanford University School of Medicine · Stanford University Hospital · 1000 Welch Road, Suite 202, Palo Alto, CA 94304 · 415-725-6458

Stephen E. Jones · Professor of Oncology, and Director, Clinical Research, Baylor University Medical Center · Sammons Cancer Center, 3330 Junius, Room 4800, Dallas, TX 75246 · 214-820-2021

Alexandra M. Levine · (AIDS Lymphomas) · Professor of Medicine, and Chief, Division of Hematology, University of Southern California School of Medicine · The Los Angeles County + University of Southern California Medical Center; Kenneth Norris, Jr. Cancer Hospital & Research Institute · 1975 Zonal Avenue, KAM-110, Los Angeles, CA 90033 · 213-224-6668

Dan L. Longo · Director of Biological Response Modifiers Program, National Cancer Institute, National Institutes of Health, Frederick Cancer Research & Development Center · Fort Detrick, Building 576, Room 100, Frederick, MD 21702-1201 · 301-846-1416

Thomas P. Miller · Professor of Medicine, The University of Arizona College of Medicine · Director of the Arizona Cancer Center Clinics, Arizona Cancer Center 1515 North Campbell Avenue, Tucson, AZ 85724 · 602-626-2667

Lee M. Nadler · Associate Professor of Medicine, Harvard Medical School · Dana-Farber Cancer Institute · 44 Binney Street, Boston, MA 02115 · 617-732-3332

Martin M. Oken · Professor of Medicine, University of Minnesota School of Medicine · Medical Director, The Virginia Piper Cancer Institute, Abbott Northwestern Hospital · 800 East 28th Street, Minneapolis, MN 55407 · 612-863-4633

Bruce A. Peterson · Professor of Medicine, & American Cancer Society Professor of Clinical Oncology, University of Minnesota School of Medicine · University of Minnesota Hospital & Clinics · Box 348 UMHC, Minneapolis, MN 55455 · 612-624-5631

Carol J. Portlock · Chief of Lymphoma, Memorial Sloan-Kettering Cancer Center · 1275 York Avenue, Howard 13, New York, NY 10021 · 212-639-8109

Saul A. Rosenberg · (Hodgkin's Disease) · Professor of Medicine and Radiation Oncology, Stanford University School of Medicine · Chief, Division of Oncology, Stanford University Hospital · 300 Pasteur Drive, Stanford, CA 94305 · 415-725-6455

Robert C. Young · President, Fox Chase Cancer Center · 7701 Burholme Avenue, Philadelphia, PA 19111 · 215-728-2781

MYELOMA

Raymond Alexanian · Professor of Medicine, The University of Texas · The University of Texas MD Anderson Cancer Center · 1515 Holcombe Boulevard, Houston. TX 77030 · 713-792-2850

Bart Barlogie · (Multiple Myeloma) · Chief of Hematology, and Professor of Medicine and Pathology, and Director of Research, Arkansas Cancer Research Center, University of Arkansas for Medical Sciences · 4301 West Markham, Slot 508, Little Rock, AR 72205 · 501-686-5222

Robert A. Kyle · (Amyloidosis) · Professor of Medicine and Laboratory Medicine, Mayo Medical School · Mayo Clinic · 200 First Street, SW, Rochester, MN 55905 507-284-2865

Martin M. Oken · Professor of Medicine, University of Minnesota School of Medicine · Medical Director, The Virginia Piper Cancer Institute, Abbott Northwestern Hospital · 800 East 28th Street, Minneapolis, MN 55407 · 612-863-4633

Sydney Salmon · (Multiple Myeloma) · Regents Professor of Medicine, The University of Arizona College of Medicine · Director, Arizona Cancer Center · 1515 North Campbell Avenue, Tucson, AZ 85724 · 602-626-7925

NEURO-ONCOLOGY
(See also Adult Neurology, Neuro-oncology; Child Neurology, Neuro-oncology; Radiation Oncology, Brain Cancer)

J. Gregory Cairncross · Professor of Clinical Neurological Sciences and Oncology, The University of Western Ontario · Attending Neurologist, London Regional Cancer Centre; Victoria Hospital · 790 Commissioners Road East, London, Ontario N6A 4L6 · 519-685-8640 x3292

Terrence Cascino · Associate Professor of Neurology, Mayo Medical School · Mayo Clinic · 200 First Street, SW, Rochester, MN 55905 · 507-284-2511

Kathleen M. Foley · (Pain Syndromes) · Chief, Pain Service, Memorial Sloan-Kettering Cancer Center · 1275 York Avenue, New York, NY 10021 · 212-639-7050

Peter C. Phillips · (Pediatric Brain Tumor) · Assistant Professor in Neurology, University of Pennsylvania School of Medicine · The Children's Hospital of Philadelphia · 34th and Civic Center Boulevard, Suite 2002, Philadelphia, PA 19104 215-590-1719

S. Clifford Schold, Jr. · (Brain Tumors) · Professor of Medicine and Assistant Professor of Pathology, Duke University School of Medicine · Duke University Medical Center · P.O. Box 3963, Durham, NC 27710 · 919-684-2662

William R. Shapiro · (Brain Tumors) · Chairman, Division of Neurology, The Barrow Neurological Institute at St. Joseph's Hospital & Medical Center · 350 West Thomas Road, Phoenix, AZ 85013 · 602-285-3895

Russell W. Walker · (Pediatric Brain Tumor) · Associate Professor of Pediatrics and Neurology, Cornell University Medical College · Associate Attending Pediatrician and Neurologist, Memorial Sloan-Kettering Cancer Center · 1275 York Avenue, New York, NY 10021 · 212-639-6597

W. K. Alfred Yung · (Brain Tumors) · Associate Professor of Neurology, The University of Texas Medical School at Houston · Deputy Chairman, Department of Neuro-oncology, The University of Texas MD Anderson Cancer Center · 1515 Holcombe Boulevard, Box 100, Houston, TX 77030 · 713-792-2573

PROSTATE CANCER

Frederick Ahmann · Associate Professor of Medicine, The University of Arizona College of Medicine · Chief, Hematology & Oncology Section, Tucson Veterans Affairs Medical Center · 3601 South Sixth Avenue, 111D, Tucson, AZ 85723 · 602-792-1450 x6600

Mario Eisenberger · Associate Professor of Medicine & Oncology, University of Maryland School of Medicine · University of Maryland Cancer Center · 22 South Greene Street, Baltimore, MD 21201 · 301-328-2565

L. Michael Glode · Professor of Medicine, Division of Medical Oncology, University of Colorado School of Medicine · University of Colorado Health Sciences Center · 4200 East Ninth Avenue, Box B-171, Denver, CO 80262 · 303-270-8801

David Johnson · Associate Professor of Medicine, Division of Medical Oncology, Vanderbilt University School of Medicine · Vanderbilt University Medical Center 1956 The Vanderbilt Clinic, Nashville, TN 37232-5536 · 615-322-4967

SOLID TUMORS

L. Michael Glode · Professor of Medicine, Division of Medical Oncology, University of Colorado School of Medicine · University of Colorado Health Sciences Center · 4200 East Ninth Avenue, Box B-171, Denver, CO 80262 · 303-270-8801

James F. Holland · Professor and Chairman, Department of Neoplastic Diseases, Mt. Sinai School of Medicine · Mt. Sinai Medical Center · One Gustave L. Levy Place, Box 1129, New York, NY 10029-6574 · 212-241-6361

Franco M. Muggia · Professor of Medicine, University of Southern California School of Medicine · Associate Director, Clinical Investigations, The Los Angeles County + University of Southern California Medical Center; Kenneth Norris, Jr. Cancer Hospital & Research Institute · 1441 Eastlake Avenue, Suite 162, Los Angeles, CA 90033 · 213-224-6677

NEPHROLOGY

DIALYSIS

William Bennett · (Hemodialysis, Drug Induced Kidney Disease) · Professor of Medicine, Oregon Health Sciences University · 3181 Southwest Sam Jackson Park Road, Portland, OR 97201 · 503-494-8490

Allan J. Collins · (Hemodialysis) · Assistant Professor of Medicine, University of Minnesota School of Medicine · Executive Director of the Metropolitan Dialysis Division, Hennepin County Medical Center, Regional Kidney Disease Program · 701 Park Avenue, D5, Minneapolis, MN 55415 · 612-347-5811

Jose A. Diaz-Buxo · (Peritoneal Dialysis, Mineral Matabolism) · Associate Clinical Professor of Medicine, University of North Carolina at Chapel Hill · Chief of Nephrology, Carolinas Medical Center · Metrolina Nephrology Associates, 928 Baxter Street, Charlotte, NC 28204 · 704-374-1321

Fredric O. Finkelstein · (Hemodialysis) · Clinical Professor of Medicine, Yale University School of Medicine · Hospital of St. Raphael, Yale-New Haven Hospital · 136 Sherman Avenue, New Haven, CT 06511 · 203-787-0117

Eli A. Friedman · (Diabetic Kidney Disease) · Professor of Medicine, State University of New York Health Science Center at Brooklyn · Director, Renal Disease, University Hospital, Brooklyn, and Kings County Hospital, Brooklyn · 1049 East 17th Street, Brooklyn, NY 11230 · 718-270-1584, 212-270-1584

Thomas Alan Golper · (Hemodialysis) · Professor of Medicine, University of Louisville School of Medicine · Director, Dialysis Related Services, Norton Hospital; Jewish Hospital; Humana Hospital University of Louisville · Kidney Disease Program, University of Louisville, Louisville, KY 40292 · 502-588-5757

Frank A. Gotch · (Hemodialysis) · Associate Clinical Professor of Medicine, University of California at San Francisco School of Medicine · Medical Director, Artificial Kidney Center, Davies Medical Center · 45 Castro Street, Suite 227, San Francisco, CA 94114 · 415-621-9616

Raymond M. Hakim · (Hemodialysis) · Professor of Medicine, Division of Nephrology, Vanderbilt University School of Medicine · 1161 Twenty-First Avenue South, Nashville, TN 37232-2373 · 615-343-4823

J. Michael Lazarus · (Hemodialysis) · Associate Professor of Medicine, Harvard Medical School · Director of Clinical Services, Nephrology Division, Brigham & Women's Hospital · 75 Francis Street, Boston, MA 02115 · 617-732-6137

Nathan W. Levin · (Hemodialysis) · Professor of Medicine, Mt. Sinai School of Medicine · Chief, Division of Nephrology & Hypertension, Beth Israel Medical Center · Division of Nephrology & Hypertension, First Avenue at 16th Street, New York, NY 10003 · 212-420-4017

Jack W. Moncrief · (Peritoneal Dialysis) · Co-Director of Hemodialysis & Transplantation, Austin Diagnostic Clinic; Brackenridge Hospital · 801 West 34th Street, Austin, TX 78705 · 512-459-1111

Allen R. Nissenson · (Hemodialysis, Peritoneal Dialysis) · Professor of Medicine and Director, Dialysis Program, University of California at Los Angeles School of Medicine · Attending Physician, UCLA Medical Center · 200 Medical Plaza, Room 565-57, Los Angeles, CA 90024-6945 · 310-825-9464

Karl D. Nolph · (Peritoneal Dialysis, Diabetic Kidney Disease) · Director of Division of Nephrology, and Broaddus Distinguished and University of Missouri Board of Curators Professor of Medicine, University of Missouri · University of Missouri Hospital & Clinics · MA436 Health Sciences Center, Columbia, MO 65212 · 314-882-7991

Dimitrios Oreopoulos · (Peritoneal Dialysis, Diabetic Kidney Disease) · Professor of Medicine, University of Toronto School of Medicine · Director, Peritoneal Dialysis Unit, The Toronto Western Hospital · 399 Bathurst Street, Toronto, Ontario M5T 2S8 · 416-364-9974

Friederich K. Port · (Hemodialysis) · Professor of Medicine and Epidemiology, The University of Michigan Medical School · Director of the Michigan Kidney

Registry, Ann Arbor Veterans Affairs Medical Center; The University of Michigan Medical Center · 315 West Huron, Suite 340, Ann Arbor, MI 48103 · 313-998-7794

Edwin A. Rutsky · (Hemodialysis) · Professor of Medicine, The University of Alabama School of Medicine · Director, Medical Dialysis Units, The University of Alabama Hospital · 614 Ziegler Building, Birmingham, AL 35294 · 205-934-5642

Michael I. Sorkin · (Hemodialysis) · Associate Professor of Medicine, and Chief, Section of Nephrology, West Virginia University School of Medicine · West Virginia University Health Sciences Center · 4101 Health Sciences Center North, Morgantown, WV 26506 · 304-293-2551

Wadi N. Suki · (Hemodialysis, Peritoneal Dyalysis) · Professor of Medicine, Molecular Physiology, and Biophysics and Chief, Renal Section, Baylor College of Medicine · Senior Attending Physician, The Methodist Hospital · 6550 Fannin Street, Suite 1273, Houston, TX 77030 · 713-790-3275

James F. Winchester · (Poisoning, CAP) · Professor of Medicine, Georgetown University School of Medicine · Acting Director, Division of Nephrology, Georgetown University Medical Center · Pasquerilla Health Care Center, Suite 6003, 3800 Reservoir Road, NW, Washington, DC 20007 · 202-687-8539

GENERAL ADULT NEPHROLOGY

Cecil H. Coggins · Associate Professor of Medicine, Harvard Medical School · Clinical Director, Renal Unit, Massachusetts General Hospital · Jackson Eight, Boston, MA 02114 · 617-726-3770

Harry R. Jacobson · Professor of Medicine and Director of the Division of Nephrology, Vanderbilt University School of Medicine · Vanderbilt University Medical Center · 1161 Twenty-First Avenue South, Division of Nephrology, Room S3223 MCN, Nashville, TN 37232-2372 · 615-322-4794

Saulo Klahr · John E. & Adaline Simon Professor of Medicine, Washington University School of Medicine · Physician-in-Chief, The Jewish Hospital of St. Louis · 216 South Kingshighway Boulevard, St. Louis, MO 63110 · 314-454-7107

Robert W. Schrier · Professor and Chairman, Department of Medicine, University of Colorado School of Medicine · Head, Division of Renal Diseases & Hypertension, University of Colorado Health Sciences Center · 4200 East Ninth Avenue, Box B-178, Denver, CO 80262 · 303-270-7765

Theodore Irving Steinman · Associate Clinical Professor of Medicine, Harvard Medical School · Director, Dialysis Unit, Beth Israel Hospital · 1101 Beacon Street, Boston, MA 02146 · 617-277-7141

Wadi N. Suki · (Hemodialysis, Peritoneal Dyalysis) · Professor of Medicine, Molecular Physiology, and Biophysics and Chief, Renal Section, Baylor College of Medicine · Senior Attending Physician, The Methodist Hospital · 6550 Fannin Street, Suite 1273, Houston, TX 77030 · 713-790-3275

GLOMERULAR DISEASES

Gerald B. Appel · Professor of Clinical Medicine, College of Physicians & Surgeons of Columbia University · Director of Clinical Nephrology, Columbia-Presbyterian Medical Center · 622 West 168th Street, Room 4128, New York, NY 10032 · 212-305-3273

David S. Baldwin · Professor of Medicine and Director, Department of Nephrology, New York University School of Medicine · Attending in Medicine, Tisch Hospital of New York University Medical Center, and Bellevue Hospital; Consultant in Nephrology, Veterans Affairs Medical Center · 20 East 68th Street, New York, NY 10021 · 212-737-8989

W. Kline Bolton · Professor of Medicine and Chief, Division of Nephrology, University of Virginia School of Medicine · University of Virginia Health Sciences Center · Box 133, Charlottesville, VA 22908 · 804-924-5125

William G. Couser · Head, Division of Nephrology, University of Washington School of Medicine · Division of Nephrology, Mail Stop RM-11, BB1265 Health Sciences Building, Seattle, WA 98195 · 206-543-3792

James V. Donadio · Professor of Medicine, Mayo Medical School · Consultant, Internal Medicine & Nephrology, Mayo Clinic · 200 First Street, SW, Rochester, MN 55905 · 507-284-3588

Ronald J. Falk · (Rapidly Progressive Glomerulonephritis, Systemic Vasculitis, Wegener's Vasculitis) · Associate Professor of Medicine, University of North Carolina School of Medicine · University of North Carolina Hospitals at Chapel Hill · 3034 Old Clinic Building, CB 7155, Chapel Hill, NC 27599 · 919-966-2561

Richard J. Glassock · Professor of Medicine, University of California at Los Angeles School of Medicine · Chairman of Medicine, Harbor-UCLA Medical Center · 1000 West Carson Street, Torrance, CA 90509 · 310-533-2401

Edmund J. Lewis · Professor of Medicine, Director, Section of Nephrology, Rush-Presbyterian-St. Luke's Medical Center · Rawson Building, 1653 West Congress Parkway, Room 503, Chicago, IL 60612 · 312-942-6685

Marc A. Pohl · Staff, Department of Hypertension & Nephrology, The Cleveland Clinic Foundation · One Clinic Center, 9500 Euclid Avenue, Desk-A101, Cleveland, OH 44195-5042 · 216-444-6776

David J. Salant · Professor of Medicine, Boston University School of Medicine · Chief, Renal Section, The University Hospital · 88 East Newton Street, E428, Boston, MA 02118 · 617-638-7480

HYPERTENSION

John H. Bauer · Professor of Medicine, University of Missouri · University of Missouri Hospital & Clinics · School of Medicine, Department of Medicine, Hypertension Section N425, One Hospital Drive, Columbia, MO 65212 · 314-882-4894

Ray W. Gifford, Jr. · Senior Vice-Chairman, Division of Medicine, and Acting Chairman, Department of Hypertension & Nephrology, The Cleveland Clinic Foundation · Department Hypertention & Nephrology, One Clinic Center, 9500 Euclid Avenue, Cleveland, OH 44195 · 216-444-6764

KIDNEY DISEASE

William Bennett · (Hemodialysis, Drug Induced Kidney Disease) · Professor of Medicine, Oregon Health Sciences University · 3181 Southwest Sam Jackson Park Road, Portland, OR 97201 · 503-494-8490

Jack W. Coburn · (Bone & Calcium Metabolism) · Adjunct Professor of Medicine, University of California, Los Angeles School of Medicine · Attending Physician, Cedars-Sinai Medical Center; University of California, Los Angeles Center for the Health Sciences; Brotman Medical Center; Century City Hospital · 9400 Brighton Way, Beverly Hills CA 90210 · 213-276-2033

Eli A. Friedman · (Diabetic Kidney Disease) · Professor of Medicine, State University of New York Health Science Center at Brooklyn · Director, Renal Disease, University Hospital, Brooklyn, and Kings County Hospital, Brooklyn · 1049 East 17th Street, Brooklyn, NY 11230 · 718-270-1584, 212-270-1584

Carl M. Kjellstrand · (Diabetic Kidney Disease) · Professor of Medicine, University of Alberta · The University of Alberta Hospitals · 2E3.31 Walter Mackenzie Center, Edmonton, Alberta T6G 2B7 · 403-492-5588

Karl D. Nolph · (Peritoneal Dialysis, Diabetic Kidney Disease) · Director of Division of Nephrology, and Broaddus Distinguished and University of Missouri Board of Curators Professor of Medicine, University of Missouri · University of

Missouri Hospital & Clinics · MA436 Health Sciences Center, Columbia, MO 65212 · 314-882-7991

Dimitrios Oreopoulos · (Peritoneal Dialysis, Diabetic Kidney Disease) · Professor of Medicine, University of Toronto School of Medicine · Director, Peritoneal Dialysis Unit, The Toronto Western Hospital · 399 Bathurst Street, Toronto, Ontario M5T 2S8 · 416-364-9974

KIDNEY TRANSPLANTATION
(See also General Surgery, Transplantation; Infectious Disease, Transplantation Infections; Urology, Kidney Transplantation)

William J. C. Amend · Professor of Clinical Medicine and Surgery, University of California at San Francisco School of Medicine · Kidney Transplant Service, University of California at San Francisco Medical Center · 505 Parnassus Avenue, Moffitt 884, San Francisco, CA 94143 · 415-476-1551

Charles B. Carpenter · Professor of Medicine, Harvard Medical School · Director of Immunogenetics, Brigham & Women's Hospital · Immunogenetics Laboratory, 75 Francis Street, Boston, MA 02115 · 617-732-5868

M. Roy First · Professor of Medicine, and Director, Section of Transplantation, Division of Nephrology, University of Cincinnati College of Medicine · University of Cincinnati Medical Center · 231 Bethesda Avenue, Cincinnati, OH 45267-0585 513-558-7001

Thomas A. Gonwa · Clinical Assistant Professor of Medicine, Southwestern Medical School · Associate Director, Transplant Services, Baylor University Medical Center, Baylor Transplant Services · 3500 Gaston Avenue, Dallas, TX 75246 · 214-820-2050

Ronald D. Guttmann · Professor of Medicine, McGill University · Director, McGill Center for Clinical Immunobiology & Transplantation · 687 Pine Avenue West, Montreal, Quebec H3A 1A1 · 514-843-1512

Barry Levin · Medical Director, Transplantation Program, California Pacific Medical Center · 2340 Clay Street, San Francisco, CA 94115 · 415-923-3450

Douglas J. Norman · Professor of Medicine, Oregon Health Sciences University Director of Transplant Medicine, and Director, Laboratory of Immunogenetics & Transplantation, Oregon Health Sciences University · 3181 Southwest Sam Jackson Park Road, MQ-360, Portland, OR 97201-3098 · 503-494-7880

Terry B. Strom · (Immunology) · Professor of Medicine, Harvard Medical School Director, Division of Clinical Immunology, Beth Israel Hospital · 330 Brookline Avenue, Research East 319, Boston, MA 02215 · 617-735-3550

Wadi N. Suki · (Hemodialysis, Peritoneal Dyalysis) · Professor of Medicine, Molecular Physiology, and Biophysics and Chief, Renal Section, Baylor College of Medicine · Senior Attending Physician, The Methodist Hospital · 6550 Fannin Street, Suite 1273, Houston, TX 77030 · 713-790-3275

Manikkam Suthanthiran · Professor of Medicine & Biochemistry, Cornell University Medical College · Director, Immunogenetics & Transplantation Center, The Rogosin Institute, The New York Hospital-Cornell Medical Center · 430 East 71st Street, New York, NY 10021 · 212-772-6735

NEUROLOGICAL SURGERY

CRANIAL NERVE SURGERY

Peter J. Jannetta · (Trigeminal Neuralgia, Acoustic Neuromas) · Professor and Chairman, Department of Neurological Surgery, University of Pittsburgh School of Medicine · Presbyterian University Hospital · 230 Lothrop Street, Room 9402 PUH, Pittsburgh, PA 15213 · 412-648-9248

Albert L. Rhoton, Jr. · (Trigeminal Neuralgia, Acoustic Neuroma) · R. D. Keene Family Professor and Chairman, Department Neurological Surgery, University of Florida College of Medicine · Box J265 JHMHC, Gainesville, FL 32610 · 904-392-4331

John M. Tew, Jr. · (Trigeminal Neuralgia) · Professor and Chairman, Department of Neurosurgery, University of Cincinnati College of Medicine · University of Cincinnati Hospital; Good Samaritan Hospital; Children's Hospital Medical Center · 231 Bethesda Avenue, ML 515, Cincinnati, OH 45267-0515 · 513-558-5387

Charles B. Wilson · (Trigeminal Neuralgia) · Professor and Chairman, Department of Neurological Surgery, University of California at San Francisco School of Medicine · University of California at San Francisco Medical Center · 505 Parnassus Avenue, Room M-787, San Francisco, CA 94143-0112 · 415-476-1087

EPILEPSY SURGERY
(See also Adult Neurology, Epilepsy; Child Neurology, Epilepsy)

Robert G. Grossman · Professor and Chairman, Department of Neurological Surgery, Baylor College of Medicine · Chief, Neurosurgical Service, The Methodist Hospital · One Baylor Plaza, Houston, TX 77030 · 713-798-4696

George A. Ojemann · Professor of Neurological Surgery, University of Washington School of Medicine · University of Washington Medical Center · 1959 Northeast Pacific Street, RI-20, Seattle, WA 98195 · 206-543-3572

Andre Olivier · Professor and Chairman, Division of Neurosurgery, McGill University, and Montreal Neurological Institute · Neurosurgeon-in-Chief, Montreal Neurologic Hospital · 3801 University Street, Suite 109, Montreal, Quebec H3A 2B4 · 514-398-1937

Dennis Spencer · Chief of Neurosurgery, Yale University School of Medicine · 333 Cedar Street, New Haven, CT 06510 · 203-785-2811

Allen R. Wyler · Professor of Neurosurgery, Anatomy and Neurobiology, The University of Tennessee at Memphis, College of Medicine · Director, Epi-Care Center, Baptist Memorial Hospital · 910 Madison, Suite 906, Memphis, TN 38103 · 901-227-5854

GENERAL NEUROLOGICAL SURGERY

Peter M. Black · Franc D. Ingraham Professor of Neurosurgery, Harvard Medical School · Neurosurgeon-in-Chief, Brigham & Women's Hospital; Children's Hospital · 75 Francis Street, Boston, MA 02115 · 617-732-6810

Ivan S. Ciric · Clinical Professor of Surgery, Northwestern University Medical School · Bennett-Tarkington Chair in Neurosurgery, and Head, Divison of Neurosurgery, Evanston Hospital; Highland Park Hospital · 2500 Ridge Avenue, Suite 208, Evanston, IL 60201 · 708-491-1100

Ralph G. Dacey, Jr. · (Cerebrovascular Disease) · Professor and Chairman, Department of Neurosurgery, Washington University School of Medicine · Barnes Hospital · 660 South Euclid Avenue, St. Louis, MO 63110 · 314-362-3571

Robert M. Levy · (AIDS) · Associate Professor of Neurological Surgery & Physiology, Northwestern University Medical School · Northwestern Memorial Hospital · 233 East Erie Street, Suite 500, Chicago, IL 60611 · 312-908-8143

Joseph C. Maroon · Clinical Professor of Neurosurgery, Medical College of Pennsylvania- Allegheny Campus · Chairman, Department of Neurosurgery, Allegheny General Hospital · 420 East North Avenue, Suite 302, Pittsburgh, PA 15212 · 412-359-4323

Russell H. Patterson, Jr. · Professor of Surgery (Neurosurgery), The New York Hospital-Cornell Medical Center · 525 East 68th Street, New York, NY 10021 · 212-746-5454

William Shucart · Chairman and Professor of Neurosurgery, Tufts University School of Medicine · Chairman, Department of Neurosurgery, New England Medical Center · 750 Washington Street, Box 178, Boston, MA 02111 · 617-956-5858

PEDIATRIC NEUROLOGICAL SURGERY

Derek A. Bruce · (Trauma, Head Injury, Brain Tumors) · Clinical Associate Professor, Department of Neurosurgery, University of Texas Southwestern Medical Center · Director, Pediatric Neurosurgical Institute, Humana Advanced Surgical Institute; Pediatric Neurosurgeon, Humana Hospital—Medical City, Dallas 7777 Forest Lane; Suite C-703, Dallas, TX 75230 · 214-788-6660

Michael S. B. Edwards · (Brain Tumors) · Professor of Neurosurgery and Pediatrics and Director, Division of Pediatric Neurosurgery, University of California at San Francisco School of Medicine · University of California at San Francisco Medical Center · 533 Parnassus Avenue, Room U-126, San Francisco, CA 94143 415-476-5711

Fred Jacob Epstein · (Brain and Spinal Tumors) · Professor and Director, Division of Pediatric Neurosurgery, New York University School of Medicine · New York University Medical Center · 550 First Avenue, Room 518, New York, NY 10016 · 212-263-6419

Harold J. Hoffman · (Brain Tumors) · Professor of Surgery, University of Toronto School of Medicine · Head, Division of Neurosurgery, The Hospital for Sick Children · 555 University Avenue, Toronto, Ontario M5G 1X8 · 416-598-6426

Robin P. Humphreys · (Vascular Pediatric Surgery, Brain Tumors, Congenital Anomalies) · Associate Professor, Department of Surgery, University of Toronto School of Medicine · Associate Surgeon-in-Chief, The Hospital for Sick Children 555 University Avenue, Suite 1504, Toronto, Ontario M5G 1X8 · 416-598-6427

J. Gordon McComb · Professor of Neurosurgery, University of Southern California School of Medicine · Head, Division of Neurosurgery, Children's Hospital of Los Angeles · 1300 North Vermont Avenue, Suite 906, Los Angeles, CA 90027 · 213-663-8128

David G. McLone · (Spina Bifida, Myelodysplasia, Hydrocephalus, Congenital Anomalies) · Professor of Neurosurgery, Northwestern University Medical School Head, Pediatric Neurosurgery, The Children's Memorial Hospital · 2300 Children's Plaza, Box 28, Chicago, IL 60614 · 312-880-4373

Arnold H. Menezes · (Cranial Cervical Stabilization Problems, Spine, Surgery of the Cranial Vertebral Junction, Transoral Surgery) · Professor, Division of Neurosurgery, The University of Iowa College of Medicine · The University of Iowa Hospitals & Clinics · Iowa City, IA 52242 · 319-356-2768

W. Jerry Oakes · (Congenital Anomalies) · Associate Professor, Division of Neurosurgery, and Assistant Professor, Department of Pediatrics, Duke University School of Medicine · Duke University Medical Center · P.O. Box 3272, Durham, NC 27710 · 919-684-5013

Warwick J. Peacock · (Seizure Surgery, Cerebral Palsy Surgery) · Professor of Surgery, Division of Neurosurgery, University of California at Los Angeles School of Medicine · Chief of Pediatric Neurosurgery, University of California at Los Angeles Center for the Health Sciences · 10833 LeConte Avenue, Los Angeles, CA 90024-6901 · 213-206-6677

Harold L. Rekate · (Brain Tumors, Hydrocephalus) · Clinical Professor of Neurosurgery, The University of Arizona · Chief of Pediatric Neurosurgery, The Barrow Neurological Institute at St. Joseph's Hospital & Medical Center · 2910 North Third Avenue, Phoenix, AZ 85013 · 602-285-3181

Robert Alex Sanford · (Brain Tumors) · Associate Professor of Neurological Surgery, The University of Tennessee at Memphis, College of Medicine · Chief of Surgery, Le Bonheur Children's Medical Center; Neurosurgery Consultant, Brain Tumor Team, St. Jude Research Hospital; Pediatric Surgeon, Semmes-Murphey Clinic · 920 Madison Avenue, Suite 201, Memphis, TN 38103 · 901-522-7700

Luis Schut · (Brain Tumors, Hydrocephalus, Congenital Spinal Anomalies) · Professor of Neurosurgery & Pediatrics, University of Pennsylvania School of Medicine · Chief of Neurosurgical Services, The Children's Hospital of Philadelphia · 34th and Civic Center Boulevard, Third Floor, Philadelphia, PA 19104 · 215-590-2780

R. Michael Scott · Associate Professor of Surgery, Harvard Medical School · Director, Section of Pediatric Neurosurgery, Children's Hospital · 300 Longwood Avenue, Bader-3, Boston, MA 02115 · 617-735-6011

Leslie N. Sutton · (Brain Tumors) · Associate Professor of Neurosurgery, University of Pennsylvania School of Medicine · Associate Neurosurgeon, The Children's Hospital of Philadelphia · 34th and Civic Center Boulevard, Philadelphia, PA 19104-4399 · 215-590-2780

Marion L. Walker · (Brain Tumors) · Associate Professor of Surgery (Neurosurgery) and Pediatrics, University of Utah School of Medicine · Chairman, Division of Pediatric Neurosurgery, Primary Children's Medical Center · 100 North Medical Drive, Salt Lake City, UT 84113 · 801-588-3400

PERIPHERAL NERVE SURGERY
(See also Hand Surgery, Peripheral Nerve Surgery; Orthopaedic Surgery, Peripheral Nerve Surgery; Plastic Surgery, Peripheral Nerve Surgery)

James N. Campbell · (Pain) · Professor of Neurosurgery, Johns Hopkins University School of Medicine · Associate Director, Department of Neurosurgery, The Johns Hopkins Medical Institutions · 600 North Wolfe Street, Meyer 7-113, Baltimore, MD 21205 · 410-955-2058

Allan H. Friedman · Associate Professor of Neurosurgery, Duke University School of Medicine · Duke University Medical Center · P.O. Box 3807, Durham, NC 27710 · 919-681-6421

Alan R. Hudson · University of Toronto School of Medicine · President and CEO, The Toronto Hospital · 585 University Avenue, Belwing 1-658, Toronto, Ontario M5G 2C4 · 416-340-3300

David G. Kline · (Electrodiagnosis) · Professor and Chairman, Department of Neurosurgery, Louisiana State University School of Medicine · Louisiana State University Medical Center · 1542 Tulane Avenue, New Orleans, LA 70112 · 504-568-6120

SPINAL SURGERY

Vallo Benjamin · Professor of Neurological Surgery, New York University School of Medicine · New York University Medical Center · 400 East 34th Street, Room 605, New York, NY 10016 · 212-263-5013

Edward S Connolly · Chief and Head of Neurosurgery, Ochsner Clinic · 1514 Jefferson Highway, New Orleans, LA 70121 · 504-838-4033

Paul Richard Cooper · Professor of Neurosurgery, New York University School of Medicine · New York University Medical Center · 550 First Avenue, New York, NY 10016 · 212-263-6514

David L. Kelly, Jr. · (Tumor Surgery) · Professor and Chairman, Department of Neurosurgery, The Bowman Gray School of Medicine of Wake Forest University North Carolina Baptist Hospital · Medical Center Boulevard, Winston-Salem, NC 27157-1029 · 919-748-4038

Sanford J. Larson · Professor and Chairman, Department of Neurosurgery, Medical College of Wisconsin · Froedtert Memorial Lutheran Hospital · 9200 West Wisconsin Avenue, Milwaukee, WI 53226 · 414-454-5407

Burton M. Onofrio · Professor, Department of Neurologic Surgery, Mayo Medical School · Mayo Clinic · 200 First Street, SW, Rochester, MN 55905 · 507-284-8167

Phanor L. Perot, Jr. · Professor and Chairman, Department of Neurological Surgery, Medical University of South Carolina · 171 Ashley Avenue, Charleston, SC 29425-2272 · 803-792-2300

Volker K. H. Sonntag · Clinical Professor of Surgery, The University of Arizona College of Medicine · Vice Chairman, Department of Neurosurgery, The Barrow Neurological Institute at St. Joseph's Hospital & Medical Center · Neurosurgical Associates, 2910 North Third Avenue, Phoenix, AZ 85013 · 602-285-3458

Narayan (Sunny) Sundaresan · Associate Professor of Neurosurgery, Mount Sinai Medical School · Chief of Neurosurgery at Doctor's Hospital (Beth Israel North); Attending Neurosurgeon, Mt. Sinai Medical Center · 53 East 67th Street, New York, NY 10021 · 212-861-2020

STEREOTACTIC RADIOSURGERY

Michael L. J. Apuzzo · Professor of Neurological Surgery, University of Southern California School of Medicine · The Los Angeles County + University of Southern California Medical Center · 1200 North State Street, Suite 5046, Los Angeles, CA 90033 · 213-226-7421

William A. Friedman · Professor of Stereotactic Neurosurgery, University of Florida College of Medicine · Shands Hospital at the University of Florida · 1600 Southwest Archer Road, Room M219, P.O. Box 100265, Gainesville, FL 32610 · 904-392-4331

Philip H. Gutin · (Neuro-oncology) · Professor of Neurological Surgery and Radiation Oncology, University of California at San Francisco School of Medicine · University of California at San Francisco Medical Center · 505 Parnassus Avenue, Box 0112, San Francisco, CA 94143-0112 · 415-476-1678

Peter Heilbrun · Professor and Head, Division of Neurosurgery, University of Utah School of Medicine · University of Utah Health Sciences Center · 50 North Medical Drive, Salt Lake City, UT 84132 · 801-581-6908

Patrick J. Kelly · (Neuro-oncology, Deep-Seated Brain Tumors) · Professor, Department of Neurologic Surgery, Mayo Medical School · Consultant, Department Neurologic Surgery, Mayo Clinic · 200 First Street, SW, Rochester, MN 55905 · 507-284-2816

L. Dade Lunsford · Professor of Neurological Surgery, Radiation Oncology and Radiology, University of Pittsburgh School of Medicine · Director, Specialized Neurosurgical Center, Presbyterian University Hospital; Montefiore University Hospital; Children's Hospital · 230 Lothrop Street, Room 9402, P.U.H., Pittsburgh, PA 15213 · 412-647-3685

Ladislau Steiner · Professor of Neurosurgery, Alumni Professor of Neurosurgery, Department of Neurological Surgery, University of Virginia School of Medicine · Director, Lars Leksell Center for Radiosurgery, University of Virginia Health Sciences Center · Hospital Drive, Room 1507, Charlottesville, VA 22980 · 804-924-5842

TRAUMA

Donald P. Becker · (Head Injury) · Professor and Chief, Division of Neurosurgery, University of California at Los Angeles School of Medicine · University of California at Los Angeles Center for the Health Sciences · 10833 LeConte Avenue, Mail Code 690118, Los Angeles, CA 90024-6901 · 310-825-5111

Lawrence F. Marshall · (Head Injury, Spinal Surgery, Complex Spine) · Professor of Surgery (Neurosurgery), University of California at San Diego School of Medicine · Chief, Neurosurgical Services, University of California at San Diego Medical Center · 225 Dickinson Street, San Diego, CA 92103-8893 · 619-543-5543

TUMOR SURGERY

Ossama Al-Mefty · (Skull-Base Surgery) · Professor of Surgery, Loyola Stritch School of Medicine · Loyola University Medical Center · 2160 South First Avenue, Division of Neurological Surgery, Maywood, IL 60153 · 708-216-8235

William F. Chandler · (Pituitary Surgery) · Professor of Neurosurgery, The University of Michigan Medical School · The University of Michigan Medical Center 2124 Taubman Center, 1500 East Medical Center Drive, Box 0338, Ann Arbor, MI 48109-0338 · 313-936-5020

Joseph H. Galicich · (Neuro-oncology) · Professor of Surgery, Cornell University Medical College · Chief, Neurosurgery Service, Memorial Sloan-Kettering Cancer Center · 1275 York Avenue, New York, NY 10021 · 212-639-7056

Philip H. Gutin · (Neuro-oncology) · Professor of Neurological Surgery and Radiation Oncology, University of California at San Francisco School of Medicine · University of California at San Francisco Medical Center · 505 Parnassus Avenue, Box 0112, San Francisco, CA 94143-0112 · 415-476-1678

Jules Hardy · (Pituitary Surgery) · Professor of Neurological Surgery, University of Montreal; McGill University · Consulting Neurosurgeon, Montreal General Hospital; Active Neurosurgeon, Notre Dame Hospital · 1560 Sherbrook Street East, Montreal, Quebec H2L 4M1 · 514-526-0419

Julian T. Hoff · (Acoustic Neuromas, Spinal Surgery) · Professor of Surgery, The University of Michigan Medical School · Chief, Section of Neurosurgery, The University of Michigan Medical Center · 1500 East Medical Center Drive, Box 0338, Ann Arbor, MI 48109-0338 · 313-936-5015

John A. Jane · (Craniofacial Surgery, Lumbar and Cervical Spine Surgery) · David D. Weaver Professor of Neurosurgery and Chairman of Neurological Surgery, University of Virginia School of Medicine · University of Virginia Health Sciences Center · Box 212, Charlottesville, VA 22908 · 804-924-8101

Peter J. Jannetta · (Acoustic Neuromas) · Professor and Chairman, Department of Neurological Surgery, University of Pittsburgh School of Medicine · Presbyterian University Hospital · 230 Lothrop Street, Room 9402 PUH, Pittsburgh, PA 15213 · 412-648-9248

Patrick J. Kelly · (Neuro-oncology, Deep-Seated Brain Tumors) · Professor, Department of Neurologic Surgery, Mayo Medical School · Consultant, Department Neurologic Surgery,Mayo Clinic · 200 First Street, SW, Rochester, MN 55905 · 507-284-2816

Edward R. Laws, Jr. · (Pituitary Surgery, Neuro-oncology) · Chairman, Department of Neurosurgery, The George Washington University School of Medicine · The George Washington University Medical Center · 2150 Pennsylvania Avenue, NW, Washington, DC 20037 · 202-994-4035

Donlin Long · (Pain Problems) · Professor and Director, Department of Neurosurgery, Johns Hopkins University School of Medicine · Neurosurgeon in Chief, The Johns Hopkins Medical Institutions · 600 North Wolfe Street, Baltimore, MD 21205 · 410-955-2252

Robert G. Ojemann · (Acoustic Neuromas, Meningiomas) · Professor of Surgery, Harvard Medical School · Massachusetts General Hospital · Department of Surgery, Boston, MA 02114 · 617-726-2936

Kalmon D. Post · (Pituitary Surgery) · Professor and Chairman, Department of Neurological Surgery, Mt. Sinai Medical Center · One Gustave Levy Place, Box 1136, New York, NY 10029 · 212-241-0933

James T. Robertson · Professor and Chairman, Department of Neurosurgery, The University of Tennessee at Memphis, College of Medicine · Chairman, Department of Neurosurgery, Baptist Memorial Hospital · 956 Court Avenue, Room A202, Memphis, TN 38163 · 901-528-6374

Laligam N. Sekhar · (Skull-Base Surgery) · Associate Professor of Neurosurgery, University of Pittsburgh School of Medicine · Co-Director, Center for Cranial Base Surgery, Presbyterian University Hospital · 230 Lothrup Street, Room 9402 PUH, Pittsburgh, PA 15213 · 412-647-6360

Bennett M. Stein · Byron Stookey Professor of Neurological Surgery, and Chairman, Department of Neurosurgery, College of Physicians & Surgeons of Columbia University · Director of Service, Neurological Institute of New York · 710 West 168th Street, Room 204, New York, NY 10032 · 212-305-5543

George T. Tindall · (Pituitary Surgery) · Professor of Surgery, and Chairman of Neurosurgery, Emory University School of Medicine · Chairman, Department of Neurosurgery, Emory University Affiliated Hospitals · 1327 Clifton Road, Atlanta, GA 30322 · 404-248-3391

Martin H. Weiss · (Pituitary Surgery) · Professor and Chairman, Department of Neurological Surgery, University of Southern California School of Medicine · Chief, Department of Neurological Surgery, The Los Angeles County + University of Southern California Medical Center; University of Southern California University Hospital · 1200 North State Street, Suite 5046, Los Angeles, CA 90033 · 213-226-7421

Charles B. Wilson · (Pituitary Surgery, Neuro-oncology) · Professor and Chairman, Department of Neurological Surgery, University of California at San Francisco School of Medicine · University of California at San Francisco Medical Center · 505 Parnassus Avenue, Room M-787, San Francisco, CA 94143-0112 · 415-476-1087

Nicholas T. Zervas · (Pituitary Surgery) · Higgins Professor of Neurosurgery, Harvard Medical School · Chief of Neurosurgery, Massachusetts General Hospital Fruit Street, White 502, Boston, MA 02114 · 617-726-8581

VASCULAR NEUROLOGICAL SURGERY

Robert M. Crowell · Associate Professor of Surgery, Harvard Medical School · Director of Cerebrovascular Surgery, Massachusetts General Hospital · 15 Parkman Street, ACC 312, Boston, MA 02114 · 617-726-5530

Arthur L. Day · Professor of Neurosurgery, University of Florida College of Medicine · Shands Hospital at the University of Florida · 1600 Southwest Archer Road, Room M215, P.O. Box J100265, Gainesville, FL 32610 · 904-392-4331

Charles G. Drake · (Aneurysms) · Professor of Neurological Surgery, The University of Western Ontario · University Hospital · 339 Windermere Road, London, Ontario N6A 5A5 · 519-663-3670

Eugene S. Flamm · (Aneurysms) · Charles Harrison Fraizer Professor and Chairman, Department of Neurosurgery, University of Pennsylvania School of Medicine · Hospital of the University of Pennsylvania · 3400 Spruce Street, Philadelphia, PA 19104 · 215-662-3483

Steven L. Giannotta · Professor, Department of Neurosurgery, University of Southern California School of Medicine · The Los Angeles County + University of Southern California Medical Center · 1200 North State Street, Room 5046, Los Angeles, CA 90033 · 213-226-7421

Roberto C. Heros · Lyle A. French Professor, and Head, Department of Neurosurgery, University of Minnesota School of Medicine · University of Minnesota Hospital & Clinics · 420 Delaware Street, SE, Minneapolis, MN 55455 · 612-626-0137

L. Nelson Hopkins · (Endovascular Neurosurgery) · Professor and Chairman, Department of Neurosurgery, State University of New York Health Science Center at Buffalo · Professor and Chairman, Department of Neurosurgery, Millard Fillmore Hospital · Three Gates Circle, Buffalo, NY 14209 · 716-887-5200, 887-5210

Richard B. Morawetz · Professor of Neurosurgery, The University of Alabama School of Medicine · Director, Division of Neurosurgery, The University of Alabama Hospital · 1813 Sixth Avenue South, MEB 512, Birmingham, AL 35294 · 205-934-7170

Sydney J. Peerless · Professor of Neurological Surgery, University of Miami School of Medicine · Director, Cerebrovascular Unit, University of Miami-Jackson Memorial Medical Center · 1501 Northwest Ninth Avenue, Miami, FL 33136 · 305-547-5896

David G. Piepgras · Professor, Department of Neurological Surgery, Mayo Medical School · Mayo Clinic · 200 First Street, SW, Rochester, MN 55905 · 507-284-3331

Donald O. Quest · (Carotid Artery Surgery) · Professor of Clinical Neurological Surgery, College of Physicians & Surgeons of Columbia University · Attending Neurological Surgery, Columbia-Presbyterian Medical Center; Neurological Institute of New York; Valley Hospital, Ridgewood, NJ · 710 West 168th Street, New York. NY 10032 · 212-305-5582

James T. Robertson · Professor and Chairman, Department of Neurosurgery, The University of Tennessee at Memphis, College of Medicine · Chairman, Department of Neurosurgery, Baptist Memorial Hospital · 956 Court Avenue, Room A202, Memphis, TN 38163 · 901-528-6374

Robert F. Spetzler · Professor, Section of Neurosurgery, The University of Arizona, Tucson · Director, The Barrow Neurological Institute; Chairman, Division of Neurological Surgery, The Barrow Neurological Institute at St. Joseph's Hospital & Medical Center · 2910 North Third Avenue, Phoenix, AZ 85013 · 602-285-3489

Bennett M. Stein · Byron Stookey Professor of Neurological Surgery, and Chairman, Department of Neurosurgery, College of Physicians & Surgeons of Columbia University · Director of Service, Neurological Institute of New York · 710 West 168th Street, Room 204, New York, NY 10032 · 212-305-5543

Thoralf M. Sundt · (Aneurysms) · Professor and Chairman, Department of Neurologic Surgery, Mayo Medical School · Mayo Clinic · 200 First Street, SW, Rochester, MN 55905 · 507-284-2611

Bryce K. A. Weir · Professor and Chief, Section of Neurosurgery, University of Chicago · Chief, Section of Neurosurgery, The University of Chicago Hospital · Section of Neurosurgery, 5841 South Maryland Avenue, Chicago, IL 60637 · 312-702-6158

Charles B. Wilson · Professor and Chairman, Department of Neurological Surgery, University of California at San Francisco School of Medicine · University of California at San Francisco Medical Center · 505 Parnassus Avenue, Room M-787, San Francisco, CA 94143-0112 · 415-476-1087

H. Richard Winn · Professor and Chairman of Neurological Surgery, University of Washington School of Medicine · Chief of Neurological Surgery, University of Washington Medical Center, and Harborview Medical Center; Children's Hospital and Medical Center · Department of Neurological Surgery, 325 Ninth Avenue (ZA-86), Seattle, WA 98104 · 206-223-3497

NEUROLOGY, ADULT

BEHAVIORAL NEUROLOGY

Martin Albert · (Geriatric Neurology, Language Disorders, Alzheimers) · Professor of Neurology, Boston University School of Medicine · Director, Behavioral Neurosciences, Boston Veterans Affairs Medical Center · Neurology Department (127), 150 South Huntington Avenue, Boston, MA 02130 · 617-232-9500

D. Frank Benson · (Language Disorders) · Augustus S. Rose Professor of Neurology, University of California, Los Angeles School of Medicine · University of California, Los Angeles Center for the Health Sciences · 710 Westwood Plaza, Los Angeles, CA 90024-1769 · 310-825-9873

Antonio Damasio · (Language Disorders, Memory Loss, Visual-Perceptual Disorders, Alzheimers) · Van Allen Professor and Head, Department of Neurology, The University of Iowa College of Medicine; The Salk Institute for Biological Studies · The University of Iowa Hospitals & Clinics · Iowa City, IA 52242 · 319-356-4295

Martha Bridge Denckla · (Specific Developmental Disabilities) · Professor of Neurology & Pediatrics, Johns Hopkins University School of Medicine · Director of Developmental Neurobehavior Clinic, and Director, Learning Disabilities Research Center, The Kennedy Institute · 707 North Broadway, Suite 501, Baltimore, MD 21205 · 410-550-9399

Albert M. Galaburda · (Developmental Dyslexia) · Associate Professor of Neurology, Harvard Medical School · Director, Dyslexia Neuroanatomical Laboratory, Beth Israel Hospital · Department of Neurology, 330 Brookline Avenue, Boston, MA 02215 · 617- 735-2698

Kenneth M. Heilman · (General, Apraxia, Memory Loss, Attentional Disorders, Language Disorders) · Professor of Neurology, University of Florida College of Medicine · Shands Hospital at the University of Florida · P.O. Box 100236, Gainesville, FL 32610-0236 · 904-392-3491

Marek-Marsel Mesulam · (General) · Professor of Neurology, Harvard Medical School · Director, Division of Neuroscience & Behavioral Neurology, Beth Israel Hospital · 330 Brookline Avenue, Boston, MA 02215 · 617-735-2075

Jonathan L. Pincus · (Violence) · Professor and Chairman, Department of Neurology, Georgetown University School of Medicine · Georgetown University Medical Center · 3800 Reservoir Road, NW, Washington, DC 20007 · 202-784-2170

CRITICAL CARE MEDICINE

Allan H. Ropper · Professor of Neurology, Tufts University School of Medicine · Chief, Division of Neurology, St. Elizabeth's Hospital of Boston · Division of Neurology, 736 Cambridge Street, Boston, MA 02135 · 617-789-3300

DEGENERATIVE DISEASES

Barry G.W. Arnason · (Amyotrophic Lateral Sclerosis) · Raymond Professor and Chairman, Department of Neurology, University of Chicago, Pritzker School of Medicine · Director, Brain Research Institute, University of Chicago Medical Center · 5841 South Maryland Avenue, Box 425, Chicago, IL 60637-1470 · 312-702-6222

Leonard Berg · (Alzheimer's) · Professor of Neurology, and Director, The Alzheimer's Disease Research Center, Washington University School of Medicine · Neurologist, Barnes Hospital · 660 South Euclid Avenue, Campus Box 8111-ADRC, St. Louis, MO 63110 · 314-362-2881

Robert H. Brown, Jr. · (Peripheral Nerve Disorders, Amyotrophic Lateral Sclerosis) · Associate Professor of Neurology, Harvard Medical School · Director, Day Neuromuscular Research Laboratory, Massachusetts General Hospital · Building 149, 13th Street, Charlestown, MA 02129 · 617-726-5750

Antonio Damasio · (Language Disorders, Memory Loss, Visual-Perceptual Disorders, Alzheimers) · Van Allen Professor and Head, Department of Neurology, The University of Iowa College of Medicine; The Salk Institute for Biological Studies · The University of Iowa Hospitals & Clinics · Iowa City, IA 52242 · 319-356-4295

David A. Drachman · (Geriatric Neurology, Alzheimers) · Professor and Chairman, Department of Neurology, University of Massachusetts Medical School · University of Massachusetts Medical Center · 55 Lake Avenue North, S5-753, Worcester, MA 01655 · 508-856-3081

Peter J. Dyck · (Peripheral Nerve Disorders, Motor-Neuron Disease) · Professor of Neurology, Mayo Medical School · Mayo Clinic · 200 First Street, SW, Rochester, MN 55905 · 507-284-3769

Sid Gilman · (Cerebellar Disease) · Professor and Chair, Department of Neurology, The University of Michigan Medical School · Chief of Services, Department of Neurology, The University of Michigan Medical Center · 1914 Taubman Center, 1500 East Medical Center Drive, Box 0316, Ann Arbor, MI 48109-0316 · 313-936-9070

John H. Growdon · (Alzheimers) · Associate Professor of Neurology, Harvard Medical School · Massachusetts General Hospital · 32 Fruit Street, ACC 7, Boston, MA 02114 · 617-726-1728

Robert Katzman · (Alzheimers) · Professor of Neurosciences, and Florence Riford Professor of Alzheimer's Disease Research, Department of Neurosciences, University of California at San Diego School of Medicine · Director, Alzheimers Disease Research Center, and Attending Neurologist, University of California at San Diego Medical Center · 9500 Gilman Drive, La Jolla, CA 92093-0624 · 619-534-1377

Richard Mayeux · (Alzheimer's Disease, Parkinson's Disease) · Professor of Neurology & Psychiatry, College of Physicians & Surgeons of Columbia University · Director, Gertrude H. Scrgievsky Center, Neurological Institute of New York · 710 West 168th Street, New York, NY 10032 · 212-305-5276

Peter J. Whitehouse · (Alzheimers) · Associate Professor, Department of Neurology, and Chief, Division of Behavioral & Geriatric Neurology, Case Western Reserve University School of Medicine · Director, Alzheimer Center, University Hospitals of Cleveland · 2074 Abington Road, Cleveland, OH 44106 · 216-844-7360

ELECTROMYOGRAPHY
(See also Physical Medicine & Rehabilitation, Electromyography)

James W. Albers · Professor, Department of Neurology, The University of Michigan Medical School · Director, Neuromuscular Program in the Department of Neurology, The University of Michigan Medical Center · 1500 East Medical Center Drive, 1C325 UH-0032, Ann Arbor, MI 48109 · 313-936-7165

Jasper R. Daube · Professor and Chair, Department of Neurology, Mayo Medical School · Mayo Clinic · 200 First Street, SW, Rochester, MN 55905 · 507-284-2675

Andrew Eisen · (Peripheral Nerve Disorders, Electrodiagnosis, Amyotrophic Lateral Sclerosis) · Professor of Neurology, The University of British Columbia · Head, Neuromuscular Disease Unit, Vancouver General Hospital · 855 West 12th Avenue, Vancouver, British Columbia V5Z 1M9 · 604-875-4405

Ludwig Gutmann · Professor and Chairman, Department of Neurology, West Virginia University School of Medicine · West Virginia University Health Sciences Center · 103G Health Sciences Center North, Morgantown, WV 26506 · 304-293-2342

Mark Hallett · (Movement Disorders) · Clinical Professor of Neurology, Uniformed Services University for the Health Sciences · Clinical Director, NINDS, National Institute of Neurological Disorders & Stroke, Division of Intramural Research, National Institutes of Health · 9000 Rockville Pike, Building 10, Room 5N226, Bethesda, MD 20892 · 301-496-1561

John Kelly · (Peripheral Neuropathies) · Professor and Chairman of Neurology, The George Washington University · Chairman, Department of Neurology, George Washington University Medical Center · 2150 Pennsylvania Avenue, NW, Seventh Floor, Room 404, Washington, DC 20037 · 202-994-4063

Robert T. Leshner · Professor of Neurology and Pediatrics, Virginia Commonwealth University, Medical College of Virginia · Medical College of Virginia Hospital · Medical College of Virginia, Box 211, Richmond, VA 23298-0211 · 804-786-0442

Janice M. Massey · Assistant Professor of Medicine, Duke University School of Medicine · Assistant Director, Electromyography Laboratory, Duke University Medical Center · P.O. Box 3403, Durham, NC 27710 · 919-684-5196

Robert Gordon Miller · Clinical Professor of Neurology, University of California at San Francisco School of Medicine · Chief, Clinical Neurology, California Pacific Medical Center · California Campus East, 3700 California Street, San Francisco, CA 94118 · 415-750-6040

Lawrence H. Phillips II · Associate Professor of Neurology, University of Virginia School of Medicine · University of Virginia Health Sciences Center · McKim Hall, Room 2001, Hospital Drive, Box 394, Charlottesville, VA 22908 · 804-924-5361

Donald B. Sanders · Duke University School of Medicine · Duke University Medical Center · Box 3403, DUMC, Durham, NC 27710 · 919-684-6078

Austin J. Sumner · (Peripheral Nerve Disorders) · Professor and Head of Neurology, Louisiana State University School of Medicine · Hotel Dieu Hospital; Charity Hospital of New Orleans · 1542 Tulane Avenue, Room 220, New Orleans, LA 70112 · 504-568-4082

Thomas R. Swift · Professor and Chairman, Department of Neurology, Medical College of Georgia · Department of Neurology, Augusta, GA 30912 · 404-721-4583

Asa J. Wilbourn · Associate Clinical Professor of Neurology, Case Western Reserve University School of Medicine · Director, EMG Laboratory, The Cleveland Clinic Foundation · Department of Neurology, 9500 Euclid Avenue, Cleveland, OH 44195 · 216-444-5548

EPILEPSY
(See also Neurological Surgery, Epilepsy Surgery)

Fredrick Anderman · Professor of Neurology and Pediatrics, McGill University · Director, Epilepsy Service, The Montreal Neurological Institute & Hospital · 3801 University Street, Montreal, Quebec H3A 2B4 · 514-398-1976

Thomas Reed Browne III · (Clinical Pharmacology, Electroencephalography) · Professor and Vice-Chairman of Neurology, Boston University School of Medicine Associate Chief of the Neurology Service, Boston Veterans Affairs Medical Center; University Hospital · 150 South Huntington Avenue, Neurology Service (127), Boston, MA 02130 · 617-739-3499

Fritz E. Dreifuss · Professor of Neurology and Vice-Chairman, Department of Neurology, University of Virginia School of Medicine · Director, Comprehensive Epilepsy Program, University of Virginia Health Sciences Center · Hospital Drive, Box 394, Charlottesville, VA 22908 · 804-924-5669

Jerome Engel, Jr. · Professor, Neurology and Anatomy & Cell Biology, University of California, Los Angeles School of Medicine · Chief, Division of Epilepsy & Clinical Neurophysiology, University of California, Los Angeles Center for the Health Sciences · Reed Neurological Research Center, 710 Westwood Plaza, Room 1250, Los Angeles, CA 90024-1769 · 310-825-5745

Ilo E. Leppik · Clinical Professor of Neurology & Pharmacy Practice, University of Minnesota School of Medicine · Director of Research, MINCEP Epilepsy Care, University of Minnesota Hospital & Clinics · 420 Delaware Street SE, Box 295 UMHC, Minneapolis, MN 55455 · 612-525-2400

Hans O. Lüders · (Electroencephalography) · Chairman, Department of Neurology, The Cleveland Clinic Foundation · One Clinic Center, 9500 Euclid Avenue, S90, Cleveland, OH 44106 · 216-444-5530

Richard Mattson · Professor, Department of Neurology, Yale University School of Medicine · Yale-New Haven Hospital · 333 Cedar Street, Room 702LCI, New Haven, CT 06510 · 203-785-4085

Timothy A. Pedley · Professor and Vice Chairman, Department of Neurology, College of Physicians & Surgeons of Columbia University · Director, Comprehensive Epilepsy Center; Associate Director, Neurology Service, Columbia-Presbyterian Medical Center · Neurological Institute, 710 West 168th Street, New York, NY 10032 · 212-305-6489

James Kiffin Penry · Professor of Neurology, and Senior Associate Dean for Research Development, The Bowman Gray School of Medicine of Wake Forest University · North Carolina Baptist Hospital · Research Development, Medical Center Boulevard, Winston-Salem, NC 27157-1023 · 919-748-2382

Roger J. Porter · Deputy Director, National Institute of Neurological Disorders & Stroke, National Institutes of Health · 9000 Rockville Pike, Building 31, Room 8A52, Bethesda, MD 20892 · 301-496-3167

David M. Treiman · Professor of Neurology, University of California at Los Angeles School of Medicine · Co-Director, Department of Veterans Affairs, Southwest Regional Epilepsy Center; Director, Neuropharmacology Research Laboratories, DVA West Los Angeles Medical Center; Reed Neurological Research Center · 710 Westwood Plaza, Los Angeles, CA 90024 · 213-824-4371

GENERAL ADULT NEUROLOGY

Arthur K. Asbury · (Peripheral Nerve Disorders) · Van Meter Professor of Neurology, and Vice Dean for Research, School of Medicine, University of Pennsylvania School of Medicine · Hospital of the University of Pennsylvania · Gates Building, 3400 Spruce Street, Third Floor, Philadelphia, PA 19104-4283 · 215-662-2629

John C. M. Brust · Professor of Clinical Neurology, College of Physicians & Surgeons of Columbia University · Director, Department of Neurology, Harlem Hospital Center · Department of Neurology, 506 Lennox Avenue, New York, NY 10029 · 212-491-1470

John R. Calverley · Warmoth Professor and Chairman, Department of Neurology, The University of Texas Medical Branch at Galveston · University of Texas Medical Branch, Galveston, TX 77550 · 409-772-2646

John J. Caronna · Professor of Clinical Neurology, Cornell University Medical College · The New York Hospital-Cornell Medical Center · 525 East 68th Street, New York, NY 10021 · 212-746-2304

Robert C. Collins · Professor and Chairman, Department of Neurology, University of California at Los Angeles School of Medicine · University of California at Los Angeles Center for the Health Sciences · 10833 LeConte Avenue, 710 Westwood Plaza, Los Angeles, CA 90024 · 310-825-5521

James N. Hayward · N. Houston Merritt Distinguished Professor and Chair, Department of Neurology, University of North Carolina School of Medicine · Attending Physician, University of North Carolina Hospitals · 751 Clinical Sciences Building, Campus Box 7025, Chapel Hill, NC 27599-7025 · 919-966-2526

William M. Landau · Professor of Neurology, Washington University School of Medicine · Barnes Hospital · Box 8111, 660 South Euclid Avenue, St. Louis, MO 63110 · 314-362-4985

Elliott L. Mancall · Professor and Chairman, Department of Neurology, Hahnemann University · Hahnemann Hospital · Broad & Vine Streets, MS423, Philadelphia, PA 19119 · 215-448-8092

E. Wayne Massey · Professor of Neurology, Duke University School of Medicine Duke University Medical Center · Box 3909, Durham, NC 27710 · 919-684-5816

John C. Mazziotta · (Nuclear Medicine, Positron Emission Tomography [PET]) Professor of Neurology and Radiological Sciences, University of California at Los Angeles School of Medicine · Vice-Chairman, Department of Neurology, and Head of the Neuroscience Section, Division of Nuclear Medicine, University of California at Los Angeles Medical Center · 10833 LeConte Avenue, B2-085, Los Angeles, CA 90024-1769 · 310-825-2699

George W. Paulson · Professor, Department of Neurology, Ohio State University College of Medicine · The Ohio State University Hospitals · 1654 Upham Drive, Room 443, Columbus, OH 43210 · 614-293-4963

Fred Plum · Professor and Chairman, Department of Neurology & Neuroscience, Cornell University Medical College · Neurologist-in-Chief, The New York Hospital-Cornell Medical Center · Department of Neurology & Neuroscience, 525 East 68th Street, New York, NY 10021 · 212-746-6141

Jerome B. Posner · (Cancer in the Nervous System) · Chairman, Department of Neurology, Memorial Sloan-Kettering Cancer Center · 1275 York Avenue, New York, NY 10021 · 212-639-7047

Thomas Daniel Sabin · Professor of Neurology & Psychiatry, Boston University School of Medicine · Chief of Neurology, Boston City Hospital · Medical Building, 818 Harrison Avenue, Ninth Floor, Boston, MA 02118 · 617-534-5230

Martin A. Samuels · Associate Professor of Neurology, Harvard Medical School · Chief of Neurology, Brigham & Women's Hospital · 75 Francis Street, Boston, MA 02115 · 617-732-5500

Burton A. Sandok · Professor of Neurology, and Dean, Mayo Medical School · Consultant, Department of Neurology,Mayo Clinic · 200 First Street, SW, Rochester, MN 55905 · 507-284-3334

HEADACHE
(See also Psychiatry, Headache)

J. Keith Campbell · Associate Professor of Neurology, Mayo Medical School · Mayo Clinic · 200 First Street, SW, Rochester, MN 55905 · 507-284-3334

John Gordon Edmeads · Professor of Medicine (Neurology), University of Toronto School of Medicine · Head of Neurology, Sunnybrook Health Science Center 2075 Bayview Avenue, Room A460, Toronto, Ontario M4N 3M5 · 416-480-4516

Ninan T. Mathew · Clinical Professor of Restorative Neurology & Neurobiology, Baylor College of Medicine · Director, Houston Headache Clinic · 1213 Hermann Drive, Suite 350, Houston, TX 77004 · 713-528-1916

Alan Mark Rapoport · Assistant Clinical Professor of Neurology, Yale University School of Medicine · Chief, Department of Neurology, Greenwich Hospital · The New England Center for Headache, 778 Long Ridge Road, Stamford, CT 06902 203-968-1799

Neil H. Raskin · (Facial Pain) · Professor and Vice-Chairman, Department of Neurology, University of California at San Francisco School of Medicine · University of California at San Francisco Medical Center · 505 Parnassus Avenue, Room 794 Moffitt, Box 0114, San Francisco, CA 94143-0114 · 415-476-1487

Joel R. Saper · Professor of Neurology, The University of Michigan Medical School · Director,, Michigan Head Pain & Neurological Institute · 3120 Professional Drive, Ann Arbor, MI 48109 · 313-973-1155

Stephen David Silberstein · Associate Professor of Neurology, Temple University School of Medicine · Germantown Hospital · One Penn Boulevard, Philadelphia, PA 19144 · 215-843-5070

Seymour Solomon · Professor of Neurology, Albert Einstein College of Medicine Director, Headache Unit, Montefiore Medical Center · 111 East 210th Street, Bronx, NY 10467 · 212-920-4203

K. Michael A. Welch · Adjunct Professor of Medical Physics, Oakland University, Rochester, MI; Professor of Clinical Neurology, University of Michigan, Ann Arbor · William T. Gossett Chair, Department of Neurology, and Vice-President for Academic Affairs, Henry Ford Medical Center · 2799 West Grand Boulevard, Detroit, MI 48202 · 313-876-3396

INFECTIOUS & DEMYELINATING DISEASES
(See also Infectious Disease)

Jack P. Antel · (Multiple Sclerosis, Degenerative Diseases) · Chairman, Department of Neurology & Neurosurgery, McGill University · Neurologist-in-Chief, The Montreal Neurological Institute & Hospital · 3801 University Street, Montreal, Quebec H3A 2B4 · 514-398-8531

Barry G. W. Arnason · (Multiple Sclerosis, Virology, Neuroimmunology) · Raymond Professor and Chairman, Department of Neurology, University of Chicago, Pritzker School of Medicine · Director, Brain Research Institute, University of Chicago Medical Center · 5841 South Maryland Avenue, Box 425, Chicago, IL 60637-1470 · 312-702-6222

Richard J. Baringer · (Infectious Diseases) · Professor of Neurology, University of Utah School of Medicine · University of Utah Health Sciences Center · 50 North Medical Drive, Salt Lake City, UT 84132 · 801-581-4283

Joseph R. Berger · (AIDS) · Professor of Neurology and Internal Medicine, University of Miami School of Medicine · Jackson Memorial Medical Center; University of Miami Hospital & Clinics · National Parkinson Foundation, 1501 Northwest Ninth Avenue, Second Floor, Miami, FL 33136 · 305-547-6732

Gary Birnbaum · (Multiple Sclerosis) · Professor of Neurology, University of Minnesota School of Medicine · Director, Multiple Sclerosis Research & Treatment Center, University of Minnesota Hospital & Clinics · Harvard Street at East River Road, Minneapolis, MN 55455 · 612-625-2633

Benjamin R. Brooks · (Multiple Sclerosis, Neuromuscular Disease) · Professor of Neurology, University of Wisconsin-Madison School of Medicine · Director, ALS Clinic and Neuromuscular Clinic, University of Wisconsin Hospital & Clinics; Chief, Neurology Service, William S. Middleton Memorial Veterans Affairs Hospital · 600 Highland Avenue, Clinical Science Center, H6-558, Madison, WI 53792-5132 · 608-263-5421, 262-7090

Jonathan L. Carter · (Multiple Sclerosis) · Assistant Professor of Neurology, Mayo Medical School, and Mayo Graduate School of Medicine · Mayo Clinic · 13400 East Shea Boulevard, Scottsdale, AZ 85259 · 602-391-8111

Larry E. Davis · (Multiple Sclerosis, Infectious Diseases) · Professor of Neurology and Microbiology, and Vice-Chairman of Neurology, The University of New Mexico School of Medicine · Chief, Neurology Service, Veterans Affairs Medical Center · 2100 Ridgecrest Drive SE, Neurology Service (127), Albuquerque, NM 87108 · 505-256-2752

George Cornell Ebers · (Multiple Sclerosis) · Professor of Neurology, the University of Western Ontario · Director of Multiple Sclerosis Clinic, University Hospital · 339 Windermere Road, London, Ontario N6A 5A5 · 519-663-3656

George W. Ellison · (Multiple Sclerosis) · Professor of Neurology, University of California at Los Angeles School of Medicine · University of California at Los Angeles Center for the Health Sciences · 10833 LeConte Avenue, Los Angeles, CA 90024-1769 · 310-825-7313, 794-1212

Robert A. Fishman · (Infectious Diseases, Metabolic Disorders) · Professor and Chairman, Department of Neurology, University of California at San Francisco School of Medicine · University of California at San Francisco Medical Center · 505 Parnassus Avenue, Room 794 Moffitt, Box 0114, San Francisco, CA 94143-0114 · 415-476-1487

Donald H. Gilden · (Degenerative Diseases, Multiple Sclerosis, Infectious Disease) · Professor and Chairman, Department of Neurology, and Professor of Microbiology and Immunology, University of Colorado School of Medicine · University of Colorado Health Sciences Center · 4200 East Ninth Avenue, Box B-182, Denver, CO 80262 · 303-270-8281

Donald E. Goodkin · (Multiple Sclerosis) · The Cleveland Clinic Foundation · One Clinic Center, 9500 Euclid Avenue, U-10, Cleveland, OH 44195-5244 · 216-444-8623

Stephen L. Hauser · (Multiple Sclerosis) · Associate Professor of Neurology, Harvard Medical School · Director, Neuroimmunology Unit, Massachusetts General Hospital · 32 Fruit Street, Boston, MA 02114 · 617-726-3787

Robert Herndon · (Multiple Sclerosis) · Professor of Neurology, Oregon Health Sciences University · Chief, Department of Neurology, Good Samaritan Hospital & Medical Center · 1040 Northwest 22nd Avenue, Suite N460, Portland, OR 97210 · 503-229-8441

Kenneth P. Johnson · (Multiple Sclerosis) · Professor and Chairman, Department of Neurology, University of Maryland School of Medicine · University of Maryland Medical Center · 22 South Greene Street, Room N4W46, Baltimore, MD 21201 · 301-328-6484

Richard T. Johnson · (Viral Infections of the Nervous System, Degenerative Diseases, Infectious Diseases, Multiple Sclerosis) · Professor and Director, Department of Neurology, Johns Hopkins University School of Medicine · Chief, Division of Neurology, The Johns Hopkins Medical Institutions · 600 North Wolfe Street, Meyer Building, Room 6113, Baltimore, MD 21205 · 410-955-5103

Robert P. Lisak · (Multiple Sclerosis) · Professor and Chairman, Department of Neurology, Wayne State University School of Medicine · Chief of Neurology, Detroit Medical Center; Harper Hospital · 4201 St. Antoine Boulevard, 6E UHC, Detroit, MI 48201 · 313-577-1249

Justin C. McArthur · (AIDS) · Associate Professor of Neurology, Johns Hopkins University School of Medicine · The Johns Hopkins Medical Institutions · 600 North Wolfe Street, Meyer 6-109, Baltimore, MD 21205 · 410-955-3730

Dale E. McFarlin · (Multiple Sclerosis) · Chief, Neuroimmunology Branch, National Institute of Neurological Disorders & Strokes, Division of Intramural Research, National Institutes of Health · 9000 Rockville Pike, Building 10, Room 5B16, Bethesda, MD 20892 · 301-496-1561

Aaron E. Miller · (Multiple Sclerosis) · Associate Professor of Clinical Neurology, State University of New York Health Science Center at Brooklyn · Director, Division of Neurology, Maimonides Medical Center · 4802 Tenth Avenue, Brooklyn, NY 11219 · 718-283-7470

Lawrence W. Myers · (Multiple Sclerosis) · Adjunct Professor of Neurology, University of California at Los Angeles School of Medicine · University of California at Los Angeles Medical Center · 10833 LeConte Avenue, Los Angeles, CA 90024-1769 · 310-825-7313

John H. Noseworthy · (Multiple Sclerosis) · Associate Professor of Neurology, Mayo Medical School · Mayo Clinic · 200 First Street, SW, Rochester, MN 55905 507-284-8533

Donald W. Paty · (Multiple Sclerosis) · Professor and Head, Division of Neurology, The University of British Columbia · Vancouver General Hospital · 2775 Heather Street, Suite 222, Vancouver, British Columbia V5Z 3J5 · 604-875-4108

Jack H. Petajan · (Multiple Sclerosis) · Professor of Neurology, University of Utah School of Medicine · University of Utah Health Sciences Center · 50 North Medical Drive, 3R210 Medical Center, Salt Lake City, UT 84132 · 801-581-2121

Richard W. Price · (AIDS) · Professor and Head, Department of Neurology, University of Minnesota School of Medicine · University of Minnesota Hospital & Clinics · 420 Delaware Street, SE, Box 295, Minneapolis, MN 55455 · 612-625-8983

Moses Rodriguez · (Multiple Sclerosis) · Professor of Neurology, Mayo Medical School · The Mayo Clinic · 200 First Street, SW, Rochester, MN 55905 · 507-284-8533

Richard A. Rudick · (Multiple Sclerosis, Neuroimmunologic Diseases) · Director, Mellen Center for Multiple Sclerosis Treatment & Research, The Cleveland Clinic Foundation · One Clinic Center, 9500 Euclid Avenue, Area U-10, Cleveland, OH 44195-5244 · 216-444-8603

Randall T. Schapiro · (Multiple Sclerosis) · Clinical Professor of Neurology, University of Minnesota School of Medicine · Director of Rehabilitation & Multiple Sclerosis, Fairview Multiple Sclerosis Center, Riverside Medical Center · Riverside and 25th Avenue, Minneapolis, MN 55454 · 612-588-0661

Labe C. Scheinberg · (Neuro Rehabilitation, Multiple Sclerosis) · Professor of Neurology, Rehabilitation and Psychiatry, Albert Einstein College of Medicine · Multiple Sclerosis Care Center · Nurses Residence, 1300 Morris Park Avenue, Bronx, NY 10461 · 212-430-2682

William A. Sibley · (Multiple Sclerosis) · Professor of Neurology, The University of Arizona College of Medicine · The University of Arizona Health Sciences Center · 1501 North Campbell Avenue, Tucson, AZ 85724 · 602-626-4541

Stanley van den Noort · (Multiple Sclerosis) · Professor and Chairman of Department of Neurology, University of California at Irvine School of Medicine · University of California at Irvine Medical Center · 107 Whitby Building, Irvine, CA 92717 · 714-856-5692

John N. Whitaker · (Multiple Sclerosis) · Chairman, Department of Neurology, The University of Alabama School of Medicine · Neurologist-in-Chief, University of Alabama Hospital; Birmingham Veterans Medical Center · Department of Neurology, University Hospital, University Station, Birmingham, AL 35294 · 205-934-2402

Leslie P. Wiener · (Degenerative Diseases, Infectious Diseases, Neurovirology) · Professor and Chairman, Department of Neurology and Micropbiology, University of Southern California School of Medicine · Chief of Neurology, The Los Angeles County + University of Southern California Medical Center; University of Southern California University Hospital · 1510 San Pablo Street, Suite 618, Los Angeles, CA 90033-4606 · 213-342-5710

Jerry S. Wolinsky · (Neurovirology, Multiple Sclerosis, Infectious Diseases) · Professor of Neurology, The University of Texas Health Science Center at Houston · Hermann Hospital · 6431 Fannin Street, Suite 7044, Houston, TX 77030 · 713-792-5777

MAGNETIC RESONANCE IMAGING
(See also Cardiovascular Disease, Magnetic Resonance Imaging; Radiology, Magnetic Resonance Imaging)

Jack O. Greenberg · Professor of Neurology, Medical College of Pennsylvania · Medical Director, Northeastern Magnetic Imaging Center · Neurological Associates, 7901 Buftleton Avenue, Suite 204, Philadelphia, PA 19152 · 215-333-0530

Donald B. Calne · (Parkinson's Disease) · Professor of Neurology, The University of British Columbia · Director, Neurodegenerative Disorders Centre, University Hospital · 2211 Wesbrook Mall, Vancouver, British Columbia V6T 1W5 · 604-822-7660

Stanley Fahn · (Parkinson's Disease, Dystonia, Tardive Dyskinesia, Myoclonus) H. Houston Merritt Professor of Neurology, College of Physicians & Surgeons of Columbia University · Attending Neurologist and Chief, Movement Disorder Clinic, and Director, Dystonia Clinical Research Center, Neurological Institute of New York · 710 West 168th Street, New York, NY 10032 · 212-305-5277

Sid Gilman · (Cerebellar Disease) · Professor and Chair, Department of Neurology, The University of Michigan Medical School · Chief of Services, Department of Neurology, The University of Michigan Medical Center · 1914 Taubman Center, 1500 East Medical Center Drive, Box 0316, Ann Arbor, MI 48109-0316 · 313-936-9070

Christopher G. Goetz · (Parkinson's Disease) · Associate Chairman, Department of Neurological Sciences, Rush-Presbyterian-St. Luke's Medical Center · 1725 West Harrison, Suite 1106, Chicago, IL 60612 · 312-942-5936

Joseph Jankovic · Professor of Neurology, Baylor College of Medicine · Senior Attending, The Methodist Hospital · 6550 Fannin Street, Suite 1801, Houston, TX 77030 · 713-798-5998

William C. Koller · (Tremor, Parkinson's Disease) · Professor and Chairman, Department of Neurology, University of Kansas School of Medicine · University of Kansas Medical Center · 39th and Rainbow Boulevard, Kansas City, KS 66103 913-588-6094

Anthony E. Lang · (Parkinson's Disease, Dystonia) · Associate Professor, University of Toronto School of Medicine · Director, Movement Disorders Clinic, The Toronto Hospital · 399 Bathurst Street, 11th Floor, Main Pavilion, Room 304, Toronto, Ontario M5T 2S8 · 416-369-6422

J. William Langston · (Parkinson's Disease) · President & Founder, California Parkinson Foundation · 2444 Morpark Avenue, Suite 316, San Jose, CA 95128 · 408-998-2722

Joseph B. Martin · (Huntington's Disease) · Professor of Neurology and Dean, School of Medicine, University of California at San Francisco School of Medicine University of California at San Francisco Medical Center · 503 Parnassus Avenue, Room S-224, San Francisco, CA 94143 · 415-476-2341

C. Warren Olanow · Professor of Neurology, and Professor of Pharmacology & Experimental Therapeutics, University South Florida College of Medicine · Tampa General Hospital · 4 Columbia Drive, Suite 410, Tampa, FL 33606 · 813-253-4455

Ira Shoulson · (Huntington's Disease, Parkinson's Disease) · Professor of Neurology, Pharmacology & Medicine, University of Rochester School of Medicine & Dentistry · Strong Memorial Hospital, University of Rochester Medical Center · 601 Elmwood Avenue, Rochester, NY 14642 · 716-275-5130

Anne B. Young · (Huntington's Disease) · Julieanne Dorn Professor of Neurology, Harvard Medical School · Chief, Neurology Service, Massachusetts General Hospital · Department of Neurology, 32 Fruit Street, Boston, MA 02114 · 617-726-2383

NEURO REHABILITATION

Fletcher H. McDowell · Associate Dean & Professor of Neurology, Cornell University Medical College · Executive Medical Director, Burke Rehabilitation Hospital; Attending Neurologist, The New York Hospital-Cornell Medical Center · 785 Mamaroneck Avenue, White Plains, NY 10605 · 914-948-0050

Steven P. Ringel · Professor of Neurology and Director, Neuromuscular Division, University of Colorado School of Medicine · University of Colorado Health Sciences Center · 4200 East Ninth Avenue, Box B-185, Denver, CO 80262 · 303-270-7221

NEURO-OPHTHALMOLOGY
(See also Ophthalmology, Neuro-Ophthalmology)

Ronald M. Burde · Professor of Ophthalmology and Neurology and Neurological Surgery, Albert Einstein College of Medicine · Chairman, Department of Ophthalmology & Visual Sciences, Montefiore Medical Center · 111 East 210th Street, Bronx, NY 10467 · 212-920-6665

Thomas J. Carlow · Adjunct Professor of Neurology, The University of New Mexico School of Medicine · 101 Hospital Loop NE, Suite 103, Albuquerque, NM 87109 · 505-883-6800

James J. Corbett · Professor and Chairman, Department of Neurology, and Professor of Ophthalmology, University of Mississippi · University of Mississippi Medical Center · Department of Neurology, 2500 North State Street, Jackson, MS 39216 · 601-984-5500

Robert B. Daroff · (Eye Movements) · The Gilbert W. Humphrey Professor and Chairman, Department of Neurology, Case Western Reserve University School of Medicine · Director, Department of Neurology, University Hospitals of Cleveland Department of Neurology, 2074 Abington Road, Cleveland, OH 44106 · 216-844-3193

Bradley K. Farris · Associate Professor of Ophthalmology, and Adjunct Associate Professor of Neurosurgery and Neurology, The University of Oklahoma College of Medicine · Neuro-Ophthalmologist, Dean A. McGee Eye Institute, and The University of Oklahoma Health Sciences Center · 608 Stanton L. Young Boulevard, Suite 205, Oklahoma City, OK 73104 · 405-271-6463

Steven L. Galetta · Assistant Professor of Neurology and Ophthalmology, University of Pennsylvania School of Medicine · Hospital of the University of Pennsylvania · Gates Building, 3400 Spruce Street, Third Floor, Philadelphia, PA 19104 · 215-662-3381

Joel S. Glaser · Professor of Ophthalmology, Neurology & Neurosurgery, University of Miami School of Medicine · Director, Neuro-Ophthalmology Unit, Bascom Palmer Eye Institute; Anne Bates Leach Eye Hospital · 900 Northwest 17th Street, Miami, FL 33136 · 305-326-6193

James A. Goodwin · Associate Professor of Neurology and Ophthalmology, The University of Illinois College of Medicine at Chicago · Director, Neuro-Ophthalmology Service, The University of Illinois Eye Center & Visual Sciences · 1855 West Taylor Street, Suite 144, Chicago, IL 60612 · 312-996-9120

Thomas R. Hedges III · Associate Professor of Ophthalmology & Neurology, Tufts University School of Medicine · Director, Neuro-ophthalmology Service, New England Medical Center · 750 Washington Street, Box 381, Boston, MA 02111 · 617-956-5488

William Hoyt · Professor of Ophthalmology, Neurology & Neurosurgery, University of California at San Francisco School of Medicine · Neuro-ophthalmology Unit, 533 Parnassus Avenue, Room U-125, San Francisco, CA 94143 · 415-476-1130

James R. Keane · Professor of Neurology, University of Southern California School of Medicine · The Los Angeles County + University of Southern California Medical Center · 1200 North State Street, Room 5640, Los Angeles, CA 90033 · 213-226-7381

Lanning B. Kline · Professor of Neuro-Ophthalmology, The University of Alabama School of Medicine · Eye Foundation Hospital; The University of Alabama Hospital · 1600 Seventh Avenue South, Suite 555, Birmingham, AL 35233 · 205-939-9778

Mark J. Kupersmith · Professor of Neurology & Ophthalmology, New York University School of Medicine · New York University Medical Center; New York Eye & Ear Infirmary · 530 First Avenue, Suite 3B, New York, NY 10016 · 212-263-7429

Patrick J. Lavin · Associate Professor, Vanderbilt University School of Medicine Vanderbilt University Medical Center · 2100 Pierce Avenue, #351, Nashville, TN 37212 · 615-322-3461

Simmons Lessell · Professor of Ophthalmology, Harvard Medical School · Director of Neuro-Ophthalmology, Massachusetts Eye & Ear Infirmary · 243 Charles Street, Boston, MA 02114 · 617-573-3412

John A. McCrary III · Professor of Ophthalmology, Neurology, & Neurosurgery, Baylor College of Medicine · Cullen Eye Institute · 6501 Fannin Street, NC-200, Houston, TX 77030 · 713-798-4914

Neil R. Miller · Professor of Ophthalmology, Johns Hopkins University School of Medicine · The Johns Hopkins Medical Institutions · 600 North Wolfe Street, Maumenee B-109, Baltimore, MD 21205 · 410-955-8679

Nancy J. Newman · Assistant Professor of Ophthalmology and Neurology, Emory University School of Medicine · Director, Neuro-ophthalmology Unit, Emory University Affiliated Hospitals · 1327 Clifton Road NE, Suite 4305, Atlanta, GA 30322 404-248-5360

Peter J. Savino · Professor of Ophthalmology at Jefferson Medical College; Clinical Professor of Ophthalmology, University of Pennsylvania School of Medicine · Chairman, Department of Ophthalmology, Graduate Hospital; Director, Neuro-Ophthalmology Service, Wills Eye Hospital · 900 Walnut Street, Philadelphia, PA 19107 · 215-928-3130

John B. Selhorst · Professor and Chairman, Department of Neurology, and Professor of Ophthalmology, St. Louis University School of Medicine · St. Louis University Medical Center · 3635 Vista Avenue at Grand Boulevard, St. Louis, MO 63110-0250 · 314-577-8026

James A. Sharpe · Professor and Head of Neurology, University of Toronto Faculty of Medicine · Head, Division of Neurology, and Director, Neuro-Ophthalmology Unit, The Toronto Hospital · 399 Bathurst Street, EC6-022, Toronto, Ontario M5T 2S8 · 416-369-5950

J. Lawton Smith · Professor of Ophthalmology, University of Miami School of Medicine · Bascom Palmer Eye Institute · 900 Northwest 17th Street, Miami, FL 33136 · 305-326-6128

Jonathan D. Trobe · Professor of Ophthalmology and Associate Professor of Neurology, The University of Michigan Medical School · Director, Neuro-Ophthalmology Service, W.K. Kellogg Eye Center, The University of Michigan Medical Center · 1000 Wall Street, Room 645, Ann Arbor, MI 48105 · 313-763-9147

B. Todd Troost · Professor and Chairman, Department of Neurology, The Bowman Gray School of Medicine of Wake Forest University · North Carolina Baptist Hospital · Medical Center Boulevard, Winston-Salem, NC 27157-1078 · 919-748-3429

Michael Wall · Associate Professor of Neurology, The University of Iowa College of Medicine · The University of Iowa Hospitals & Clinics · 200 Hawkins Drive, Iowa City, IA 52242-1009 · 319-356-2932

Jonathan D. Wirtschafter · (Optic Nerve Compressions, Graves Disease, Eyelid Spasms) · Professor of Ophthalmology and Neurology, University of Minnesota School of Medicine · Director, Neuro-ophthalmology, Orbit & Oculoplastic Service, University of Minnesota Hospital & Clinics · 516 Delaware SE, Box 493, Minneapolis, MN 55455 · 612-625-4400

Shirley H. Wray · Associate Professor of Neurology, Harvard Medical School · Director, Unit for Neurovisual Disorders, Massachusetts General Hospital · 15 Parkman Street, Suite ACC-837, Boston, MA 02114 · 617-726-5537

Robert D. Yee · Professor and Chairman, Department of Ophthalmology, Indiana University School of Medicine · Indiana University Medical Center · 702 Rotary Circle, Room 344, Indianapolis, IN 46202 · 317-274-7101

NEUROGENETICS

Thomas D. Bird · Professor of Medicine, and Professor of Neurology and Medical Genetics, University of Washington School of Medicine · Chief, Neurology Service, Department of Veterans Affairs Medical Center · Neurology (127), 1660 South Columbian Way, Seattle, WA 98108 · 206-764-2021

Roger N. Rosenberg · Professor and Chairman, Department of Neurology, The University of Texas Southwestern Medical Center at Dallas · 5323 Harry Hines Boulevard, Dallas, TX 75235 · 214-688-3239

NEUROMUSCULAR DISEASE

Arthur K. Asbury · (Peripheral Nerve Disorders) · Van Meter Professor of Neurology, and Vice Dean for Research, School of Medicine, University of Pennsylvania School of Medicine · Hospital of the University of Pennsylvania · Gates Building, 3400 Spruce Street, Third Floor, Philadelphia, PA 19104-4283 · 215-662-2629

Walter G. Bradley · (Peripheral Nerve Disorders, Memory Disorders, Dementia) Professor and Chairman, Department of Neurology, University of Miami School of Medicine · Chief, Neurology Service, University of Miami-Jackson Memorial Medical Center · 1501 Northwest Ninth Avenue, P.O. Box 016960, Miami, FL 33101 · 305-547-6718

Michael H. Brooke · Professor of Neurology, University of Alberta · Director, Division of Neurology, Walter C. Mackenzie Health Sciences Center · 8440 One Hundred Twelfth Street, 2E3-12, Edmonton, Alberta T6G 2B7 · 403-492-8822

Robert H. Brown, Jr. · (Peripheral Nerve Disorders, Amyotrophic Lateral Sclerosis) · Associate Professor of Neurology, Harvard Medical School · Director, Day Neuromuscular Research Laboratory, Massachusetts General Hospital · Building 149, 13th Street, Charlestown, MA 02129 · 617-726-5750

David Michael Dawson · (Peripheral Nerve Disorders) · Professor of Neurology, Harvard Medical School · Chief of Neurology, Brockton-West Roxbury Veterans Affairs Medical Center · 45 Francis Street, Boston, MA 02115 · 617-732-5771

Peter J. Dyck · (Peripheral Nerve Disorders, Motor-Neuron Disease) · Professor of Neurology, Mayo Medical School · Mayo Clinic · 200 First Street, SW, Rochester, MN 55905 · 507-284-3769

Andrew Eisen · (Peripheral Nerve Disorders, Electrodiagnosis, Amyotrophic Lateral Sclerosis) · Professor of Neurology, The University of British Columbia · Head, Neuromuscular Disease Unit, Vancouver General Hospital · 855 West 12th Avenue, Vancouver, British Columbia V5Z 1M9 · 604-875-4405

Andrew G. Engel · 3M—McKnight Professor of Neuroscience, Mayo Medical School · Director, Neuromuscular Research Laboratory, Mayo Clinic · 200 First Street, SW, Rochester, MN 55905 · 507-284-5102

John W. Griffin · (Peripheral Nerve Disorders) · Professor and Associate Director, Department of Neurology, Johns Hopkins University School of Medicine · The Johns Hopkins Medical Institutions · 600 North Wolfe Street, Meyer 6-109, Baltimore, MD 21205 · 410-955-2227

Robert C. Griggs · Professor and Chairman, Department of Neurology, University of Rochester School of Medicine & Dentistry · Strong Memorial Hospital, University of Rochester Medical Center · Department of Neurology, 601 Elmwood Avenue, Box 673, Rochester, NY 14642 · 716-275-6375

Ludwig Gutmann · Professor and Chairman, Department of Neurology, West Virginia University School of Medicine · West Virginia University Health Sciences Center · 103G Health Sciences Center North, Morgantown, WV 26506 · 304-293-2342

George Karpati · Isaac Walton Killam Professor of Neurology and Professor of Pediatrics, McGill University · Director, Neuromuscular Research Labs, The Montreal Neurological Institute & Hospital · Room 633, 3801 University Street, Montreal, Quebec H3A 2B4 · 514-398-8528

Robert B. Layzer · Professor of Neurology, University of California at San Francisco School of Medicine · University of California at San Francisco Medical Center · 505 Parnassus Avenue, Room M-794, San Francisco, CA 94143 · 415-476-1487

Phillip A. Low · (Peripheral Nerve Disorders, Autonomic Nervous Systems) · Professor of Neurology, Mayo Medical School · Consultant in Neurology, Mayo Clinic · 200 First Street SW, Rochester, MN 55905 · 507-284-2511

Janice M. Massey · Assistant Professor of Medicine, Duke University School of Medicine · Assistant Director, Electromyography Laboratory, Duke University Medical Center · P.O. Box 3403, Durham, NC 27710 · 919-684-5196

Jerry R. Mendell · (Peripheral Nerve Disorders) · Professor of Neurology, and Director, Neuromuscular Disease Center, Ohio State University College of Medicine · The Ohio State University Hospitals · 1654 Upham Drive, 473 Means Hall, Columbus, OH 43210 · 614-293-4962

Robert Gordon Miller · Clinical Professor of Neurology, University of California at San Francisco School of Medicine · Chief, Clinical Neurology, California Pacific Medical Center · California Campus East, 3700 California Street, San Francisco, CA 94118 · 415-750-6040

Theodore L. Munsat · Professor of Neurology and Pharmacology, Tufts University School of Medicine · Director, Neuromuscular Research Unit, New England Medical Center · Box 273, 750 Washington Street, Boston, MA 02111 · 617-956-5855

Audrey S. Penn · Professor of Neurology, College of Physicians & Surgeons of Columbia University · Attending Neurology, Columbia-Presbyterian Medical Center · Neurological Institute, 710 West 168th Street, New York, NY 10032 · 212-305-3533

David E. Pleasure · (Peripheral Nerve Disorders) · Professor of Neurology and Pediatrics, University of Pennsylvania School of Medicine · Director of Neurology Research, The Children's Hospital of Philadelphia · 3400 Civic Center Boulevard, Room 6128, Philadelphia, PA 19104 · 215-590-2090

Steven P. Ringel · Professor of Neurology and Director, Neuromuscular Division, University of Colorado School of Medicine · University of Colorado Health Sciences Center · 4200 East Ninth Avenue, Box B-185, Denver, CO 80262 · 303-270-7221

Lewis P. Rowland · Henry & Lucy Moses Professor and Chairman, Department of Neurology, College of Physicians & Surgeons of Columbia University · Director, Neurological Service, Neurological Institute of New York, Presbyterian Hospital · 710 West 168th Street, Room 1406, New York, NY 10032 · 212-305-8551

Donald B. Sanders · Duke University School of Medicine · Duke University Medical Center · Box 3403, DUMC, Durham, NC 27710 · 919-684-6078

Herbert H. Schaumburg · (Peripheral Nerve Disorders) · Professor and Chairman, Department of Neurology, Albert Einstein College of Medicine · Albert Einstein University Hospital · Department of Neurology, 1300 Morris Park Avenue, Bronx, NY 10461 · 212-430-3166

Thomas R. Swift · Professor and Chairman, Department of Neurology, Medical College of Georgia · Department of Neurology, Augusta, GA 30912 · 404-721-4583

Anthony J. Windebank · (Peripheral Nerve Disorders) · Consultant in Neurology, and Professor of Neurology, Mayo Medical School · Mayo Clinic · 200 First Street, SW, Rochester, MN 55905 · 507-284-2511

NEURO-ONCOLOGY
(See also Child Neurology, Neuro-oncology; Medical Oncology & Hematology, Neuro-oncology; Radiation Oncology, Brain Cancer)

J. Gregory Cairncross · Professor of Clinical Neurological Sciences and Oncology, The University of Western Ontario · Attending Neurologist, London Regional Cancer Centre; Victoria Hospital · 790 Commissioners Road East, London, Ontario N6A 4L6 · 519-685-8640 x3292

Terrence Cascino · Associate Professor of Neurology, Mayo Medical School · Mayo Clinic · 200 First Street, SW, Rochester, MN 55905 · 507-284-2511

Kathleen M. Foley · (Pain Syndromes) · Chief, Pain Service, Memorial Sloan-Kettering Cancer Center · 1275 York Avenue, New York, NY 10021 · 212-639-7050

Harry S. Greenberg · (Brain Tumors) · Professor of Neurology, The University of Michigan Medical School · The University of Michigan Medical Center · 1914 Taubman Center, 1500 East Medical Center Drive, Box 0316, Ann Arbor, MI 48109-0316 · 313-936-9055

Fred H. Hochberg · (Brain Tumors) · Associate Professor of Neurology, Harvard Medical School · Attending Neurologist, Massachusetts General Hospital · One Hawthorne Place, Suite 103, Boston, MA 02114 · 617-726-8657

Victor A. Levin · (Brain and Spinal Tumors) · Professor and Chairman, Department of Neuro-oncology, The University of Texas MD Anderson Cancer Center Neuro-oncologist, The University of Texas MD Anderson Cancer Center · 1515 Holcombe Boulevard, Houston, TX 77030 · 713-792-2121

Jerome B. Posner · (Cancer in the Nervous System) · Chairman, Department of Neurology, Memorial Sloan-Kettering Cancer Center · 1275 York Avenue, New York, NY 10021 · 212-639-7047

S. Clifford Schold, Jr. · (Brain Tumors) · Professor of Medicine and Assistant Professor of Pathology, Duke University School of Medicine · Duke University Medical Center · P.O. Box 3963, Durham, NC 27710 · 919-684-2662

William R. Shapiro · (Brain Tumors) · Chairman, Division of Neurology, The Barrow Neurological Institute at St. Joseph's Hospital & Medical Center · 350 West Thomas Road, Phoenix, AZ 85013 · 602-285-3895

Nicholas A. Vick · Professor of Neurology, Northwestern University Medical School · Head, Division of Neurology, Evanston Hospital · 2650 Ridge, Room 309 Burch Hall, Evanston, IL 60201 · 708-570-2025

W. K. Alfred Yung · (Brain Tumors) · Associate Professor of Neurology, The University of Texas Medical School at Houston · Deputy Chairman, Department of Neuro-oncology, The University of Texas MD Anderson Cancer Center · 1515 Holcombe Boulevard, Box 100, Houston, TX 77030 · 713-792-2573

NEUROPSYCHIATRY
(See also Psychiatry, Neuropsychiatry)

Jeffrey Lee Cummings · (Neuropsychiatric Aspects of Alzheimer's Disease and Dementias) · Director, UCLA Alzheimer's Disease Center, and Associate Professor of Neurology and Psychiatry, University of California at Los Angeles · Chief, Behavioral Neuroscience Section, Psychiatry Service, West Los Angeles Veterans Affairs Medical Center · Sawtelle & Wilshire Boulevard, Neurobehavior, Building 256B, 691/B111, Los Angeles, CA 90073 · 213-824-3166

Daniel R. Weinberger · Chief, Clinical Brain Disorders Branch, National Institute of Mental Health, National Institutes of Health · Neuroscience Center, 2700 Martin Luther King, Jr., Avenue, SE, Room 500, Washington DC 20032 · 202-373-6228

STROKES

Harold P. Adams, Jr. · (Subarachnoid Hemorrhage) · Professor of Neurology, The University of Iowa College of Medicine · Director, Division of Cerebrovascular Diseases, The University of Iowa Hospitals & Clinics · 200 Hawkins Drive, Iowa City, IA 52242 · 319-356-8755

Henry J. Barnett · (Stroke-Prevention) · President and Scientific Director, The John P. Robarts Research Institute · 100 Perth Drive, London, Ontario N6A 5K8 519-663-3678

José Biller · Professor of Neurology, Northwestern University Medical School · Director, Stroke Program, Northwestern Memorial Hospital · 233 East Erie Street, Suite 500, Chicago, IL 60611 · 312-908-8737

Thomas G. Brott · Associate Professor of Neurology, University of Cincinnati College of Medicine · Director, Stroke Program, University of Cincinnati Hospital 231 Bethesda Avenue, 4010 Medical Science Building, Cincinnati, OH 45267-0525 · 513-558-5431

Louis R. Caplan · Chairman and Professor, Department of Neurology, Tufts University School of Medicine · Neurologist-in-Chief, New England Medical Center · 750 Washington Street, Boston, MA 02111 · 617-956-5854

Bruce Dobkin · (Rehabilitation of Strokes) · Professor of Clinical Neurology, University of California at Los Angeles School of Medicine · Director, Comprehensive Rehabilitation Program, University of California at Los Angeles Medical Center · 300 UCLA Medical Plaza, Suite B-200, Los Angeles, CA 90024-6975 · 213-206-6500

Mark L. Dyken · Professor and Chairman, Department of Neurology, Indiana University School of Medicine · Indiana University Medical Center · 545 Barnhill Drive, Room 125, Indianapolis, IN 46202 · 317-274-4455

J. Donald Easton · Professor and Chairman, Department of Neurology, Brown University School of Medicine · Neurologist-in-Chief, Rhode Island Hospital · 110 Lockwood Street, Providence, RI 02903 · 401-277-8795

C. Miller Fisher · Professor of Neurology Emeritus, Harvard Medical School · Physician, Massachusetts General Hospital · Department of Neurology, ? Fruit Street, Boston, MA 02114 · 617-726-3895

Anthony J. Furlan · Head, Section of Adult Neurology, Department of Neurology, The Cleveland Clinic Foundation · One Clinic Center, 9500 Euclid Avenue, Cleveland, OH 44195-5227 · 216-444-5535

James Grotta · Professor of Neurology, Director of Stroke Unit, The University of Texas · 6655 Travis Street, Suite 930, Houston, TX 77030 · 713-794-5236

Vladimir C. Hachinski · Richard and Beryl Ivey Professor and Chairman, Department of Clinical Neurological Sciences, The University of Western Ontario · University Hospital · 339 Windermere Road, P.O. Box 5339, London, Ontario N6A 5A5 · 519-663-3000

Robert G. Hart · Associate Professor of Medicine (Neurology), The University of Texas Health Science Center at San Antonio · Audie L. Murphy Memorial Veterans Hospital · 7703 Floyd Curl Drive, San Antonio, TX 78284 · 512-617-5161

Carlos S. Kase · Professor of Neurology, Boston University School of Medicine · Visiting Neurologist, The University Hospital · 80 East Concord Street, Room B605, Boston, MA 02118 · 617-638-5102

J. P. Mohr · Sciarra Professor of Clinical Neurology, College of Physicians & Surgeons of Columbia University · Director, Stroke Center, Neurological Institute of New York · 710 West 168th Street, New York, NY 10032 · 212-305-8033

Fred Plum · Professor and Chairman, Department of Neurology & Neuroscience, Cornell University Medical College · Neurologist-in-Chief, The New York Hospital-Cornell Medical Center · Department of Neurology & Neuroscience, 525 East 68th Street, New York, NY 10021 · 212-746-6141

William J. Powers · Associate Professor of Neurology & Radiology, Washington University School of Medicine · Neurologist-in-Chief, The Jewish Hospital of St. Louis · 216 South Kingshighway Boulevard, St. Louis, MO 63110 · 314-454-5605

Thomas R. Price · Professor of Neurology, University of Maryland School of Medicine · University of Maryland Medical Center · Department of Neurology, 22 South Greene Street, Baltimore, MD 21201 · 301-328-5080

David Sherman · Professor and Chief, Department of Neurology, The University of Texas Health Science Center at San Antonio · Medicine—Neurology, 7703 Floyd Curl Drive, San Antonio, TX 78284-7883 · 512-617-5161

James F. Toole · Teagle Professor of Neurology and Professor of Public Health Sciences, The Bowman Gray School of Medicine of Wake Forest University · Director, Stroke Center, North Carolina Baptist Hospital · Medical Center Boulevard, Winston-Salem, NC 27157-1069 · 919-748-2338

K. Michael A. Welch · Adjunct Professor of Medical Physics, Oakland University, Rochester, MI; Professor of Clinical Neurology, University of Michigan, Ann Arbor · William T. Gossett Chair, Department of Neurology, and Vice-President for Academic Affairs, Henry Ford Medical Center · 2799 West Grand Boulevard, Detroit, MI 48202 · 313-876-3396

Jack P. Whisnant · Professor of Neurology, Mayo Medical School · Chairman, Department of Health Sciences Research, Mayo Clinic · 200 First Street, SW, Rochester, MN 55905 · 507-284-2720

Frank M. Yatsu · Professor and Chairman, Department of Neurology, The University of Texas Medical School at Houston · Hermann Hospital · Department of Neurology, 6431 Fannin Street, Suite 7044-MSMB, Houston, TX 77030 · 713-792-5777

NEUROLOGY, CHILD

AIDS
(See also Infectious Disease, AIDS; Medical Oncology & Hematology,
AIDS; Pulmonary & Critical Care Medicine, AIDS)

Leon G. Epstein · Professor of Neurology, Pediatrics, Microbiology, and Immunology, University of Rochester School of Medicine & Dentistry · Unit Chief, Pediatric Neurology, Strong Memorial Hospital, University of Rochester Medical Center · 601 Elmwood Avenue, Box 631, Rochester, NY 14642 · 716-275-0613

CENTRAL NERVOUS SYSTEM INFECTIONS

William Bell · Professor, Department of Pediatrics, Division of Child Neurology, The University of Iowa College of Medicine · The University of Iowa Hospitals & Clinics · Iowa City, IA 52242 · 319-356-2833

CHILD DEVELOPMENT

Gerald S. Golden · Professor of Pediatrics & Neurology, The University of Tennessee at Memphis, College of Medicine · LeBonheur Children's Medical Center 711 Jefferson Avenue, Memphis, TN 38105 · 901-528-6512

Peter R. Huttenlocher · (Brain Development) · Professor, Department of Pediatrics and Neurology, University of Chicago, Pritzker School of Medicine · University of Chicago Medical Center · 5841 South Maryland Avenue, Box 228, Chicago, IL 60637-1470 · 312-702-6487

Isabelle Rapin · (Language Disorders) · Professor of Neurology & Pediatrics (Neurology), Albert Einstein College of Medicine · 1410 Pelham Parkway South, Kennedy Center, Room 807, Bronx, NY 10461 · 212-430-2478

Lawrence T. Taft · (Developmental Disabilities, Neurodevelopmental Pediatrics) Professor of Pediatrics, and Co-Director, Center for Human Development & Developmental Disabilities, Robert Wood Johnson Medical School-University of Medicine & Dentistry of New Jersey · Robert Wood Johnson University Hospital 97 Patterson Street, New Brunswick, NJ 08903 · 908-937-7888

EPILEPSY
(See also Neurological Surgery, Epilepsy Surgery)

Fredrick Anderman · Professor of Neurology and Pediatrics, McGill University · Director, Epilepsy Service, The Montreal Neurological Institute & Hospital · 3801 University Street, Montreal, Quebec H3A 2B4 · 514-398-1976

W. Edwin Dodson · Professor of Pediatrics and Neurology, and Associate Dean, Admissions, Washington University School of Medicine · St. Louis Children's Hospital · 400 South Kingshighway Boulevard, St. Louis, MO 63110 · 314-454-6120

Fritz E. Dreifuss · Professor of Neurology and Vice-Chairman, Department of Neurology, University of Virginia School of Medicine · Director, Comprehensive Epilepsy Program, University of Virginia Health Sciences Center · Hospital Drive, Box 394, Charlottesville, VA 22908 · 804-924-5669

John M. Freeman · Professor of Neurology and Pediatrics, and Lederer Professor of Pediatric Neurology, Johns Hopkins University School of Medicine · Director of Pediatric Epilepsy Center, The Johns Hopkins Medical Institutions · 600 North Wolfe Street, CMSC 1-141, Baltimore, MD 21205 · 410-955-9100

Gregory L. Holmes · Associate Professor of Neurology, Harvard Medical School Director of Clinical Neurophysiology Laboratory, and Director of Epilepsy Program, Children's Hospital · 300 Longwood Avenue, Boston, MA 02115 · 617-735-7970

O. Carter Snead III · Professor of Pediatrics, Professor and Vice-Chairman, Department of Neurology, and Professor of Toxicology & Pharmacology, University of Southern California School of Medicine · Chief, Division of Neurology, Children's Hospital of Los Angeles · 4650 Sunset Boulevard, Los Angeles, CA 90027 213-669-2498

Elaine Wiley · Head, Pediatric Epilepsy Program, The Cleveland Clinic Foundation · One Clinic Center, 9500 Euclid Avenue, Cleveland, OH 44195 · 216-444-2095

GENERAL CHILD NEUROLOGY

Bruce O. Berg · Professor of Neurology, and Director of Child Neurology, Department of Pediatrics, University of California at San Francisco School of Medicine · University of California at San Francisco Medical Center · 505 Parnassus Avenue, Room 651 Moffitt, Box 0106, San Francisco, CA 94143-0106 · 415-476-1625

Ian J. Butler · (Tourette Syndrome) · Professor and Director, Division of Child Neurology & Developmental Pediatrics, The University of Texas Medical School at Houston · Attending Staff, Hermann Hospital; The University of Texas MD Anderson Cancer Center; Shriner Hospital · 6431 Fannin Street, Suite 7044, Houston, TX 77030 · 713-792-5777 x35

Abraham M. Chutorian · Professor, Departments of Pediatrics & Neurology, Cornell University Medical College · Chief, Department of Pediatric Neurology, The New York Hospital-Cornell Medical Center · 525 East 68th Street, New York, NY 10021 · 212-746-3278

John M. Freeman · Professor of Neurology and Pediatrics, and Lederer Professor of Pediatric Neurology, Johns Hopkins University School of Medicine · Director of Pediatric Epilepsy Center, The Johns Hopkins Medical Institutions · 600 North Wolfe Street, CMSC 1-141, Baltimore, MD 21205 · 410-955-9100

Peter R. Huttenlocher · (Brain Development) · Professor, Department of Pediatrics and Neurology, University of Chicago, Pritzker School of Medicine · University of Chicago Medical Center · 5841 South Maryland Avenue, Box 228, Chicago, IL 60637-1470 · 312-702-6487

Merton Richard Koenigsberger · Associate Professor of Neuroscience & Pediatrics, University of Medicine & Dentistry of New Jersey · Director, Division of Pediatric Neurology, University Hospital; Children's Hospital; Newark Beth Israel Medical Center · 185 South Orange Avenue, MSB-H506, Newark, NJ 07103 201-456-5204

Robert T. Leshner · (Electromyography) · Professor of Neurology and Pediatrics, Virginia Commonwealth University, Medical College of Virginia · Medical College of Virginia Hospital · Medical College of Virginia, Box 211, Richmond, VA 23298-0211 · 804-786-0442

John H. Menkes · Professor Emeritus of Neurology and Pediatrics, University of California at Los Angeles School of Medicine · Attending Physician, Center for the Health Sciences, University of California at Los Angeles; Cedars-Sinai Medical Center · 9320 Wilshire Boulevard, Beverly Hills, CA 90212 · 310-277-6568

Arthur L. Prensky · Professor of Pediatrics and Neurology, and Allen P. & Josephine B. Green Professor of Pediatric Neurology, Washington University School of Medicine · St. Louis Children's Hospital · 400 South Kingshighway Boulevard, St. Louis, MO 63110 · 314-454-6085

Sanford Schneider · Professor of Pediatrics and Neurology, Loma Linda University School of Medicine · Head, Division of Child Neurology, Loma Linda University Medical Center · 11262 Campus Street, West Hall, Room 150, Loma Linda, CA 92354 · 714-824-0800 x2212

INHERITED BIOCHEMICAL DISORDERS

John H. Menkes · Professor Emeritus of Neurology and Pediatrics, University of California at Los Angeles School of Medicine · Attending Physician, Center for the Health Sciences, University of California at Los Angeles; Cedars-Sinai Medical Center · 9320 Wilshire Boulevard, Beverly Hills, CA 90212 · 310-277-6568

Kenneth F. Swaiman · Professor of Neurology and Pediatrics and Director, Division of Pediatric Neurology, University of Minnesota School of Medicine · University of Minnesota Hospital & Clinics · 420 Delaware Street, SE, Minneapolis, MN 55455 · 612-625-7466

METABOLIC DISEASES
(See also Pediatrics, Metabolic Diseases)

Darryl C. De Vivo · Sidney Carter Professor of Neurology, and Professor of Pediatrics, College of Physicians & Surgeons of Columbia University · Attending Neurologist, and Attending Pediatrician, and Director of Pediatric Neurology, Columbia-Presbyterian Medical Center · Neurological Institute, 710 West 168th Street, New York, NY 10032 · 212-305-5244

MOVEMENT DISORDER

Ian J. Butler · (Tourette Syndrome) · Professor and Director, Division of Child Neurology & Developmental Pediatrics, The University of Texas Medical School at Houston · Attending Staff, Hermann Hospital; The University of Texas MD Anderson Cancer Center; Shriner Hospital · 6431 Fannin Street, Suite 7044, Houston, TX 77030 · 713-792-5777 x35

NEONATAL NEUROLOGY

Merton Richard Koenigsberger · Associate Professor of Neuroscience & Pediatrics, University of Medicine & Dentistry of New Jersey · Director, Division of Pediatric Neurology, University Hospital; Children's Hospital; Newark Beth Israel Medical Center · 185 South Orange Avenue, MSB-H506, Newark, NJ 07103 201-456-5204

Joseph J. Volpe · Bronson Crothers Professor of Neurology, Harvard Medical School · Neurologist-in-Chief, Children's Hospital · 300 Longwood Avenue, Boston, MA 02115 · 617-735-6386

NEUROMUSCULAR DISEASE

Merton Richard Koenigsberger · Associate Professor of Neuroscience & Pediatrics, University of Medicine & Dentistry of New Jersey · Director, Division of Pediatric Neurology, University Hospital; Children's Hospital; Newark Beth Israel Medical Center · 185 South Orange Avenue, MSB-H506, Newark, NJ 07103 201-456-5204

Robert Gordon Miller · Clinical Professor of Neurology, University of California at San Francisco School of Medicine · Chief, Clinical Neurology, California Pacific Medical Center · California Campus East, 3700 California Street, San Francisco, CA 94118 · 415-750-6040

Richard T. Moxley III · Professor of Neurology and Pediatrics, University of Rochester School of Medicine & Dentistry · Director, Neuromuscular Disease Center, Strong Memorial Hospital, University of Rochester Medical Center · 601 Elmwood Avenue, Box 673, Rochester, NY 14642 · 716-275-5006

NEURO-ONCOLOGY
(See also Adult Neurology, Neuro-oncology; Medical Oncology & Hematology, Neuro-oncology; Radiation Oncology, Brain Cancer)

Jeffrey C. Allen · (Pediatric Brain Tumor) · Associate Professor of Neurology, New York University School of Medicine · New York University Medical Center 550 First Avenue, New York, NY 10016 · 212-263-6989

Michael E. Cohen · (Pediatric Brain Tumor) · Professor and Chairman, Department of Neurology, State University of New York at Buffalo School of Medicine & Biomedical Sciences · Director of Neurology, Children's Hospital of Buffalo · 219 Bryant Street, Buffalo, NY 14222 · 716-878-7848

Patricia Kressel Duffner · (Pediatric Brain Tumor) · Professor of Neurology and Pediatrics, State University of New York at Buffalo School of Medicine & Biomedical Sciences · Associate Director, Division of Child Neurology, Children's Hospital of Buffalo · 219 Bryant Street, Buffalo, NY 14222 · 716-878-7840

Roger Packer · (Pediatric Brain Tumor) · Professor of Neurology and Pediatrics, George Washington University · Chairman, Neurology, Children's National Medical Center · 111 Michigan Avenue NW, Washington, DC 20010 · 202-745-2120

Peter C. Phillips · (Pediatric Brain Tumor) · Assistant Professor in Neurology, University of Pennsylvania School of Medicine · The Children's Hospital of Philadelphia · 34th and Civic Center Boulevard, Suite 2002, Philadelphia, PA 19104 215-590-1719

Russell W. Walker · (Pediatric Brain Tumor) · Associate Professor of Pediatrics and Neurology, Cornell University Medical College · Associate Attending Pediatrician and Neurologist, Memorial Sloan-Kettering Cancer Center · 1275 York Avenue, New York, NY 10021 · 212-639-6597

NEUROVIROLOGY

Leon G. Epstein · Professor of Neurology, Pediatrics, Microbiology, and Immunology, University of Rochester School of Medicine & Dentistry · Unit Chief, Pediatric Neurology, Strong Memorial Hospital, University of Rochester Medical Center · 601 Elmwood Avenue, Box 631, Rochester, NY 14642 · 716-275-0613

NUCLEAR MEDICINE

BONE

B. David Collier · Associate Professor, and Chief of Nuclear Medicine & Radiology, Medical College of Wisconsin · Director of Nuclear Medicine, Milwaukee County Medical Complex · 8700 West Wisconsin Avenue, Box 104, Milwaukee, WI 53226 · 414-257-5971

BRAIN

Abass Alavi · (Positron Emission Tomography [PET]) · Professor of Radiology, Neurology & Psychiatry, University of Pennsylvania School of Medicine · Chief, Division of Nuclear Medicine, Hospital of the University of Pennsylvania · One Donner, 3400 Spruce Street, Philadelphia, PA 19104 · 215-662-3069

Frederick J. Bonte · Professor of Radiology, and Director of the Nuclear Medicine Center, The University of Texas Southwestern Medical Center at Dallas · Parkland Memorial Hospital · 5323 Harry Hines Boulevard, Dallas, TX 75235-9061 · 214-688-2025

Ralph Edward Coleman · (Positron Emission Tomography [PET]) · Professor of Radiology, Duke University School of Medicine · Director of Nuclear Medicine, Duke University Medical Center · P.O. Box 3949, Durham, NC 27710 · 919-660-2711

J. James Frost · (Positron Emission Tomography [PET]) · Associate Professor of Radiology and Neuroscience, Johns Hopkins University School of Medicine · The Johns Hopkins Medical Institutions · Tower Basement Building, 600 North Wolfe Street, Room B1-130, Baltimore, MD 21205 · 410-955-8449

Randall Hawkins · (Positron Emission Tomography [PET]) · Section Head, Clinical Nuclear Medicine, and Associate Professor of Radiological Sciences, Division of Nuclear Medicine & Biophysics, Department of Radiological Sciences, University of California at Los Angeles School of Medicine · Nuclear Medicine Clinic, AR-250, CHS, 10833 LeConte Avenue, Los Angeles, CA 90024 · 310-825-7361

Peter Herscovitch · (Positron Emission Tomography [PET]) · National Institutes of Health · Chief, Positron Emission Tomography Imaging Section, Clinical Center, National Institutes of Health · 9000 Rockville Pike, Buildign 10, Room 1C-401, Bethesda, MD 20892 · 301-496-5675

B. Leonard Holman · Philip H. Cook Professor of Radiology, Harvard Medical School · Chairman of Radiology, Brigham & Women's Hospital · 75 Francis Street, Boston, MA 02115 · 617-732-6273

David E. Kuhl · (Positron Emission Tomography [PET]) · Professor of Internal Medicine and Radiology, The University of Michigan Medical School · Chief, Division of Nuclear Medicine, The University of Michigan Medical Center · 1500 East Medical Center Drive, Ann Arbor, MI 48109-0028 · 313-936-5388

John C. Mazziotta · (Positron Emission Tomography [PET]) · Professor of Neurology and Radiological Sciences, University of California at Los Angeles School of Medicine · Vice-Chairman, Department of Neurology, and Head of the Neuroscience Section, Division of Nuclear Medicine, University of California at Los Angeles Medical Center · 10833 LeConte Avenue, B2-085, Los Angeles, CA 90024-1769 · 310-825-2699

Mark A. Mintun · (Positron Emission Tomography [PET]) · Associate Professor of Diagnostic Radiology, University of Pittsburgh School of Medicine · Medical Director of the PET Facility, Presbyterian University Hospital · 4880 Main Tower, DeSoto at O'Hara Streets, Pittsburgh, PA 15213 · 412-647-7291

Henry N. Wagner, Jr. · (Positron Emission Tomography [PET]) · Professor of Medicine, Radiology and Environmental Health Sciences, and Director, Nuclear

Medicine, Johns Hopkins University School of Medicine; Director, Division of Radiation Health Sciences, Johns Hopkins University School of Hygiene & Public Health · Director, Nuclear Medicine, The Johns Hopkins Medical Institutions · 615 North Wolfe Street, Room 2001, Baltimore, MD 21205-2179 · 410-955-3350

GENERAL NUCLEAR MEDICINE

Abass Alavi · (Positron Emission Tomography [PET]) · Professor of Radiology, Neurology & Psychiatry, University of Pennsylvania School of Medicine · Chief, Division of Nuclear Medicine, Hospital of the University of Pennsylvania · One Donner, 3400 Spruce Street, Philadelphia, PA 19104 · 215-662-3069

Naomi P. Alazraki · Professor of Radiology, Emory University School of Medicine Co-Director, Division of Nuclear Medicine, Department of Radiology, Emory University Affiliated Hospitals · 1364 Clifton Road, NE, Atlanta, GA 30322 · 404-727-4843

Philip O. Alderson · Professor and Chairman, Department of Radiology, College of Physicians & Surgeons of Columbia University · Columbia-Presbyterian Medical Center · Milstein Hospital, 622 West 168th Street, Second Floor, Room 131, New York, NY 10032 · 212-305-8994

William L. Ashburn · Professor of Radiology, University of California at San Diego School of Medicine · Chief, Nuclear Medicine Division, University of California at San Diego Medical Center · 225 Dickinson Street, Mail Code 8758, San Diego, CA 92103-8758 · 619-543-6682

Harold L. Atkins · Professor of Radiology, and Chief, Division of Nuclear Medicine, State University of New York Health Science Center at Stony Brook · SUNY at Stony Brook Hospital · Room 092, Stony Brook, NY 11794-8460 · 516-444-2431

William H. Beierwaltes · (Thyroidology) · Professor of Medicine (Emeritus); and Director of Thyroid Clinic and Nuclear Medicine Division (Emeritus), The University of Michigan Medical School · Staff Member, St. John Hospital & Medical Center; Eastside Nuclear Medicine · Department of Nuclear Medicine, 22101 Moross Road, Detroit, MI 48236 · 313-343-3015

Manuel L. Brown · Professor of Diagnostic Radiology, University of Pittsburgh School of Medicine · Director of Diagnostic Nuclear Medicine, Presbyterian University Hospital · 4880 Main Tower, DeSoto at O'Hara Streets, Pittsburgh, PA 15213 · 412-647-7260

Ralph Edward Coleman · (Positron Emission Tomography [PET]) · Professor of Radiology, Duke University School of Medicine · Director of Nuclear Medicine, Duke University Medical Center · P.O. Box 3949, Durham, NC 27710 · 919-660-2711

Glenn V. Dalrymple · Professor of Radiology and Internal Medicine, University of Nebraska College of Medicine · Director of Nuclear Medicine, University of Nebraska Medical Center · 600 South 42nd Street, Omaha, NE 68198-1045 · 402-559-5280

Howard J. Dworkin · Clinical Assistant Professor, Department of Medicine, Wayne State University Medical School; Assistant Clinical Professor, Department of Radiology, Michigan State University College of Human Medicine; Clinical Professor, Department of Medical Physics, Oakland University · Director, Department of Nuclear Medicine, William Beaumont Hospital · 3601 West Thirteen Mile Road, Royal Oak, MI 48073 · 313-551-4128

Leonard M. Freeman · Professor of Nuclear Medicine and Radiology, Albert Einstein College of Medicine · Director of Nuclear Medicine, Montefiore Medical Center · 111 East 210th Street, Bronx, NY 10467 · 212-920-6060

Stanley J. Goldsmith · Professor of Medicine, Mt. Sinai School of Medicine · Mt. Sinai Medical Center · One Gustave Levy Place, Box 1141, New York, NY 10029 212-241-7888

Robert E. Henkin · Professor of Radiology, and Director of Nuclear Medicine, Loyola Stritch School of Medicine · Foster G. McGaw Hospital · 2160 South First Avenue, Maywood, IL 60153 · 708-216-3779

Paul B. Hoffer · Professor of Diagnostic Radiology, and Director, Section of Nuclear Medicine, Yale University School of Medicine · Yale-New Haven Hospital · Department of Diagnostic Radiology, 333 Cedar Street, New Haven, CT 06510 · 203-785-2384

B. Leonard Holman · Philip H. Cook Professor of Radiology, Harvard Medical School · Chairman of Radiology, Brigham & Women's Hospital · 75 Francis Street, Boston, MA 02115 · 617-732-6273

John W. Keyes, Jr. · (Computer) · Professor of Radiology, and Director of the PET Center, The Bowman Gray School of Medicine of Wake Forest University · North Carolina Baptist Hospital · Medical Center Boulevard, Winston-Salem, NC 27157 · 919-748-7461

Peter T. Kirchner · Professor of Radiology and Medicine, The University of Iowa College of Medicine · Director, Division of Nuclear Medicine, The University of Iowa Hospitals & Clinics · 200 Hawkins Drive, Iowa City, IA 52242 · 319-356-4302

Leon S. Malmud · Herbert M. Stauffer Professor and Chairman, Department of Diagnostic Imaging, Temple University School of Medicine · Vice-President for

Health Sciences, Temple University Hospital · Broad and Ontario Streets, Philadelphia, PA 19140 · 215-221-4638

C. Douglas Maynard · Professor and Chairman, Department of Radiology, The Bowman Gray School of Medicine of Wake Forest University · North Carolina Baptist Hospital · Medical Center Boulevard, Winston-Salem, NC 27157-1088 · 919-748-2466

Kenneth A. McKusick · Associate Professor of Radiology, Harvard Medical School Radiologist, Massachusetts General Hospital · Nuclear Medicine Division, Tilton 2, 32 Fruit Street, Boston, MA 02114 · 617-726-8356

Wil B. Nelp · Professor of Medicine and Radiology, University of Washington School of Medicine · Director, Division of Nuclear Medicine, University of Washington Medical Center · 1959 Northeast Pacific Street, RC-70, Seattle, WA 98195 206-548-4240

Dennis David Patton · Professor of Radiology, The University of Arizona College of Medicine · Director, Division of Nuclear Medicine, The University of Arizona Health Sciences Center · 1501 North Campbell Avenue, Tucson, AZ 85724 · 602-626-7709

Louis A. Perez · Director, Department of Radiology, Lawrence Hospital · 55 Palmer Avenue, Bronxville, NY 10708 · 914-337-7300 x1007

Richard C. Reba · Professor of Radiology, University of Chicago School of Medicine · Chief, Nuclear Medicine Section, Department of Radiology, University of Chicago Hospitals · 5841 South Maryland Avenue, UC Hospital, Box429, Chicago, IL 60637 · 312-702-5968

Ralph G. Robinson · (Radioisotopic Therapy) · Professor of Diagnostic Radiology, and Head, Division of Nuclear Medicine, University of Kansas School of Medicine · University of Kansas Medical Center · 3901 Rainbow Boulevard, Kansas City, KS 66160-7234 · 913-588-6810

Barry A. Siegel · Professor of Radiology and Medicine, Washington University School of Medicine · Director of Division of Nuclear Medicine, Mallinckrodt Institute of Radiology, Barnes Hospital; St. Louis Children's Hospital · 510 South Kingshighway Boulevard, St. Louis, MO 63110 · 314-362-2809

Edward B. Silberstein · Professor of Radiology & Medicine, University of Cincinnati College of Medicine · Attending Physician, University of Cincinnati Hospital, and The Jewish Hospital of Cincinnati · 234 Goodman, ML 577, Cincinnati, OH 45267 · 513-558-4282, 569-2291

Stewart M. Spies · Professor of Radiology, and Associate Dean of the Honors Program in Medical Education, Northwestern University Medical School · Director, Nuclear Medicine, Northwestern Memorial Hospital · 250 East Superior Street, Suite 484, Chicago, IL 60611 · 312-908-2514

James H. Thrall · The Juan M. Taveras Professor of Radiology, Harvard Medical School · Radiologist-in-Chief, Massachusetts General Hospital · 55 Fruit Street, Boston, MA 02114 · 617-726-5244

Henry N. Wagner, Jr. · (Positron Emission Tomography [PET]) · Professor of Medicine, Radiology and Environmental Health Sciences, and Director, Nuclear Medicine, Johns Hopkins University School of Medicine; Director, Division of Radiation Health Sciences, Johns Hopkins University School of Hygiene & Public Health · Director, Nuclear Medicine, The Johns Hopkins Medical Institutions · 615 North Wolfe Street, Room 2001, Baltimore, MD 21205-2179 · 410-955-3350

Alan D. Waxman · Director of Nuclear Medicine, Cedars-Sinai Medical Center · 8700 Beverly Boulevard, Room A042, Los Angeles, CA 90048 · 213-855-4216

Henry N. Wellman · Professor of Medicine and Radiology, Indiana University School of Medicine · Director, Division of Nuclear Medicine, Indiana University Medical Center · 926 West Michigan Street, UHP16, Indianapolis, IN 46202 · 317-274-8832

KIDNEY

M. Donald Blaufox · Professor of Nuclear Medicine and Medicine, Albert Einstein College of Medicine · Attending, Montefiore Medical Center · 1300 Morris Park Avenue, Mazer Dorm 324, Bronx, NY 10461 · 212-904-4011

Eva V. Dubovsky · Professor of Radiology, The University of Alabama School of Medicine · Director of Nuclear Medicine, The University of Alabama Hospital; The Department of Veterans Affairs Medical Center-Birmingham · 619 South 19th Street, Birmingham, AL 35233 · 205-934-2140

Andrew Taylor, Jr. · Professor of Radiology, Emory University School of Medicine · Co-Director, Division of Nuclear Medicine, Emory University Affiliated Hospitals · 1364 Clifton Road, NE, Atlanta, GA 30322 · 404-727-4852

NUCLEAR CARDIOLOGY
(See also Cardiovascular Disease, Nuclear Cardiology)

Daniel S. Berman · Professor of Medicine, University of California at Los Angeles School of Medicine · Director, Nuclear Cardiology, Cedars-Sinai Medical Center 8700 Beverly Boulevard, Room A-042, Los Angeles, CA 90048 · 213-855-4223

Elias H. Botvinick · Professor of Medicine and Radiology, University of California at San Francisco School of Medicine · University of California at San Francisco Medical Center · 505 Parnassus Avenue, Room L-340, San Francisco, CA 94143 415-476-1521

Ernest Gordon DePuey · Associate Professor of Radiology, College of Physicians & Surgeons of Columbia University · Director of Nuclear Medicine, St. Luke's-Roosevelt Hospital Center · Amsterdam Avenue at 114th Street, New York, NY 10025 · 212-523-3398

Raymundo Tiu Go · (Cardiac Positron Emission Tomography [PET]) · Chairman, Department of Nuclear Medicine, Division of Radiology, The Cleveland Clinic Foundation · One Clinic Center, 9500 Euclid Avenue, Cleveland, OH 44195-5047 216-444-2665

Jamshid Maddahi · (Positron Emission Tomography [PET]) · Professor of Radiological Sciences, University of California at Los Angeles School of Medicine · Director, Clinical Positron Emission Tomography (PET) Center, University of California at Los Angeles Medical Center · 10833 LeConte Avenue, AR175, Los Angeles, CA 90024-1721 · 213-206-9896

Roderic I. Pettigrew · (Magnetic Resonance Imaging) · Associate Professor of Radiology, Emory University School of Medicine · Director of Cardiovascular NMR, Emory University Affiliated Hospitals · 1364 Clifton Road, NE, Atlanta, GA 30322 · 404-727-4807

Ralph G. Robinson · (Radioisotopic Therapy) · Professor of Diagnostic Radiology, and Head, Division of Nuclear Medicine, University of Kansas School of Medicine · University of Kansas Medical Center · 3901 Rainbow Boulevard, Kansas City, KS 66160-7234 · 913-588-6810

Alan Rozanski · (Preventive Cardiology) · Associate Professor of Medicine, College of Physicians & Surgeons of Columbia University · Director of Nuclear Cardiology & Cardiac Stress Testing, St. Luke's-Roosevelt Hospital Center · 114th Street and Amsterdam Avenue, New York, NY 10025 · 212-523-4011

Heinrich R. Schelbert · (Cardiac Positron Emission Tomography [PET]) · Professor of Radiological Sciences, University of California at Los Angeles School of Medicine · Head, Cardiovascular Section, Division of Nuclear Medicine & Biophysics, University of California at Los Angeles Center for the Health Sciences · 10833 LeConte Avenue, Room B2-085C CHS, Los Angeles, CA 90024-1721 · 310-825-3076

Markus Schwaiger · (Cardiac Positron Emission Tomography [PET]) · Professor of Internal Medicine, The University of Michigan Medical School · Director of Cardiovascular Nuclear Medicine, The University of Michigan Medical Center ·

1500 East Medical Center Drive, Room UHB1G505, Box 0028, Ann Arbor, MI 48109-0028 · 313-936-5385

H. William Strauss · Professor of Radiology, Harvard Medical School · Director, Division of Nuclear Medicine, Massachusetts General Hospital · Tilton 2, 32 Fruit Street, Boston, MA 02114 · 617-726-8353

Raymond Taillefer · Professor of Radiology, University of Montreal · Chief of Department of Nuclear Medicine, Hotel-Dieu de Montreal · 3840, Rue St-Urbain, Montreal, Quebec H2W 1T8 · 514-843-2680

James L. Tatum · Professor of Radiology and Cardiology, Virginia Commonwealth University, Medical College of Virginia · Director, Nuclear Cardiology, Medical College of Virginia Hospital · 1300 East Marshall Street, North Hospital 7-022, Richmond, VA 23298 · 804-786-8263

ONCOLOGY

Janet F. Eary · Associate Professor of Radiology and Pathology, University of Washington School of Medicine · University of Washington Medical Center · 1959 Northeast Pacific Street, RC-70, Seattle, WA 98195 · 206-548-4240

Randall Hawkins · (Positron Emission Tomography [PET]) · Section Head, Clinical Nuclear Medicine, and Associate Professor of Radiological Sciences, Division of Nuclear Medicine & Biophysics, Department of Radiological Sciences, University of California at Los Angeles School of Medicine · Nuclear Medicine Clinic, AR-250, CHS, 10833 LeConte Avenue, Los Angeles, CA 90024 · 310-825-7361

Thomas Powell Haynie · James E. Anderson Professor of Nuclear Medicine, The University of Texas MD Anderson Cancer Center · Chairman, Department of Nuclear Medicine, The University of Texas MD Anderson Cancer Center · 1515 Holcombe Boulevard, Box 83, Houston, TX 77030 · 713-792-3007

William D. Kaplan · Associate Professor, Radiology, Harvard Medical School · Chief, Oncologic Nuclear Medicine, Dana-Farber Cancer Institute · 44 Binney Street, Boston, MA 02115 · 617-732-3223

E. Edmund Kim · (Positron Emission Tomography [PET]) · Professor of Radiology and Medicine, and Chief, Section of Experimental Nuclear Medicine, and Director of Metabolic and Experimental Imaging, The University of Texas MD Anderson Cancer Center · Department of Nuclear Medicine, 1515 Holcombe Boulevard, Box 59, Houston, TX 77030 · 713-794-1052

Steven Mark Larson · (Positron Emission Tomography [PET]) · Professor of Radiology, Cornell University Medical College · Chief, Nuclear Medicine Service, Department of Medical Imaging, Memorial Sloan-Kettering Cancer Center 1275 York Avenue, New York, NY 10021 · 212-639-7373

Richard L. Wahl · Professor of Internal Medicine and Radiology, The University of Michigan Medical School · Director of General Nuclear Imaging, Division of Nuclear Medicine, Department of Internal Medicine, The University of Michigan Medical Center · 1500 East Medical Center Drive, UHB1G505, Box 0028, Ann Arbor, MI 48109-0028 · 313-936-5384

Alan D. Waxman · Director of Nuclear Medicine, Cedars-Sinai Medical Center · 8700 Beverly Boulevard, Room A042, Los Angeles, CA 90048 · 213-855-4216

PEDIATRIC

James J. Conway · Professor of Radiology, Northwestern University Medical School · Chief, Division of Nuclear Medicine, Children's Memorial Hospital · 2300 Children's Plaza, Box 42, Chicago, IL 60614 · 312-880-4411

David L. Gilday · Professor of Radiology, University of Toronto School of Medicine · Director for Nuclear Medicine, The Hospital for Sick Children · 555 University Avenue, Toronto, Ontario M5G 1X8 · 416-598-6038

Sydney Heyman · Professor of Radiology, University of Pennsylvania School of Medicine · Director, Division of Nuclear Medicine, The Children's Hospital of Philadelphia · 34th Street and Civic Center Boulevard, Philadelphia, PA 19104 · 215-590-2587

Salvadore Treves · Professor of Radiology, Harvard Medical School · Chief, Division of Nuclear Medicine, Children's Hospital · 300 Longwood Avenue, Boston, MA 02115 · 617-735-7935

PULMONARY

Philip O. Alderson · Professor and Chairman, Department of Radiology, College of Physicians & Surgeons of Columbia University · Columbia-Presbyterian Medical Center · Milstein Hospital, 622 West 168th Street, Second Floor, Room 131, New York, NY 10032 · 212-305-8994

RADIATION ACCIDENTS

Henry D. Royal · Associate Professor of Radiology, Washington University School of Medicine · Associate Director of Nuclear Medicine, Mallinckrodt Institute of Radiology · 510 South Kingshighway Boulevard, St. Louis, MO 63110 · 314-362-2809

THYROID
(See also Endocrinology & Metabolism, Thyroid)

David V. Becker · Professor of Radiology & Medicine, Cornell University Medical College · Director of Nuclear Medicine, The New York Hospital-Cornell Medical Center · 525 East 68th Street, Room Starr 221, New York, NY 10021 · 212-746-4583

James R. Hurley · Associate Professor of Radiology & Medicine, Cornell University Medical College · Associate Director, Division of Nuclear Medicine, The New York Hospital-Cornell Medical Center · 525 East 68th Street, Room Starr 221, New York, NY 10021 · 212-746-4584

OBSTETRICS & GYNECOLOGY

GENETICS

Mary E. D'Alton · Associate Professor of Obstetrics & Gynecology, Tufts University School of Medicine · Director, Maternal & Fetal Medicine, St. Margaret's Hospital for Women · 90 Cushing Avenue, MSM Department, Boston, MA 02125 617-436-8600

Sherman Elias · Professor of Obstetrics & Gynecology, and Director, Division of Reproductive Genetics, The University of Tennessee at Memphis, College of Medicine · 853 Jefferson Street, Room E102, Memphis, TN 38103 · 901-577-4905

Mitchell S. Golbus · Professor of Obstetrics, Gynecology & Reproductive Sciences, and Professor of Pediatrics, University of California at San Francisco School of Medicine · University of California at San Francisco Medical Center · 533 Parnassus Avenue, Room U-262, San Francisco, CA 94143-0720 · 415-476-4157

Michael T. Mennuti · Professor and Chairman, Department of Obstetrics & Gynecology, University of Pennsylvania School of Medicine · Professor and Chairman, Department of Obstetrics & Gynecology, Hospital of the University of Pennsylvania · 3400 Spruce Street, Four Gibson Building, Philadelphia, PA 19104-4283 · 215-662-3234

Joe Leigh Simpson · Faculty Professor and Chairman of Obstetrics & Gynecology, The University of Tennessee, Memphis, College of Medicine · Regional Medical Center at Memphis · 853 Jefferson Street, Room E102, Memphis, TN 38163 · 901-528-5340

GENITAL DERMATOLOGICAL DISEASE
(See also Dermatology, Genital Dermatological Disease)

Raymond H. Kaufman · (Vulvar Disease) · Chairman and Professor, Department of Obstetrics & Gynecology, Baylor College of Medicine · The Methodist Hospital; St. Luke's Episcopal Hospital · One Baylor Plaza, Houston, TX 77030 · 713-798-7500

Stanley C. Marinoff · (Vulvar Disease) · Clinical Professor of Obstetrics & Gynecology, The George Washington University School of Medicine · Attending Physician, George Washington University Hospital; Columbia Hospital for Women · Three Washington Circle, NW, Suite 110, Washington, DC 20037 · 202-659-6480

GYNECOLOGIC CANCER
(See also Medical Oncology & Hematology, Gynecologic Cancer)

Hervy E. Averette · American Cancer Society Professor of Clinical Oncology/Sylvester Professor and Director, Division of Gynecologic Oncology, University of Miami School of Medicine · University of Miami-Jackson Memorial Medical Center · East Tower Building, Suite 7007, 1611 Northwest 16th Avenue, Miami, FL 33136 · 305-585-7985

Jonathan S. Berek · Professor and Vice-Chairman, Department of Obstetrics & Gynecology, University of California at Los Angeles (UCLA) School of Medicine · Chief of Gynecology, Director, Gynecologic Oncology Service, University of California at Los Angeles (UCLA) Medical Center · Department of Obstetrics & Gynecology, Los Angeles, CA 90024-1740 · 310-825-7786

Michael L. Berman · Professor, Division of Gynecologic Oncology, University of California, Irvine School of Medicine · University of California, Irvine Medical Center; Long Beach Memorial Hospital · 2880 Atlantic Avenue, Long Beach, CA 90806; 101 The City Drive, Building 22A, Orange, CA 92668 · 714-634-6570, 213-595-2463

Richard C. Boronow · Clinical Professor of Gynecology, University of Mississippi Mississippi Baptist Medical Center · 1190 North State Street, Suite 402, Jackson, MS 39202 · 601-944-0220

John G. Boyce · Professor and Chairman, Department of Obstetrics & Gynecology, State University of New York Health Science Center at Brooklyn · Director of Gynecologic Oncology, University Hospital of Brooklyn; Chief of Obstetrics & Gynecology, Kings County Hospital Center · 450 Clarkson Avenue, Brooklyn, NY 11203 · 718-270-2057

Patricia S. Braly · Associate Professor, Department of Reproductive Medicine, University of California at San Diego School of Medicine · Director, Divison of Gynecologic Oncology, University of California at San Diego Medical Center · 225 Dickinson Street, San Diego, CA 92103-8433 · 619-543-6905

Daniel L. Clarke-Pearson · Professor of Gynecologic Oncology, Duke University School of Medicine · Director of Gynecologic Oncology, Duke University Medical Center · P.O. Box 3079, Durham, NC 27710 · 919-684-3765

Carmel Cohen · Professor and Vice-Chairman, Obstetrics, Gynecology & Reproductive Science, Mt. Sinai School of Medicine · Director, Division of Gynecologic Oncology, Mt. Sinai Medical Center · 1176 Fifth Avenue, Box 1173, New York, NY 10029 · 212-241-6554

Larry J. Copeland · Professor, Department of Obstetrics & Gynecology, and Director, Division of Gynecologic Oncology, Ohio State University College of Medicine · The Ohio State University Hospitals · 1654 Upham Drive, N500 Means Hall, Columbus, OH 43210 · 614-293-8737

William T. Creasman · Sims-Hester Professor and Chairman, Department of Obstetrics & Gynecology, Medical University of South Carolina · Medical University of South Carolina · Medical University of South Carolina, 171 Ashley Avenue, Charleston, SC 29425-2233 · 803-792-4509

Stephen L. Curry · (Complicated Surgical Gynecology, Vulvar Disease) · Professor of Obstetrics & Gynecology, University of Connecticut School of Medicine; Adjunct Professor of Maternal & Child Health, Dartmouth Medical School · Director, Department of Obstetrics & Gynecology, Hartford Hospital · 80 Seymour Street, Hartford, CT 06115 · 203-524-2795

Amodio Dennis DePetrillo · Professor and Director of Gynecologic Oncology, University of Toronto School of Medicine · Chief, Surgical Oncology, Princess Margaret Hospital · 500 Sherbourne Street, Toronto, Ontario M4X 1K9 · 416-926-6583

Philip J. DiSaia · The Dorothy Marsh Chair in Reproductive Biology; and Professor, Department of Obstetrics & Gynecology, University of California, Irvine School of Medicine · Director, Division of Gynecologic Oncology, University of California, Irvine Medical Center; Long Beach Memorial Medical Center · 101 The City Drive, Building 26, Orange, CA 92668 · 714-634-5220

Wesley C. Fowler, Jr. · Palumbo Professor and Associate Chair, Department of Obstetrics & Gynecology, Division of Oncology, University of North Carolina School of Medicine · University of North Carolina Hospitals · Campus Box 7570, Chapel Hill, NC 27599-7570 · 919-966-1196

David M. Gershenson · Professor of Gynecology, The University of Texas · The University of Texas MD Anderson Cancer Center · 1515 Holcombe Boulevard, Houston, TX 77030 · 713-792-2770

Kenneth D. Hatch · Professor of Obstetrics & Gynecology, The University of Arizona College of Medicine · Director of Obstetrics & Gynecology Division, The University of Arizona Health Sciences Center · 1501 North Campbell Avenue, Tucson, AZ 85724 · 602-626-2719

Arthur L. Herbst · Joseph Bolivar DeLee Distinguished Service Professor, and Chairman of Obstetrics & Gynecology, University of Chicago, Pritzker School of Medicine · University of Chicago Medical Center · 5841 South Maryland Avenue, Box 446, Chicago, IL 60637 · 312-702-6127

Howard D. Homesley · Professor and Section Head, Department of Gynecology/Oncology, The Bowman Gray School of Medicine of Wake Forest University · North Carolina Baptist Hospital · Medical Center Boulevard, Winston-Salem, NC 27157-1065 · 919-748-4022

William J. Hoskins · Chief of Gynecology, Memorial Sloan-Kettering Cancer Center · 1275 York Avenue, New York, NY 10021 · 212-639-7766

Leo D. Lagasse · Professor of Obstetrics & Gynecology, University of California at Los Angeles School of Medicine · Director, Division of Gynecologic Oncology, Cedars-Sinai Medical Center · 8700 Beverly Boulevard, Suite 1738, Los Angeles, CA 90048 · 213-855-3373

John L. Lewis, Jr. · Professor of Obstetrics & Gynecology, Cornell University Medical College · Attending Surgeon, Memorial Sloan-Kettering Cancer Center · 1275 York Avenue, New York, NY 10021 · 212-639-7664

Francis J. Major · Associate Professor of Obstetrics & Gynecology, University of Colorado School of Medicine · Chief, Gynecology Tumor Service, Presbyterian-St. Luke's Medical Center · 1955 Pennsylvania Street, Suite 208, Denver, CO 80203 · 303-860-0246

John J. Mikuta · Franklin Payne Professor of Gynecologic Oncology, University of Pennsylvania School of Medicine · Director, Gynecologic Oncology, Hospital of the University of Pennsylvania · Courtyard Building, 3400 Spruce Street, Suite 1000, Philadelphia, PA 19104 · 215-662-3313

George W. Morley · The University of Michigan Medical School · The University of Michigan Medical Center · 1500 East Medical Center Drive, Ann Arbor, MI 48109 · 313-764-8125

C. Paul Morrow · Professor of Gynecology, University of Southern California School of Medicine · Director of Gynecologic Oncology, The Los Angeles County + University of Southern California Medical Center; University of Southern California Kenneth Norris, Jr. Cancer Hospital · 1240 North Mission Road, Room L903, Los Angeles, CA 90033 · 213-226-3397

Karl C. Podratz · Professor of Obstetrics & Gynecology, and Joseph & Barbara Ashkins Professor of Surgery, Mayo Graduate School of Medicine · Chairman, Department of Obstetrics & Gynecology, Mayo Clinic · 200 First Street, SW, Rochester, MN 55905 · 507-284-2715

Carolyn D. Renowicz · Director of Gynecologic Oncology, Albert Einstein College of Medicine · Weiler Hospital of the Albert Einstein College of Medicine · Belfer Building, 1300 Morris Park Avenue, Room 50, New York, NY 10461 · 212-430-3582

Neil B. Rosenshein · (Epidemiology) · Associate Professor, Johns Hopkins University School of Medicine · The Johns Hopkins Medical Institutions · 550 North Broadway, Baltimore, MD 21205 · 410-955-5478

Peter E. Schwartz · Professor of Obstetrics & Gynecology, and Director of Gynecologic Oncology, Yale University School of Medicine · Attending Physician, Yale-New Haven Hospital · 333 Cedar Street, 316FMB, New Haven, CT 06510 203-785-4176

Hugh M. Shingleton · J. Marion Sims Professor and Chairman, Department of Obstetrics & Gynecology, The University of Alabama School of Medicine · Obstetrician-Gynecologist-in-Chief, The University of Alabama Hospital · 618 South 20th Street, Room 560 Old Hillman Building, Birmingham, AL 35233-7333 205-934-3394

Frederick D. Stehman · Professor of Obstetrics & Gynecology, Indiana University School of Medicine · Chief of Obstetrics & Gynecology Services, Wishard Memorial Hospital; Indiana University Medical Center · 1001 West 10th Street, Indianapolis, IN 46202 · 317-630-7837

Leo B. Twiggs · Professor and Interim Head, Department of Obstetrics & Gynecology, University of Minnesota School of Medicine · University of Minnesota Hospital & Clinics · 420 Delaware Street SE, Box 395 UMHC, Minneapolis, MN 55455 · 612-626-6220

Paul Underwood, Jr. · The W. N. Thornton, Jr. Professor of Obstetrics & Gynecology, and Chair, Department of Obstetrics & Gynecology, University of Virginia School of Medicine · University of Virginia Health Sciences Center · Box 387, Charlottesville, VA 22908 · 804-924-9937

John R. van Nagell · Professor and Director, Division of Gynecologic Oncology, University of Kentucky College of Medicine · University of Kentucky Medical Center · Department of Obstetrics & Gynecology, Room MN308, 800 Rose Street, Lexington, KY 40536 · 606-233-5553

J. Taylor Wharton · Professor and Chairman of Gynecology, The University of Texas · The University of Texas MD Anderson Cancer Center · 10 Tokeneke Trail, Houston, TX 77024 · 713-792-2770

INFECTIOUS DISEASE
(See also Infectious Disease)

Marvin S. Amstey · Professor of Obstetrics & Gynecology, University of Rochester School of Medicine & Dentistry · Chief, Department of Obstetrics & Gynecology, Highland Hospital · 1000 South Avenue, Rochester, NY 14620 · 716-461-6730

W. Patrick Duff · Professor of Obstetrics & Gynecology, University of Florida College of Medicine · Shands Hospital at the University of Florida · 1600 Southwest Archer Road, Room M373, P.O. Box 100294, Gainesville, FL 32610 · 904-392-3222

David Eschenbach · (Sexually Transmitted Disease) · Professor of Obstetrics & Gynecology, University of Washington School of Medicine · University of Washington Medical Center · 1959 Northeast Pacific Street, Seattle, WA 98195 · 206-543-3423

Sebastian Faro · Professor and Vice-Chairman, Department of Obstetrics & Gynecology, Baylor College of Medicine · The Methodist Hospital; St. Luke's Episcopal Hospital; Harris County Hospital District · 6550 Fannin Street, Suite 701, Houston, TX 77030 · 713-798-7500

Ronald S. Gibbs · (Sexually Transmitted Disease) · Professor and Chairman, Department of Obstetrics & Gynecology, University of Colorado School of Medicine · University of Colorado Health Sciences Center · 4200 East Ninth Avenue, Box B-198, Denver, CO 80262 · 303-270-7616

William J. Ledger · Given Foundation Professor of Obstetrics & Gynecology, Cornell University Medical College · Obstetrician & Gynecologist-in-Chief, The New York Hospital-Cornell Medical Center · 525 East 68th Street, Room M-036, New York, NY 10021 · 212-746-3009

James A. McGregor · Professor of Obstetrics & Gynecology, University of Colorado School of Medicine · University of Colorado Health Sciences Center · 4200 East Ninth Avenue, B198, Denver, CO 80262 · 303-270-7924

Philip B. Mead · Clinical Professor, Department of Obstetrics & Gynecology, University of Vermont School of Medicine · Hospital Epidemiologist, Medical Center Hospital of Vermont · MCHV Infection Control, Adams Building, Burlington, VT 05401 · 802-656-2760

Howard L. Minkoff · Professor of Obstetrics & Gynecology, and Director of Maternal & Fetal Medicine, State University of New York Health Science Center at Brooklyn · 14519 Newport Avenue, Brooklyn, NY 11203 · 718-270-2072

David E. Soper · Associate Professor of Department of Obstetrics & Gynecology, Virginia Commonwealth University, Medical College of Virginia · Medical College of Virginia Hospital · 12th and Marshall, Eighth Floor, Room 220, Richmond, VA 23298-0034 · 804-371-8612

Richard L. Sweet · (Sexually Transmitted Disease) · Professor and Vice-Chairman, Department of Obstetrics, Gynecology & Reproductive Sciences, University of California at San Francisco School of Medicine · Chief of Obstetrics & Gynecology, San Francisco General Hospital · 1001 Potrero Avenue, OB-GYN Ward 6D, Room 14, San Francisco, CA 94110 · 415-821-8358

MATERNAL & FETAL MEDICINE
(See also Pediatrics, Neonatal-Perinatal Medicine)

Garland D. Anderson · (Perinatology) · Gennie Sealy Smith Professor of Obstetrics & Gynecology, The University of Texas Medical Branch at Galveston · Chairman, Department of Obstetrics & Gynecology, The University of Texas Medical Branch at Galveston · 301 University Boulevard, Route E-87, Galveston, TX 77550 · 409-772-1572

Thomas J. Benedetti · (Perinatology) · Professor of Obstetrics & Gynecology, University of Washington School of Medicine · Director, Perinatal Medicine, University of Washington Medical Center · Department of OB/GYN, Mail Stop RH-20, Seattle, WA 98195 · 206-543-3729

Richard Berkowitz · Professor and Chairman, Department of Obstetrics & Gynecology, Mt. Sinai School of Medicine · Mt. Sinai Medical Center · One Gustave L. Levy Place, Box 1171, New York, NY 10029 · 212-241-5681

Frank H. Boehm · Director of Maternal & Fetal Medicine, Vanderbilt University School of Medicine · Vanderbilt University Medical Center · B1100 Medical Center North, Nashville, TN 37232-2519 · 615-322-2071

Watson A. Bowes, Jr. · Professor Of Obstetrics & Gynecology, University of North Carolina School of Medicine · University of North Carolina Hospitals · Campus Box 7570, Chapel Hill, NC 27599-7570 · 919-966-4688

M. Shannon Burke · Clinical Instructor, University of Colorado Health Sciences Center · Medical Director, Perinatal Resource Center, Swedish Medical Center · 601 East Hampden Avenue, Suite 430, Englewood, CO 80110-2764 · 303-788-8550

Micki L. Cabaniss · Associate Professor of Obstetrics & Gynecology, University of North Carolina School of Medicine; Mountain Area Health Education Center, Department of Obstetrics & Gynecology · Mountain Area Women's Health Service; Memorial Mission Hospital · 60 Livingston Street, Suite 100, Asheville, NC 28801 · 704-258-1202

Steve N. Caritis · Professor of Obstetrics & Gynecology, University of Pittsburgh School of Medicine · Director, Division of Maternal & Fetal Medicine, Magee-Womens Hospital, University of Pittsburgh Medical Center · 300 Halket Street, Pittsburgh, PA 15213 · 412-647-4874

Dru E. Carlson · Assistant Professor of Obstetrics & Gynecology, University of California at Los Angeles School of Medicine · Director, Reproductive Genetics, Cedars-Sinai Medical Center · 8700 Beverly Boulevard, Suite 1738, Los Angeles, CA 90048 · 213-855-4410

Robert C. Cefalo · Professor of Obstetrics & Gynecology, and Director of Maternal & Fetal Medicine, University of North Carolina School of Medicine · Assistant Dean, Head Office of Graduate Medical Education, University of North Carolina Hospitals · 214 MacNider Building, Campus Box 7570, Chapel Hill, NC 27599-7570 · 919-966-1601

Curtis L. Cetrulo · Professor of Obstetrics & Gynecology, Tufts University School of Medicine · Director, Maternal & Fetal Medicine, St. Margaret's Hospital for Women · 90 Cushing Avenue, Boston, MA 02125 · 617-436-2195

Frank A. Chervenak · (Ultrasound, Ethics) · Associate Professor of Obstetrics & Gynecology, Cornell University Medical College · Director of Obstetrics, and Director, Division of Maternal-Fetal Medicine, The New York Hospital-Cornell

Medical Center · 525 East 68th Street, Room M036, New York, NY 10021 · 212-746-3184

Ronald A. Chez · Professor of Obstetrics & Gynecology, and Professor of Community & Family Helath, University South Florida College of Medicine · Director, Genesis Program, Tampa General Hospital · Four Columbia Drive, Suite 529, Tampa, FL 33606 · 813-254-7774

Steven L. Clark · Professor of Obstetrics & Gynecology, University of Utah School of Medicine · Director, Perinatal Centers for Intermountain Health Care, Latter Day Saints Hospital · Eighth Avenue and C Street, Salt Lake City, UT 84143 · 801-321-3446

William H. Clewell · Associate Director, Department of Maternal & Fetal Medicine, Good Samaritan Hospital · 1300 North 12th Street, Suite 320, Phoenix, AZ 85006 · 602-239-2647

David B. Cotton · Professor and Chairman, Department of Obstetrics & Gynecology, Wayne State University School of Medicine · Chief, Department of Obstetrics & Gynecology, Detroit Medical Center-Hutzel Hospital · 4707 St. Antoine Boulevard, Detroit, MI 48201 · 313-745-7283

Larry M. Cousins · Director, Maternal & Fetal Medicine, Sharp Perinatal Center 8010 Frost Street, Suite M, San Diego, CA 92123 · 619-541-6872

Don Coustan · Professor and Chairman of Obstetrics & Gynecology, Brown University School of Medicine · Chief of Obstetrics & Gynecology, Women & Infants Hospital · 101 Dudley Street, Providence, RI 02905 · 401-274-1100

Robert K. Creasy · Professor and Chairman of Obstetrics & Gynecology, The University of Texas Health Science Center at Houston · Hermann Hospital · 6431 Fannin Street, Suite 3204, Houston, TX 77030 · 713-792-5362

Marion Carlyle Crenshaw, Jr. · Professor and Chairman of Obstetrics & Gynecology, University of Maryland School of Medicine · Clinical Chief, Obstetrics & Gynecology, University of Maryland Medical Center · 22 South Greene Street, Sixth Floor North, Baltimore, MD 21201 · 410-328-5966

Dwight P. Cruikshank IV · McMahon Professor and Chairman, Department of Obstetrics & Gynecology, Medical College of Wisconsin · Milwaukee County Medical Complex · 8700 West Wisconsin Avenue, Box 121, Milwaukee, WI 53226 414-257-5560

Mary E. D'Alton · Associate Professor of Obstetrics & Gynecology, Tufts University School of Medicine · Director, Maternal & Fetal Medicine, St. Margaret's Hospital for Women · 90 Cushing Avenue, MSM Department, Boston, MA 02125 617-436-8600

Bonnie J. Dattel · Assistant Professor of Obstetrics, Gynecology & Reproductive Sciences, Division of Maternal & Fetal Medicine, University of California at San Francisco School of Medicine · Medical Director, San Francisco Rape Treatment Center, San Francisco General Hospital · 1001 Potrero Avenue, Ward 6D, San Francisco, CA 94110 · 415-821-5108

O. Richard Depp · Professor of Obstetrics & Gynecology, Jefferson Medical College of Thomas Jefferson University · Chairman, Department of Obstetrics & Gynecology, Thomas Jefferson University Hospital · 1025 Walnut Street, Room 310, Philadelphia, PA 19107 · 215-955-6920

Lawrence D. Devoe · Professor of Obstetrics & Gynecology, and Director, Maternal & Fetal Medicine, Medical College of Georgia · 1120 Fifteenth Street, Room CJ134, Augusta, GA 30912 · 404-721-3556

Sharon Lee Dooley · Associate Professor, Northwestern University Medical School · Prentice Women's Hospital · 333 East Superior Street, Room 410, Chicago, IL 60611 · 312-908-7519

Maurice L. Druzin · Professor of Gynecology & Obstetrics, Stanford University School of Medicine · Chief, Section of Maternal & Fetal Medicine, and Director of Perinatal Diagnostic Center, Stanford University Hospital · 300 Pasteur Drive, A-342, Stanford, CA 94305-5317 · 415-725-8623

W. Patrick Duff · Professor of Obstetrics & Gynecology, University of Florida College of Medicine · Shands Hospital at the University of Florida · 1600 Southwest Archer Road, Room M373, P.O. Box 100294, Gainesville, FL 32610 · 904-392-3222

Thomas R. Easterling · Assistant Professor of Obstetrics & Gynecology, University of Washington School of Medicine · University of Washington Medical Center 1959 Northeast Pacific Street, RH-20, Seattle, WA 98195 · 206-543-1521

Joseph McDonald Ernest · Associate Professor of Obstetrics & Gynecology, The Bowman Gray School of Medicine of Wake Forest University · North Carolina Baptist Hospital · Medical Center Boulevard, Winston-Salem, NC 27157-1066 · 919-748-4291

Roger K. Freeman · Professor of Obstetrics & Gynecology, University of California at Irvine School of Medicine · Senior Vice-President, Women's Services, Long Beach Memorial Medical Center · 2801 Atlantic Avenue, Long Beach, CA 90801 · 213-595-3145

Fredric D. Frigoletto · William Lambert Richardson Professor of Obstetrics, Harvard Medical School · Vice Chairman of Obstetrics & Gynecology, Brigham & Women's Hospital · 75 Francis Street, Boston, MA 02115 · 617-732-5445

Steven G. Gabbe · Professor and Chairman, Department of Obstetrics & Gynecology, Ohio State University College of Medicine · The Ohio State University Hospitals · 1654 Upham Drive, Room 505 Means Hall, Columbus, OH 43210 · 614-293-8697

Norman F. Gant, Jr. · Professor of Obstetrics & Gynecology, The University of Texas Southwestern Medical Center at Dallas · Attending Staff, Parkland Memorial Hospital · 5323 Harry Hines Boulevard, Dallas, TX 75235-9032 · 214-688-3755

Thomas J. Garite · Professor and Chairman, Department of Obstetrics & Gynecology, University of California, Irvine School of Medicine · UCI Medical Center 101 The City Drive, Orange, CA 92668 · 714-634-5968

Larry C. Gilstrap III · Professor of Obstetrics & Gynecology, and Director of Maternal & Fetal Medicine Fellowship & Clinical Genetics, The University of Texas Southwestern Medical Center at Dallas · Attending Physician, Parkland Memorial Hospital; St. Paul's Medical Center · 5323 Harry Hines Boulevard, Dallas, TX 75235 · 214-688-2646

Bernard Gonik · Associate Professor of Obstetrics & Gynecology, Division of Maternal & Fetal Medicine, The University of Texas Medical School at Houston Hermann Hospital · 6431 Fannin Street, Suite 3.204, Houston, TX 77030 · 713-792-5360

Gary D. V. Hankins · Chairman, Department of Obstetrics & Gynecology, Uniformed Services of the Health Sciences Center · Wilford Hall, United States Air Force Medical Center · Lackland Air Force Base, San Antonio, TX 78236 · 512-670-6136

John C. Hauth · Director of the Division of Maternal & Fetal Medicine, The University of Alabama School of Medicine · Director of Maternal-Fetal Medicine, The University of Alabama Hospital · Old Hillman Building, 619 South Twentieth Street, Suite 458, Birmingham, AL 35233-7333 · 205-934-5612

John C. Hobbins · (Ultrasound) · Professor of Obstetrics & Gynecology & Diagnostic Radiology, Yale University School of Medicine · Director of Obstetrics, Yale-New Haven Hospital · Department of OBGYN, 333 Cedar Street, New Haven, CT 06510 · 203-785-6755

John F. Huddleston · Professor of Obstetrics & Gynecology, Emory University School of Medicine · Director of Maternal & Fetal Medicine, Crawford W. Long Memorial Hospital; Grady Memorial Hospital · 20 Linden Avenue, Suite 4701, Atlanta, GA 30308 · 404-686-8121

Robert W. Huff · Professor and Deputy Chairman, Department of Obstetrics & Gynecology, The University of Texas Health Science Center at San Antonio · The University of Texas Health Science Center at San Antonio · 7703 Floyd Curl Drive, San Antonio, TX 78284 · 512-567-5008

Jay D. Iams · Professor, Department of Obstetrics & Gynecology, Ohio State University College of Medicine · Attending Physician; Director, Prematurity Prevention Program; Director, Prenatal Diagnosis Program, The Ohio State University Hospitals · 4775 Knightsbridge Boulevard, Columbus, OH 43214 · 614-442-5763

John W. C. Johnson · Professor of Obstetrics & Gynecology, University of Florida College of Medicine · Shands Hospital at the University of Florida · 1600 Southwest Archer Road, Room M318, P.O. Box 100294, Gainesville, FL 32610 · 904-392-3306

Allen Killam · Professor, Department of Obstetrics & Gynecology, and Director, Maternal & Fetal Medicine Program, Duke University School of Medicine · Duke University Medical Center · Box 3122, DUMC, Durham, NC 27710 · 919-684-2876

G. Eric Knox · Clinical Associate Professor of Obstetrics & Gynecology, University of Minnesota School of Medicine · Director, Perinatal Center, Abbott Northwestern Hospital · 800 East 28th Street, Minneapolis, MN 55407 · 612-863-5030

Neil K. Kochenour · University of Utah School of Medicine · University of Utah Health Sciences Center · 50 North Medical Drive, Suite 2B-200, Salt Lake City, UT 84132 · 801-581-7260

Kathleen A. Kuhlman · Assistant Professor of Obstetrics & Gynecology, Jefferson Medical College of Thomas Jefferson University · Director, Reproductive Ultrasound, Thomas Jefferson University Hospital · 1025 Walnut Street, Room 310, Philadelphia, PA 19107 · 215-955-7996

Oded Langer · (Diabetes) · Jane & Roland Blumberg Professor in Obstetrics & Gynecology, The University of Texas Health Science Center at San Antonio · Medical Center Hospital · 7703 Floyd Curl Drive, San Antonio, TX 78284-7836 · 512-567-5009

Russell K. Laros, Jr. · Professor and Vice-Chairman, Department of Obstetrics, Gynecology & Reproductive Sciences, University of California at San Francisco School of Medicine · University of California at San Francisco Medical Center · 400 Parnassus Avenue, Box 0346, San Francisco, CA 94143-0346 · 415-476-3223

Richard I. Lowensohn · Associate Professor of Obstetrics & Gynecology, Oregon Health Sciences University · Chief of Obstetrics, Oregon Health Sciences University · 3181 Southwest Sam Jackson Park Road, Portland, OR 97201-3098 · 503-494-7968

Denise M. Main · Director, Perinatal Diagnosis Center, and Associate Chief, Perinatal Services, California Pacific Medical Center · 2100 Webster Street, Suite 300, San Francisco, CA 94115 · 415-923-3046

Frank A. Manning · Professor and Chairman, Department of Obstetrics & Gynecology, University of Manitoba School of Medicine · Women's Centre of the Health Sciences Centre · 735 Notre Dame Avenue, Suite WR-120, Winnipeg, Manitoba R3E 0L8 · 204-787-3175

Paul J. Meis · Section Head and Professor of Obstetrics & Gynecology, The Bowman Gray School of Medicine of Wake Forest University · Forsyth Memorial Hospital · Medical Center Boulevard, Winston-Salem, NC 27157-1066 · 919-748-4595

Michael T. Mennuti · Professor and Chairman, Department of Obstetrics & Gynecology, University of Pennsylvania School of Medicine · Professor and Chairman, Department of Obstetrics & Gynecology, Hospital of the University of Pennsylvania · 3400 Spruce Street, Four Gibson Building, Philadelphia, PA 19104-4283 · 215-662-3234

Frank C. Miller · Professor and Chairman of Obstetrics & Gynecology, University of Kentucky Medical Center · 800 Rose Street, MN318, Lexington, KY 40536-0084 · 606-233-5345

Thomas R. Moore · Director, Division of Perinatal Medicine, Department of Reproductive Medicine, University of California at San Diego School of Medicine · University of California at San Diego Medical Center · 225 Dickinson Street, Mail Code 8433, San Diego, CA 92103-8433 · 619-543-5400

Mark A. Morgan · Assistant Professor in Residence, University of California at Irvine School of Medicine · University of California at Irvine Medical Center · 101 The City Drive, Building 25, Orange, CA 92668 · 714-634-6618

John Morrison · Professor of Obstetrics & Gynecology, and Pediatrics, University of Mississippi · Vice-Chairman and Director of Research, Department of Obstetrics & Gynecology, University of Mississippi Medical Center · 2500 North State Street, Jackson, MS 39216-4505 · 601-984-1010

David Augustus Nagey · Associate Professor of Obstetrics & Gynecology, and Adjunct Associate Professor in Electrical Engineering, University of Maryland School of Medicine · Director, Division of Maternal-Fetal Medicine, University of

Maryland Medical Center · 419 West Redwood Street, Suite 500, Baltimore, MD 21201 · 410-328-6640

Roger B. Newman · Associate Professor of Obstetrics & Gynecology, and Director, Maternal & Fetal Medicine, Medical University of South Carolina · 171 Ashley Avenue, Charleston, SC 29425 · 803-792-7100

Jennifer R. Niebyl · Professor of Obstetrics & Gynecology, The University of Iowa College of Medicine · Chairman, Department of Obstetrics & Gynecology, The University of Iowa Hospitals & Clinics · 200 Hawkins Drive, Iowa City, IA 52242 · 319-356-1976

David J. Nochimson · Professor of Obstetrics & Gynecology, and Vice-Chairman, Department of Obstetrics, and Associate Dean, Medical Affairs, University of Connecticut School of Medicine · John Dempsey Hospital · 263 Farmington Avenue, Room C2165, Farmington, CT 06030 · 203-679-3267

William F. O'Brien · Professor of Obstetrics & Gynecology, and Director of Obstetrics/Maternal Fetal Medicine, University South Florida College of Medicine · Tampa General Hospital · 12901 Bruce B. Downs Boulevard, Box 18, Tampa, FL 33612 · 813-254-7774

Valerie M. Parisi · Associate Professor of Obstetrics, Gynecology & Reproductive Sciences, and Pediatrics, The University of Texas Medical School at Houston · Director, Division of Maternal & Fetal Medicine, Hermann Hospital; Lyndon Baines Johnson Hospital · 6431 Fannin Street, Suite 3.204, Houston, TX 77030 · 713-792-5360 x727

Roy H. Petrie · (Perinatology) · Professor of Obstetrics & Gynecology, Washington University School of Medicine · Barnes Hospital · 4911 Barnes Hospital Plaza, St. Louis, MO 63110 · 314-362-1016

Roy M. Pitkin · Professor and Chairman, Department of Obstetrics & Gynecology, University of California at Los Angeles School of Medicine · University of California at Los Angeles Center for the Health Sciences · 10833 LeConte Avenue, Los Angeles, CA 90024-1740 · 213-206-2056

Richard P. Porreco · Associate Clinical Professor, University of Colorado School of Medicine · Presbyterian-St. Luke's Medical Center · 601 East 19th Avenue, Denver, CO 80203 · 303-869-2086

Manuel Porto · Associate Professor of Obstetrics & Gynecology, University of California, Irvine School of Medicine · Director, Maternal & Fetal Medicine, University of California, Irvine Medical Center · 101 The City Drive, Building 25, Orange, CA 92668 · 714-634-5967

John P. Queenan · Professor and Chairman, Department of Obstetrics & Gynecology, Georgetown University School of Medicine · Georgetown University Medical Center · Pasquerilla Health Care Center, Third Floor, 3800 Reservoir Road, NW, Washington, DC 20007 · 202-687-8531

J. Gerald Quirk, Jr. · Professor and Chairman, Department of Obstetrics & Gynecology, University of Arkansas for Medical Sciences · 4301 West Markham Street, Little Rock, AR 72205 · 501-686-5380

Kathryn L. Reed · Associate Professor of Obstetrics & Gynecology, The University of Arizona College of Medicine · The University of Arizona Health Sciences Center · 1501 North Campbell Avenue, Tucson, AZ 85724 · 602-626-6174

Robert Resnik · Professor and Chairman, Department of Reproductive Medicine, University of California at San Diego School of Medicine · Chief of Obstetrics & Gynecology, University of California at San Diego Medical Center · 225 Dickinson Street, Box 8433, San Diego, CA 92103 · 619-543-6960

J. W. Knox Ritchie · Professor of Obstetrics & Gynecology, University of Toronto School of Medicine · Obstetrician & Gynecologist-in-Chief, Mt. Sinai Hospital · 600 University Avenue, Room 465, Toronto, Ontario M5G 1X5 · 416-586-5309

Roberto Romero · Associate Professor and Director of Perinatal Research, Yale University School of Medicine · Yale-New Haven Hospital · 333 Cedar Street, New Haven, CT 06510 · 203-785-6598

Mortimer G. Rosen · Willard C. Rappleye Professor of Obstetrics,and Chairman, Department of Obstetrics & Gynecology, College of Physicians & Surgeons of Columbia University · Columbia-Presbyterian Medical Center · 622 West 168th Street, PH16-28, New York, NY 10032 · 212-305-2377

John Seeds · Professor of Obstetrics & Gynecology, and Director, Division of Maternal & Fetal Medicine, and Residency Program Director, Department of Obstetrics & Gynecology, The University of Arizona Health Sciences Center · 1501 North Campbell Avenue, Tucson, AZ 85724 · 602-626-5995

Michael L. Socol · Associate Professor and Head, Section of Maternal Fetal Medicine, Department of Obstetrics & Gynecology, Northwestern University Medical School · Chief, Division of Obstetrics, Prentice Women's Hospital & Maternity Center of Northwestern Memorial Hospital · 333 East Superior Street, Room 410, Chicago, IL 60611 · 312-908-7518

Robert J. Sokol · (Fetal-Alcohol Syndrome, Addicted Pregnant Women) · Dean, School of Medicine, and Professor of Obstetrics & Gynecology, Wayne State University Medical Center · Chairman of the Medical Board, Detroit Medical Center · 540 East Canfield, Detroit, MI 48201 · 313-577-1335

William N. Spellacy · Professor and Chairman, Obstetrics & Gynecology, University South Florida College of Medicine · Four Columbia Drive, Suite 529, Tampa, FL 33606 · 813-254-7774

James A. Thorp · Assistant Professor of Obstetrics & Gynecology, University of Missouri at Kansas City School of Medicine · Associate Director of Maternal & Fetal Medicine, St. Luke's Perinatal Center · 4400 Wornall Road, Kansas City, MO 64111 · 816-932-3585

J. Peter VanDorsten · Professor of Obstetrics & Gynecology, Virginia Commonwealth University, Medical College of Virginia · Director of Maternal & Fetal Medicine, Medical College of Virginia Hospital · Box 34, MCV Station, Richmond, VA 23298-0034 · 804-786-5938

Isabelle A. Wilkins · Assistant Professor, Department of Obstetrics, Gynecology & Reproductive Sciences, and Assistant Professor, Department of Pediatrics, The University of Texas Medical School at Houston · Director of Antepartum Testing Unit, Hermann Hospital; Director, Obstetrical Ultrasound, and Director, Prenatal Diagnosis Program, Houston Medical Center · 6431 Fannin Street, Suite 3.204, Houston, TX 77030 · 713-792-5360

James R. Woods · (High-Risk Pregnancies) · Professor of Obstetrics & Gynecology, University of Rochester School of Medicine & Dentistry · Associate Chair, Department of Obstetrics & Gynecology, and Director of Obstetrics & Maternal & Fetal Medicine, Strong Memorial Hospital, University of Rochester Medical Center · 601 Elmwood Avenue, Box 668, Rochester, NY 14642 · 716-275-7824

John D. Yeast · Associate Professor of Obstetrics & Gynecology, University of Missouri at Kansas City School of Medicine · Director, Maternal & Fetal Medicine, St. Luke's Hospital of Kansas City · Outpatient Center, 4400 Wornall Road, Kansas City, MO 64111 · 816-932-3585

Margaret Lynn Yonekura · (Addicted Pregnant Women) · Associate Professor of Obstetrics & Gynecology, University of California at Los Angeles School of Medicine · Harbor-UCLA Medical Center · 1000 West Carson Street, Box 3, Torrance, CA 90509 · 213-533-3565

William P. Young · (Perinatology) · Associate Professor of Obstetrics & Gynecology, Oregon Health Sciences University · Chief of Obstetrics & Gynecology, Emanuel Hospital & Health Center · 2801 North Gantenbein Avenue, Portland, OR 97227 · 503-280-4658

PEDIATRIC & ADOLESCENT GYNECOLOGY
(See also Pediatrics, Pediatric & Adolescent Gynecology)

S. Jean Emans · Associate Professor of Pediatrics, Harvard Medical School · Associate Chief, Division of Adolescent/Young Adult Medicine, Children's Hospital · 300 Longwood Avenue, Boston, MA 02115 · 617-735-6000

Alvin F. Goldfarb · (Reproductive Endocrinology) · Professor of Obstetrics & Gynecology, and Director, Medical Education of Department of Obstetrics & Gynecology, Jefferson Medical College of Thomas Jefferson University · Thomas Jefferson University Hospital · 1025 Walnut Street, Room 310, Philadelphia, PA 19107 · 215-955-8461

John A. Rock · (Reproductive Surgery, Endometriosis) · Professor, Department of Gynecology & Obstetrics, Johns Hopkins University School of Medicine · Chairman, Department of Gynecology & Obstetrics, The Union Memorial Hospital; The Johns Hopkins Medical Institutions · The Union Memorial Hospital, 201 East University Parkway, Baltimore, MD 21218 · 301-554-2940

Joseph S. Sanfilippo · Associate Professor of Obstetrics & Gynecology, University of Louisville School of Medicine · Chief of Obstetrics & Gynecology, Norton Hospital; Chief of Gynecology, Kosair Children's Hospital · 601 South Floyd Street, Louisville, KY 40202 · 502-583-3845

REPRODUCTIVE ENDOCRINOLOGY

Eli Y. Adashi · Professor of Obstetrics & Gynecology, University of Maryland School of Medicine · Director, Division of Reproductive Endocrinology, University of Maryland Medical Center · 405 West Redwood Street, Third Floor, Baltimore, MD 21201 · 301-328-2304

E. James Aiman · Professor of Obstetrics & Gynecology, Medical College of Wisconsin · Medical College of Wisconsin Affiliated Hospitals · 8700 West Wisconsin Avenue, Milwaukee, WI 53226 · 414-257-5568

Ricardo H. Asch · (Assisted Reproductive Technology) · Professor of Obstetrics & Gynecology, University of California at Irvine School of Medicine · Director, Center for Reproductive Health · 101 The City Drive, Pavilion Two, Orange, CA 92668 · 714-634-5800

Robert L. Barbieri · Professor and Chairman, Department of Obstetrics & Gynecology, State University of New York Health Science Center at Stony Brook · Chief, Obstetrics & Gynecology, SUNY at Stony Brook Hospital · Health Science Center, T-9, Room 020, Stony Brook, NY 11794-8091 · 516-444-2734

Richard Edgar Blackwell · Professor of Obstetrics & Gynecology, and Director, Division of Reproductive Biology & Endocrinology, The University of Alabama School of Medicine · Old Hillman Building, 619 South 20th Street, Room 555, Birmingham, AL 35233-7333 · 205-934-6090

John E. Buster · (Infertility) · Professor and Director, Division of Reproductive Endocrinology and Infertility, The University of Tennessee at Memphis, College of Medicine · University of Tennessee Bowld Hospital; Baptist Memorial Hospital 956 Court Avenue, Room D-324, Memphis, TN 38163 · 901-528-5859

Bruce R. Carr · Paul C. MacDonald Professor of Obstetrics & Gynecology; and Director, Division of Reproductive Endocrinology, The University of Texas Southwestern Medical Center at Dallas · Attending Physician, Zale-Lipshy University Hospital; Parkland Memorial Hospital · 5323 Harry Hines Boulevard, Dallas, TX 75235-9032 · 214-688-4747

Sandra A. Carson · Associate Professor of Obstetrics & Gynecology, The University of Tennessee at Memphis, College of Medicine · University of Tennessee Health Science Center · 956 Court Avenue, Room D-324, Memphis, TN 38163 · 901-528-5859

R. Jeffrey Chang · University of California, Davis School of Medicine · Stockton Boulevard, Sacramento, CA 95817 · 916-734-6930

Alan H. De Cherney · Louis E. Phaneuf Professor, Tufts University School of Medicine · Chairman, Department of Obstetrics & Gynecology, New England Medical Center · 750 Washington Street, Boston, MA 02110 · 617-956-6063

Celso-Ramón García · (Infertility, Reproductive Surgery, Menopause) · Professor of Obstetrics & Gynecology, and the William Shippen, Jr. Professor of Human Reproduction, University of Pennsylvania School of Medicine · Consultant, Pennsylvania Hospital; Hospital of the University of Pennsylvania · 3400 Spruce Street, Philadelphia, PA 19104 · 215-662-2974

Jairo E. Garcia · (Fertility & Reproductive Endocrinology, Assisted Reproductive Technology) · Director, Woman's Hospital Fertility Center, Greater Baltimore Medical Center · 6565 North Charles Street, Suite 207, Baltimore, MD 21204 · 410-828-2484

Charles B. Hammond · Professor and Chairman, Department of Obstetrics & Gynecology, Duke University School of Medicine · Chief of Staff, Duke University Medical Center · P.O. Box 3853, Durham, NC 27710 · 919-684-3008

Mary G. Hammond · Associate Professor of Obstetrics & Gynecology, University of North Carolina School of Medicine · University of North Carolina Hospitals · Manning Drive, Campus Box 7570, Chapel Hill, NC 27599-7570 · 919-966-5283

Arthur F. Haney · Professor of Obstetrics & Gynecology, Duke University School of Medicine · Chief of Reproductive Endocrinology, Duke University Medical Center · P.O. Box 2971, Durham, NC 27710 · 919-684-5327

Robert B. Jaffe · Professor and Chairman, Department of Obstetrics, Gynecology & Reproductive Sciences; and Director, Reproductive Endocrinology Center, University of California, San Francisco School of Medicine · 505 Parnassus Avenue, M-1490, Box 0132, San Francisco, CA 94143-0132 · 415-476-2564

Georgeanna Seegar Jones · Professor of Obstetrics & Gynecology, Eastern Virginia Medical School · Sentara Hospitals · 825 Fairfax Avenue, Sixth Floor, Norfolk, VA 23507 · 804-446-8935

Howard W. Jones · (Assisted Reproductive Technology) · Professor of Obstetrics & Gynecology, Eastern Virginia Medical School · Sentara Hospitals · 601 Colley Avenue, Norfolk, VA 23507 · 804-446-8935

William Richard Keye, Jr. · Chief, Division of Reproductive Endocrinology & Infertility, William Beaumont Hospital · 3535 West Thirteen Mile Road, Suite 344, Royal Oaks, MI 48073 · 313-551-0515

Moon H. Kim · (Infertility) · The Richard L. Meiling Chair Professor and Vice-Chairman, Department of Obstetrics & Gynecology, Ohio State University College of Medicine · The Ohio State University Hospitals; Mt. Carmel Hospital · 1654 Upham Drive, Room 535, Columbus, OH 43210 · 614-293-8511

Oscar A. Kletzky · Professor of Obstetrics & Gynecology, University of California at Los Angeles School of Medicine · Chief, Division of Reproductive Endocrinology, Harbor-UCLA Medical Center · 21840 South Normandie Avenue, Suite 1000, Torrance, CA 90502 · 310-783-5125

James H. Liu · Associate Professor, Department of Obstetrics & Gynecology, and Director, Division of Reproductive Endocrinology & Infertility, University of Cincinnati College of Medicine · University of Cincinnati Hospital · 231 Bethesda Avenue, ML 526, Cincinnati, OH 45267 · 513-558-6560

Rogerio A. Lobo · Professor of Obstetrics & Gynecology, University of Southern California School of Medicine · Chief, Division of Reproductive Endocrinology & Infertility, The Los Angeles County + University of Southern California Medical Center, University of Southern California University Hospital · 1240 North Mission Road, Room 1M2, Los Angeles, CA 90033 · 213-226-3026

L. Russell Malinak · (Endometriosis) · Professor, Department of Obstetrics & Gynecology, Baylor College of Medicine · Medical Director, Center for Reproductive Medicine & Surgery, The Methodist Hospital;, St. Luke's Episcopal

Hospital · 6550 Fannin Street, Smith Tower, Suite 801, Houston, TX 77030 · 713-798-7686

Charles M. March · Professor of Obstetrics & Gynecology, University of Southern California School of Medicine · University of Southern California University Hospital, Saint Joseph Medical Center · 1560 East Chevy Chase Drive, Glendale, CA 91206 · 818-242-9933

Richard P. Marrs · (Assisted Reproductive Technology) · Loma Linda University School of Medicine · Director for Institute of Reproductive Research, Hospital of the Good Samaritan · 1245 Wilshire Boulevard, Suite 905, Los Angeles, CA 90017 213-482-4552

Mary C. Martin · Associate Professor, Department of Obstetrics, Gynecology & Reproductive Sciences, University of California at San Francisco School of Medicine · Director, In Vitro Fertilization Program, University of California at San Francisco Medical Center · 505 Parnassus Avenue, Box 0132, San Francisco, CA 94143-0132 · 415-476-2224

Luigi Mastroianni, Jr. · (Infertility) · The William Goodell Professor of Obstetrics & Gynecology and Director, Division of Human Reproduction, University of Pennsylvania School of Medicine · Hospital of the University of Pennsylvania · 3400 Spruce Street, Suite 106 Dulles, Philadelphia, PA 19104-4283 · 215-662-2951

Paul G. McDonough · Professor of Obstetrics & Gynecology, and Chief, Reproductive Endocrine Section, and Section Director of the Genetics Program, Medical College of Georgia · 1120 Fifteenth Street, Room CK159, Augusta, GA 30912 404-721-3832

David Roy Meldrum · (Assisted Reproductive Technology) · Clinical Professor, University of California at Los Angeles School of Medicine · Director, South Bay Center for Advanced Reproductive Care · 510 North Prospect Avenue, Suite 202, Redondo Beach, CA 90277 · 213-318-4741

Daniel R. Mishell, Jr. · The Lyle G. McNeile Professor and Chairman, Department of Obstetrics & Gynecology, University of Southern California School of Medicine · Chief of Professional Services, Women's Hospital; The Los Angeles County + University of Southern California Medical Center; University of Southern California University Hospital · 1240 North Mission Road, Los Angeles, CA 90033 · 213-226-3416

Mary Lake Polan · Professor and Chairman, Department of Gynecology & Obstetrics, Stanford University School of Medicine · Stanford University Medical Clinic · 300 Pasteur Drive, Room A-342, Stanford, CA 94305 · 415-723-5505

Robert William Rebar · George B. Riley Professor and Director, Department of Obstetrics & Gynecology, University of Cincinnati College of Medicine · Chief of Obstetrics & Gynecology, University Hospital, Children's Hospital, Good Samaritan Hospital, Christ Hospital · 231 Bethesda Avenue, ML 526, Cincinnati, OH 45267 · 513-558-8440

Daniel H. Riddick · Professor and Chairman, Department of Obstetrics & Gynecology, University of Vermont College of Medicine · Chief, Obstetrics & Gynecology, Medical Center Hospital of Vermont · Shepardson-4 South, Burlington, VT 05401-1435 · 802-656-1235

John A. Rock · (Endometriosis) · Professor, Department of Gynecology & Obstetrics, Johns Hopkins University School of Medicine · Chairman, Department of Gynecology & Obstetrics, The Union Memorial Hospital; The Johns Hopkins Medical Institutions · The Union Memorial Hospital, 201 East University Parkway, Baltimore, MD 21218 · 301-554-2940

Zev Rosenwaks · (Assisted Reproductive Technology) · Professor of Obstetrics & Gynecology, Cornell University Medical College · Director, The Center for Reproductive Medicine & Infertility, The New York Hospital-Cornell Medical Center · 505 East 70th Street, HT300, P.O. Box One, New York, NY 10021 · 212-746-1743

Kenneth J. Ryan · Kate Macy Ladd Professor and Chairman, Department of Obstetrics & Gynecology & Reproductive Biology; and Director, Laboratory of Human Reproduction & Reproductive Biology, Harvard Medical School · Chairman, Department of Obstetrics & Gynecology, Brigham & Women's Hospital · 75 Francis Street, Boston, MA 02115 · 617-732-5444

Cecilia L. Schmidt · (Infertility) · Professor of Obstetrics & Gynecology, and Director, Reproductive Endocrinology & Infertility, New York University Medical Center · 530 First Avenue, Suite 5F, New York, NY 10016 · 212-263-7566

James R. Schreiber · Professor and Head, Department of Obstetrics & Gynecology, Washington University School of Medicine · Obstetrician-Gynecologist-in-Chief, Barnes Hospital; The Jewish Hospital of St. Louis; St. Louis Regional Medical Center · 4911 Barnes Hospital Plaza, St. Louis, MO 63110 · 314-362-7139

Antonio Scommegna · Professor and Head of Obstetrics & Gynecology, The University of Illinois College of Medicine at Chicago · Chief of Service, Obstetrics & Gynecology, University of Illinois Hospital & Clinics; Humana Hospital-Michael Reese · 840 South Wood Street (M/C 808), Chicago, IL 60612 · 312-996-0222, 440-5180

Michael Roy Soules · (Infertility) · Professor of Obstetrics & Gynecology, University of Washington School of Medicine · Director, Division of Reproductive Endocrinology & Infertility, University of Washington Medical Center · Department of Obstetrics & Gynecology, 1959 Northeast Pacific Street, RH-20, Seattle, WA 98195 · 206-543-4693

Leon Speroff · Professor of Obstetrics & Gynecology, Oregon Health Sciences University · 3181 Southwest Sam Jackson Park Road, Portland, OR 97201-3098 · 503-494-4469

Robert J. Stillman · Professor of Obstetrics & Gynecology, The George Washington University School of Medicine · George Washington University Medical Center · 2150 Pennsylvania Avenue, NW, Washington, DC 20037 · 202-994-4614

Luther Marcus Talbert · University of North Carolina School of Medicine · University of North Carolina Hospitals · Department of OB-GYN, Campus Box 7570, Chapel Hill, NC 27599 · 919-966-5438

Edward E. Wallach · Professor and Chairman, Department of Gynecology & Obstetrics, and The Dorothy Edwards Professor of Gynecology, Johns Hopkins University School of Medicine · Director, Department of Gynecology & Obstetrics, The Johns Hopkins Hospital · Hauck Building, 600 North Wolfe Street, Room 264, Baltimore, MD 21205 · 410-955-7800

Gerson Weiss · Professor and Chairman, Department of Obstetrics & Gynecology, University of Medicine & Dentistry of New Jersey · Chief of Services, Department of Obstetrics & Gynecology, University Hospital · 185 South Orange Avenue, Newark, NJ 07103 · 201-456-5266

Samuel S. C. Yen · (Infertility) · Professor and Director of Productive Endocrinology & Infertility, University of California, San Diego School of Medicine · Director, Division of Reproductive Endocrinology & Infertility, University of California, San Diego Medical Center · Department of Reproductive Medicine (0802), University of California, San Diego School of Medicine, 9500 Gilman Drive, La Jolla, CA 92093-0802 · 619-543-3718

Howard Zacur · Vice-Chairman, Department of Gynecology & Obstetrics, and Director, Division of Reproductive Endocrinology, and Associate Professor of Gynecology & Obstetrics, Johns Hopkins University School of Medicine · The Johns Hopkins Medical Institutions · 600 North Wolfe Street, Houck 247, Baltimore, MD 21205 · 410-955-7294

Paul W. Zarutskie · (Fertility & Reproductive Endocrinology, Assisted Reproductive Technology) · Associate Professor of Obstetrics & Gynecology, University of Washington School of Medicine · Medical Director, Fertility and Endocrine Center; University of Washington Medical Center · 1959 Northeast Pacific Street, RH-20, Seattle, WA 98195 · 206-543-0670

REPRODUCTIVE SURGERY

Celso-Ramón García · Professor of Obstetrics & Gynecology, and the William Shippen, Jr. Professor of Human Reproduction, University of Pennsylvania School of Medicine · Consultant, Pennsylvania Hospital; Hospital of the University of Pennsylvania · 3400 Spruce Street, Philadelphia, PA 19104 · 215-662-2974

Ray A. Lee · Professor of Obstetrics & Gynecology, Mayo Medical School · Head, Section of Gynecologic Surgery, Mayo Clinic · 200 First Street, SW, Rochester, MN 55905 · 507-284-2511

L. Russell Malinak · Professor, Department of Obstetrics & Gynecology, Baylor College of Medicine · Medical Director, Center for Reproductive Medicine & Surgery, The Methodist Hospital;, St. Luke's Episcopal Hospital · 6550 Fannin Street, Smith Tower, Suite 801, Houston, TX 77030 · 713-798-7686

Charles M. March · Professor of Obstetrics & Gynecology, University of Southern California School of Medicine · University of Southern California University Hospital, Saint Joseph Medical Center · 1560 East Chevy Chase Drive, Glendale, CA 91206 · 818-242-9933

Daniel Clyde Martin · (Operative Laparoscopy) · Clinical Associate Professor of Obstetrics & Gynecology, The University of Tennessee at Memphis, College of Medicine · Reproductive Surgeon, Baptist Memorial Hospital · 910 Madison Avenue, Suite 805, Memphis, TN 38103 · 901-227-7287

John A. Rock · (Endometriosis) · Professor, Department of Gynecology & Obstetrics, Johns Hopkins University School of Medicine · Chairman, Department of Gynecology & Obstetrics, The Union Memorial Hospital; The Johns Hopkins Medical Institutions · The Union Memorial Hospital, 201 East University Parkway, Baltimore, MD 21218 · 301-554-2940

Morton A. Stenchever · (Infertility, Repairative Surgery) · Professor and Chair, Department of Obstetrics & Gynecology, University of Washington School of Medicine · Chief, Obstetrics & Gynecology, University of Washington Medical Center · 1959 Northeast Pacific Street, RH-20, Seattle, WA 98195 · 206-543-3045

OPHTHALMOLOGY

ANTERIOR SEGMENT (CATARACT SURGERY)

Charles H. Bechert II · Holy Cross Hospital · Sight Foundation, 4750 North Federal Highway, First Floor, Fort Lauderdale, FL 33308 · 305-771-4451

Ralph G. Berkeley · (Refractive Surgery) · Clinical Assistant Professor of Ophthalmology, The University of Texas Health Science Center at Houston · The Houston Eye Clinic; Houston Microsurgical Center · 1200 Binz, Suite 1000, Houston, TX 77004 · 713-526-1600

Stephen F. Brint · Assistant Clinical Professor of Ophthalmology, Tulane University School of Medicine · Pendleton Memorial Methodist Hospital · 5640 Read Boulevard, Suite 900, New Orleans, LA 70127 · 504-246-2136

Henry M. Clayman · Clinical Associate Professor of Ophthalmology, University of Miami School of Medicine · Chief of Ophthalmology, St. Francis Hospital; Bascom Palmer Eye Institute · 18999 Biscayne Boulevard, Miami, FL 33180 · 305-945-7433

Alan S. Crandall · Professor of Ophthalmology, University of Utah School of Medicine · University of Utah Health Sciences Center · 50 North Medical Drive, Salt Lake City, UT 84132 · 801-581-2769

Jack M Dodick · Associate Clinical Professor of Ophthalmology, College of Physicians & Surgeons of Columbia University · Chairman, Department of Ophthalmology, Manhattan Eye, Ear & Throat Hospital · 535 Park Avenue, New York, NY 10021 · 212-288-7638

David D. Dulaney · Dulaney Eye Clinic, 9425 West Bell Road, Sun City, AZ 85351 · 602-974-1000

I. Howard Fine · Clinical Assistant Professor of Ophthalmology, Oregon Health Sciences University; Adjunct Professor of Health Education, University of Oregon Co-Founder, Oregon Eye Surgery Center at the Oregon Eye Institute; Sacred Heart General Hospital; McKenzie Willamette General Hospital · 1550 Oak Street, Suite Five, Eugene, OR 97401 · 503-687-2110, 484-3883

Howard V. Gimbel · (Refractive Surgery) · Clinical Assistant Professor, University of Calgary Faculty of Medicine, Division of Ophthalmology · Foothills Hospital · Gimbel Eye Centre, 4935 Fortieth Avenue NW, Suite 450, Calgary, Alberta T3A 2N1 · 403-286-3022

John D. Hunkeler · Associate Clinical Professor of Ophthalmology, University of Kansas School of Medicine · St. Luke's Hospital of Kansas City · Hunkeler Eye Clinic, 4321 Washington Street, Suite 6000, Kansas City, MO 64111 · 816-931-4733

Stephen H. Johnson · Hoag Memorial Hospital Presbyterian · 1441 Avocado Avenue, Suite 206, Newport Beach, CA 92660 · 714-760-9007

Leeds (Jack) Katzen · Clinical Professor of Ophthalmology, University of Maryland School of Medicine; Assistant Clinical Professor of Ophthalmology, New York Medical College · Chief, Department of Ophthalmology, Mercy Medical Center · 1306 Bellona Avenue, Lutherville, MD 21093; Mercy Medical Center Professional Office Building, 301 St. Paul Place, Suite 902, Baltimore, MD 21202 301-821-9490

Douglas D. Koch · Associate Professor of Ophthalmology, Cullen Eye Institute, Baylor College of Medicine, Department of Ophthalmology · Attending Staff, The Methodist Hospital · 6501 Fannin Street, Suite NC200, Houston, TX 77030 713-798-6443

Paul S. Koch · Chief of Ophthalmology, Kent County Memorial Hospital · 566 Tollgate Road, Warwick, RI 02886 · 401-738-4800

Manus C. Kraff · (Refractive Surgery) · Professor of Clinical Ophthalmology, Northwestern University School of Medicine · Our Lady of the Resurrection Hospital; Lutheran General Hospital; 25 East Same Day Surgery · 25 East Washington Street, Chicago, IL 60602; Kraff Eye Institute, 5600 West Addison Street, Fourth Floor, Chicago, IL 60634 · 312-777-4444, 444-1111

Stephen S. Lane · Associate Clinical Professor, Department of Ophthalmology, University of Minnesota School of Medicine · Assistant Chief of Ophthalmology, Minnesota Veterans Affairs Medical Center · 232 North Main Street, Stillwater, MN 55082 · 612-439-8500

James H. Little · Associate Clinical Professor of Ophthalmology, The University of Oklahoma College of Medicine · Chief of Staff, Department of Ophthalmology, South Community Hospital · Southwest Eye Clinic, 1240 Southwest 44th Street, Oklahoma City, OK 73109 · 405-631-1527

Andrew W. Lyle · The Eye Institute · 755 East 3900 South, Salt Lake City, UT 84107 · 801-266-2283

Robert G. Martin · (Refractive Surgery) · Carolina Eye Associates · 2170 Midland Road, Southern Pines, NC 28387 · 919-295-2100

Samuel Masket · Associate Clinical Professor of Ophthalmology, Jules Stein Eye Institute; University of California, Los Angeles Center for the Health Sciences · Humana West Hills Hospital; Motion Picture Hospital; University of California, Los Angeles Medical Center · 7230 Medical Center Drive, Suite 204, West Hills, CA 91307 · 818-348-5166

David J. McIntyre · University of Washington School of Medicine · McIntyre Eye Clinic · 1920 116th Avenue NE, Bellevue, WA 98004 · 206-454-3937

David D. Michaels · Professor of Ophthalmology, University of California at Los Angeles School of Medicine · University of California at Los Angeles Medical Center; Jules Stein Eye Institute · 1441 West Seventh Street, San Pedro, CA 90732 · 213-833-1311

Albert C. Neumann · Medical Director, Newmann Eye Institute · 801 North Stone Street, De Land, FL 32720 · 904-734-4431

Stephen A. Obstbaum · Director, Department of Ophthalmology, Lenox Hill Hospital · 115 East 39th Street, New York, NY 10016 · 212-687-4106

Robert H. Osher · Medical Director, Cincinnati Eye Institute · 10494 Montgomery Road, Cincinnati, OH 45242 · 513-984-5133

John A. Retzlaff · Medical Eye Center · 2727 East Barnett Road, Medford, OR 97504 · 503-779-4711

Steven P. Shearing · Assistant Clinical Professor, University of Nevada Medical School in Reno · Valley Hospital · The Shearing Institute, 2575 Lindell Road, Las Vegas, NV 89102 · 702-362-3937

John H. Sheets · Associate Clinical Professor of Ophthalmology, The University of Texas Southwestern Medical School · Medical Center Hospital · 155 East Loop, Suite 100, Odessa, TX 79762 · 915-367-7241

John R. Shepherd · Clinical Associate Professor, University of Utah School of Medicine · Humana Hospital Sunrise · 3575 Pecos McLeod, Las Vegas, NV 89121 702-731-2088

Robert Sinskey · 2232 Santa Monica Boulevard, P.O. Box 4031, Santa Monica, CA 9044-0031 · 213-453-8911

Walter J. Stark · Professor of Ophthalmology, and Director, Corneal Service, Johns Hopkins University School of Medicine · The Johns Hopkins Medical Institutions · 600 North Wolfe Street, Maumenee 327, Baltimore, MD 21205 · 410-955-5490

Roger Steinert · (Refractive Surgery, Phacoemulsification, Cataracts) · Professor of Ophthalmology, Tufts University School of Medicine; Assistant Clinical Professor, Harvard Medical School · Massachusetts Eye & Ear Infirmary; New England Medical Center · Ophthalmic Consultants of Boston, 50 Staniford Street, Boston, MA 02114 · 617-367-4800

Spencer Phillips Thornton · Director of Cataract & Cornea Service, Baptist Hospital · 2010 Church Street, Suite 207, Nashville, TN 37203 · 615-329-7890

CORNEAL DISEASES & TRANSPLANTATION

Jules L. Baum · (Infectious Diseases) · Research Professor of Ophthalmology, Tufts University School of Medicine · Massachusetts Eye & Ear Infirmary · 16

Webster Street, Brookline, MA 02146 and Boston Eye Associates, One Brookline Place, Suite 623, Brookline, MA 02146 · 617-739-8929, 735-8810

Perry S. Binder · (Corneal Transplantation, Refractive Surgery, Cataracts) · Associate Clinical Professor, Department of Ophthalmology, University of California at San Diego · Member, Mericos Eye Institute, Scripps Memorial Hospital; Director, Ophthalmic Surgery and Research, Sharp Cabrillo Hospital · 9834 Gennesse, Suite 200, La Jolla, CA 92037 · 619-457-3050

S. Arthur Boruchoff · (Infectious Diseases) · Associate Professor of Ophthalmology, Harvard Medical School · Surgeon in Ophthalmology, Massachusetts Eye & Ear Infirmary · The Massachusetts Eye and Ear Associates, 50 Staniford Street, Third Floor, Boston, MA 02114 · 617-573-5550

William M. Bourne · (Corneal Transplantation) · Professor of Ophthalmology, Mayo Medical School · Mayo Clinic · 200 First Street, SW, Rochester, MN 55905 507-284-3614

John Chandler · (Transplantation, Infectious Diseases) · Professor & Head of Ophthalmology & Visual Sciences, The University of Illinois College of Medicine at Chicago · Chief of Ophthalmology, The University of Illinois Hospitals · 1855 West Taylor Street, Suite 2.50, Chicago, IL 60612 · 312-996-6590

Daniel S. Durrie · (Corneal Transplantation, Refractive Surgery) · Clinical Associate Professor of Ophthalmology, University of Nebraska Medical Center · St. Luke's Hospital of Kansas City; The Children's Mercy Hospital; Trinity Lutheran Hospital · The Hunkeler Eye Clinic, 4321 Washington Street, Suite 6000, Kansas City, MO 64111 · 816-931-4733

Gary I. Foulks · Duke University School of Medicine · Duke University Medical Center · P.O. Box 5802, Durham, NC 27710 · 919-684-6322

Dan B. Jones · (Infectious Diseases) · Professor and Chairman, Department of Ophthalmology, Cullen Eye Institute, Baylor College of Medicine, Department of Ophthalmology · Chief, Ophthalmology Service, The Methodist Hospital · 6501 Fannin Street, NC200, Houston, TX 77030 · 713-798-5951

Herbert E. Kaufman · (Corneal Transplantation, Refractive Surgery) · Boyd Professor of Ophthalmology, Pharmacology & Experimental Therapeutics, and Head, Department of Ophthalmology, Louisiana State University Eye Center, Louisiana State University School of Medicine · Staff Member, Hotel Dieu Hospital · 2020 Gravier Street, Suite B, New Orleans, LA 70112. · 504-568-6700 x303

Richard H. Keates · Professor and Chair, Department of Ophthalmology, University of California at Irvine School of Medicine · University of California at Irvine Medical Center · Medical Plaza Building, Room 2004, Irvine, CA 92717 · 714-856-8610

Kenneth R. Kenyon · (Dry Eyes) · Associate Professor of Ophthalmology, Harvard Medical School · Surgeon in Ophthalmology, Massachusetts Eye & Ear Infirmary · Cornea Consultants, 100 Charles River Plaza, Boston, MA 02114; and Eye Health Associates, 540 Hawthorn Street, North Dartmouth, MA 02747 · 617-742-1020; 508-997-1271

Jay H. Krachmer · Professor of Ophthalmology, The University of Iowa College of Medicine · Director, Iowa Lions Cornea Center, The University of Iowa Hospitals & Clinics · Iowa City, IA 52242 · 319-356-2861

Steven G. Kramer · (Transplantation) · Professor and Chairman, Department of Ophthalmology, University of California at San Francisco School of Medicine · University of California at San Francisco Medical Center · 10 Kirkham Street, Room K-301, San Francisco, CA 94143 · 415-476-1921

Peter R. Laibson · (General, Infectious Diseases) · Professor of Ophthalmology, Jefferson Medical College of Thomas Jefferson University · Director, Cornea Service, Wills Eye Hospital · 900 Walnut Street, Philadelphia, PA 19107 · 215-928-3180

Jonathan H. Lass · University Hospitals of Cleveland · Department of Ophthalmology, 2074 Abington Road, Cleveland, OH 44106 · 216-844-3601

Michael A. Lemp · (Dry Eyes) · Professor & Chairman, Department of Ophthalmology, Georgetown University School of Medicine · Center for Sight, Georgetown University Medical Center · 3800 Reservoir Road, NW, Washington, DC 20007 · 202-687-4968

Thomas John Liesegang · (External Disease) · Chairman of Ophthalmology, and Consultant in Ophthalmology, The Mayo Clinic—Jacksonville · Chairman, Ophthalmology, St. Luke's Hospital · Davis Building, 4500 San Pablo Road, Jacksonville, FL 32224 · 904-223-2232

Richard L. Lindstrom · (Refractive Surgery, Cataracts) · Clinical Professor of Ophthalmology, University of Minnesota School of Medicine · Phillips Eye Institute, Abbott Northwestern, St. Paul Ramsey, United Hospital, University of Minnesota, Fairview Southdale, Minneapolis Veterans Medical Center · Park Avenue Medical Office Building, 710 East 24th Street, Suite 106, Minneapolis, MN 55404 · 612-336-5493

Scott M. MacRae · (Corneal and External Disease) · Associate Professor of Ophthalmology, Oregon Health Sciences University · Oregon Health Sciences University; Casey Eye Institute; St. Vincent Hospital · The Casey Eye Institute, 3375 Southwest Terwilliger Boulevard, Portland, OR 97201-3098 · 503-494-7674

Leo J. Maguire · (Refractive Surgery) · Assistant Professor of Ophthalmology, Mayo Medical School · Mayo Clinic · 200 First Street, SW, Rochester, MN 55905 507-284-4152

James P. McCulley · Professor and Chairman of Ophthalmology, The University of Texas Southwestern Medical Center at Dallas · Parkland Memorial Hospital · 5323 Harry Hines Boulevard, Dallas, TX 75235 · 214-688-3407

Marguerite B. McDonald · (Refractive Surgery) · Professor of Ophthalmology, and Director of the Cornea Service, Louisiana State University Eye Center, Louisiana State University School of Medicine · Hotel Dieu Hospital · 2020 Gravier Street, Suite B, New Orleans, LA 70112 · 504-568-6700 x306

David M. Meisler · Staff Physician, The Cleveland Clinic Foundation · One Clinic Center, 9500 Euclid Avenue, Cleveland, OH 44195-5024 · 216-444-8102

Roger F. Meyer · (Corneal Transplantation) · Professor of Ophthalmology, The University of Michigan Medical School · W.K. Kellogg Eye Center, The University of Michigan Medical Center · 1000 Wall Street, Ann Arbor, MI 48105 · 313-763-5506

Anthony B. Nesburn · (Infectious Diseases) · Clinical Professor of Ophthalmology, Jules Stein Eye Institute, University of California at Los Angeles School of Medicine · Director, Ophthalmology Research Department, Cedars-Sinai Medical Center · 8700 Beverly Boulevard, Halper Room 111, Los Angeles, CA 90048 · 310-855-6455, 652-1133

Denis M. O'Day · (Infectious Disease) · Michael J. Hogan Professor of Ophthalmology, Vanderbilt University School of Medicine · Department of Ophthalmology, D5217, Nashville, TN 37232-2540 · 615-322-2046

Randall J. Olson · (Refractive Surgery, Cataract Surgery) · Chairman and Professor, Department of Ophthalmology, University of Utah School of Medicine · University of Utah Health Sciences Center · Department of Ophthalmology, 50 North Medical Drive, Salt Lake City, UT 84132 · 801-581-2702

Francis W. Price, Jr. · (Corneal Transplantation) · Clinical Professor of Ophthalmology, Indiana University School of Medicine · St. Vincent Hospital & Health Care Center; Community Hospitals Indianapolis · 9002 North Meridan Street, Suite 100, Indianapolis, IN 46260 · 317-844-5530

Larry F. Rich · Associate Professor of Ophthalmology, Oregon Health Sciences University · Chief of Cornea & External Disease Service, Oregon Health Sciences University · The Casey Eye Institute, 3375 Southwest Terwilliger Boulevard, Portland, OR 97201-3098 · 503-494-7674

J. James Rowsey · (Refractive Surgery) · Professor and Chairman, Department of Ophthalmology, University South Florida College of Medicine · University Community Ambulatory Surgery Center, Tampa General Hospital · 12901 Bruce B. Downs Boulevard, Box 21, Tampa, FL 33612 · 813-974-3820

David J. Schanzlin · Professor and Chairman of Ophthalmology, St. Louis University School of Medicine · President and CEO, Bethesda Eye Institute · 3655 Vista Avenue, St. Louis, MO 63110 · 314-577-8265

Ronald E. Smith · (Infectious Diseases) · Professor and Vice-Chairman, Department of Ophthalmology, University of Southern California School of Medicine · Doheny Eye Institute · 1355 San Pablo Street, Los Angeles, CA 90033 · 213-342-6424

Walter J. Stark · (Cornea Transplantation) · Professor of Ophthalmology, and Director, Corneal Service, Johns Hopkins University School of Medicine · The Johns Hopkins Medical Institutions · 600 North Wolfe Street, Maumenee 327, Baltimore, MD 21205 · 410-955-5490

Roger Steinert · (Transplantation, Refractive Surgery, Phacoemulsification, Cataracts) · Professor of Ophthalmology, Tufts University School of Medicine; Assistant Clinical Professor, Harvard Medical School · Massachusetts Eye & Ear Infirmary; New England Medical Center · Ophthalmic Consultants of Boston, 50 Staniford Street, Boston, MA 02114 · 617-367-4800

R. Doyle Stulting · (Transplantation) · Associate Professor of Ophthalmology, Emory University School of Medicine · Emory Eye Center · 1327 Clifton Road, NE, Atlanta, GA 30322 · 404-248-5818

Alan Sugar · Professor of Ophthalmology, The University of Michigan Medical School · The University of Michigan Medical Center · 1000 Wall Street, Ann Arbor, MI 48105 · 313-763-5506

Joel Sugar · Professor of Ophthalmology, The University of Illinois College of Medicine at Chicago · The University of Illinois Hospital · 1855 West Taylor Street, Suite 3164, Chicago, IL 60612 · 312-996-8937

George O. Waring III · (Refractive Surgery) · Professor of Ophthalmology and Director of Refractive Surgery, Emory University School of Medicine · Emory

University Hospital; Egleston Hospital for Children; Crawford W. Long Hospital; Veteran's Administration Hospital in Atlanta · The Emory Eye Center, 1327 Clifton Road, Atlanta, GA 30322 · 404-248-3244

GLAUCOMA

Jorge A. Alvarado · Professor of Ophthalmology, University of California at San Francisco School of Medicine · Director of Glaucoma Service, University of California at San Francisco Medical Center · 503 Parnassus Avenue, Room K-331, San Francisco, CA 94143-0730 · 415-476-3944

Douglas R. Anderson · Professor of Ophthalmology, University of Miami School of Medicine · Bascom Palmer Eye Institute, Anne Bates Leach Eye Hospital · 900 Northwest 17th Street, Miami, FL 33136 · 305-326-6146

A. Robert Bellows · Assistant Clinical Professor, Harvard Medical School · Massachusetts Eye & Ear Infirmary · 50 Staniford Street, Boston, MA 02114 · 617-367-4800

Reay H. Brown · Associate Professor of Ophthalmology, Emory University School of Medicine · Director of Glaucoma Services, Emory Eye Center · 1365 Clifton Road, NE, Atlanta, GA 30322 · 404-248-5805

Richard Brubaker · Mayo Medical School · Mayo Clinic · 200 First Street, SW, Rochester, MN 55905 · 507-284-3760

Gordon Douglas · Associate Professor of Ophthalmology, The University of British Columbia · Vancouver General Hospital · 2550 Willow Street, Vancouver, British Columbia V5Z 3N9 · 604-875-4375

Stephen M. Drance · Professor of Ophthalmology, The University of British Columbia · University Hospital · Eye Care Center, 2550 Willow Street, Vancouver, British Columbia V5Z 3N9 · 604-875-4365

David L. Epstein · Associate Professor of Ophthalmology, Harvard Medical School Director of the Glaucoma Service, Massachusetts Eye & Ear Infirmary · 243 Charles Street, Boston, MA 02114 · 617-573-3674

Max Forbes · Professor of Clinical Ophthalmology, College of Physicians & Surgeons of Columbia University · Columbia-Presbyterian Medical Center · 635 West 165th Street, New York, NY 10032 · 212-927-1854

John N. Hetherington, Jr. · Clinical Professor of Ophthalmology, University of California at San Francisco School of Medicine · St. Mary's Hospital & Medical Center · 490 Post Street, Suite 640, San Francisco, CA 94102 · 415-986-0220

Dale K. Heuer · Associate Professor of Ophthalmology, University of Southern California School of Medicine · Doheny Eye Institute, The Los Angeles County + University of Southern California Medical Center · 1355 San Pablo Street, Suite 312, Los Angeles, CA 90033 · 213-342-6412

Eve J. Higginbotham · Associate Professor of Ophthalmology, The University of Michigan Medical School · W.K. Kellogg Eye Center, The University of Michigan Medical Center · 1000 Wall Street, Room 539, Ann Arbor, MI 48105 · 313-763-3732

H. Dunbar Hoskins, Jr. · Clinical Professor of Ophthalmology, University of California at San Francisco School of Medicine · University of California at San Francisco Medical Center · 490 Post Street, Suite 640, San Francisco, CA 94102 415-986-0220

B. Thomas Hutchinson · Associate Clinical Professor of Ophthalmology, Harvard Medical School · Surgeon in Ophthalmology, Massachusetts Eye & Ear Infirmary 50 Staniford Street, Boston, MA 02114 · 617-367-4800

Murray Johnstone · Consultant, University of Washington School of Medicine · Swedish Hospital Medical Center · 1221 Madison Street, Suite 1124, Seattle, WA 98104 · 206-682-3447

Michael A. Kass · Professor of Ophthalmology, Washington University School of Medicine · Barnes Hospital/Washington University Eye Center · Department of Ophthalmology & Visual Sciences, Campus Box 8096, 660 South Euclid Avenue, St. Louis, MO 63110 · 314-362-5713

Allan E. Kolker · Professor of Ophthalmology, Washington University School of Medicine · Barnes Hospital; Washington University Eye Center · 660 South Euclid Avenue, Box 8096, St. Louis, MO 63110 · 314-362-3937

Theodore Krupin · Professor of Ophthalmology, Northwestern University Medical School · Northwestern Memorial Hospital · 303 East Chicago Avenue, Ward 2-186, Chicago, IL 60611 · 312-503-9866

William E. Layden · Professor, Department of Ophthalmology, University South Florida College of Medicine · University Community Hospital · 13550 North 31st Street, #250, Tampa, FL 33613 · 813-972-9040

Raymond P. Le Blanc · Professor and Head of Ophthalmology, Dalhousie University · Halifax Infirmary · Nova Scotia Eye Center, 1335 Queen Street, Halifax, Nova Scotia B3J 2H6 · 902-428-4343

Paul R. Lichter · F. Bruce Fralick Professor and Chairman, The University of Michigan Medical School · The University of Michigan Medical Center · 1000 Wall Street, Ann Arbor, MI 48105 · 313-764-6468

Richard P. Mills · (Neuro-opthalmology) · Professor and Vice-Chair, Department of Ophthalmology, University of Washington School of Medicine · University of Washington Medical Center · 1959 Northeast Pacific Street, RJ-10, Seattle, WA 98195 · 206-685-2089

Donald S. Minckler · Professor of Ophthalmology, University of Southern California School of Medicine · Doheny Eye Institute · 1355 San Pablo Street, Los Angeles, CA 90033 · 213-342-6434

Paul F. Palmberg · Professor of Ophthalmology, University of Miami School of Medicine · Bascom Palmer Eye Institute · 900 Northwest 17th Street, Miami, FL 33136 · 305-326-6386

Richard K. Parrish II · Associate Professor of Ophthalmology, University of Miami School of Medicine · Bascom Palmer Eye Institute · 900 Northwest 17th Street, Miami, FL 33136 · 305-326-6389

Steven M. Podos · Professor and Chairman, Department of Ophthalmology, Mt. Sinai School of Medicine · Mt. Sinai Medical Center · One Gustave L. Levy Place, Box 1183, New York, NY 10029 · 212-241-6752

Irvin P. Pollack · Professor of Ophthalmology, Johns Hopkins University School of Medicine · Chief of Ophthalmology, The Krieger Eye Institute, Sinai Hospital of Baltimore · Belvedere at Greenspring, Baltimore, MD 21215-5271 · 410-578-5900

Harry A. Quigley · Professor of Ophthalmology, Johns Hopkins University School of Medicine · The Johns Hopkins Medical Institutions · 600 North Wolfe Street, Wilmer 120, Baltimore, MD 21205 · 410-955-2777

M. Bruce Shields · Professor of Ophthalmology, Duke University School of Medicine · Duke Eye Center, Duke University Medical Center · P.O. Box 3802, Durham, NC 27710 · 919-684-2841

Richard Simmons · Associate Clinical Professor Ophthalmology, Harvard Medical School · Chief of Ophthalmology, Hahnemann Hospital; Surgeon in Ophthalmology, Massachusetts Eye & Ear Infirmary · Simmons Eye Associates, 100 Charles River Plaza, Boston, MA 02114 · 617-742-1020

George L. Spaeth · Professor of Ophthalmology, Jefferson Medical College of Thomas Jefferson University · Director, William & Anna Goldberg Glaucoma Service & Research Laboratories, Wills Eye Hospital; Attending, Chestnut Hill Hospital, Thomas Jefferson University Hospital, Wills Eye Hospital · Ninth and Walnut Streets, Philadelphia, PA 19107-5599 · 215-928-3197

Robert L. Stamper · Chairman, Department of Ophthalmology, California Pacific Medical Center · 2340 Clay Street, Fifth Floor, San Francisco, CA 94115 · 415-923-3930

E. Michael Van Buskirk · Chenoweth Chair of Ophthalmology, Devers Eye Institute · Good Samaritan Hospital & Medical Center · 1040 Northwest 22nd Avenue, Suite N320, Portland, OR 97210-3065 · 503-229-8184

Robert N. Weinreb · Professor and Vice-Chairman, Department of Ophthalmology, University of California at San Diego School of Medicine · Chief, Glaucoma, Shiley Eye Center, University of California at San Diego Medical Center · Shiley Eye Center, 9415 Campus Point Drive, 0946, La Jolla, CA 92093-0946 · 619-534-8824, 534-6290

Jacob T. Wilensky · Professor of Ophthalmology, and Associate Head of Ophthalmology, The University of Illinois College of Medicine at Chicago · Director, Glaucoma Service, The University of Illinois Eye Center · 1855 West Taylor Street, Room 278, Chicago, IL 60612 · 312-996-7030

Richard P. Wilson · Associate Professor of Ophthalmology, Jefferson Medical College of Thomas Jefferson University · Attending Surgeon, Wills Eye Hospital; Lankenau Hospital · 900 Walnut Street, Philadelphia, PA 19107 · 215-928-3129

MEDICAL RETINAL DISEASES

Thomas Marshall Aaberg · (Vitreoretinal Diseases and Surgery) · Professor and Chairman of Ophthalmology, and F. Phinizy Calhoun, Sr. Professor, Emory University School of Medicine · Attending, Emory University Affiliated Hospitals; Egleston Hospital for Children; Crawford W. Long Memorial Hospital; Veterans Administration Hospital; Grady Memorial Hospital · 1327 Clifton Road NE, Atlanta, GA 30322 · 404-248-4456

Lloyd M. Aiello · (Diabetic Retinopathy) · Associate Professor of Ophthalmology, Harvard Medical School · Joslin Diabetes Center · One Joslin Place, Boston, MA 02215 · 617-732-2520

George W. Blankenship, Jr. · (Vitreoretinal Diseases and Surgery, Diabetic Retinopathy, Vascular Occlusions, Laser Surgery) · Professor and Chairman, Department of Ophthalmology, Pennsylvania State University · The Milton S. Hershey Medical Center · 500 University Drive, P.O. Box 850, Hershey, PA 17033 · 717-531-8783

Mark S. Blumenkranz · (Vitreoretinal Diseases and Surgery) · Adjunct Associate Professor of Ophthalmology, The Eye Research Institute of Oakland University · Attending Physician, and Vitreoretinal Fellowship Director, William Beaumont Eye Institute, William Beaumont Hospital · 3535 West Thirteen Mile Road, Suite 632, Royal Oak, MI 48073 · 313-288-2280

George H. Bresnick · (Diabetic Retinopathy) · Professor and Acting Chairman, Department of Ophthalmology, University of Wisconsin-Madison School of Medicine · University of Wisconsin-Madison Hospital & Clinics · 600 Highland Avenue, Room F4-334, Madison, WI 53792 · 608-263-9797

Alexander J. Brucker · (Diabetic Retinopathy, Macular Degeneration, Vascular Occlusions, Laser Surgery, Vitreoretinal Surgery) · Associate Professor of Ophthalmology, University of Pennsylvania School of Medicine · Chief, Retina & Vitreous Service, Scheie Eye Institute; Presbyterian Medical Center; Hospital of the University of Pennsylvania; Graduate Hospital · Myrin Circle, 51 North 39th Street, Philadelphia, PA 19104 · 215-662-8675

John G. Clarkson · (Vitreoretinal Diseases and Surgery, Diabetic Retinopathy, Macular Degeneration, Vascular Occlusions, Laser Surgery,) · Professor of Ophthalmology, University of Miami School of Medicine · Chairman, Department of Ophthalmology, Bascom Palmer Eye Institute · 900 Northwest 17th Street, Miami, FL 33136 · 305-326-6116

Stuart L. Fine · (Diabetic Retinopathy, Macular Degeneration, Vascular Occlusions, Laser Surgery) · Professor and Chairman, Department of Ophthalmology, University of Pennsylvania School of Medicine · Scheie Eye Institute · 51 North 39th Street, Philadelphia PA 19104 · 215-662-8657

J. Donald M. Gass · (Macular Degeneration) · Professor of Ophthalmology, University of Miami School of Medicine · Bascom Palmer Eye Institute · 900 Northwest 17th Street, Miami, FL 33136 · 305-326-6198

Kurt A. Gitter · (Diabetic Retinopathy, Macular Degeneration, Vascular Occlusions, Laser Surgery, Vitreoretinal Surgery) · Louisiana State University School of Medicine · Touro Eye Research Laboratory · 3525 Prytania Street, Suite 320, New Orleans, LA 70115 · 504-895-3961

Lee M. Jampol · (Diabetic Retinopathy, Macular Degeneration, Vascular Occlusions, Laser Surgery) · Feinberg Professor and Chairman, Department of Ophthalmology, Northwestern University Medical School · Northwestern Memorial Hospital, The Children's Memorial Hospital, Evanston Hospital · 303 East Chicago Avenue, Ward 2-186, Chicago, IL 60611-3008 · 312-908-8152

Hilel Lewis · (Vitreoretinal Diseases and Surgery, Diabetic Retinopathy, Macular Degeneration, Vascular Occlusions, Laser Surgery) · Assistant Professor of Ophthalmology, University of California at Los Angeles School of Medicine · The Charles Kenneth Feldman Scholar, Jules Stein Eye Institute · 100 Stein Plaza, Los Angeles, CA 90024-7007 · 213-206-3110

Richard A. Lewis · Professor of Ophthalmology, Medicine, Pediatrics, and The Institute for Molecular Genetics, Baylor College of Medicine · Cullen Eye Institute · One Baylor Plaza, Suite NC206, Houston, TX 77030 · 713-798-3030

David H. Orth · (Diabetic Retinopathy, Macular Degeneration, Vascular Occlusions, Laser Surgery) · Professor, Department of Ophthalmology, Rush-Presbyterian-St. Luke's Medical Center · Medical Director, Irwin Retina Center, Ingalls Hospital, Harvey, IL; Illinois Retina Associates · 71 West 156th Street, Suite 400, Harvey, IL 60426 · 708-596-8710

Dennis M. Robertson · (Diabetic Retinopathy, Macular Degeneration, Vascular Occlusions, Laser Surgery) · Professor of Ophthalmology, Mayo Medical School · Mayo Clinic · 200 First Street, SW, Rochester, MN 55905 · 507-284-3721

Andrew P. Schachat · (Melanoma) · Associate Professor of Ophthalmology, Johns Hopkins University School of Medicine · The Johns Hopkins Medical Institutions 600 North Wolfe Street, Maumenee 713, Baltimore, MD 21205 · 410-955-7411

Howard Schatz · (Macular Degeneration, Diabetic Retinopathy, Macular and Retinal Vascular Diseases, Laser Surgery) · Director, Retina Research Fund, St. Mary's Hospital and Medical Center; and Clinical Professor of Ophthalmology, University of California Medical Center, San Francisco · One Daniel Burnham Court, Suite 210, San Francisco, CA 94109 · 415-441-0906

Jerry A. Shields · (Melanoma, Retinoblastoma) · Professor of Ophthalmology, Jefferson Medical College of Thomas Jefferson University · Consulting Ophthalmologist, Lankenau Hospital and Children's Hospital; Director, Oncology Service, Wills Eye Hospital; Thomas Jefferson University Hospital · 900 Walnut Street, Philadelphia, PA 19107 · 215-928-3105

Lawrence J. Singerman · (Diabetic Retinopathy, Macular Degeneration, Vascular Occlusions, Laser Surgery, Vitreoretinal Surgery) · Clinical Professor of Surgery (Ophthalmology), Case Western Reserve University School of Medicine · Director, Retinal Institute & Retinal Service, The Mt. Sinai Medical Center · 26900 Cedar Road, Suite 303, Cleveland, OH 44122 · 216-831-5700

Lawrence A. Yannuzzi · (Diabetic Retinopathy, Macular Degeneration, Vascular Occlusions, Laser Surgery) · Vice-Chairman, Department of Ophthalmology, and Associate Professor of Ophthalmology, Columbia University Medical Center · Director of Retinal Services, Manhattan Eye, Ear & Throat Hospital · 519 East 72nd Street, Suite 203, New York, NY 10021 · 212-861-9797

NEURO-OPHTHALMOLOGY
(See also Adult Neurology, Neuro-Ophthalmology)

Roy W. Beck · Professor of Ophthalmology and Neurology, University South Florida College of Medicine · Tampa General Hospital · Department of Ophthalmology, 12901 Bruce B. Downs Boulevard, Box 21, Tampa, FL 33612 · 813-978-5915

Myles M. Behrens · Professor of Clinical Ophthalmology, College of Physicians & Surgeons of Columbia University · Columbia-Presbyterian Medical Center · 635 West 165th Street, Room 114, New York, NY 10032 · 212-305-5415

Ronald M. Burde · Professor of Ophthalmology and Neurology and Neurological Surgery, Albert Einstein College of Medicine · Chairman, Department of Ophthalmology & Visual Sciences, Montefiore Medical Center · 111 East 210th Street, Bronx, NY 10467 · 212-920-6665

Thomas J. Carlow · Adjunct Professor of Neurology, The University of New Mexico School of Medicine · 101 Hospital Loop NE, Suite 103, Albuquerque, NM 87109 · 505-883-6800

Bradley K. Farris · Associate Professor of Ophthalmology, and Adjunct Associate Professor of Neurosurgery and Neurology, The University of Oklahoma College of Medicine · Neuro-Ophthalmologist, Dean A. McGee Eye Institute, and The University of Oklahoma Health Sciences Center · 608 Stanton L. Young Boulevard, Suite 205, Oklahoma City, OK 73104 · 405-271-6463

John W. Gittinger, Jr. · Professor of Surgery and Neurology, University of Massachusetts Medical School · Chairman, Division of Ophthalmology, University of Massachusetts Medical Center · 55 Lake Avenue, North, Worcester, MA 01655 · 508-856-2289

Joel S. Glaser · Professor of Ophthalmology, Neurology & Neurosurgery, University of Miami School of Medicine · Director, Neuro-Ophthalmology Unit, Bascom Palmer Eye Institute; Anne Bates Leach Eye Hospital · 900 Northwest 17th Street, Miami, FL 33136 · 305-326-6193

Thomas R. Hedges III · Associate Professor of Ophthalmology & Neurology, Tufts University School of Medicine · Director, Neuro-ophthalmology Service, New England Medical Center · 750 Washington Street, Box 381, Boston, MA 02111 · 617-956-5488

Robert S. Hepler · Professor of Ophthalmology, University of California at Los Angeles School of Medicine · Division Chief of Neuro-Ophthalmology, University of California at Los Angeles Medical Center · 100 Stein Plaza, Los Angeles, CA 90024-7005 · 310-825-5695

James R. Keane · Professor of Neurology, University of Southern California School of Medicine · The Los Angeles County + University of Southern California Medical Center · 1200 North State Street, Room 5640, Los Angeles, CA 90033 · 213-226-7381

John L. Keltner · Chairman, Department of Ophthalmology, and Professor of Ophthalmology, Neurology and Neurological Surgery, University of California at Davis School of Medicine · University of California at Davis Medical Center · 1603 Alhambra Boulevard, Sacramento, CA 95816 · 916-734-6073

Lanning B. Kline · Professor of Neuro-Ophthalmology, The University of Alabama School of Medicine · Eye Foundation Hospital; The University of Alabama Hospital · 1600 Seventh Avenue South, Suite 555, Birmingham, AL 35233 · 205-939-9778

Mark J. Kupersmith · Professor of Neurology & Ophthalmology, New York University School of Medicine · New York University Medical Center; New York Eye & Ear Infirmary · 530 First Avenue, Suite 3B, New York, NY 10016 · 212-263-7429

Simmons Lessell · Professor of Ophthalmology, Harvard Medical School · Director of Neuro-Ophthalmology, Massachusetts Eye & Ear Infirmary · 243 Charles Street, Boston, MA 02114 · 617-573-3412

John A. McCrary III · Professor of Ophthalmology, Neurology, & Neurosurgery, Baylor College of Medicine · Cullen Eye Institute · 6501 Fannin Street, NC-200, Houston, TX 77030 · 713-798-4914

Neil R. Miller · Professor of Ophthalmology, Johns Hopkins University School of Medicine · The Johns Hopkins Medical Institutions · 600 North Wolfe Street, Maumenee B-109, Baltimore, MD 21205 · 410-955-8679

Nancy J. Newman · Assistant Professor of Ophthalmology and Neurology, Emory University School of Medicine · Director, Neuro-ophthalmology Unit, Emory University Affiliated Hospitals · 1327 Clifton Road NE, Suite 4305, Atlanta, GA 30322 · 404-248-5360

Peter J. Savino · Professor of Ophthalmology at Jefferson Medical College; Clinical Professor of Ophthalmology, University of Pennsylvania School of Medicine · Chairman, Department of Ophthalmology, Graduate Hospital; Director, Neuro-Ophthalmology Service, Wills Eye Hospital · 900 Walnut Street, Philadelphia, PA 19107 · 215-928-3130

Norman Schatz · Professor of Clinical Ophthalmology and Neurology, University of Miami School of Medicine · Bascom Palmer Eye Institute · 900 Northwest 17th Street, Miami, FL 33136 · 305-326-6193

Robert C. Sergott · Clinical Associate Professor of Ophthalmology and Neurology, University of Pennsylvania; Clinical Associate Professor of Ophthalmology and Neurology, Scheie Eye Institute · Attending Neuro-Ophthalmologist, Wills Eye Hospital, and Children's Hospital of Philadelphia, and Pennsylvania Hospital; Attending Ophthalmoligist, Lankenau Hospital, and Graduate Hospital of the University of Pennsylvania; Scheie Eye Institute · Ninth And Walnut Streets, Philadelphia, PA 19107 · 215-928-3130

William Thomas Shults · Clinical Associate Professor of Ophthalmology and Clinical Associate Professor of Neurology, Oregon Health Sciences University · Chief of Neuro-Ophthalmology, Devers Eye Institute; Good Samaritan Hospital & Medical Center · 1040 Northwest 22nd Avenue, Suite 320, Portland, OR 97210 503-229-7249, 800-433-3122 x7429

J. Lawton Smith · Professor of Ophthalmology, University of Miami School of Medicine · Bascom Palmer Eye Institute · 900 Northwest 17th Street, Miami, FL 33136 · 305-326-6128

H. Stanley Thompson · (Pupillary Problems) · Professor of Ophthalmology, The University of Iowa College of Medicine · Director of Neuro-ophthalmology Unit, The University of Iowa Hospitals & Clinics · Iowa City, IA 52242 · 319-356-2868

Jonathan D. Trobe · Professor of Ophthalmology and Associate Professor of Neurology, The University of Michigan Medical School · Director, Neuro-Ophthalmology Service, W.K. Kellogg Eye Center, The University of Michigan Medical Center · 1000 Wall Street, Room 645, Ann Arbor, MI 48105 · 313-763-9147

B. Todd Troost · Professor and Chairman, Department of Neurology, The Bowman Gray School of Medicine of Wake Forest University · North Carolina Baptist Hospital · Medical Center Boulevard, Winston-Salem, NC 27157-1078 · 919-748-3429

Michael Wall · Associate Professor of Neurology, The University of Iowa College of Medicine · The University of Iowa Hospitals & Clinics · 200 Hawkins Drive, Iowa City, IA 52242-1009 · 319-356-2932

Joel M. Weinstein · Associate Professor of Ophthalmology, Neurology and Neurosurgery, University of Wisconsin-Madison School of Medicine · University of Wisconsin Hospital & Clinics · 600 Highland Avenue, Room F4-340, Madison, WI 53792 · 608-263-2052

Jonathan D. Wirtschafter · (Optic Nerve Compressions, Graves Disease, Eyelid Spasms) · Professor of Ophthalmology and Neurology, University of Minnesota School of Medicine · Director, Neuro-ophthalmology, Orbit & Oculoplastic Service, University of Minnesota Hospital & Clinics · 516 Delaware SE, Box 493, Minneapolis, MN 55455 · 612-625-4400

Robert D. Yee · Professor and Chairman, Department of Ophthalmology, Indiana University School of Medicine · Indiana University Medical Center · 702 Rotary Circle, Room 344, Indianapolis, IN 46202 · 317-274-7101

Brian R. Younge · Mayo Clinic · 200 First Street, SW, Rochester, MN 55905 · 507-284-4152

OCULAR ONCOLOGY

James Augsburger · (Melanoma, Retinoblastoma, Intraocular & Conjunctival Tumors) · Associate Clinical Professor of Ophthalmology, Jefferson Medical College of Thomas Jefferson University · Attending Surgeon, Wills Eye Hospital · Retina Oncology Unit, 900 Walnut Street, Second Floor, Philadelphia, PA 19107 215-928-3221

Devron H. Char · (Melanoma, Retinoblastoma, Thyroid Eye Disease) · Professor of Ophthalmology & Radiation Oncology, and Professor, Francis I. Proctor Foundation, University of California at San Francisco School of Medicine · Director, Ocular Oncology Unit, University of California at San Francisco Medical Center · Eight Kirkham Street, Box 0730, San Francisco, CA 94143 · 415-476-4096

Robert M. Ellsworth · (Retinoblastoma) · Professor of Ophthalmology, Cornell University Medical College · Vice-Chairman, Department of Ophthalmology, The New York Hospital-Cornell Medical Center · Department of Ophthalmology, 525 East 68th Street, New York, NY 10021 · 212-746-2490

Evangelos S. Gragoudas · (Melanoma) · Associate Professor of Ophthalmology, Harvard Medical School · Director of the Retina Service, Massachusetts Eye & Ear Infirmary · 243 Charles Street, Boston, MA 02114 · 617-573-3515

Jerry A. Shields · (Melanoma, Retinoblastoma) · Professor of Ophthalmology, Jefferson Medical College of Thomas Jefferson University · Consulting Ophthalmologist, Lankenau Hospital and Children's Hospital; Director, Oncology Service, Wills Eye Hospital; Thomas Jefferson University Hospital · 900 Walnut Street, Philadelphia, PA 19107 · 215-928-3105

OCULOPLASTIC & ORBITAL SURGERY
(See also Plastic Surgery, Oculoplastic & Orbital Surgery)

Richard L. Anderson · Professor of Ophthalmology, and Chief, Division of Ophthalmic Plastic Orbital & Reconstructive Surgery, University of Utah School of Medicine · University of Utah Health Sciences Center; Holy Cross Hospital; L.D.S. Hospital; Primary Childrens Hospital · 1002 East South Temple, Suite 308, Salt Lake City, UT 84102 · 801-363-3355

Henry I. Baylis · (Blepharoplasty) · Clinical Professor of Ophthalmology, University of California at Los Angeles School of Medicine · Jules Stein Eye Institute · 11470 Olympic, Los Angeles, CA 90064 · 213-207-0300

Michael A. Callahan · Associate Professor of Ophthalmology, The University of Alabama School of Medicine · Eye Foundation Hospital · 700 Eighteenth Street South, Suite 511, Birmingham, AL 35233 · 205-933-6888

Richard P. Carroll · Clinical Professor of Ophthalmology, University of Minnesota School of Medicine · Phillips Eye Institute; Midway Hospital; Abbott Northwestern Hospital · 1690 University Avenue, Suite 200, St. Paul, MN 55104 · 612-646-2581

Richard K. Dortzbach · Clinical Professor of Ophthalmology, University of Wisconsin-Madison School of Medicine · University of Wisconsin Hospital & Clinics University Station Clinics, 2880 University Avenue, Madison, WI 53705 · 608-263-1468

Jonathan J. Dutton · Associate Professor of Oculoplastic, Orbital and Ophthalmic Oncology Surgery, Duke University School of Medicine · Duke Eye Center, Duke University Medical Center · P.O. Box 3802-200, Durham, NC 27710 · 919-684-4224

Joseph C. Flanagan · Professor of Ophthalmology, Jefferson Medical College of Thomas Jefferson University · Head of Oculoplastic Department, Wills Eye Hospital; Chief of Ophthalmology, Lankenau Hospital; Jefferson Park Hospital · Lankenau Medical Building, Suite 256, Wynnewood, PA 19096 · 215-649-1970

Bartley R. Frueh · Professor of Ophthalmology, The University of Michigan Medical School · Co-Director of Eye Plastic & Orbital Surgery, W.K. Kellogg Eye Center, The University of Michigan Medical Center · 1000 Wall Street, Ann Arbor, MI 48105 · 313-763-9146

Russell S. Gonnering · Assistant Clinical Professor of Ophthalmology, University of Wisconsin-Madison School of Medicine · St. Luke's Medical Center; St. Joseph's Hospital; Children's Hospital of Wisconsin · 2600 North Mayfair Road, Suite 950, Milwaukee, WI 53226 · 414-257-0170

Arthur S. Grove, Jr. · Assistant Clinical Professor of Ophthalmology, Harvard Medical School · Associate Surgeon In Ophthalmology, Massachusetts Eye & Ear Infirmary; Director of Ophthalmic Plastic and Orbital Surgery, Beth Israel Hospital · 50 Staniford Street, Third Floor, Boston, MA 02114 · 617-523-5206

Gerald J. Harris · Professor of Ophthalmology, Medical College of Wisconsin · Head, Orbit & Oculoplastic Section, The Eye Institute, The Milwaukee County Medical Complex · 8700 West Wisconsin Avenue, Milwaukee, WI 53226 · 414-257-5055

Albert Hornblass · Clinical Professor of Ophthalmology, State University of New York Health Science Center at Brooklyn · Chief of Ophthalmic Plastic, Orbital & Reconstructive Surgery, Manhattan Eye, Ear & Throat Hospital; Director of Ophthalmic Plastic Surgery, Lenox Hill Hospital · 130 East 67th Street, New York, NY 10021 · 212-879-6824

Jeffrey J. Hurwitz · (Lacrimal Surgery) · Associate Professor of Ophthalmology, and Director of the Oculoplastic Division, University of Toronto School of Medicine · Chief of Ophthalmology, Mt. Sinai Hospital · 600 University Avenue, Room 3408, Toronto, Ontario M5G 1X5 · 416-586-5134

Nicholas T. Iliff · Associate Professor of Ophthalmology, Johns Hopkins University School of Medicine · The Johns Hopkins Medical Institutions · The Wilmer Eye Institute, 600 North Wolfe Street, Maumenee 127, Baltimore, MD 21205 · 410-955-1112

Glenn W. Jelks · Associate Professor of Ophthalmology and Plastic Surgery, New York University Medical Center · Manhattan Eye, Ear & Throat Hospital; New York Eye & Ear Infirmary; Valley Hospital, Ridgewood, NJ · 830 Park Avenue, New York, NY 10021 · 212-988-3303

James A. Katowitz · Associate Professor of Ophthalmology, University of Pennsylvania School of Medicine · The Children's Hospital of Philadelphia; The Scheie Eye Institute; Presbyterian Hospital; Hospital of the University of Pennsylvania · 1624 Locust Street, Suite 400, Philadelphia, PA 19103 · 215-561-2340

John S. Kennerdell · (Orbital Surgery) · Clinical Professor of Ophthalmology & Neurology, University of Pittsburgh School of Medicine · Chairman, Department of Ophthalmology, Allegheny General Hospital · 420 East North Avenue, Suite 116, Pittsburgh, PA 15212 · 412-359-6300

John V. Linberg · Associate Professor of Ophthalmology, West Virginia University School of Medicine · West Virginia University Health Sciences Center · Morgantown, WV 26506 · 304-293-3757

Richard D. Lisman · Associate Clinical Professor of Ophthalmology, New York University Medical Center · Surgeon Director, Manhattan Eye, Ear & Throat Hospital, and New York University Medical Center · 140 East 56th Street, New York, NY 10022 · 212-755-0699

Clinton D. McCord · Attending, Piedmont Hospital, and Metropolitan Hospital 1938 Peachtree Road, Suite 300, Atlanta, GA 30309 · 404-351-2643

Jeffrey A. Nerad · Associate Professor of Ophthalmology, The University of Iowa College of Medicine · Director of Oculoplastic, Orbital & Oncology Surgery, Department of Ophthalmology, The University of Iowa Hospitals & Clinics · Iowa City, IA 52242 · 319-356-2590

James C. Orcutt · Associate Professor of Ophthalmology, University of Washington School of Medicine · University of Washington Medical Center · 1959 Northeast Pacific Street, RJ-10, Seattle, WA 98195 · 206-543-3883

James R. Patrinely · Associate Professor of Ophthalmology & Plastic Surgery, Cullen Eye Institute, Baylor College of Medicine · Clinical Assistant Surgeon of Ophthalmology, and Clinical Assistant Professor in the Division of Surgery, Department of Head & Neck Surgery, University of Texas, MD Anderson Cancer Center; The Methodist Hospital; St. Luke's Episcopal Hospital; Texas Children's Hospital · 6501 Fannin Street, NC205, Houston, TX 77030 · 713-798-5870

Allen Putterman · Professor of Clinical Ophthalmology, The University of Illinois College of Medicine at Chicago · Chief of Oculoplastic Surgery Service, The University of Illinois Eye Center & Visual Sciences; Humana Hospital; Michael Reese Hospital · 111 North Wabash, Chicago, IL 60602 · 312-372-2256

Jack Rootman · (Orbital Tumors, Orbital Diseases, Thyroid Orbitopathy) · Professor of Ophthalmology & Pathology, The University of British Columbia · Head, Department of Ophthalmology, Vancouver General Hospital · 2550 Willow Street, Vancouver, British Columbia V5Z 3N9 · 604-875-4555

John W. Shore · Assistant Professor of Ophthalmology, Harvard Medical School Associate Chief of Ophthalmology; Director of Eye Plastics & Orbit Service, Massachusetts Eye & Ear Infirmary · 50 Staniford Street, Third Floor, Boston, MA 02114 · 617-573-5534

Norman Shorr · Clinical Professor of Ophthalmology, University of California at Los Angeles School of Medicine · Jules Stein Eye Institute · 100 Stein Plaza, Los Angeles, CA 90024-7007 · 213-278-1839

Stephen Lewis Trokel · (Thyroid Eye Disease) · Professor of Clinical Ophthalmology, College of Physicians & Surgeons of Columbia University · Columbia-Presbyterian Medical Center · 635 West 165th Street, New York, NY 10032 · 212-305-5477

David T. Tse · Associate Professor of Ophthalmology, University of Miami School of Medicine · Bascom Palmer Eye Institute · 900 Northwest 17th Street, Miami, FL 33136 · 305-326-6086

Robert Benson Wilkins · Clinical Associate Professor of Ophthalmology, The University of Texas Medical Branch at Galveston · Hermann Hospital; Diagnostic Center Hospital; Park Plaza Hospital · 2855 Gramercy Street, Houston, TX 77025 713-668-6828

John L. Wobig · Professor Lester T. Jones Oculoplastic Chair, Oregon Health Sciences University · Casey Eye Institute and Devers Memorial Eye Clinic · The Casey Eye Institute, 3375 Southwest Terwilliger Boulevard, Portland, OR 97201 503-494-3010

Allan E. Wulc · Assistant Professor of Ophthalmology, University of Pennsylvania School of Medicine · Chief, Oculoplastic & Orbital Services, Scheie Eye Institute 51 North 39th Street, Philadelphia, PA 19104 · 215-662-8652

OPHTHALMIC GENETICS

J. Bronwyn Bateman · Professor of Ophthalmology, University of California, Los Angeles School of Medicine · Jules Stein Eye Institute · 200 Stein Plaza, Los Angeles, CA 90024 · 310-206-6349

John R. Heckenlively · (Retinitis Pigmentosa, and Related) · Professor of Ophthalmology, University of California at Los Angeles School of Medicine · Jules Stein Eye Institute · 100 Stein Plaza, Retina Division, Los Angeles, CA 90024-7007 · 310-825-6089

Richard A. Lewis · Professor of Ophthalmology,Medicine, Pediatrics, and The Institute for Molecular Genetics, Baylor College of Medicine · Cullen Eye Institute · One Baylor Plaza, Suite NC206, Houston, TX 77030 · 713-798-3030

Irene H. Maumenee · Professor of Ophthalmology, Johns Hopkins University School of Medicine · The Johns Hopkins Medical Institutions · 600 North Wolfe Street, Maumenee 321, Baltimore, MD 21205 · 410-955-5214

A. Linn Murphree · Professor of Ophthalmology and Pediatrics and Acting Chairman, Department of Ophthalmology, University of Southern California School of Medicine · Head, Division of Ophthalmology, Children's Hospital of Los Angeles 4650 Sunset Boulevard, Los Angeles, CA 90027 · 213-342-6444

Edwin M. Stone · Assistant Professor of Ophthalmology, The University of Iowa College of Medicine · Director, Molecular Ophthalmology Laboratory, The University of Iowa Hospitals & Clinics · 200 Hawkins Drive, Iowa City, IA 52242 · 319-335-8270

Richard Gordon Weleber · Professor of Ophthalmology & Medical Genetics, Oregon Health Sciences University · Good Samaritan Hospital · The Casey Eye Institute, 3375 Southwest Terwilliger Boulevard, Portland, OR 97201 · 503-494-8386

OPTICS & REFRACTION

David L. Guyton · (Pediatric Optics & Refraction, Strabismus) · Professor of Ophthalmology, Johns Hopkins University School of Medicine · The Johns Hopkins Medical Institutions · 600 North Wolfe Street, Wilmer Institute, Baltimore, MD 21205 · 410-955-8314

Jack T. Holladay · A. G. McNeese Professor of Ophthalmology, The University of Texas Medical School at Houston · Staff Surgeon, Hermann Hospital; Park Plaza Hospital; St. Joseph Hospital · 6411 Fannin Street, Houston, TX 77030 · 713-797-1777

David D. Michaels · Professor of Ophthalmology, University of California at Los Angeles School of Medicine · University of California at Los Angeles Medical Center; Jules Stein Eye Institute · 1441 West Seventh Street, San Pedro, CA 90732 · 213-833-1311

Benjamin Milder · (Lacrimal) · Professor of Ophthalmology, Washington University School of Medicine · Barnes Hospital; The Jewish Hospital of St. Louis · 2821 North Ballas Road, Suite 120, St. Louis, MO 63131 · 314-432-7010

PEDIATRIC OPHTHALMOLOGY

Edward G. Buckley · (Strabismus) · Associate Professor of Ophthalmology and Assistant Professor of Pediatrics, Duke University School of Medicine · Duke Eye Center, Duke University Medical Center · P.O. Box 3802, Durham, NC 27710 · 919-684-6084

Forrest D. Ellis · (Strabismus) · Professor of Ophthalmology, Indiana University School of Medicine · Co-Director, Section of Pediatric Ophthalmology, Indiana University Medical Center · 702 Rotary Circle, Indianapolis, IN 46202 · 317-274-7919

John T. Flynn · (Strabismus) · Professor of Ophthalmology, University of Miami School of Medicine · Bascom Palmer Eye Institute, Anne Bates Leach Eye Hospital · 900 Northwest 17th Street, Miami, FL 33136 · 305-326-6050

David L. Guyton · (Pediatric Optics & Refraction, Strabismus) · Professor of Ophthalmology, Johns Hopkins University School of Medicine · The Johns Hopkins Medical Institutions · 600 North Wolfe Street, Wilmer Institute, Baltimore, MD 21205 · 410-955-8314

Eugene M. Helveston · (Strabismus) · Professor of Ophthalmology, Indiana University School of Medicine · Chief, Section of Pediatric Ophthalmology, Indiana University Medical Center · 702 Rotary Circle, Indianapolis, IN 46202-5175 · 317-274-1214

Creig S. Hoyt · (Neuro-Ophthalmology) · Professor and Vice-Chairman, Department of Ophthalmology, University of California at San Francisco School of Medicine · Director of Pediatric Ophthalmology, University of California at San Francisco Medical Center · 400 Parnassus Avenue, Room 704-A, San Francisco, CA 94143 · 415-476-1289

Malcolm R. Ing · (Strabismus) · Professor and Chief of Ophthalmology, John A. Burns School of Medicine, University of Hawaii · 1319 Punahou Street, Suite 1110, Honolulu, HI 96826 · 808-955-5951

Arthur Jampolsky · (Strabismus) · Executive Director, Smith-Kettlewell Eye Research Institute, California Pacific Medical Center · California Pacific Medical Center · 2232 Webster Street, Suite 500, San Francisco, CA 94115 · 415-923-3671

Burton J. Kushner · (Strabismus) · Clinical Professor of Ophthalmology, University of Wisconsin-Madison School of Medicine · Davis-Duehr Eye Associates; University of Wisconsin Clinical Science Center · 1025 Regent Street, Madison, WI 53705 · 608-258-4520

Malcolm L. Mazow · (Strabismus) · Clinical Professor of Ophthalmology, The University of Texas Health Science Center at Houston · Hermann Hospital; Texas Children's Hospital; Park Plaza Hospital · 2855 Gramercy Street, Houston, TX 77025 · 713-668-6828

Henry S. Metz · (Strabismus) · Professor and Chairman, Department of Ophthalmology, University of Rochester School of Medicine & Dentistry · Strong Memorial Hospital, University of Rochester Medical Center · 601 Elmwood Avenue, Box 659, Rochester, NY 14642 · 716-275-3256

Marshall M. Parks · (Strabismus) · Professor of Ophthalmology, The George Washington University School of Medicine · Children's National Medical Center 3400 Massachusetts Avenue, NW, Washington, DC 20007 · 202-338-3680

John Pratt-Johnson · (Strabismus) · Professor and Head, Department of Pediatric Ophthalmology, The University of British Columbia · Children's Hospital · 4480 Oak Street, Vancouver, British Columbia V6H 3V4 · 604-874-0644

Robert D. Reinecke · (Strabismus, Neuro-ophthalmology, Nystagmus) · Professor of Ophthalmology, Jefferson Medical College of Thomas Jefferson University · Attending Surgeon, Pediatric Ophthalmology Service, and Director, Foerderer Eye Movement Center for Children, Wills Eye Hospital · Ninth and Walnut Streets, Philadelphia, PA 19107 · 215-928-3149

Arthur L. Rosenbaum · (Strabismus) · Professor and Vice-Chairman, Department of Ophthalmology, University of California at Los Angeles School of Medicine · Chief, Division of Pediatric Ophthalmology, Jules Stein Eye Institute · 100 Stein Plaza, Los Angeles, CA 90024-7001 · 310-825-2872

Alan B. Scott · (Strabismus) · Senior Scientist, Smith-Kettlewell Eye Research Institute · California Pacific Medical Center · 2100 Webster Street, Suite 222, San Francisco, CA 94115 · 415-923-3120

William E. Scott · (Strabismus) · Professor of Ophthalmology, The University of Iowa College of Medicine · The University of Iowa Hospitals & Clinics · Iowa City, IA 52242 · 319-356-2877

David R. Stager · (Strabismus) · Clinical Professor, Southwestern Medical School Director of Ophthalmology Service, Children's Medical Center of Dallas · 8226 Douglas Street, Suite 805, Dallas, TX 75225 · 214-369-6434

Gunter K. von Noorden · (Strabismus) · Professor of Ophthalmology and Pediatrics, Baylor College of Medicine · Chief of Ophthalmology, Texas Children's Hospital · 6621 Fannin Street, Houston, TX 77030 · 713-770-3230

ULTRASOUND

Yale L. Fisher · Assistant Professor of Ophthalmology, Cornell University Medical College · Attending Surgeon, Manhattan Eye, Ear & Throat Hospital · 519 East 72nd Street, Suite 203, New York, NY 10021 · 212-861-9797

UVEITIS
(See also Rheumatology, Uveitis)

William Culbertson · Associate Professor of Ophthalmology, University of Miami School of Medicine · Chief of Cornea Service, Bascom Palmer Eye Institute · 900 Northwest 17th Street, Miami, FL 33136 · 305-326-6364

C. Stephen Foster · Associate Professor of Ophthalmology, Harvard Medical School · Director, Immunology Service, Massachusetts Eye & Ear Infirmary · 243 Charles Street, Boston, MA 02114 · 617-573-3591

Rudolph M. Franklin · Mercy Hospital; Hotel Dieu Hospital; Eye, Ear, Nose & Throat Hospital; Slidell Memorial Hospital; Terrebonne General Medical Center Mercy Medical Plaza, Suite 350, 319 North Genois Street, New Orleans, LA 70119 · 504-486-5353

Gary N. Holland · (Ocular Infectious Diseases) · Associate Professor of Ophthalmology, University of California at Los Angeles School of Medicine · Director, UCLA Ocular Inflammatory Disease Center, Jules Stein Eye Institute · 100 Stein Plaza, UCLA, Los Angeles, CA 90024-7003 · 310-825-9508

Douglas A. Jabs · Associate Professor of Ophthalmology and Medicine, Johns Hopkins University School of Medicine · Johns Hopkins Hospital, Wilmer Ophthalmological Institute · 850 North Broadway, Suite 700, Baltimore, MD 21205 · 410-955-1966

Henry J. Kaplan · (Macular Disease) · Professor and Chairman, Department of Ophthalmology and Visual Sciences, Washington University School of Medicine · Attending Physician, Barnes Hospital, St. Louis Children's Hospital, and The Jewish Hospital of St. Louis · Box 8096, 660 South Euclid Avenue, St. Louis, MO 63110 · 314-362-3937

David M. Meisler · Staff Physician, The Cleveland Clinic Foundation · One Clinic Center, 9500 Euclid Avenue, Cleveland, OH 44195-5024 · 216-444-8102

Robert A. Nozik · Clinical Professor of Ophthalmology, University of California, San Francisco School of Medicine · Chief, Uveitis Clinic, Francis I. Proctor Foundation, California Pacific Medical Center, Merritt Peralta Medical Center, University of California, San Francisco Medical Center · 513 Parnassus Avenue, Room S-315, San Francisco, CA 94143-0412 · 415-476-1441, 871-8856

Robert B. Nussenblatt · Clinical Director, and Acting Scientific Director, and Director of Laboratory of Immunology, National Eye Institute, National Institutes of Health · 9000 Rockville Pike, Building 10, Room 10N202, Bethesda, MD 20892 · 301-496-3123

E. Mitchel Opremcak · Assistant Professor, Department of Ophthalmology, Ohio State University College of Medicine · The Ohio State University Hospitals; Columbus Children's Hospital · 456 West 10th Avenue, Columbus, OH 43210 · 614-293-4358

Alan G. Palestine · Clinical Associate Professor of Ophthalmology, Georgetown University School of Medicine · Georgetown University Medical Center · 1145 Nineteenth Street, NW, Suite 607, Washington, DC 20036 · 202-833-1668

Ronald E. Smith · (Infectious Diseases) · Professor and Vice-Chairman, Department of Ophthalmology, University of Southern California School of Medicine · Doheny Eye Institute · 1355 San Pablo Street, Los Angeles, CA 90033 · 213-342-6424

VITREO-RETINAL SURGERY

Thomas Marshall Aaberg · (Vitreoretinal Diseases and Surgery) · Professor and Chairman of Ophthalmology, and F. Phinizy Calhoun, Sr. Professor, Emory University School of Medicine · Attending, Emory University Affiliated Hospitals; Egleston Hospital for Children; Crawford W. Long Memorial Hospital; Veterans Administration Hospital; Grady Memorial Hospital · 1327 Clifton Road NE, Atlanta, GA 30322 · 404-248-4456

Gary W. Abrams · (Vitreoretinal Diseases and Surgery) · Professor of Ophthalmology and Head, Vitreoretinal Service, Medical College of Wisconsin · The Eye Institute, Milwaukee County Medical Complex · 8700 West Wisconsin Avenue, Milwaukee, WI 53226 · 414-257-5343

William E. Benson · Professor of Ophthalmology, Jefferson Medical College of Thomas Jefferson University · Wills Eye Hospital · 910 East Willow Grove Avenue, Philadelphia, PA 19118 · 215-233-4300

George W. Blankenship, Jr. · (Vitreoretinal Diseases and Surgery, Diabetic Retinopathy, Vascular Occlusions, Laser Surgery) · Professor and Chairman, Department of Ophthalmology, Pennsylvania State University · The Milton S. Hershey Medical Center · 500 University Drive, P.O. Box 850, Hershey, PA 17033 · 717-531-8783

Mark S. Blumenkranz · (Vitreoretinal Diseases and Surgery) · Adjunct Associate Professor of Ophthalmology, The Eye Research Institute of Oakland University · Attending Physician, and Vitreoretinal Fellowship Director, William Beaumont Eye Institute, William Beaumont Hospital · 3535 West Thirteen Mile Road, Suite 632, Royal Oak, MI 48073 · 313-288-2280

Alexander J. Brucker · (Diabetic Retinopathy, Macular Degeneration, Vascular Occlusions, Laser Surgery, Vitreoretinal Surgery) · Associate Professor of Ophthalmology, University of Pennsylvania School of Medicine · Chief, Retina & Vitreous Service, Scheie Eye Institute; Presbyterian Medical Center; Hospital of the University of Pennsylvania; Graduate Hospital · Myrin Circle, 51 North 39th Street, Philadelphia, PA 19104 · 215-662-8675

Stanley Chang · (Vitreoretinal Diseases and Surgery) · Associate Professor of Ophthalmology, Cornell University Medical College · The New York Hospital-Cornell Medical Center · 520 East 70th Street, Suite Starr 817, New York, NY 10021 · 212-746-2470

Steven Thomas Charles · Clinical Associate Professor of Ophthalmology, and Chief, Vitreo-Retinal Service, The University of Tennessee at Memphis, College of Medicine · Chief, Vitreo-Retinal Service, Baptist Memorial Hospital · 6401 Poplar Avenue, Suite 190, Memphis, TN 38119 · 901-767-4499

John G. Clarkson · (Vitreoretinal Diseases and Surgery, Diabetic Retinopathy, Macular Degeneration, Vascular Occlusions, Laser Surgery,) · Professor of Ophthalmology, University of Miami School of Medicine · Chairman, Department of Ophthalmology, Bascom Palmer Eye Institute · 900 Northwest 17th Street, Miami, FL 33136 · 305-326-6116

D. Jackson Coleman · (Vitreoretinal Diseases and Surgery; Ultrasound) · Professor and Chairman, Department of Ophthalmology, Cornell University Medical College · The New York Hospital-Cornell Medical Center · 525 East 68th Street, New York, NY 10021 · 212-746-5588

Donald J. D'Amico · (Vitreoretinal Diseases and Surgery) · Associate Professor of Ophthalmology, Harvard Medical School · Associate Chief of Ophthalmology for Clinical Affairs, and Director, Diabetic Retinopathy Unit, Massachusetts Eye & Ear Infirmary · 243 Charles Street, Boston, MA 02114 · 617-573-3291

Jay L. Federman · (Vitreoretinal Diseases and Surgery) · Professor of Ophthalmology, Jefferson Medical College of Thomas Jefferson University · Wills Eye Hospital; Lankenau Hospital · 160 Lankenau Medical Building, East, Wynnewood, PA 19096 · 215-896-0768

Harry Weisiger Flynn, Jr. · (Diabetic Retinopathy) · Associate Professor of Ophthalmology, University of Miami School of Medicine · Bascom Palmer Eye Institute · 900 Northwest 17th Street, Miami, FL 33136 · 305-326-6118

Hal MacKenzie Freeman · Associate Clinical Professor of Ophthalmology, Harvard Medical School · Massachusetts Eye & Ear Infirmary · The Retina Associates, 100 Charles River Plaza, Boston, MA 02114 · 617-523-7810

Bert M. Glaser · (Vitreoretinal Diseases and Surgery) · Saint Joseph Hospital · The Retina Center at Saint Joseph Hospital, P.O. Box 20000, Baltimore, MD 21284 · 301-337-4500

Allan E. Kreiger · Professor of Ophthalmology, University of California at Los Angeles School of Medicine · Chief, Retina Division, Jules Stein Eye Institute · 100 Stein Plaza, Los Angeles, CA 90024-7007 · 310-825-5477

John S. Lean · Saddleback Hospital; Western Medical Center · 23521 Paseo de Valencia, Suite 207, Laguna Hills, CA 92653 · 714-717-5125

Hilel Lewis · (Vitreoretinal Diseases and Surgery, Diabetic Retinopathy, Macular Degeneration, Vascular Occlusions, Laser Surgery) · Assistant Professor of Ophthalmology, University of California at Los Angeles School of Medicine · The Charles Kenneth Feldman Scholar, Jules Stein Eye Institute · 100 Stein Plaza, Los Angeles, CA 90024-7007 · 213-206-3110

Robert Machemer · (Vitreoretinal Diseases and Surgery) · Helena Rubinstein Foundation Professor of Ophthalmology, Duke University School of Medicine · Duke Eye Center, Duke University Medical Center · P.O. Box 3802, Durham, NC 27710 · 919-684-3891

Brooks Walton McCuen II · (Vitreoretinal Diseases and Surgery) · Professor of Ophthalmology, Duke University School of Medicine · Chief, Vitreo-Retinal Division, Duke Eye Center, Duke University Medical Center · P.O. Box 3802, Durham, NC 27710 · 919-684-6749

Travis A. Meredith · (Vitreoretinal Diseases and Surgery) · Clinical Professor of Ophthalmology, Bethesda Eye Institute; St. Louis University School of Medicine Attending Staff, St. Luke's Hospital of Kansas City; Clinical Professor of Ophthalmology, Bethesda Eye Institute · One Barnes Hospital Plaza, Suite 17413, East Pavilion, St. Louis, MO 63110 · 314-367-1181

Kirk H. Packo · Assistant Professor of Ophthalmology, Rush Medical College · Director, Retina Program, Ingalls Memorial Hospital · The Retina Center, 71 West 156th Street, Suite 400, Harvey, IL 60426 · 708-333-2300

Thomas A. Rice · Associate Clinical Professor of Surgery (Ophthalmology), Case Western Reserve University School of Medicine · University Hospitals of Cleveland; St. Luke's Hospital; The Mt. Sinai Medical Center; Lakewood Hospital · 26900 Cedar Road, Suite 303, Cleveland, OH 44122 · 216-831-5700

Dennis M. Robertson · (Diabetic Retinopathy, Macular Degeneration, Vascular Occlusions, Laser Surgery) · Professor of Ophthalmology, Mayo Medical School · Mayo Clinic · 200 First Street, SW, Rochester, MN 55905 · 507-284-3721

Stephen J. Ryan · (Vitreoretinal Diseases and Surgery) · Professor and Chairman, Department of Ophthalmology, University of Southern California School of Medicine · The Los Angeles County + University of Southern California Medical Center · 1355 San Pablo Street, Los Angeles, CA 90033 · 213-342-6444

George A. Williams · Associate Clinical Professor of Ophthalmology, and Associate Clinical Professor of Biomedical Sciences, The Eye Research Institute of Oakland University, Wayne State University · Attending Staff, William Beaumont Hospital · 632 William Beaumont Medical Building, 3535 West Thirteen Mile Road, Royal Oak, MI 48073 · 313-288-2280

ORTHOPAEDIC SURGERY

FOOT & ANKLE SURGERY

Donald E. Baxter · (Runners' Injuries) · Clinical Professor of Orthopaedic Surgery, Baylor College of Medicine, and The University of Texas · The Methodist Hospital; Southwest Memorial Hospital · 7500 Beechnut Street, Suite 175, Houston, TX 77074 · 713-772-5000

R. Luke Bordelon · Clinical Professor of Orthopaedic Surgery, Louisiana State University School of Medicine · Director, Foot Clinic, Doctors Hospital of Opelousas · The Opelousas Orthopaedic Clinic, 5069 Highway I-49 South, Opelousas, LA 70570 · 318-942-6503

Michael Coughlin · University of Idaho · 901 North Curtis Road, Boise, ID 83706 208-377-1000

Andrea Cracchiolo · Professor of Orthopaedic Surgery, University of California, Los Angeles School of Medicine · University of California, Los Angeles Center for the Health Sciences · 10833 LeConte Avenue, Room 76-139, Los Angeles, CA 90024 · 310-825-0804

John Samuel Gould · Professor and Chairman, Department of Orthopaedic Surgery, Medical College of Wisconsin · 8700 West Wisconsin Avenue, Milwaukee, WI 53226 · 414-257-6655

William G. Hamilton · (Dance) · Associate Clinical Professor of Orthopaedic Surgery, College of Physicians & Surgeons of Columbia University · Senior Orthopaedic Attending Surgeon, St. Luke's-Roosevelt Hospital Center · 345 West 58th Street, New York, NY 10019 · 212-765-2262

Sigvard T. Hansen, Jr. · Professor of Orthopaedics, University of Washington School of Medicine · Department of Orthopaedics, Harborview Medical Center · 325 Ninth Avenue, Seattle, WA 98104 · 206-223-4487

Kenneth A. Johnson · Professor of Orthopaedic Surgery, Mayo Medical School · Head of Section, Section of Orthopaedic Surgery, Mayo Clinic Scottsdale · 13400 East Shea Boulevard, Scottsdale, AZ 85259 · 602-391-8000

Roger A. Mann · Associate Clinical Professor of Orthopaedic Surgery, University of California at San Francisco School of Medicine · Chief of Foot Surgery, Samuel Merritt Hospital · 3300 Webster Street, Suite 1200, Oakland, CA 94609 · 510-483-2500

Francesca M. Thompson · Clinical Assistant Professor of Orthopaedics, College of Physicians & Surgeons of Columbia University · Chief, Adult Orthopaedic Foot Clinic; St. Luke's-Roosevelt Hospital Center; Co-Director, Combined Foot & Ankle Fellowship; The Hospital for Special Surgery · 345 West 58th Street, New York, NY 10019 · 212-765-2373

Theodore R. Waugh · (Ankle) · Professor of Orthopaedic Surgery, New York University School of Medicine · New York University Medical Center · 550 First Avenue, New York, NY 10016 · 212-263-7279

HIP SURGERY

Harlan C. Amstutz · (Hip Replacements) · Professor Emeritus, University of California at Los Angeles School of Medicine · Medical Director of Joint Replacement Institute, Orthopaedic Hospital · 2400 South Flower Street, Loman Outpatient Wing, Third Floor, Los Angeles, CA 90007 · 213-742-1075

John M. Cuckler · Associate Professor of Orthopaedic Surgery, University of Pennsylvania School of Medicine · Director, Bone Bank, Hospital of the University of Pennsylvania · 3400 Spruce Street, Second Floor, Silverstein Pavilion, Philadelphia, PA 19104 · 215-662-3340

Harold K. Dunn · Chairman and Professor, Division of Orthopaedics, University of Utah School of Medicine · University of Utah Health Sciences Center · 50 North Medical Drive, Salt Lake City, UT 84132 · 801-581-7601

Charles Engh · Clinical Assistant Professor in Orthopaedic Surgery, Georgetown University School of Medicine; University of Maryland School of Medicine · National Hospital for Orthopaedics & Rahabilitation · Anderson Clinic, 2445 Army Navy Drive, Arlington, VA 22206 · 703-892-6500

Robert H. Fitzgerald, Jr. · Professor and Chairman, Department of Orthopaedic Surgery, Wayne State University School of Medicine · Orthopaedic Surgeon-in-Chief, Detroit Medical Center; Chief, Department of Orthopaedic Surgery, Hutzel Hospital; Detroit Receiving Hospital; Harper Hospital · 4707 St. Antoine Boulevard, Detroit, MI 48201 · 313-745-6953

William H. Harris · Clinical Professor of Orthopaedic Surgery, Harvard Medical School · Chief, Hip & Implant Unit, Massachusetts General Hospital · 15 Parkman Street, ACC Building, Suite 533, Boston, MA 02114 · 617-726-3556

Eduardo A. Salvati · (Joint Replacement) · Clinical Professor of Orthopaedics, Cornell University Medical College · Chief, Hip Clinic, The Hospital for Special Surgery · 535 East 70th Street, New York, NY 10021 · 212-606-1472

Hugh S. Tullos · Wilhelmina Barnhart Chairman, Department of Orthopaedic Surgery, Baylor College of Medicine · Chief of Orthopaedic Surgery Services, The Methodist Hospital · 6550 Fannin Street, Suite 2625, Houston, TX 77030 · 713-790-3112

Roderick H. Turner · Clinical Professor of Orthopaedic Surgery, Tufts University School of Medicine · Senior Attending Staff, New England Baptist Hospital · 70 Parker Hill Avenue, Suite 500, Boston, MA 02120 · 617-738-5467

Jerome D. Wiedel · (Hemophilia) · Professor and Chairman, Department of Orthopaedics, University of Colorado School of Medicine · University of Colorado Health Sciences Center · 4701 East Ninth Avenue, Box E203, Denver, CO 80262 · 303-272-1254

KNEE SURGERY

Harold K. Dunn · Chairman and Professor, Division of Orthopaedics, University of Utah School of Medicine · University of Utah Health Sciences Center · 50 North Medical Drive, Salt Lake City, UT 84132 · 801-581-7601

John Nevil Insall · Professor of Orthopaedic Surgery, Cornell University Medical College · Attending Orthopaedic Surgeon, Beth Israel Hospital North; Director, Insall Scott Kelly Institute for Orthopaedics and Sports Medicine, Beth Israel Hospital North · 170 East End Avenue at 87th Street, Fourth Floor, New York, NY 10128 · 212-472-5975

Leonard Marmor · St. John's Hospital & Health Center · 10921 Wilshire Boulevard, Suite 911, Los Angeles, CA 90024 · 213-208-4441

Frank Noyes · Director, Cincinnati Sportsmedicine & Orthopaedic Center; Clinical Professor of Orthopaedic Surgery, and Adjunct Professor, Department of Engineering, University of Cincinnati · Director, Research & Education, Deaconess Hospital; Bethesda Hospital; St. Elizabeth Hospital · Cincinnati Sportsmedicine & Orthopaedic Center, One Lytle Place, Cincinnati OH 45202 · 513-421-5100

Jerome D. Wiedel · (Hemophilia) · Professor and Chairman, Department of Orthopaedics, University of Colorado School of Medicine · University of Colorado Health Sciences Center · 4701 East Ninth Avenue, Box E203, Denver, CO 80262 303-272-1254

PEDIATRIC ORTHOPAEDIC SURGERY

David S. Bradford · (Spine Deformities) · Professor and Chairman, Department of Orthopaedic Surgery, University of California, San Francisco School of Medicine · University of California, San Francisco Medical Center · 533 Parnassus Avenue, U-471, Box 0728, San Francisco, CA 94143-0728 · 415-476-4010

Harold Michael Dick · (Musculoskeletal Tumor Surgery) · Professor and Chairman, Department of Orthopaedic Surgery, College of Physicians & Surgeons of Columbia University · Director, Orthopaedic Surgery, Columbia-Presbyterian Medical Center · 161 Fort Washington Avenue, New York, NY 10032 · 212-305-5561

Denis S. Drummond · (Spine Deformities) · Professor of Orthopaedic Surgery, University of Pennsylvania School of Medicine · Chairman, Pediatric Orthopaedic Surgery, The Children's Hospital of Philadelphia · Department of Orthopaedics, 34th and Civic Center Boulevard, Philadelphia, PA 19104 · 215-590-1527

Robert Gillespie · Professor and Chairman, Department of Orthopaedics, State University of New York Health Science Center at Buffalo · Children's Hospital of Buffalo · 219 Bryant Street, Buffalo, NY 14222 · 716-878-7563

Neil E. Green · Professor and Vice-Chairman, Department of Orthopaedic Surgery, and Head of Pediatric Orthopaedics, Vanderbilt University School of Medicine · Department of Orthopaedics and Rehabilitation, Nashville, TN 37232 · 615-322-7133

Paul P. Griffin · Professor of Orthopaedic Surgery, Medical University of South Carolina · 171 Ashley Avenue, Charleston, SC 29425 · 803-792-9435

John E. Hall · (Spine) · Professor of Orthopaedic Surgery, Harvard Medical School Orthopaedic Surgeon in Chief, Children's Hospital · 300 Longwood Avenue, Boston, MA 02115 · 617-735-6756

Robert N. Hensinger · Professor of Surgery, The University of Michigan Medical School · Chief, Section of Pediatric Orthopaedics, C.S. Mott Children's Hospital, The University of Michigan Medical Center · 1500 East Medical Center Drive, Box 0328, Ann Arbor, MI 48109-0328 · 313-936-5715

G. Dean MacEwen · (Spine & Hip Problems in Children) · Professor of Orthopaedics, Louisiana State University School of Medicine · Chairman, Department of Pediatric Orthopaedic Surgery, Children's Hospital of New Orleans · 200 Henry Clay Avenue, New Orleans, LA 70118 · 504-891-7067

Raymond T. Morrissy · Clinical Professor of Orthopaedic Surgery, Emory University School of Medicine · Medical Director and Chief of Orthopaedics, Scottish Rite Children's Medical Center · 1001 Johnson Ferry Road, Atlanta, GA 30363 · 404-250-2022

Robert B. Salter · (Hip Surgery) · Professor of Orthopaedic Surgery, University of Toronto School of Medicine · Senior Orthopaedic Surgeon, The Hospital for Sick Children · 555 University Avenue, Room 1254, Toronto, Ontario M5G 1X8 · 416-598-6435

Lynn T. Staheli · (Pediatric, Hip Surgery) · Professor of Orthopaedic Surgery, University of Washington · Director, Department of Orthopaedics, Children's Hospital & Medical Center · 4800 Sand Point Way NE, P.O. Box C5371, Seattle, WA 98105 · 206-526-2108

Vernon Thorpe Tolo · Professor of Orthopaedic Surgery, University of Southern California School of Medicine · Head, Division of Orthopaedic Surgery, Children's Hospital of Los Angeles · 4650 Sunset Boulevard, Los Angeles, CA 90027 213-669-4658

John H. Wedge · (Hip Surgery) · R. S. McLaughlin Professor and Chairman, Department of Surgery, University of Toronto Faculty of Medicine · Head, Division of Orthopaedic Surgery, The Hospital for Sick Children · 555 University Avenue, Toronto, Ontario M5G 1X8 · 416-598-6944

PERIPHERAL NERVE SURGERY
(See also Hand Surgery, Peripheral Nerve Surgery; Neurological Surgery, Peripheral Nerve Surgery; Plastic Surgery, Peripheral Nerve Surgery)

Frank William Bora, Jr. · Professor of Orthopaedic Surgery, University of Pennsylvania School of Medicine · Chief, Hand Surgery, Hospital of the University of Pennsylvania · Penn Tower Hotel, 34th Street and Civic Center Boulevard, Eighth Floor, Philadelphia, PA 19104 · 215-662-6106

Richard M. Braun · Board Member, Rehabilitation Committee, Sharp Memorial Hospital; Chairman, Orthopaedic Department, Alvarado Hospital · 6699 Alvarado Road, Suite 2302, San Diego, CA 92120 · 619-287-4477

Richard H. Gelberman · Professor of Orthopaedic Surgery, Harvard Medical School · Chief, Hand Surgery Service, Department of Orthopaedic Surgery, Massachusetts General Hospital · 15 Parkman Street, WACC 527, Boston, MA 02114 · 617-726-2946

George E. Omer · Professor Emeritus, the University of New Mexico School of Medicine · The University Hospital · University of New Mexico Medical Center, Department of Orthopaedics, Albuquerque NM 87131-5296 · 505-272-4107

Morton Spinner · (Nerve Compression Lesions) · Clinical Professor of Orthopaedic Surgery, Albert Einstein College of Medicine · Consultant in Hand Surgery, Franklin Hospital Medical Center; North Shore University Hospital; Long Island Jewish Medical Center · 557 Central Avenue, Cedarhurst, NY 11516 · 516-569-6323

Jack W. Tupper · Clinical Professor of Orthopaedic Surgery, University of California at San Francisco School of Medicine · Director, Hand Clinic, Children's Hospital of the East Bay, Samuel Merritt Hospital · 2938 Webster Street, Oakland, CA 94609 · 510-893-9589

Virchel E. Wood · Professor of Orthopaedic Surgery, Loma Linda University School of Medicine · Chief of Hand Surgery Service, Loma Linda University Medical Center · 11234 Anderson Street, Room A519, Loma Linda, CA 92350 · 714-824-4413

RECONSTRUCTIVE SURGERY
(See also Hand Surgery, Reconstructive Surgery; Plastic Surgery, Reconstructive Surgery)

Louis Urban Bigliani · (Shoulder) · Assistant Professor of Orthopaedic Surgery, College of Physicians & Surgeons of Columbia University · Columbia-Presbyterian Medical Center · 161 Fort Washington Avenue, New York, NY 10032 · 212-305-5564

Lester S. Borden · (Hip, Knee) · Head, Section of Joint Replacement & Arthritis Surgery, The Cleveland Clinic Foundation · One Clinic Center, 9500 Euclid Avenue, Cleveland, OH 44195-5001 · 216-444-2627

Michael W. Chapman · (Adult Leg Length Discrepancy, Trauma Reconstruction, Nonunions & Malunions) · Professor and Chairman, Department of Orthopaedics, University of California, Davis School of Medicine · University of California, Davis Medical Center · 2230 Stockton Boulevard, Sacramento, CA 95817 · 916-734-2709

Robert H. Cofield · (Shoulder) · Professor of Orthopaedic Surgery, Mayo Medical School · Mayo Clinic · 200 First Street, SW, Rochester, MN 55905 · 507-284-2995

Clifford W. Colwell · (Hip, Knee) · Head, Division of Orthopaedic Surgery, Scripps Clinic & Research Foundation · 10666 North Torrey Pines Road, La Jolla, CA 92037 · 619-554-8852

Ralph W. Coonrad · (Elbow Reconstruction, Hand Reconstruction, Wrist Reconstruction) · Associate Clinical Professor of Orthopaedic Surgery, Duke University School of Medicine · Durham General Hospital · 1828 Hillandale Road, Durham, NC 27705 · 919-220-5593

Richard D. Coutts · (Hip, Knee) · Associate Clinical Professor of Orthopaedics, University of California at San Diego School of Medicine · Adjunct Professor, Department of Orthopaedics & Rehabilitation, University of California at San Diego Medical Center; Sharp Memorial Hospital · 7910 Frost Street, Suite 202, San Diego, CA 92123 · 619-278-8300

Lawrence D. Dorr · (Hip, Knee) · Clinical Professor of Orthopaedic Surgery, University of California at Irvine School of Medicine; University of Southern California School of Medicine · Kerlan-Jobe Clinic · 501 East Hardy Street, Suite 200, Inglewood, CA 90301 · 213-674-5200

Nas S. Eftekhar · (Hip, Knee) · Professor of Clinical Orthopaedic Surgery, College of Physicians & Surgeons of Columbia University · Director, Implant Service, Columbia-Presbyterian Medical Center · 161 Fort Washington Avenue, 234, New York, NY 10032 · 212-305-5368

Frederick C. Ewald · (Elbow) · Associate Professor of Orthopaedic Surgery, Harvard Medical School · Orthopaedic Surgeon, Brigham & Women's Hospital · 75 Francis Street, Boston, MA 02115 · 617-732-5382

Jorge O. Galante · (Hip, Knee) · The Wiliam A. Hark M.D.-Susanne G. Swift Professor and Chairman, Rush Medical College · Rush-Presbyterian-St. Luke's Medical Center · Jelke Building, 1750 West Harrison Street, Suite 1471, Chicago, IL 60612 · 312-942-5850

Victor M. Goldberg · (Hip, Knee) · Professor and Chairman, Department of Orthopaedic Surgery, Case Western Reserve University School of Medicine · Director, Department of Orthopaedics, University Hospitals of Cleveland · 2078 Abington Road, Cleveland, OH 44106 · 216-844-3044

Richard J. Hawkins · (Shoulder) · Clinical Professor, Department of Orthopaedics, University of Colorado School of Medicine · Orthopaedic Consultant, Vail Valley Medical Center · Steadman-Hawkins Clinic, 181 West Meadow Drive, Suite 400, Vail, CO 81657 · 303-476-1100

Anthony K. Hedley · (Hip, Knee) · Director of Surgical Research, Harrington Arthritis Research Center · Chairman, Department of Orthopaedics, St. Luke's Medical Center · 3320 North Second Street, Phoenix, AZ 85012 · 602-266-6390

David S. Hungerford · (Hip, Knee) · Professor of Orthopaedic Surgery, Johns Hopkins University School of Medicine · Chief, Division of Arthritis Surgery, Good Samaritan Hospital; The Johns Hopkins Medical Institutions · Good Samaritan Professional Building, Suite G1, 5601 Loch Raven Boulevard, Baltimore, MD 21239 · 301-532-4732

Allan E. Inglis · (Elbow) · Professor of Clinical Surgery, and Professor of Clinical Anatomy In Cell Biology & Anatomy, Cornell University Medical College · Director, Reconstructive & Surgical Arthritis Center, Beth Israel Hospital North; The Hospital for Special Surgery · 1725 York Avenue, New York, NY 10128 · 212-410-2379

Kenneth A. Krackow · (Hip, Knee) · Professor of Orthopaedic Surgery, Johns Hopkins University School of Medicine · The Johns Hopkins Medical Institutions; The Good Samaritan Hospital; Childrens Hospital of Baltimore; Union Memorial Hospital; Sinai Hospital of Baltimore · Good Samaritan Professional Building, Suite G1, 5601 Loch Raven Boulevard, Baltimore, MD 21239 · 410-955-4734

Paul A. Lotke · (Hip, Knee) · Professor of Orthopaedic Surgery and Medicine, University of Pennsylvania, School of Medicine; Professor of Orthopaedic Surgery, Hospital of the University of Pennsylvania · Chief, Implant Service, Hospital of the University of Pennsylvania · 3400 Spruce Street, Second Floor, Silverstein Pavilion, Philadelphia, PA 19104 · 215-662-3349

Thomas H. Mallory · (Hip, Knee) · Assistant Clinical Professor, Department of Orthopaedic Surgery, Ohio State University College of Medicine · Chairman, Section of Joint Implant Surgery, Grant Medical Center · 720 East Broad Street, Columbus, OH 43215 · 614-221-6331

Frederick A. Matsen III · (Shoulder) · Professor and Chairman, Department of Orthopaedics, University of Washington School of Medicine · University of Washington Medical Center · 1959 Northwest Pacific Street, RK-10, Seattle, WA 98195 206-543-5450

Robert William McGraw · (Hip, Knee) · Professor and Head, Department of Orthopaedics, The University of British Columbia · Vancouver General Hospital 910 West 10th Avenue, Third Floor, Vancouver, British Columbia V5Z 4E3 · 604-875-4595

John R. Moreland · (Hip, Knee) · Assistant Clinical Professor of Orthopaedic Surgery, University of California at Los Angeles School of Medicine · Attending Staff, St. John's Hospital & Health Center · 2021 Santa Monica Boulevard, Suite 710E, Santa Monica, CA 90404 · 213-453-1911

Bernard F. Morrey · (Hip, Knee, Elbow) · Professor and Chairman, Department of Orthopaedics, Mayo Medical School · Consultant, Orthopaedic Surgery, Mayo Clinic · 200 First Street, SW, Rochester, MN 55905 · 507-284-3659

Shawn W. O'Driscoll · (Elbow, Shoulder, Cartilage Regeneration) · Assistant Professor of Orthopaedic Surgery, University of Toronto School of Medicine · Director, Cartilage & Connective Tissue Research Laboratory, St. Michael's Hospital · 55 Queen Street East, Suite 800, Toronto, Ontario M5C 1R6 · 416-864-6003

Chitranjan S. Ranawat · (Hip, Knee) · Professor of Orthopaedic Surgery, Cornell University Medical College · Attending Surgeon and Chief, Surgical Arthritis Service, The Hospital for Special Surgery · 535 East 70th Street, Room 354, New York, NY 10021 · 212-606-1494

James A. Rand · (Hip, Knee) · Associate Professor of Orthopaedic Surgery, Mayo Medical School · Consultant in Orthopaedic Surgery, Mayo Clinic · 200 First Street, SW, Rochester, MN 55905 · 507-284-3957

Charles A. Rockwood, Jr. · (Shoulder) · Professor and Chairman Emeritus, The University of Texas Medical School & Health Science Center at San Antonio · Medical Center Hospital · 7703 Floyd Curl Drive, San Antonio, TX 78284 · 512-567-5125

Richard H. Rothman · (Hip, Knee) · James Edwards Professor and Chairman, Department of Orthopaedic Surgery, Jefferson Medical College of Thomas Jefferson University · Chairman, The Rothman Institute, Pennsylvania Hospital · 800 Spruce Street, Philadelphia, PA 19107 · 215-829-3458

Richard David Scott · (Hip, Knee) · Associate Clinical Professor of Orthopaedic Surgery, Harvard Medical School · Brigham & Women's Hospital · 125 Parker Hill Avenue, Boston, MA 02120 · 617-738-9151

Clement Blount Sledge · (Hip, Knee) · John B. & Buckminster Brown Professor of Orthopaedic Surgery, Harvard Medical School · Chairman, Department of Orthopaedic Surgery, Brigham & Women's Hospital · 75 Francis Street, Boston, MA 02115 · 617-732-5358

Richard N. Stauffer · (Hip, Knee) · Robinson Professor of Orthopaedic Surgery, Johns Hopkins University School of Medicine · Chief, Department of Orthopaedic Surgery, The Johns Hopkins Medical Institutions · 600 North Wolfe Street, Harvey 611, Baltimore, MD 21205 · 410-955-9300

Bernard N. Stulberg · (Hip, Knee) · Associate Professor of Orthopaedics, Case Western Reserve University School of Medicine · Head, Division of Arthritis & Joint Implant Surgery, University Hospitals of Cleveland · 2074 Abington Road, Cleveland, OH 44106 · 216-844-3007

David Stulberg · (Hip, Knee) · Associate Professor of Orthopaedic Surgery, Northwestern University Medical School · Director, The Joint Reconstruction & Implant Service, Northwestern Memorial Hospital · 211 East Chicago Avenue, Suite 1336, Chicago, IL 60611 · 312-440-1340

Thomas Thornhill · (Hip, Knee) · Associate Clinical Professor of Orthopaedic Surgery, Harvard Medical School · Brigham & Women's Hospital · 75 Francis Street, Boston, MA 02115 · 617-732-5383

Robert E. Tooms · (Hip, Knee) · Professor of Orthopaedic Surgery, The University of Tennessee at Memphis, College of Medicine · Active Staff and Chief of Staff, Campbell Clinic, Baptist Hospital · 869 Madison Avenue, Memphis, TN 38103 · 901-577-9524

James R. Urbaniak · Virginia Flowers Baker Professor of Orthopaedic Surgery, and Chief, Division of Orthopaedic Surgery, Duke University School of Medicine Duke University Medical Center · P.O. Box 2912, Duke University Medical Center, Durham, NC 27710 · 919-684-2476

Robert G. Volz · (Hip, Knee) · Professor of Surgery, The University of Arizona College of Medicine · Chief, Section of Orthopaedic Surgery, The University of Arizona Health Sciences Center · 1501 North Campbell Avenue, Tucson, AZ 85724 · 602-626-7644

Alan H. Wilde · (Hip, Knee) · Professor of Orthopaedic Surgery, Case Western Reserve University School of Medicine · University Orthopaedic Associates; University Hospitals of Cleveland · 2074 Abington Road, Cleveland, OH 44106 · 216-844-3219

Virchel E. Wood · (Thoracic Outlet Disorders, Congenital Anomalies) · Professor of Orthopaedic Surgery, Loma Linda University School of Medicine · Chief of Hand Surgery Service, Loma Linda University Medical Center · 11234 Anderson Street, Room A519, Loma Linda, CA 92350 · 714-824-4413

RHEUMATOID ARTHRITIS

Andrea Cracchiolo · Professor of Orthopaedic Surgery, University of California, Los Angeles School of Medicine · University of California, Los Angeles Center for the Health Sciences · 10833 LeConte Avenue, Room 76-139, Los Angeles, CA 90024 · 310-825-0804

William H. Thomas · Associate Clinical Professor of Orthopaedic Surgery, Harvard Medical School · Orthopaedic Surgeon, Brigham & Women's Hospital · 75 Francis Street, Boston, MA 02115 · 617-732-5384

SHOULDER SURGERY

Robert D. Leffert · (Thoracic Outlet Disorders) · Professor of Orthopaedic Surgery, Harvard Medical School · Chief, Surgical Upper Extremity Rehabilitation Unit, Massachusetts General Hospital · 32 Fruit Street, Boston, MA 02114 · 617-726-2954

SPINE SURGERY

Joseph S. Barr, Jr. · Associate Clinical Professor of Orthopaedic Surgery, Harvard Medical School · Visiting Orthopaedic Surgeon, Massachusetts General Hospital · Zero Emerson Place, Suite 120, Boston, MA 02114 · 617-536-3750

Henry Hubert Bohlman · Professor of Orthopaedic Surgery, Case Western Reserve University School of Medicine · Chief, Reconstructive & Traumatic Spine Surgery, University Hospitals of Cleveland · 2078 Abington Road, Cleveland, OH 44106 · 216-844-1025

David S. Bradford · (Pediatric) · Professor and Chairman, Department of Orthopaedic Surgery, University of California, San Francisco School of Medicine · University of California, San Francisco Medical Center · 533 Parnassus Avenue, U-471, Box 0728, San Francisco, CA 94143-0728 · 415-476-4010

Denis S. Drummond · (Spine Deformities, Pediatric) · Professor of Orthopaedic Surgery, University of Pennsylvania School of Medicine · Chairman, Pediatric Orthopaedic Surgery, The Children's Hospital of Philadelphia · Department of Orthopaedics, 34th and Civic Center Boulevard, Philadelphia, PA 19104 · 215-590-1527

John E. Hall · (Pediatric) · Professor of Orthopaedic Surgery, Harvard Medical School · Orthopaedic Surgeon in Chief, Children's Hospital · 300 Longwood Avenue, Boston, MA 02115 · 617-735-6756

SPORTS MEDICINE

James R. Andrews · (Knee, Shoulder, Arthroscopic Procedures) · Orthopaedic Surgeon, American Sports Medicine Institute · Alabama Sports Medicine & Orthopaedic Center · 1222 Fourteenth Avenue South, Birmingham, AL 35205 · 205-933-7422

Donald E. Baxter · (Runners' Injuries) · Clinical Professor of Orthopaedic Surgery, Baylor College of Medicine, and The University of Texas · The Methodist Hospital; Southwest Memorial Hospital · 7500 Beechnut Street, Suite 175, Houston, TX 77074 · 713-772-5000

John A. Bergfeld · (Knee) · Head, Section of Sports Medicine in the Department of Orthopaedic Surgery, The Cleveland Clinic Foundation · One Clinic Center, 9500 Euclid Avenue, Cleveland, OH 44195-5027 · 216-444-2618

Rich Caspari · (Knee, Shoulder, Arthroscopic Procedures) · Associate Professor of Orthopaedic Surgery, Virginia Commonwealth University, Medical College of Virginia · St. Mary's Hospital · 4405 Cox Road, Suite 120, Glen Allen, VA 23060 804-346-1000

William Clancy · (Knee Surgery) · 1201 Eleventh Avenue South, Birmingham, AL 35205 · 205-930-0061

Dale Daniel · (Knee) · Attending, Kaiser Permanente · Kaiser Clinic, 250 Travelodge Drive, El Cajon, CA 92020 · 619-441-0067

Kenneth E. DeHaven · (Arthroscopic Procedures) · Professor and Associate Chairman, Department of Orthopaedics, and Director of Athletic Medicine, University of Rochester School of Medicine & Dentistry · Strong Memorial Hospital, University of Rochester Medical Center · 601 Elmwood Avenue, Box 665, Rochester, NY 14642 · 716-275-2970

David Drez, Jr. · (Knee) · Clinical Professor of Orthopaedics, and Director, Louisiana State University Knee & Sports Medicine Fellowship, Louisiana State University School of Medicine · Lake Charles Memorial Hospital · 2615 Enterprise Boulevard, Lake Charles, LA 70601 · 318-439-0385

John A. Feagin · (Knee) · Associate Professor of Surgery, Duke University School of Medicine · Duke University Medical Center · P.O. Box 3672, Durham, NC 27710 · 919-684-3591

Marc Jay Friedman · (Knee, Arthroscopic Procedures) · Assistant Clinical Professor of Orthopaedic Surgery, University of California at Los Angeles School of Medicine · Fellowship Director, Southern California Orthopedic Institute Medical Group; Valley Presbyterian Hospital · 6815 Noble Avenue, Van Nuys, CA 91405-3730 · 818-901-6600

John Calvin Garrett · (Knee, Arthroscopic Procedures) · Piedmont Hospital; St. Joseph's Hospital · 5671 Peachtree Dunwoody Road NE, Suite 900, Atlanta, GA 30342 · 404-847-9999

William E. Garrett, Jr. · (Arthroscopic Procedures) · Associate Professor of Orthopaedic Surgery, Duke University School of Medicine · Research Director, Sports Medicine Center, Duke University Medical Center · P.O. Box 3435, Durham, NC 27710 · 919-684-6658

William G. Hamilton · (Dance) · Associate Clinical Professor of Orthopaedic Surgery, College of Physicians & Surgeons of Columbia University · Senior Orthopaedic Attending Surgeon, St. Luke's-Roosevelt Hospital Center · 345 West 58th Street, New York, NY 10019 · 212-765-2262

Douglas W. Jackson · (Knee) · Medical Director, Southern California Center for Sports Medicine; Sports Medicine Fellowship Director, Long Beach Memorial Medical Center · 2760 Atlantic Avenue, Long Beach, CA 90806 · 213-424-6666

Frank W. Jobe · (Elbow, Shoulder) · Clinical Professor, Department of Orthopaedics, University of Southern California School of Medicine · Kerlan-Jobe Orthopaedic Clinic · 501 East Hardy Street, Inglewood, CA 90301 · 213-674-5200

Lanny Leo Johnson · (Knee, Arthroscopic Procedures) · Clinical Professor of Surgery, Michigan State University College of Human Medicine · Ingham Medical Center · 4528 South Hagadorn, East Lansing, MI 48823 · 517-351-7450

Robert J. Johnson · (Knee Surgery) · Professor, Department of Orthopaedics, University of Vermont School of Medicine · Medical Center Hospital of Vermont 125 College Parkway, Suite 101, Colchester, VT 05446 · 802-655-4914

John B. McGinty · (Arthroscopic Procedures) · Professor and Chairman, Department of Orthopaedic Surgery, Medical University of South Carolina · 171 Ashley Avenue, Charleston, SC 29425 · 803-792-3856

Thomas D. Rosenberg · (Knee, Arthroscopic Procedures) · Clinical Assistant Professor of Orthopaedic Surgery, University of Utah School of Medicine · The Orthopedic Specialty Hospital · 5848 South 300 East, Salt Lake City UT 84107 · 801-269-4100

W. Norman Scott · (Knee) · Beth Israel Hospital North · 170 East End Avenue, New York, NY 10128 · 212-472-7701

J. Richard Steadman · (Knee) · Clinical Professor, University of Texas Southwest Medical School · Vail Valley Medical Center · 181 West Meadow Drive, Suite 400, Vail, CO 81657 · 303-476-1100

Joseph S. Torg · (Knee) · Professor of Orthopaedic Surgery, University of Pennsylvania School of Medicine · Director, Sports Medicine, Sports Medicine Center of the University of Pennsylvania · Weightman Hall, 235 South 33rd Street, Philadelphia, PA 19104 · 215-662-4090

Russell F. Warren · (Knee, Shoulder, Arthroscopic Procedures) · Professor of Orthopaedic Surgery, Cornell University Medical College · Director of Sports Medicine, The Hospital for Special Surgery · 535 East 70th Street, New York, NY 10021 · 212-606-1178

Bertram Zarins · (Knee) · Assistant Clinical Professor of Orthopaedic Surgery, Harvard Medical School · Chief, Sports Medicine Unit, Massachusetts General Hospital · 15 Parkman Street, Suite 514, Boston, MA 02114 · 617-726-3421

TRAUMA

Fred Behrens · (Major Fractures, Trauma Reconstruction, Bone Infections, Leg Length Discrepancies) · Professor, Department of Orthopaedic Surgery, Case Western Reserve University School of Medicine · Chief, Orthopaedic Traumatology, MetroHealth Medical Center · 3395 Scranton Road, Cleveland, OH 44109 · 216-459-3890

Lawrence Brunton Bone · Assistant Professor of Orthopaedic Surgery, State University of New York Health Science Center at Buffalo · Erie County Medical Center · 462 Grider Street, Buffalo, NY 14215 · 716-898-3810

Michael J. Bosse · Associate Professor of Orthopaedic Surgery, University of Maryland School of Medicine · Attending Orthopaedic Traumatologist, Maryland Shock Trauma Center · 22 South Greene Street, Baltimore, MD 21201 · 301-328-6280

Bruce D. Browner · (Osteomyelitis, Nonunion, Malunion) · Professor and Director, Department of Orthopaedic Surgery, The University of Texas Health Science Center at Houston · Chief of Orthopaedics, Hermann Hospital; Lyndon B. Johnson General Hospital · 6431 Fannin Street, Room 6154, Houston, TX 77030 713-792-5636

Robert Brumback · (Complicated Multiple Trauma, Intramedullary Nailing) · Associate Professor of Surgery, University of Maryland School of Medicine, Johns Hopkins University School of Medicine · University of Maryland Medical Center Shock Trauma Center, 22 South Greene Street, Baltimore, MD 21201 · 301-328-6280

Robert W. Bucholz · Professor and Chairman, Department of Orthopaedic Surgery, The University of Texas Southwestern Medical Center at Dallas · Parkland Memorial Hospital; Zale-Lipshy Hospital; Children's Medical Center of Dallas; Dallas Veterans Administration Hospital; Dallas Rehabilitation Institute; Texas Scottish Rite Hospital · 5323 Harry Hines Boulevard, Dallas, TX 75235-8883 · 214-688-3871

Andrew R. Burgess · Assistant Professor of Surgery, University of Maryland School of Medicine, Johns Hopkins University School of Medicine · Director, Orthopaedic Traumatology, University of Maryland Medical Center · Shock Trauma Center, 22 South Greene Street, Baltimore, MD 21201 · 301-328-6280

Michael W. Chapman · (Adult Leg Length Discrepancy, Trauma Reconstruction, Nonunions & Malunions) · Professor and Chairman, Department of Orthopaedics, University of California, Davis School of Medicine · University of California, Davis Medical Center · 2230 Stockton Boulevard, Sacramento, CA 95817 · 916-734-2709

James A. Goulet · Assistant Professor of Orthopaedic Surgery, The University of Michigan Medical School · The University of Michigan Medical Center · 2914 Taubman Center, 1500 East Medical Center Drive, Box 0328, Ann Arbor, MI 48109-0328 · 313-936-5690

Sigvard T. Hansen, Jr. · Professor of Orthopaedics, University of Washington School of Medicine · Department of Orthopaedics, Harborview Medical Center · 325 Ninth Avenue, Seattle, WA 98104 · 206-223-4487

David L. Helfet · Associate Professor of Orthopaedic Surgery, Cornell University Medical College · Director, Orthopaedic Trauma, The Hospital for Special Surgery, The New York Hospital · 535 East 70th Street, New York, NY 10021 · 212-606-1888

James L. Hughes · M. Beckett Howorth Professor and Chairman, Department of Orthopaedics, University of Mississippi · University of Mississippi Medical Center 2500 North State Street, Room U2020, Jackson, MS 39216 · 601-984-5135

Kenneth D. Johnson · (Intramedullary Nailing) · Associate Professor of Orthopaedic Surgery, Vanderbilt University School of Medicine · Chief, Division of Orthopaedic Trauma, Vanderbilt University Medical Center · 21st and Garland Avenue, T4311 Medical Center North, Nashville, TN 37232 · 615-322-7173

Richard F. Kyle · (Total Joint Replacement) · Associate Professor of Orthopaedic Surgery, University of Minnesota School of Medicine · Chairman, Department of Orthopaedic Surgery, Hennepin County Medical Center · 701 Park Avenue South, Minneapolis, MN 55415 · 612-347-2812

Jeffrey W. Mast · (Pelvis, Acetabulum, Deformities of the Long Bones, Conservative Surgery of Arthrosis, Hip Dysplasia in the Adult) · Associate Clinical Professor, Wayne State University School of Medicine · Staff Orthopaedic Surgeon, Hutzel Hospital, and Detroit Receiving Hospital · Teitge Orthopaedic Associates, 4050 East Twelve Mile Road, Suite 110, Warren, MI 48092 · 313-573-3100

Joel M. Matta · (Pelvis) · Associate Professor of Clinical Orthopaedics, University of Southern California School of Medicine · Director of Acetablum & Pelvic Fracture Service, LAC/USC Medical Center; Good Samaritan Hospital · 637 South Lucas Street, Suite 605, Los Angeles, CA 90017 · 213-977-4177

Dana Christopher Mears · (Pelvis, Acetabulum, Intramedullary Nailing) · Chairman, Department of Orthopaedic Surgery, Shadyside Hospital · 580 South Aiken Avenue, Suite 320, Pittsburgh, PA 15212 · 800-448-1348, 412-623-3902

Robert Norman Meek · Clinical Professor of Orthopaedic Surgery, The University of British Columbia · Head, Orthopaedic Trauma Division, Vancouver General Hospital · 943 West Broadway, Suite 150, Vancouver, British Columbia V5Z 4E2 · 604-731-4611

Michael E. Miller · (Pelvis, Acetabulum, Intramedullary Nailing) · Associate Clinical Professor of Orthopaedic Surgery, Emory University School of Medicine St. Joseph's Hospital; Piedmont Hospital · 5671 Peachtree Dunwoody Road, NE, Suite 900, Atlanta, GA 30342 · 404-355-3344

Berton R. Moed · Chief of Orthopaedic Trauma, and Vice-Chief of Orthopaedics, Henry Ford Medical Center · Orthopaedics Floor K-12, 2799 West Grand Boulevard, Detroit, MI 48202 · 313-876-7960

Attila Poka · Assistant Professor of Surgery, Division of Orthopaedic Surgery, Johns Hopkins University School of Medicine; University of Maryland School of Medicine · University of Maryland Medical System; The Shock Trauma Center/ Maryland Institute for Emergency Medical Services Systems · The Shock Trauma Center, 22 South Greene Street, Baltimore, MD 21201 · 410-328-6280

Thomas A. Russell · (Intramedullary Nailing) · Associate Professor of Orthopaedic Surgery, The University of Tennessee at Memphis, College of Medicine · Chief of Orthopaedics, Regional Medical Center at Memphis; William F. Bowld Hospital · Campbell Clinic, 869 Madison Avenue, Memphis, TN 38103 · 901-577-9523

Roy W. Sanders · Assistant Professor of Clinical Orthopaedic Surgery, University South Florida College of Medicine · Director, Orthopaedic Trauma Service, and Chief, Department of Orthopaedics, Tampa General Hospital · Florida Orthopaedic Institute, 4175 East Fowler Avenue, Tampa, FL 33617-2011 · 813-978-9700

Joseph Schatzker · Professor of Surgery, University of Toronto School of Medicine · Chief of Orthopaedic Surgery, Sunnybrook Health Science Center · 2075 Bayview Avenue, Room 315, Toronto, Ontario M4N 3M5 · 416-480-4999

Marc F. Swiontkowski · Professor of Orthopaedics, University of Washington School of Medicine · Chief, Orthopaedic Traumatology, Harborview Medical Center · 325 Ninth Avenue, Seattle, WA 98104 · 206-223-5414

Marvin Tile · (Pelvic and Acetabular Fractures) · Professor of Surgery, University of Toronto School of Medicine · Surgeon-in-Chief, Sunnybrook Health Science Center · 2075 Bayview Avenue, Room A333, Toronto, Ontario M4N 3M5 · 416-480-4910

Peter G. Trafton · Associate Professor of Orthopaedic Surgery, Brown University School of Medicine · Surgeon-in-Charge, Division of Orthopaedic Trauma, Rhode Island Hospital · 593 Eddy Street, Providence, RI 02903 · 401-277-8400

Robert A. Winquist · (Pelvis, Acetabulum, Intramedullary Nailing, Hip Fractures, Femoral & Tibial Fractures) · Clinical Professor of Orthopaedic Surgery, University of Washington · Chief of Orthopaedic Surgery, Swedish Hospital & Medical Center · Orthopaedic Physicians Incorporated, 1229 Madison Street, Suite 1600, Seattle, WA 98104 · 206-386-2600

Donald A. Wiss · (Fractures, Trauma Reconstruction) · Clinical Professor of Orthopaedic Surgery, University of Southern California School of Medicine · Director Orthopaedic Trauma Service, Orthopaedic Hospital; Valley Presbyterian Hospital · 2300 South Flower Street, Suite 301, Los Angeles, CA 90007; Southern California Orthopaedic Institute, 6815 Noble Avenue, Van Nuys, CA 91405-3730 213-742-1000; 818-901-6600 x3885

TUMOR SURGERY

Jeffrey J. Eckardt · Professor of Orthopaedic Surgery, University of California, Los Angeles School of Medicine · University of California, Los Angeles Center for the Health Sciences · 10833 LeConte Avenue, Los Angeles, CA 90024 · 310-206-6503

James O. Johnston · Professor of Clinical Orthopaedics, University of California at San Francisco School of Medicine · University of California at San Francisco Medical Center · 533 Parnassus Avenue, Room U-471, San Francisco, CA 94143 415-476-2495

Joseph M. Lane · (Cartiledge Metabolism) · Professor of Orthopaedic Surgery, Cornell University Medical College · Chief, Orthopaedic Oncology, Metabolic Bone Disease, Hospital for Special Surgery; Memorial Sloan-Kettering Cancer Center · 535 East 70th Street, New York, NY 10021 · 212-606-1172

Michael M. Lewis · Chairman, Department of Orthopaedic Surgery, and Orthopaedic Surgeon-In-Chief, Mt. Sinai Medical Center · Guggenheim Hall, Five East 98th Street, Ninth Floor, New York, NY 10029 · 212-241-1660

Martin Miles Malawer · (Limb-sparing Surgery) · Consultant, Surgery Branch, National Cancer Institute, National Institutes of Health; and Professor of Orthopaedic Surgery, George Washington University School of Medicine · Director, Orthopaedic Oncology, The Cancer Institute, Washington Hospital Center; Children's National Medical Center; George Washington University Medical Center · 110 Irving Street NW, Washington, DC 20010 · 202-877-3970

Henry J. Mankin · Edith M. Ashley Professor of Surgery, Harvard Medical School Chief of Orthopaedic Surgery, Massachusetts General Hospital · 32 Fruit Street, Boston, MA 02114 · 617-726-2943

Eugene R. Mindell · Professor of Orthopaedic Surgery, State University of New York at Buffalo School of Medicine · Director of Orthopaedic Oncology, Buffalo General Hospital; Orthopaedic Consultant, Roswell Park Memorial Institute · Buffalo General Hospital, 100 High Street, Room 280, Buffalo, NY 14203 · 716-845-1531

John A. Murray · Professor of Surgery and Chief of Orthopaedics, The University of Texas · The University of Texas MD Anderson Cancer Center · 1515 Holcombe Boulevard, Box 106, Houston, TX 77030 · 713-792-8828

James R. Neff · Professor and Chairman, Department of Orthopaedic Surgery & Rehabilitation, University of Nebraska College of Medicine · University of Nebraska Medical Center · 600 South 42nd Street, Omaha, NE 68198-1080 · 402-559-8000

Douglas Jack Pritchard · Professor of Orthopaedic Surgery and Professor of Oncology, Mayo Medical School and Mayo Clinic · Rochester Methodist Hospital 200 First Street, SW, Rochester, MN 55905 · 507-284-2511

Franklin H. Sim · Professor of Orthopaedic Surgery, Mayo Medical School · Mayo Clinic · 200 First Street, SW, Rochester, MN 55905 · 507-284-3661

Michael A. Simon · Professor of Surgery and Chairman, Section of Orthopaedic Surgery and Rehabilitation Medicine, University of Chicago, Pritzker School of Medicine · University of Chicago Medical Center · 5841 South Maryland Avenue, Box 421, Chicago, IL 60637-1470 · 312-702-6144

Dempsey S. Springfield · Associate Professor of Orthopaedic Surgery, Harvard Medical School · Visiting Orthopaedic Surgeon, Massachusetts General Hospital · 32 Fruit Street, Boston, MA 02114 · 617-726-2943

Roby Calvin Thompson, Jr. · (Reconstructive Hip Surgery) · Professor and Head, Department of Orthopaedic Surgery, University of Minnesota School of Medicine University of Minnesota Hospital & Clinics · 420 Delaware Street, SE, Box 492, Minneapolis, MN 55455 · 612-625-5648

OTOLARYNGOLOGY

FACIAL PLASTIC SURGERY

Ferdinand Francis Becker · (Facial Skin Cancer) · Clinical Assistant Professor of Surgery, University of Florida College of Medicine · Indian River Memorial Hospital · 777 Thirty-Seventh Street, Suite C101, Vero Beach, FL 32960 · 407-567-1164

Roger L. Crumley · Professor and Chairman, Department of Otolaryngology-Head & Neck Surgery, University of California at Irvine School of Medicine · University of California at Irvine Medical Center · 101 City Drive, Building 25, Route 81, Orange, CA 92668 · 714-634-5750

Calvin M. Johnson, Jr. · (Rhinoplasty, Secondary Rhinoplasty) · Associate Clinical Professor of Otolaryngology, Tulane University School of Medicine · Hedgewood Surgical Center · 2427 St. Charles Avenue, New Orleans, LA 70130 · 504-895-7642

Frank M. Kamer · Clinical Professor of Head & Neck Surgery, University of California at Los Angeles School of Medicine · Lasky Clinic · 201 South Lasky Drive, Beverly Hills, CA 90212 · 213-556-8155

Charles J. Krause · Professor and Chairman, Department of Otolaryngology, and Senior Associate Dean for Clinical Affairs, The University of Michigan Medical School · The University of Michigan Medical Center · 1500 East Medical Center Drive, Box 0312, Ann Arbor, MI 48109-0312 · 313-936-7483

Norman Joseph Pastorek · (Rhinoplasty) · Clinical Professor of Otolaryngology, Cornell University Medical College · The New York Hospital-Cornell Medical Center · 29 A East 63rd Street, New York, NY 10021 · 212-421-3636

David E. Schuller · Professor & Chairman, Department of Otolaryngology, and Director, Comprehensive Cancer Center-Arthur G. James Cancer Hospital & Research Institute, Ohio State University College of Medicine · Director, Comprehensive Cancer Center, Arthur G. James Cancer Hospital & Research Institute · 300 West 10th Avenue, Room 521, Columbus, OH 43210 · 614-293-8074

M. Eugene Tardy, Jr. · (Rhinoplasty, Facelift) · Professor of Clinical Otolaryngology, The University of Illinois College of Medicine at Chicago; Director, Division of Facial Plastic & Reconstructive Surgery, Indiana University School of Medicine; Instructor, Northwestern University, St. Joseph's Hospital · 2900 North Lake Shore Drive, Chicago, IL 60657 · 312-472-7559

J. Regan Thomas · Assistant Clinical Professor, Department of Otolaryngology, Head & Neck Surgery, Washington University School of Medicine · Director, Facial Plastic Surgery Center, Barnes Hospital; Barnes West County Hospital; Missouri Baptist Hospital; St. Luke's Hospital · Facial Plastic Surgery Center, 3009 North Ballas, Suite 269, St. Louis, MO 63131 · 314-997-4651

HEAD & NECK SURGERY
(See also Plastic Surgery, Head & Neck Surgery)

Byron J. Bailey · (Laryngeal Cancer, Laryngeal Reconstruction) · Wiess Professor and Chairman, Department of Otolaryngology-Head & Neck Surgery, University of Texas Medical Branch at Galveston · Director, Otolaryngology-Head & Neck Surgery, University of Texas Medical Branch Hospitals at Galveston · 7.104 John Sealy Hospital Building, Galveston, TX 77550 · 409-772-2704

Hugh F. Biller · Professor and Chairman, Department of Otolaryngology, Mt. Sinai School of Medicine · Mt. Sinai Medical Center · One Gustave L. Levy Place, Box 1189, New York, NY 10029 · 212-241-6141

Thomas C. Calcaterra · Professor of Surgery, University of California, Los Angeles School of Medicine · University of California, Los Angeles Medical Center 10833 LeConte Avenue, Room 62-158, Los Angeles, CA 90024 · 310-825-6740

Robert W. Cantrell · Fitz-Hugh Professor and Chairman, Department of Otolaryngology, Head & Neck Surgery, University of Virginia School of Medicine · University of Virginia Health Sciences Center · Box 430, Charlottesville, VA 22908 804-924-5700

Nicholas John Cassisi · Professor and Chairman of Otolaryngology, University of Florida College of Medicine · Shands Hospital at the University of Florida · 1600 Southwest Archer Road, Box 100264, Gainesville, FL 32610 · 904-392-4461

Charles W. Cummings · Andelot Professor and Director, Department of Otolaryngology-Head & Neck Surgery, Johns Hopkins University School of Medicine The Johns Hopkins Medical Institutions · Carnegie Building, 600 North Wolfe Street, Room 466, Baltimore, MD 21205 · 410-955-7400

Paul J. Donald · Professor and Vice-Chairman, Department of Otolaryngology-Head & Neck Surgery, University of California, Davis School of Medicine · Director, UCDMC Center for Skull Base Surgery, University of California, Davis Medical Center · 2500 Stockton Boulevard, Sacramento, CA 95817 · 916-734-2832

Willard E. Fee, Jr. · Professor and Chairman, Division of Otolaryngology, Head & Neck Surgery, Stanford University School of Medicine · Stanford University Hospital · 300 Pasteur Drive, Stanford, CA 94305-5328 · 415-725-6500

John M. Fredrickson · (Free Flap Reconstruction) · Lindburg Professor and Head of Otolaryngology, Washington University School of Medicine · Otolaryngolist-in-Chief, Barnes Hospital · 517 South Euclid Avenue, Room 9906, St. Louis, MO 63110 · 314-362-7550

Jack Louis Gluckman · Chairman, Department of Otolaryngology, University of Cincinnati College of Medicine · Associate Dean of Clinical Affairs, University of Cincinnati Hospital · 231 Bethesda Avenue, ML 528, Cincinnati, OH 45267-0528 513-558-4152

Helmuth Goepfert · Professor and Chairman, Department of Head & Neck Surgery, The University of Texas · The University of Texas MD Anderson Cancer Center · 1515 Holcombe Boulevard, Houston, TX 77030 · 713-792-6925

W. Jarrard Goodwin, Jr. · Chandler Professor and Chairman, Department of Otolaryngology, University of Miami School of Medicine · Chief of Otolaryngology, Jackson Memorial Hospital; Chief of Head & Neck Site Group, Sylvester Cancer Center; Attending Physician, Miami Veterans Affairs Medical Center; University of Miami/Jackson Memorial Medical Center; Miami Veterans Administration Medical Center; Anne Bates Leach Eye Hospital · Building ACC East, Room 306, 1666 Northwest 10th Avenue, Miami, FL 33136; Otolaryngology (D-48), P.O. Box 016960, Miami, FL 33101 · 305-585-6101

Patrick Joseph Gullane · Professor of Otolaryngology, University of Toronto School of Medicine · Otolaryngologist-in-Chief and Director, Head & Neck Program, The Toronto Hospital · 200 Elizabeth Street, Eaton Building North, Seventh Floor, Room 242, Toronto, Ontario M5G 2C4 · 416-340-4356

Jonas T. Johnson · Professor and Vice Chairman, Department of Otolaryngology, and Professor of Radiation Oncology, University of Pittsburgh School of Medicine Director, Division of Head & Neck Oncology & Immunology, The Eye & Ear Institute Pavilion of Montefiore University Hospital · The Eye & Ear Institute, Suite 500, Pittsburgh, PA 15213 · 412-647-2100

Charles J. Krause · Professor and Chairman, Department of Otolaryngology, and Senior Associate Dean for Clinical Affairs, The University of Michigan Medical School · The University of Michigan Medical Center · 1500 East Medical Center Drive, Box 0312, Ann Arbor, MI 48109-0312 · 313-936-7483

Paul A. Levine · Professor and Vice-Chairman, Department of Otolaryngology-Head & Neck Surgery, University of Virginia School of Medicine · Director, Head & Neck Surgical Oncology, University of Virginia Health Sciences Center · Box 430, Charlottesville, VA 22908 · 804-924-5593

Michael Maves · (Reconstructive Surgery, Voice Disorders) · Professor & Chairman of Otolaryngology-Head & Neck Surgery, St. Louis University School of Medicine · St. Louis University Medical Center · 3635 Vista Avenue at Grand Boulevard, P.O. Box 15250, St. Louis, MO 63110-0250 · 314-577-8887

William Frederick McGuirt · Professor of Otolaryngology, The Bowman Gray School of Medicine of Wake Forest University · North Carolina Baptist Hospital Medical Center Boulevard, Winston-Salem, NC 27157 · 919-748-4161

Jesus Edilberto Medina · Professor & Chairman, Department of Otorhinolaryngology, The University of Oklahoma College of Medicine · The University of Oklahoma Health Sciences Center · P.O. Box 26901, 3SP224, Oklahoma City, OK 73190 · 405-271-5504

Robert H. Miller · Professor and Chairman, Department of Otolaryngology, Head & Neck Surgery, Tulane University School of Medicine · Vice Chief of Staff, Tulane University Medical Center · 1430 Tulane Avenue, New Orleans, LA 70112-2699 · 504-588-5661

Eugene M. Myers · Professor and Chairman, Department of Otolaryngology, University of Pittsburgh School of Medicine · Eye and Ear Institute Pavilion, Montefiore University Hospital · 203 Lothrop Street, Suite 500, Pittsburgh, PA 15213 · 412-647-2110

H. Bryan Neel III · Professor of Otolaryngology, Mayo Medical School · Mayo Clinic · 200 First Street, SW, Rochester, MN 55905 · 507-284-2369

Harold C. Pillsbury III · Thomas J. Dark Distinguished Professor of Surgery and Professor and Chief, Division of Otolaryngology-Head & Neck Surgery, University of North Carolina School of Medicine · University of North Carolina Hospitals 610 Burnett-Womack Building, Manning Drive, Campus Box 7070, Chapel Hill, NC 27599-7070 · 919-966-3341

Dale H. Rice · Tiber/Alpert Professor and Chairman, Department of Otolaryngology, Head & Neck Surgery, University of Southern California School of Medicine Chief Physician, The Los Angeles County + University of Southern California Medical Center; University of Southern California University Hospital · 1200 North State Street, Room GH-4136, Los Angeles, CA 90033 · 213-226-7315, 342-5790

William J. Richtsmeier · Associate Professor of Otolaryngology, Johns Hopkins University School of Medicine · The Johns Hopkins Medical Institutions · Carnegie Building, 600 North Wolfe Street, Room 469, Baltimore, MD 21205 · 410-955-2307

Gary L. Schechter · Professor and Chairman, Department of Otolaryngology, Head & Neck Surgery, Eastern Virginia Medical School · Sentara Hospitals; DePaul Medical Center; The Children's Hospital of the King's Daughters · 825 Fairfax Avenue, Suite 510, Norfolk, VA 23507 · 804-446-5934

Victor L. Schramm · (Skull-Base Surgery) · Associate Professor, Department of Otolaryngology, University of Colorado Health Sciences Center · Presbyterian-St. Luke's Medical Center · 501 East 19th Avenue, Suite 100, Denver, CO 80203 · 303-832-0050

David E. Schuller · Professor & Chairman, Department of Otolaryngology, and Director, Comprehensive Cancer Center-Arthur G. James Cancer Hospital & Research Institute, Ohio State University College of Medicine · Director, Comprehensive Cancer Center, Arthur G. James Cancer Hospital & Research Institute · 300 West 10th Avenue, Room 521, Columbus, OH 43210 · 614-293-8074

Roy B. Sessions · Professor and Chairman, Department of Otolaryngology, Head & Neck Surgery, Georgetown University School of Medicine · Georgetown University Medical Center · 3800 Reservoir Road, NW, Washington, DC 20007 · 202-687-8186

James Y. Suen · Professor and Chairman of Otolaryngology-Head & Neck Surgery, University of Arkansas for Medical Sciences · The University Hospital of Arkansas; Arkansas Cancer Research Center; Arkansas Children's Hospital; John L. McClellan Veterans Hospital · 4301 West Markham, Slot 543, Little Rock, AR 72205 · 501-686-5140

Paul H. Ward · Professor Emeritus, University of California at Los Angeles School of Medicine · Distinguished Professor of the Veterans Administration, University of California at Los Angeles Center for the Health Sciences; Sepulveda Veterans Affairs Hospital · 10833 LeConte Avenue, Room 62-132 CHS, Los Angeles, CA 90024 · 310-825-5179

Ernest A. Weymuller · Professor and Acting Chairman, Department of Otolaryngology, University of Washington School of Medicine · University of Washington Medical Center · 1959 Northeast Pacific Street, RL-30, Seattle, WA 98195 · 206-543-5230

LARYNGOLOGY

Byron J. Bailey · (Laryngeal Cancer, Laryngeal Reconstruction) · Wiess Professor and Chairman, Department of Otolaryngology-Head & Neck Surgery, University of Texas Medical Branch at Galveston · Director, Otolaryngology-Head & Neck Surgery, University of Texas Medical Branch Hospitals at Galveston · 7.104 John Sealy Hospital Building, Galveston, TX 77550 · 409-772-2704

Hugh F. Biller · Professor and Chairman, Department of Otolaryngology, Mt. Sinai School of Medicine · Mt. Sinai Medical Center · One Gustave L. Levy Place, Box 1189, New York, NY 10029 · 212-241-6141

Andrew Blitzer · Professor of Clinical Otolaryngology, and Acting Chairman, Department of Otolaryngology, College of Physicians & Surgeons of Columbia University · Director, Department of Otolaryngology, Columbia-Presbyterian Medical Center · 630 West 168th Street, PH11-131 Stem, New York, NY 10032 · 212-305-5314, 305-5820

Thomas C. Calcaterra · Professor of Surgery, University of California, Los Angeles School of Medicine · University of California, Los Angeles Medical Center 10833 LeConte Avenue, Room 62-158, Los Angeles, CA 90024 · 310-825-6740

Roger L. Crumley · Professor and Chairman, Department of Otolaryngology-Head & Neck Surgery, University of California at Irvine School of Medicine · University of California at Irvine Medical Center · 101 City Drive, Building 25, Route 81, Orange, CA 92668 · 714-634-5750

Charles W. Cummings · (Bronchoesophegology) · Andelot Professor and Director, Department of Otolaryngology-Head & Neck Surgery, Johns Hopkins University School of Medicine · The Johns Hopkins Medical Institutions · Carnegie Building, 600 North Wolfe Street, Room 466, Baltimore, MD 21205 · 410-955-7400

Herbert H. Dedo · Professor and Vice-Chairman of Otolaryngology, University of California at San Francisco School of Medicine · University of California at San Francisco Medical Center · 400 Parnassus Avenue, San Francisco, CA 94143 · 415-476-2792

Charles N. Ford · Professor of Otolaryngology, University of Wisconsin-Madison School of Medicine · University of Wisconsin Hospital & Clinics · 600 Highland Avenue, Room H4-320, Madison, WI 53792 · 608-263-0192

David G. Hanson · Professor & Chairman, Department of Otolaryngology-Head & Neck Surgery, Northwestern University Medical School · Chairman, Otolaryngology-Head & Neck Surgery, Northwestern Memorial Hospital · 707 North Fairbanks Court, Suite 922, Chicago, IL 60611 · 312-908-8182

Haskins K. Kashima · Professor of Otolaryngology, Head & Neck Surgery, Johns Hopkins University School of Medicine · The Johns Hopkins Medical Institutions 600 North Wolfe Street, Carnegie 469, Baltimore, MD 21205 · 410-955-3400

Charles J. Krause · Professor and Chairman, Department of Otolaryngology, and Senior Associate Dean for Clinical Affairs, The University of Michigan Medical School · The University of Michigan Medical Center · 1500 East Medical Center Drive, Box 0312, Ann Arbor, MI 48109-0312 · 313-936-7483

Bernard R. Marsh · (Bronchoesophegology) · Professor of Otolaryngology, Johns Hopkins University School of Medicine · The Johns Hopkins Medical Institutions Osler Building, 600 North Wolfe Street, Room 421, Baltimore, MD 21205 · 410-955-3628

William Montgomery · Professor of Otolaryngoglogy, Harvard Medical School · Senior Surgeon in Otolaryngology, Massachusetts Eye & Ear Infirmary · 243 Charles Street, Boston, MA 02114 · 617-573-3669

H. Bryan Neel III · Professor of Otolaryngology, Mayo Medical School · Mayo Clinic · 200 First Street, SW, Rochester, MN 55905 · 507-284-2369

Nels R. Olson · The University of Michigan Medical Center · Active Staff, St. Joseph Mercy Hospital; Attending Staff, Ann Arbor V.A. Hospital; Clinical Professor, The University of Michigan Medical Center · 5333 McAuley Drive, Suite R4016, Ypsilanti, MI 48197 · 313-434-3341

Robert H. Ossoff · Guy M. Maness Professor and Chairman, Department of Otolaryngology, Vanderbilt University School of Medicine · S-2100 Medical Center North, Nashville, TN 37232-2559 · 615-322-7267

Bruce W. Pearson · Serene M. & Francis C. Durling Professor of Otolaryngology, Mayo Medical School · Chairman, Department of Otolaryngology, Mayo Clinic Jacksonville · 4500 San Pablo Road, Jacksonville, FL 32224 · 904-223-2000

Harold C. Pillsbury III · Thomas J. Dark Distinguished Professor of Surgery, and Professor and Chief, Division of Otolaryngology-Head & Neck Surgery, University of North Carolina School of Medicine · University of North Carolina Hospitals 610 Burnett-Womack Building, Manning Drive, Campus Box 7070, Chapel Hill, NC 27599-7070 · 919-966-3341

Clarence T. Sasaki · OHSE Professor of Surgery, and Chief, Section of Otolaryngology, Yale University School of Medicine · Yale-New Haven Hospital · 333 Cedar Street, P.O. Box 3333, New Haven, CT 06510 · 203-785-2592

Robert Thayer Sataloff · (Voice) · Professor of Otolaryngology, Jefferson Medical College of Thomas Jefferson University · Thomas Jefferson University Hospital · 1721 Pine Street, Philadelphia, PA 19103 · 215-545-3322

Joyce A. Schild · (Bronchoesophegology) · Professor of Otolaryngology, The University of Illinois College of Medicine at Chicago · The University of Illinois Eye Center & Visual Sciences · 1855 West Taylor Street, Suite 242, Chicago, IL 60612 · 312-996-6582

David E. Schuller · Professor & Chairman, Department of Otolaryngology, and Director, Comprehensive Cancer Center-Arthur G. James Cancer Hospital & Research Institute, Ohio State University College of Medicine · Director, Comprehensive Cancer Center, Arthur G. James Cancer Hospital & Research Institute · 300 West 10th Avenue, Room 521, Columbus, OH 43210 · 614-293-8074

Roy B. Sessions · Professor and Chairman, Department of Otolaryngology, Head & Neck Surgery, Georgetown University School of Medicine · Georgetown University Medical Center · 3800 Reservoir Road, NW, Washington, DC 20007 · 202-687-8186

Stanley M. Shapshay · (Bronchoesophegology) · Professor of Otolaryngology, Boston University School of Medicine · Chairman, Department of Otolaryngology, Head & Neck Surgery, Lahey Clinic Medical Center · 41 Mall Road, Burlington, MA 01805 · 617-273-8450

Mark I. Singer · Professor of Otolaryngology-Head & Neck Surgery, University of California at San Francisco School of Medicine · Mount Zion Medical Center of University of California at San Francisco · 2356 Sutter Street, Seventh Floor, San Francisco, CA 94115 · 415-885-7528

Paul H. Ward · (Bronchoesophegology) · Professor Emeritus, University of California at Los Angeles School of Medicine · Distinguished Professor of the Veterans Administration, University of California at Los Angeles Center for the Health Sciences; Sepulveda Veterans Affairs Hospital · 10833 LeConte Avenue, Room 62-132 CHS, Los Angeles, CA 90024 · 310-825-5179

Gayle E. Woodson · Associate Professor of Surgery, University of California at San Diego School of Medicine · Chief, Head & Neck Surgery Section, San Diego Veterans Administration Medical Center; Scripps Memorial Hospital · 3350 La Jolla Village Drive,112C, La Jolla, CA 92161 · 619-552-8585 x3405

OTOLOGY

Bruce Allen Feldman · Clinical Professor of Otolaryngology, The George Washington University School of Medicine · Children's National Medical Center; Sibley Memorial Hospital; Washington Hospital Center · 1145 Nineteenth Street NW, Suite 402, Washington, DC 20036 · 202-466-7747

Simon C. Parisier · Chairman, Department of Otolaryngology, Manhattan Eye, Ear & Throat Hospital · 210 East 64th Street, New York, NY 10021 · 212-605-3789

Rodney Perkins · Clinical Associate Professor of Surgery, Stanford University School of Medicine · El Camino Hospital · California Ear Institute, 801 Welch Road, Palo Alto, CA 94304 · 415-494-1000

M. Coyle Shea, Jr. · Baptist Memorial Hospital; Methodist Hospital; St. Francis Hospital · 6027 Walnut Grove Road, Suite 411, Memphis, TN 38120 · 901-767-7750

James L. Sheehy · Clinical Professor of Otolaryngology, University of Southern California School of Medicine · House Ear Clinic, Inc.; St. Vincent Medical Center · 2100 West Third Street, Los Angeles, CA 90057 · 213-483-9930

George Terrell Singleton · Professor of Otolaryngology, University of Florida College of Medicine · Shands Hospital at the University of Florida; Gainesville Veterans Affairs Medical Center · 1600 Southwest Archer Road, Gainesville, FL 32610-0264 · 904-392-4461

OTOLOGY/NEUROTOLOGY

Bobby R. Alford · Chairman, Department of Otolaryngology, and Dean, Baylor College of Medicine · The Methodist Hospital · One Baylor Plaza, Houston, TX 77030 · 713-798-5906

Thomas J. Balkany · Professor and Vice-Chairman, Department of Otolaryngology, and Chief, Otology & Neurotology, University of Miami School of Medicine Director, University of Miami Ear Institute; Bascom Palmer Eye Institute; University of Miami-Jackson Memorial Medical Center · 1666 Northwest 10th Avenue, Building ACC East, Department of Otolaryngology (D-48), Box 016960, Miami, FL 33101 · 305-585-6101

Loren J. Bartels · Associate Professor of Surgery, Neurology, and Radiology, University South Florida College of Medicine · Otologist, Tampa General Hospital; James Haley Veterans Hospital; H. Lee Moffitt Cancer Center · 12901 Bruce B. Downs Boulevard, Box 16, Tampa, FL 33612 · 813-974-2411

James E. Benecke, Jr. · Associate Professor & Chief of Otology/Neurotology, St. Louis University School of Medicine · St. Louis University Medical Center · 3635 Vista Avenue at Grand Boulevard, P.O. Box 15250, St. Louis, MO 63110-0250 · 314-577-8884

Derald E. Brackmann · (Acoustic Neuroma) · Clinical Professor of Otolaryngology, University of Southern California · President, House Ear Clinic, Inc., St. Vincent Medical Center · 2100 West Third Street, First Floor, Los Angeles, CA 90057 · 213-483-9930

B. Hill Britton, Jr. · HCA Presbyterian Hospital · 711 Stanton L. Young Boulevard, Suite 513, Oklahoma City, OK 73104 · 405-232-6262

Kenneth H. Brookler · Clinical Professor of Otolaryngology, New York Medical College · Lenox Hill Hospital; Manhattan Eye, Ear & Throat Hospital · 111 East 77th Street, New York, NY 10021 · 212-861-6900

Noel L. Cohen · Professor and Chairman, Department of Otolaryngology, New York University School of Medicine · Director, Otolaryngology, Tisch Hospital and Bellevue Hospital; New York University Medical Center · 530 First Avenue, Suite 3C, New York, NY 10016 · 212-263-7373

Newton J. Coker · Associate Professor, Department of Otorhinolaryngology & Communicative Sciences, Baylor College of Medicine · The Methodist Hospital One Baylor Plaza, Houston, TX 77030 · 713-798-5900

Antonio De La Cruz · (Congenital Atresia) · Director of Education, House Ear Institute; and Clinical Professor of Otolaryngology, University of Southern California · St. Vincent Medical Center; House Ear Clinic, Inc. · 2100 West Third Street, First Floor, Los Angeles, CA 90057 · 213-483-9930

John Roddey Edwards Dickins · Visiting Assistant Professor, University of Arkansas for Medical Science · St. Vincent Infirmary Medical Center; Baptist Medical Center · 1200 Medical Tower Building, Little Rock, AR 72205 · 501-227-5050

Robert A. Dobie · Professor and Chairman of Otolaryngology-Head & Neck Surgery, The University of Texas Health Science Center at San Antonio · Chief of Otolaryngology-Head & Neck Surgery, Medical Center Hospital · 7703 Floyd Curl Drive, San Antonio, TX 78284-7777 · 512-567-5655

Bruce J. Gantz · Professor, Department of Otolaryngology, The University of Iowa College of Medicine · The University of Iowa Hospitals & Clinics · Iowa City, IA 52242 · 319-356-2173

Gale Gardner · Clinical Professor, Department of Otolaryngology, University of Tennessee, Memphis · Consultant, Neurodiagnostic Department, Baptist Memorial Hospital/Medical Center · 899 Madison Avenue, Suite 602A, Memphis, TN 38013 · 901-526-5167

Michael E. Glasscock III · Associate Professor, Department of Neurosurgery, Vanderbilt University School of Medicine · Baptist Hospital · 1811 State Street, Nashville, TN 37203 · 615-327-3040

Donald W. Goin · Swedish Medical Center; University of Colorado Health Sciences Center · 601 E. Hampden Avenue, Suite 340, Englewood, CO 80110 · 303-788-7880

Malcolm D. Graham · Clinical Professor of Otorhinolaryngology, University of Michigan Medical School · President, Michigan Ear Institute; Director of Otology, Neurotology and Skull Base Surgery, Providence Hospital · 27555 Middlebelt Road, Farmington Hills, MI 48334; 16001 West Nine Mile Road, Southfield, MI 48075 · 313-476-4622, 424-3000

A. Julianna Gulya · Associate Professor of Otolaryngology, Head & Neck Surgery, Georgetown University School of Medicine · Associate Surgeon, Georgetown University Medical Center · Department of Otolaryngology, 3800 Reservoir Road, NW, Washington, DC 20007 · 202-687-8186

Michael J. Holliday · Associate Professor of Otolaryngology, Johns Hopkins University School of Medicine · The Johns Hopkins Medical Institutions · 600 North Wolfe Street, Carnegie Building, Room 484, Baltimore, MD 21205 · 410-955-3492

Melton Jay Horwitz · Clinical Assistant Professor, Baylor College of Medicine · Diagnostic Center Hospital · 6624 Fannin Street, Suite 1500, Houston, TX 77030 713-795-0111

John W. House · Clinical Associate Professor of Otolaryngology, University of Southern California School of Medicine, and University of California at Irvine School of Medicine, and House Ear Institute · St. Vincent Medical Center; The Hospital of the Good Samaritan; Huntington Memorial Hospital; Children's Hospital of Los Angeles; Los Angeles County + University of Southern California

Medical Center · 2100 West Third Street, Fifth Floor, Los Angeles, CA 90057 · 213-483-4431

William F. House · Hoag Memorial Hospital Presbyterian; St. Vincent's Hospital 361 Hospital Road, Suite 327, Newport Beach, CA 92663 · 714-631-4327

Gordon Blackistone Hughes · Director of Education, Otology & Neurotology, Department of Otolaryngology & Communicative Disorders, The Cleveland Clinic Foundation · One Clinic Center, 9500 Euclid Avenue, Cleveland, OH 44195-5034 · 216-444-5375

Robert K. Jackler · Associate Professor, Department of Otolaryngology, University of California at San Francisco School of Medicine · University of California at San Francisco Medical Center · 350 Parnassus Avenue, Suite 210, San Francisco, CA 94117 · 415-476-3856

C. Gary Jackson · Clinical Professor, Department of Surgery, Division of Otolaryngology, Head & Neck Surgery (Otology & Neurotology), University of North Carolina School of Medicine, Chapel Hill; Clinical Professor, Department of Otolaryngology, Head & Neck Surgery (Otology & Neurotology), and Clinical Professor of Hearing & Speech Sciences, Vanderbilt University School of Medicine · Baptist Hospital · The Otology Group, 1811 State Street, Nashville, TN 37203 · 615-327-3040

Carol A. Jackson · Associate Professor of Neurotology, University of California at Irvine School of Medicine · Chairman of Otolaryngology Department, Western Medical Center-Santa Ana; University of California at Irvine Medical Center · 999 North Tustin Avenue, Suite 15, Santa Ana, CA 92705 · 714-953-3328

Robert A. Jahrsdoerfer · (Congenital Atresia) · Professor and Chairman, Department of Otolaryngology, Head & Neck Surgery, The University of Texas at Houston · Chief of Service, Hermann Hospital · Box 20708, Houston, TX 77030 713-792-5866

Herman A. Jenkins · Professor and Vice-Chairman, Department of Otolaryngology & Communicative Sciences, Baylor College of Medicine · The Methodist Hospital · One Baylor Plaza, NA102, Houston, TX 77030 · 713-798-5900

Glen Dwight Johnson · Associate Professor of Clinical Surgery (Otology & Neurotology), Dartmouth Medical School · Dartmouth-Hitchcock Medical Center · One Medical Center Drive, Lebanon, NH 03756 · 603-646-8124

Donald B. Kamerer · Professor of Otolaryngology, University of Pittsburgh School of Medicine · Director, Division of Otology/Neurotology, University of Pittsburgh Medical Center · Eye & Ear Institute, Suite 500, 203 Lothrop Street, Pittsburgh, PA 15213 · 412-647-2115

Jack M. Kartush · Staff Physician, Providence Hospital · Michigan Ear Institute, 27555 Middlebelt Road, Farmington Hills, MI 48334 · 313-476-4622

John L. Kemink · Professor of Otolaryngology, The University of Michigan Medical School · Director, Division of Otology/Neurotology, The University of Michigan Medical Center · 1904 Taubman Center, 1500 East Medical Center Drive, Box 0312, Ann Arbor, MI 48109-0312 · 313-936-8006

Sam E. Kinney · Head, Section of Otology & Neurotology, Department of Otolaryngology & Communicative Disorders, The Cleveland Clinic Foundation · One Clinic Center, 9500 Euclid Avenue, Cleveland, OH 44195-5034 · 216-444-6696

John Kveton · Associate Professor of Surgery/Otolaryngology, Yale University School of Medicine · Attending Surgeon, Yale-New Haven Hospital · 333 Cedar Street, P.O. Box 3333, New Haven, CT 06510 · 203-785-2593

John P. Leonetti · Assistant Professor of Neurotology, Otology & Skull Base Surgery, Loyola Stritch School of Medicine · Loyola University Medical Center · 2160 South First Avenue, Building 105, Room 1870, Maywood, IL 60153 · 708-216-9000

Samuel C. Levine · Assistant Professor of Otolaryngology, University of Minnesota School of Medicine · Clinic Director, Department of Otolaryngology, University of Minnesota Hospital & Clinics; Minnesota Veterans Affairs Medical Center · Harvard Street at East River Road, Box 396, Minneapolis, MN 55455 · 612-625-3200

Charles M. Luetje II · Assistant Professor of Otolaryngology, University of Missouri; President and Founder, Midwest Ear Institute · Trinity Lutheran Hospital; St. Luke's Hospital of Kansas City · Otologic Center, Inc., 3100 Broadway, Suite 509, Kansas City, MO 64111 · 816-531-7373

William M. Luxford · Clinical Assistant Professor of Otolaryngology, University of Southern California School of Medicine · House Ear Clinic, Inc. · 2100 West Third Street, First Floor, Los Angeles, CA 90057 · 213-483-9930

Serge Anthony Martinez · Professor of Surgery, and Director of Otolaryngology, University of Louisville School of Medicine · Norton Hospital; Kosair Children's Hospital; Humana Hospital University of Louisville · 601 South Floyd Street, Suite 604, Louisville, KY 40202 · 502-583-8303

Douglas E. Mattox · Associate Professor of Otolaryngology-Head & Neck Surgery, Johns Hopkins University School of Medicine · The Johns Hopkins Medical Institutions · Carnegie Building, 600 North Wolfe Street, Room 434, Baltimore, MD 21205 · 410-955-7137

Robert E. Mischke · University of Colorado School of Medicine · Swedish Medical Center; Porter Memorial Hospital · 601 East Hampden Avenue, Suite 340, Inglewood, CO 80110 · 303-788-7880, 321-1298

Richard T. Miyamoto · Arilla DeVault Professor and Chairman, Department of Otolaryngology, Head & Neck Surgery, Indiana University School of Medicine · James Whitcomb Riley Hospital for Children; Indiana University Medical Center 702 Barnhill Drive, P.O. Box 66063, Indianapolis IN 46202 · 317-274-3556

Joseph B. Nadol, Jr. · Professor and Chairman, Department of Otology & Laryngology, Harvard Medical School · Chief of Otolaryngology, Massachusetts Eye & Ear Infirmary · 243 Charles Street, Boston, MA 02114 · 617-573-3632

J. Gail Neely · Professor, Department of Otorhinolaryngology, The University of Oklahoma College of Medicine · P.O. Box 26901, 3SP-226, Oklahoma City, OK 73190 · 405-271-5504

James Edward Olsson · Clinical Professor of Otolaryngology, The University of Texas Health Science Center at San Antonio · Southwest Texas Methodist Hospital · 7711 Louis Pasteur, Suite 504, San Antonio, TX 78229 · 512-614-1046

Fred D. Owens · Baylor University Medical Center · 3600 Gaston Avenue, Suite 1103, Dallas, TX 75246 · 214-742-2194

Dennis G. Pappas · Clinical Professor of Otology, The University of Alabama School of Medicine · Brookwood Medical Center · 2937 Seventh Avenue South, Suite 200, Birmingham, AL 35233 · 205-251-7169

Myles L. Pensak · Associate Professor and Director, Division of Otology & Neurotology, University of Cincinnati College of Medicine · University of Cincinnati Hospital, Children's Hospital, Good Samaritan Hospital, Bethesda Hospital, Jewish Hospital, Holmes Hospital, Veteran's Hospital, Christ Hospital · 231 Bethesda Avenue, ML 528, Cincinnati, OH 45267-0528 · 513-558-5143

Mitchell K. Schwaber · Assistant Professor, Department of Otolaryngology, Vanderbilt University School of Medicine · Vanderbilt University Medical Center Vanderbilt Medical Center, Room S2100 MCN, Nashville, TN 37232-2559 · 615-343-6106

Herbert Silverstein · Clinical Professor of Surgery, Division of Otolaryngology, University of South Florida, Tampa · President, Ear Research Foundation; Florida Otologic Center · 1901 Floyd Street, Sarasota, FL 34239 · 813-366-9222, 366-1148

Mansfield F. W. Smith · Clinical Professor of Surgery (Otology), Stanford University School of Medicine · Stanford University Hospital · 2120 Forest Avenue, San Jose, CA 95128 · 408-288-7777

Peter G. Smith · St. John's Mercy Medical Center; Barnes Hospital; St. Louis Children's Hospital; The Jewish Hospital of St. Louis · Midwest Otologic Group, 621 South New Ballas, Suite 597, St. Louis, MO 63141 · 314-432-5151

Bradley S. Thedinger · University of Kansas Medical Center; Trinity Lutheran Hospital; St. Luke's Hospital of Kansas City; Menorah Medical Center · Otologic Center, Inc., 3100 Broadway, Suite 509, Kansas City, MO 64111 · 816-531-7373

Richard J. Wiet · Professor of Clinical Otolaryngology, and Associate Professor of Clinical Neurosurgery, Northwestern University Medical School · Hinsdale Hospital; Northwestern Memorial Hospital; Children's Memorial · 950 York Road, Suite 102, Hinsdale, IL 60521 · 708-789-3110

PEDIATRIC OTOLARYNGOLOGY

James E. Arnold · Assistant Professor, Department of Pediatrics, and Assistant Professor, Department of Otolaryngology, Head & Neck Surgery, Case Western Reserve University School of Medicine · Director, Division of Pediatric Otolaryngology, Rainbow Babies & Childrens Hospital · 2074 Abington Road, Cleveland, OH 44106 · 216-844-5202

Walter M. Belenky · Children's Hospital of Michigan · Harper Professional Building, 4160 John, Suite 1008, Detroit, MI 48201 · 313-745-9048

Charles D. Bluestone · Professor, Department of Otolaryngology, University of Pittsburgh School of Medicine · Director, Department of Pediatric Otolaryngology, Children's Hospital of Pittsburgh · 3705 Fifth Avenue, Pittsburgh, PA 15213 · 412-692-6220

Linda S. Brodsky · Associate Professor of Otolaryngology and Pediatrics, State University of New York Health Science Center at Buffalo · Co-Head, Department of Pediatric Otolaryngology, Children's Hospital of Buffalo · 219 Bryant Street, Buffalo, NY 14222 · 716-878-7569

Orval E. Brown · Associate Professor of Otolaryngology, The University of Texas Southwestern Medical Center at Dallas · Children's Medical Center of Dallas · 5323 Harry Hines Boulevard, Dallas, TX 75235-9035 · 214-688-3103

Robin T. Cotton · (Laryngobronchoesophegology) · Professor, Department of Otolaryngology & Maxillofacial Surgery, University of Cincinnati College of Medicine · Director, Department of Pediatric Otolaryngology & Maxillofacial Surgery,

Children's Hospital Medical Center · Elland & Bethesda Avenues, Cincinnati, OH 45229 · 513-559-4355

William S. Crysdale · Professor of Otolaryngology, University of Toronto School of Medicine · Chief of Otolaryngology, The Hospital for Sick Children · 555 University Avenue, Suite 6126, Toronto, Ontario M5G 1X8 · 416-598-6557

James P. Cuyler · Associate Professor of Surgery, University of Alberta · University of Alberta Hospital; Alexandra Hospital; Glenrose Rehabilitation Center · 8215 One Hundred Twelfth Street, Room 405, Edmonton, Alberta T6G 2C8 · 403-432-9595

John Donaldson · Lee Memorial Hospital · 3487 Broadway, Fort Myers, FL 23901 · 813-939-2621

Ellen M. Friedman · (Congenital Airway Problems, Congenital Malformations of the Head & Neck) · Associate Professor of Otolaryngology and Pediatrics, Baylor College of Medicine · Chief of Service, Department of Pediatric Otolaryngology, Texas Children's Hospital · 6621 Fannin Street, Suite 340, Houston, TX 77030 · 713-770-3268

Steven D. Gray · Assistant Professor of Otolaryngology, University of Utah School of Medicine · University of Utah Health Sciences Center · 50 North Medical Drive, Salt Lake City, UT 84132 · 801-581-7514

Charles W. Gross · (Pediatric Sinus Disease) · Professor of Otolaryngology-Head & Neck Surgery, and Pediatrics, University of Virginia School of Medicine · University of Virginia Health Sciences Center · Box 430, Charlottesville, VA 22908 · 804-924-5700

Kenneth Martin Grundfast · (Pediatric Otology) · Professor of Otolaryngology and Pediatrics, The George Washington University School of Medicine · Chairman, Department of Otolaryngology, Children's National Medical Center · 111 Michigan Avenue NW, Washington, DC 20010 · 202-745-2159

Donald B. Hawkins · (Bronchoesophegology) · Professor of Otolaryngology-Head & Neck Surgery, Los Angeles County-University of Southern California Medical Center · Director, Pediatric Otolaryngology, Los Angeles County-University of Southern California Medical Center · 1200 North State Street, Box 296, Los Angeles, CA 90033 · 213-226-7315

Gerald B. Healy · (Laryngobronchoesophegology) · Professor of Otology and Laryngology, Harvard Medical School · Otolaryngologist in Chief, Children's Hospital · 300 Longwood Avenue, Boston, MA 02115 · 617-735-6417

Lauren D. Holinger · (Pediatric Bronchoesophegology) · Professor of Otolaryngology, Northwestern University Medical School · Head, Division of Pediatric Otolaryngology & Communicative Disorders, The Children's Memorial Hospital 2300 Children's Plaza, Box 25, Chicago, IL 60614 · 312-880-4457

Andrew Jay Hotaling · Assistant Professor and Chief, Section of Pediatric Otolaryngology, Loyola Stritch School of Medicine · 2160 South First Avenue, Building 105, Room 1870, Maywood, IL 60153 · 708-216-9000

Rodney P. Lusk · (Pediatric Bronchoesophegology) · Associate Professor and Director, Division of Pediatric Otolaryngology, Washington University School of Medicine · Otolaryngologist-in-Chief, St. Louis Children's Hospital · 400 South Kingshighway, St. Louis, MO 63110 · 314-454-2333

Trevor McGill · Associate Professor of Otolaryngology, Harvard Medical School · Associate Professor of Otolaryngology, Children's Hospital · 300 Longwood Avenue, Boston, MA 02115 · 617-735-6408

Robert H. Miller · Professor and Chairman, Department of Otolaryngology, Head & Neck Surgery, Tulane University School of Medicine · Vice Chief of Staff, Tulane University Medical Center · 1430 Tulane Avenue, New Orleans, LA 70112-2699 · 504-588-5661

Harlan R. Muntz · Associate Professor of Otolaryngology, Washington University School of Medicine · St. Louis Children's Hospital · 400 South Kingshighway, Suite S35, St. Louis, MO 63110 · 314-454-6162

Charles M. Myer III · Associate Professor, Department of Otolaryngology & Maxillofacial Surgery, University of Cincinnati College of Medicine · Children's Hospital Medical Center · Elland & Bethesda Avenues, Cincinnati, OH 45229 · 513-559-8911

Robert M. Naclerio · (Allergy) · Associate Professor of Otolaryngology, Johns Hopkins University School of Medicine · The Johns Hopkins Medical Institutions Johns Hopkins Hospital, Department of Otolaryngology, P. O. Box 41402, Baltimore, MD 21203-6402 · 410-955-7083

David S. Parsons · Clinical Professor of Otolaryngology, The University of Texas Health Science Center at San Antonio · Director, Residency Training Program, Wilford Hall, United States Air Force Medical Center · Lackland Air Force Base, San Antonio, TX 78236-5300 · 512-670-5623

William P. Potsic · Associate Professor, Department of Otolaryngology & Human Communication, Hospital of the University of Pennsylvania School of Medicine · Director, Division of Otolaryngology & Human Communication, The Children's

Hospital of Philadelphia · The Richard D. Wood Building, 34th Street and Civic Center Boulevard, First Floor, Philadelphia, PA 19104 · 215-590-3450

Seth Marc Pransky · Assistant Clinical Professor of Otolaryngology-Head & Neck Surgery, University of California, San Diego School of Medicine · Attending Pediatric Otolaryngologist, Children's Hospital & Health Center · 3030 Children's Way, Suite 402, San Diego, CA 92123 · 619-576-4085

James S. Reilly · Professor of Surgery, The University of Alabama School of Medicine · Otolaryngologist-in-Chief, Children's Hospital of Alabama · 1600 Seventh Avenue South, Birmingham, AL 35233 · 205-939-9834

Mark A. Richardson · Professor, University of Washington · Associate Director, Department of Surgery, and Chief, Division of Otolaryngology, Children's Hospital & Medical Center · 4800 Sand Point Way NE, Seattle, WA 98105 · 206-526-2115

Robert J. Ruben · Professor and Chairman, Department of Otolaryngology, and Professor, Department of Pediatrics, Albert Einstein College of Medicine · Chairman, Department of Otolaryngology, Montefiore Medical Center · 111 East 210th Street, VCA-4, Bronx, NY 10467 · 212-920-2991

Allan B. Seid · Associate Clinical Professor of Otolaryngology-Head & Neck Surgery, University of California, San Diego School of Medicine · Attending Pediatric Otolaryngologist, Children's Hospital & Health Center · 3030 Children's Way, Suite 402, San Diego, CA 92123 · 619-576-4085

Sylvan E. Stool · Professor of Otolaryngology and Pediatrics, University of Pittsburgh School of Medicine · Director of Education, Department of Pediatric Otolaryngology, Children's Hospital of Pittsburgh · 3705 Fifth Avenue at DeSoto Street, Pittsburgh, PA 15213 · 412-692-8577

Jerome W. Thompson · Assistant Clinical Professor of Otolaryngology, University of Southern California School of Medicine · Chairman, Credentials Committee, Children's Hospital of Los Angeles · 1300 North Vermont Avenue, Suite 502, Los Angeles, CA 90027 · 213-666-4670

John A. Tucker · (Pediatric Bronchoesophegology) · Professor of Pediatric Otolaryngology, Temple University School of Medicine; Professor of Otolaryngology, Hahnemann University · Chairman, Division of Otolaryngology, and Chief of Pediatric Otolaryngology, Albert Einstein Medical Center; St. Christopher's Hospital for Children; Hahnemann University; Temple University · Paley Building, Second Floor, 5501 Old York Road, Philadelphia, PA 19141 · 215-456-7140, 673-1356

Ralph F. Wetmore · Associate Professor of Otolaryngology, University of Pennsylvania School of Medicine · Associate Surgeon, The Children's Hospital of Philadelphia · The Wood Building, 34th and Civic Center Boulevard, Philadelphia, PA 19104 · 215-590-3458

Benjamin White · Section Chief for Otolaryngology, and Chief of Surgery, Scottish Rite Children's Medical Center · 5455 Meridan Mark Drive, Suite 130, Atlanta, GA 30342 · 404-255-2033

SINUS & NASAL SURGERY

Charles W. Gross · (Pediatric Sinus Disease) · Professor of Otolaryngology-Head & Neck Surgery, and Pediatrics, University of Virginia School of Medicine · University of Virginia Health Sciences Center · Box 430, Charlottesville, VA 22908 804-924-5700

David W. Kennedy · Professor and Chairman, Department of Otorhinolaryngology & Head & Neck Surgery, University of Pennsylvania School of Medicine · Otolaryngologist-in-Chief, Hospital of the University of Pennsylvania · 3400 Spruce Street, Silverstein Five, Philadelphia, PA 19104 · 215-662-2777

Eugene B. Kern · (Cosmetic, Nasal Breathing Problems) · Professor of Otorhinolaryngology, Mayo Medical School · Mayo Clinic · 200 First Street, SW, Rochester, MN 55905 · 507-284-3578

William Lawson · Professor of Otolaryngology, Mt. Sinai School of Medicine · Mt. Sinai Medical Center · Five East 98th Street, Eighth Floor, New York, NY 10029 · 212-241-9430

Howard L. Levine · Director, The Mt. Sinai Nasal-Sinus Center, The Mt. Sinai Medical Center · The Mt. Sinai Nasal-Sinus Center, 29001 Cedar Road, Suite 307, Cleveland, OH 44124 · 216-442-1200, 800-24-SINUS

Rodney P. Lusk · Associate Professor and Director, Division of Pediatric Otolaryngology, Washington University School of Medicine · Otolaryngologist-in-Chief, St. Louis Children's Hospital · 400 South Kingshighway, St. Louis, MO 63110 · 314-454-2333

Robert H. Miller · Professor and Chairman, Department of Otolaryngology, Head & Neck Surgery, Tulane University School of Medicine · Vice Chief of Staff, Tulane University Medical Center · 1430 Tulane Avenue, New Orleans, LA 70112-2699 · 504-588-5661

William Montgomery · Professor of Otolarynoglogy, Harvard Medical School · Senior Surgeon in Otolaryngology, Massachusetts Eye & Ear Infirmary · 243 Charles Street, Boston, MA 02114 · 617-573-3669

Dale H. Rice · Tiber/Alpert Professor and Chairman, Department of Otolaryngology, Head & Neck Surgery, University of Southern California School of Medicine Chief Physician, The Los Angeles County + University of Southern California Medical Center; University of Southern California University Hospital · 1200 North State Street, Room GH-4136, Los Angeles, CA 90033 · 213-226-7315, 342-5790

Frank N. Ritter · Clinical Professor of Otolaryngology-Head & Neck Surgery, The University of Michigan Medical Center · Active Staff, St. Joseph Mercy Hospital, and The University of Michigan Hospital · 5333 McAuley Drive, Suite R4016, Ypsilanti, MI 48197 · 313-434-3341

Steven Schaefer · Professor, Department of Otolaryngology, The University of Texas Southwestern Medical Center at Dallas · Staff Physician & Surgeon, University Hospital; Parkland Memorial Hospital · Department of Otolaryngology, 5323 Harry Hines Boulevard, Dallas, TX 75235-9035 · 214-688-3051, 688-3071

William King Stubbs, Jr. · (Pediatric Sinus Disease) · Courtesy-Clinical Assistant Professor, Department of Otolaryngology, University of Florida School of Medicine · Chief, Head & Neck Surgery, Indian River Memorial Hospital · 777 Thirty-Seventh Street, Suite C-101, Vero Beach, FL 32960 · 407-567-1164

Ernest A. Weymuller · Professor and Acting Chairman, Department of Otolaryngology, University of Washington School of Medicine · University of Washington Medical Center · 1959 Northeast Pacific Street, RL-30, Seattle, WA 98195 · 206-543-5230

SKULL-BASE SURGERY

Roger L. Crumley · Professor and Chairman, Department of Otolaryngology-Head & Neck Surgery, University of California at Irvine School of Medicine · University of California at Irvine Medical Center · 101 City Drive, Building 25, Route 81, Orange, CA 92668 · 714-634-5750

Paul J. Donald · Professor and Vice-Chairman, Department of Otolaryngology-Head & Neck Surgery, University of California, Davis School of Medicine · Director, UCDMC Center for Skull Base Surgery, University of California, Davis Medical Center · 2500 Stockton Boulevard, Sacramento, CA 95817 · 916-734-2832

Patrick Joseph Gullane · Professor of Otolaryngology, University of Toronto School of Medicine · Otolaryngologist-in-Chief and Director, Head & Neck Program, The Toronto Hospital · 200 Elizabeth Street, Eaton Building North, Seventh Floor, Room 242, Toronto, Ontario M5G 2C4 · 416-340-4356

Michael J. Holliday · Associate Professor of Otolaryngology, Johns Hopkins University School of Medicine · The Johns Hopkins Medical Institutions · 600 North Wolfe Street, Carnegie Building, Room 484, Baltimore, MD 21205 · 410-955-3492

Peter G. Smith · St. John's Mercy Medical Center; Barnes Hospital; St. Louis Children's Hospital; The Jewish Hospital of St. Louis · Midwest Otologic Group, 621 South New Ballas, Suite 597, St. Louis, MO 63141 · 314-432-5151

PATHOLOGY

BONE PATHOLOGY

Robert E. Fechner · Professor of Pathology and Director of Anatomic Pathology, University of Virginia School of Medicine · University of Virginia Health Sciences Center · Box 214, Charlottesville, VA 22908 · 804-924-5127

BREAST PATHOLOGY

James L. Connolly · Associate Professor of Pathology, Harvard Medical School · Pathologist, Beth Israel Hospital · 330 Brookline Avenue, Boston, MA 02215 · 617-735-4344

William H. Hartmann · Professor-in-Residence, University of California, Irvine · Medical Director, Department of Pathology, Long Beach Memorial Medical Center · 2801 Atlantic Avenue, Long Beach, CA 90801-1428 · 213-595-2217

Michael D. Lagios · Assistant Professor of Pathology, University of California at San Francisco School of Medicine · Senior Surgical Pathologist, California Pacific Medical Center · 3700 California Street, San Francisco, CA 94118 · 415-387-8700 x5515

Henry J. Norris · Chairman, Department of Gynecologic & Breast Pathology, Armed Forces Institute of Pathology · Building 54, Washington, DC 20306-6000 202-576-2981

Harold A. Oberman · Professor of Pathology, The University of Michigan Medical School · The University of Michigan Medical Center; University Hospitals Blood Bank & Transfusion Service · The University Hospital, Room 2G322, Box 0054, 1500 East Medical Center Drive, Ann Arbor, MI 48109-0054 · 313-936-6767

David L. Page · Professor of Pathology and Director of Anatomic Pathology, Vanderbilt University School of Medicine · Vanderbilt University Medical Center Vanderbilt University Medical Center North, Room C3321, Nashville, TN 37232 615-322-2102

Paul Peter Rosen · Professor of Pathology, Cornell University Medical College · Attending Pathologist and Member, Memorial Sloan-Kettering Cancer Center · 1275 York Avenue, New York, NY 10021 · 212-639-5905

Stuart J. Schnitt · Assistant Professor, Pathology, Harvard Medical School · Pathologist, Beth Israel Hospital · 330 Brookline Avenue, Boston, MA 02215 · 617-735-4344

Fattaneh Tavassoli · Consultant, National Institutes of Health · Assistant Chairman, Department of Gynecologic & Breast Pathology, Armed Forces Institute of Pathology · Washington, DC 20306-6000 · 202-576-2981

DERMATOPATHOLOGY
(See also Dermatology, Dermatopathology)

A. Bernard Ackerman · Professor, Department of Dermatology & Pathology; and Director of Dermatopathology, New York University School of Medicine · New York University Medical Center · 530 First Avenue, Suite 7J, New York, NY 10016 · 212-263-7250

John T. Headington · (Hair Disorders) · Professor of Pathology and Dermatology, The University of Michigan Medical School · The University of Michigan Medical Center · Medical Science I, 1301 Catherine, M5242/0602, Box 0602, Ann Arbor, MI 48109-0602 · 313-936-1874

ENT PATHOLOGY

Leon Barnes, Jr. · Associate Professor of Pathology & Otolaryngology, University of Pittsburgh School of Medicine · Director of Anatomic Pathology, University of Pittsburgh Medical Center · DeSoto at O'Hara Streets, Suite 684, Pittsburgh, PA 15213 · 412-647-3730

John G. Batsakis · Head, Division of Pathology, The University of Texas · Chairman, Department of Pathology, The University of Texas MD Anderson Cancer Center · 1515 Holcombe Boulevard, Houston, TX 77030 · 713-792-3100

Robert E. Fechner · Professor of Pathology and Director of Anatomic Pathology, University of Virginia School of Medicine · University of Virginia Health Sciences Center · Box 214, Charlottesville, VA 22908 · 804-924-5127

Stacey E. Mills · Professor of Pathology, University of Virginia School of Medicine Director, Immunohistochemical Laboratory, University of Virginia Health Sciences Center · Hospital Drive, Room 1885, Box 214, Charlottesville, VA 22908 · 804-924-5127

GYNECOLOGIC PATHOLOGY

Henry J. Norris · Chairman, Department of Gynecologic & Breast Pathology, Armed Forces Institute of Pathology · Building 54, Washington, DC 20306-6000 202-576-2981

Robert E. Scully · Professor of Pathology at the Massachusetts General Hospital, Harvard Medical School · Pathologist, Massachusetts General Hospital · Pathology Department, 33 Fruit Street, Boston, MA 02114 · 617-726-3956

Edward J. Wilkinson · Professor of Pathology and Associate Chairman, Department of Pathology and Laboratory Medicine, University of Florida College of Medicine · Shands Hospital at the University of Florida · 1600 Southwest Archer Road, Room M649, P.O. Box 100275, Gainesville, FL 32610 · 904-395-0208

HEMATOPATHOLOGY

Peter M. Banks · Director of Anatomic Pathology, and Frank M. Townsend Professor of Pathology, The University of Texas Health Science Center at San Antonio · Medical Center Hospital; Veterans Affairs Hospital · 7703 Floyd Curl Drive, San Antonio, TX 78284-7750 · 512-567-4034

Costan W. Berard · Professor of Pathology, University of Tennessee at Memphis, College of Medicine · Chairman, Department of Pathology and Laboratory Medicine, St. Jude Children's Research Hospital · 332 North Lauderdale, Memphis, TN 38105 · 901-522-0530

Raul C. Braylan · Professor and Chief of Hematopathology Section, University of Florida College of Medicine · Shands Hospital at the University of Florida · Department of Pathology, Box 100275 JHMHC, Gainesville, FL 32610 · 904-392-3477

Richard D, Brunning · Professor and Director of Hematopathology, University of Minnesota School of Medicine · University of Minnesota Hospital & Clinics · Mayo Building, Room D-223, 420 Delaware Street, SE, Box 198, Minneapolis, MN 55455 · 612-626-5704

James Johnson Butler · Professor of Pathology, The University of Texas · Pathologist, The University of Texas MD Anderson Cancer Center · 1515 Holcombe Boulevard, Houston, TX 77030 · 713-792-3130

Robert D. Collins · Professor of Pathology, Vanderbilt University School of Medicine · 1611 Twenty-First Avenue South, Room C3321,Medical Center North, Nashville, TN 37232-2561 · 615-322-0994

Jeffrey Cossman · Professor and Chairman, Department of Pathology, Georgetown University School of Medicine · Pathologist-in-Chief, Georgetown University Medical Center · 119 Basic Science Building, 3900 Reservoir Road, NW, Washington, DC 20007 · 202-687-1704

Ronald F. Dorfman · Professor of Pathology, Stanford University School of Medicine · Co-Director of Surgical Pathology, Stanford University Hospital · 300 Pasteur Drive, Stanford, CA 94305 · 415-723-5303

M. Kathryn Foucar · Professor of Pathology, The University of New Mexico School of Medicine · Director, Pathology Service, The University Hospital · 2211 Lomas Boulevard NE, Albuquerque, NM 87106 · 505-843-2440

Glauco Frizzera · Chairman, Department of Hematologic & Lymphatic Pathology, Armed Forces Institute of Pathology · 6825 Sixteenth Street, NW, Washington, DC 20306 · 202-576-2128

Thomas M. Grogan · Professor of Pathology, The University of Arizona College of Medicine · The University of Arizona Health Sciences Center · 1501 North Campbell Avenue, Tucson, AZ 85724 · 602-626-6100

Nancy Harris · Department of Pathology, Massachusetts General Hospital · Fruit Street, Warren-2, Boston, MA 02114 · 617-726-5155

Elaine S. Jaffe · Chief, Hematopathology Section, and Deputy Chief, Laboratory of Pathology, National Cancer Institute, National Institutes of Health · 9000 Rockville Pike, Building 10, Room 2N202, Bethesda, MD 20892 · 301-496-0183

Marshall Edward Kadin · Associate Professor of Pathology, Harvard Medical School · Director, Hematopathology, Beth Israel Hospital · 330 Brookline Avenue, Yamins 309, Boston, MA 02215 · 617-735-3648

Carl R. Kjeldsberg · Professor of Pathology, and Head, Division of Clinical Pathology, and Senior Associate Chairman, Department of Pathology, University of Utah School of Medicine · University of Utah Health Sciences Center · Department of Hematopathology, 50 North Medical Drive, Salt Lake City, UT 84132 · 801-581-5854

Daniel M. Knowles · Professor of Pathology, College of Physicians & Surgeons of Columbia University · Director, Division of Surgical Pathology, Columbia-Presbyterian Medical Center · 630 West 168th Street, VC 14th Floor, Room 209, New York, NY 10032 · 212-305-5697

Robert J. Lukes · Emeritus Professor of Pathology, University of Southern California School of Medicine · Senior Consultant, Division of Hematopathology, Scripps Clinic & Research Foundation · 10666 North Torrey Pines Road, La Jolla, CA 92037 · 619-554-9937

Robert W. McKenna · John Childers Professor and Vice-Chairman, Department of Pathology, The University of Texas Southwestern Medical Center at Dallas · Parkland Memorial Hospital; Children's Medical Center of Dallas; Zale-Lipshy University Medical Center · 5323 Harry Hines Boulevard, Room F2.118, Dallas, TX 75235-9072 · 214-688-3347

Bharat N. Nathwani · Professor of Pathology, University of Southern California School of Medicine · Chief of Hematopathology, The Los Angeles County + University of Southern California Medical Center · University of Southern California School of Medicine, 2011 Zonal Avenue, Hoffman 204, Los Angeles, CA 90033 · 213-226-7064

Geraldine S. Pinkus · Associate Professor of Pathology, Harvard Medical School Director, Hematopathology Division, Brigham & Women's Hospital · 75 Francis Street, Boston, MA 02115 · 617-732-7519

Henry Rappaport · Professor of Pathology Emeritus, University of Chicago · Distinguished Physician, City of Hope National Medical Center · 1500 East Duarte Road, Room 2204, Duarte, CA 91010-0269 · 818-359-8111 x2552

James W. Vardiman · Assistant Professor of Pathology, University of Chicago, Pritzker School of Medicine · University of Chicago Medical Center · 5841 South Maryland Avenue, Box 84, Chicago, IL 60637-1470 · 312-702-6196

Roger A. Warnke · Professor of Pathology, Stanford University School of Medicine · Co-Director of Immunopathology, Stanford University Hospital · 300 Pasteur Drive, Stanford, CA 94305 · 415-723-5303

LIVER PATHOLOGY

Jurgen Ludwig · Professor of Pathology, Mayo Medical School · Mayo Clinic · 200 First Street, SW, Rochester, MN 55905 · 507-284-3867

NEUROPATHOLOGY

Laurence E. Becker · (Pediatric) · Professor of Pathology, University of Toronto School of Medicine · Head, Division of Neuropathology, The Hospital for Sick Children · 555 University Avenue, Room 3110, Toronto, Ontario M5G 1X8 · 416-598-6595

Peter C. Burger · (Brain Tumor) · Professor of Pathology, Duke University School of Medicine · Director of Neuropathology, Duke University Medical Center · P.O. Box 3712, Durham, NC 27710 · 919-684-6667

Richard L. Davis · Professor of Pathology, University of California at San Francisco School of Medicine · Director of Neuropathology, University of California at San Francisco Medical Center · 505 Parnassus Avenue, San Francisco, CA 94143-0506 · 415-476-5236

Floyd H. Gilles · (Pediatric) · Children's Hospital of Los Angeles · Department of Neuropathology, 4650 Sunset Boulevard, Los Angeles CA 90027 · 213-660-2450

E. Tessa Hedley-Whyte · Associate Professor of Pathology, Harvard Medical School · Massachusetts General Hospital · Department of Pathology, Boston, MA 02114 · 617-726-5154

John J. Kepes · (Brain Tumors) · Professor of Pathology, University of Kansas School of Medicine · University of Kansas Medical Center · 39th Street & Rainbow Boulevard, Kansas City, KS 66103 · 913-588-5000

Lucy B. Rorke · (Pediatric) · Adjunct Professor, The Wistar Institute; Clinical Professor of Pathology & Neurology, University of Pennsylvania School of Medicine · The Children's Hospital of Philadelphia · 34th Street and Civic Center Boulevard, Philadelphia, PA 19104 · 215-590-1728

Bernd W. Scheithauer · (Tumor) · Professor of Pathology, Mayo Medical School · Head, Section of Surgical Pathology, Mayo Clinic · 200 First Street, SW, Rochester, MN 55905 · 507-284-2511

SURGICAL PATHOLOGY

John G. Batsakis · Head, Division of Pathology, The University of Texas · Chairman, Department of Pathology, The University of Texas MD Anderson Cancer Center · 1515 Holcombe Boulevard, Houston, TX 77030 · 713-792-3100

George M. Farrow · Professor of Pathology, Mayo Medical School · Mayo Clinic 200 First Street, SW, Rochester, MN 55905 · 507-284-2511

Cecilia M. Fenoglio-Preiser · Professor and Director, Department of Pathology & Laboratory Medicine, University of Cincinnati College of Medicine · Director of Hospital Laboratories, University of Cincinnati Hospital · 231 Bethesda Avenue, ML 529, Cincinnati, OH 45267-0529 · 513-558-4500

Juan Rosai · Professor of Pathology, Cornell University Medical College · Chairman, Department of Pathology, Memorial Sloan-Kettering Cancer Center · 1275 York Avenue, New York, NY 10021 · 212-639-8410

Lester E. Wold · Associate Professor of Pathology, Mayo Medical School · Vice-Chair, Department of Laboratory Medicine & Pathology, and Consultant, Section for Surgical Pathology, Mayo Clinic · 200 First Street, SW, Rochester, MN 55905 507-284-2511

PEDIATRICS

ABUSED CHILDREN
(See also Psychiatry, Child Abuse)

Randell C. Alexander · Associate Professor of Pediatrics, The University of Iowa
College of Medicine · The University of Iowa Hospitals & Clinics · 209 Hospital
School, University of Iowa, Iowa City, IA 52242 · 319-353-6136

Jan Bays · Medical Director of Cares Program, Emanuel Hospital & Health Center · 2801 North Gantenbein Avenue, Portland, OR 97227 · 503-280-4943

Carol D. Berkowitz · Professor of Clinical Pediatrics, University of California, Los Angeles School of Medicine · Acting Chair, Department of Pediatrics, Harbor-UCLA Medical Center · 1000 West Carson Street, Torrance, CA 90509 · 213-533-3091

David L. Chadwick · Adjunct Associate Professor of Pediatrics, University of California at San Diego School of Medicine · Director, Center for Child Protection, Children's Hospital & Health Center · 8001 Frost Street, Center for Child Protection, San Diego, CA 92123 · 619-576-5814

Kenneth W. Feldman · Clinical Professor of Pediatrics, University of Washington School of Medicine · Children's Hospital & Medical Center; Odessa Brown Children's Clinic · 2101 East Yesler Way, Seattle, WA 98122 · 206-329-7870

Martin A. Finkel · (Sexually Abused Children) · Associate Professor of Clinical Pediatrics, University of Medicine & Dentistry of New Jersey School of Osteopathic Medicine · Medical Director, Center for Children's Support, Kennedy Memorial Hospital-University Medical Center · 301 South Central Plaza, Laurel Road, Suite 3400, Stratford, NJ 08084 · 609-346-7036

Astrid H. Heger · Professor of Pediatrics, University of Southern California School of Medicine · Director, Sexual Child Abuse & Neglect Clinic, Pediatric Pavilion, The Los Angeles County + University of Southern California Medical Center · 1129 North State Street, Los Angeles, CA 90033 · 213-226-3961

Ray E. Helfer · Professor of Pediatrics and Human Development, Michigan State University College of Human Medicine · B240 Life Sciences, East Lansing, MI 48824-1317 · 517-353-4585

Carole Jenny · Associate Professor of Pediatrics, University of Colorado School of Medicine · Director, Child Advocacy & Protection Team, The Children's Hospital · 1056 East 19th Avenue, B-138, Denver, CO 80218 · 303-861-6919

Charles Felzen Johnson · (Child Development) · Professor of Pediatrics, Ohio State University College of Medicine · Medical Director, Child Abuse Program, Columbus Children's Hospital · 700 Children's Drive, Columbus, OH 43205 · 614-461-6888

Richard D. Krugman · Professor of Pediatrics and Acting Dean, School of Medicine, University of Colorado School of Medicine · Director, C. Henry Kempe National Center for the Prevention & Treatment of Child Abuse & Neglect, University of Colorado School of Medicine · 4200 East Ninth Avenue, Box C-290, Denver, CO 80262 · 303-270-7563

Howard B. Levy · Associate Professor of Pediatrics, Chicago Medical School · Chairman, Department of Pediatrics, Mt. Sinai Hospital Center · California at 15th Avenue, Chicago, IL 60608 · 312-542-2000

Stephen Ludwig · Professor of Pediatrics, University of Pennsylvania School of Medicine · Division Chief, General Pediatrics, The Children's Hospital of Philadelphia · 34th and Civic Center Boulevard, Suite 2011, Philadelphia, PA 19104 215-590-2162

Margaret T. McHugh · Associate Professor of Clinical Pediatrics, New York University School of Medicine · Director, Adolescent Medicine, and Director, Child Protection Team, New York University Medical Center, Bellevue Hospital · Pediatrics, 1 South 6 Bellevue Hospital Center, 462 First Avenue, New York, NY 10016 · 212-561-6321

William M. Palmer · Associate Professor of Pediatrics, University of Utah School of Medicine · Medical Director, Child Protection Team, Primary Children's Medical Center · 100 North Medical Drive, Salt Lake City, UT 84113 · 801-588-3650

Jan E. Paradise · Assistant Professor of Pediatrics, Boston University School of Medicine · Director, Child Protection Program, Boston City Hospital · Dowling One North, 818 Harrison Avenue, Boston, MA 02118 · 617-534-7902

Robert M. Reece · Associate Professor, Department of Pediatrics, Case Western Reserve University School of Medicine · Director, Child Protection Program, Rainbow Babies & Childrens Hospital · 2074 Abington Road, Cleveland, OH 44106 · 216-844-3761

Lawrence R. Ricci · Associate Professor, Department of Clinical Community & Family Medicine, and Chairperson, Section on Child Abuse & Neglect, American Academy of Pediatrics, Dartmouth Medical School · Medical Director, Diagnostic Program for Child Abuse, Mid-Maine Medical Center · Seton Unit, Chase Avenue, Waterville, ME 04901 · 207-872-4286

Sara Elizabeth Schuh · (Neglect) · Associate Professor of Pediatrics, Medical University of South Carolina · Medical University of South Carolina Hospital · Sixth Floor, Children's Hospital, 171 Ashley Avenue, Charleston, SC 29425 · 803-792-5345

Jay M. Whitworth · Associate Professor of Pediatrics, University of Florida · Executive Medical Director, Children's Crisis Center, Inc. · 655 West Eighth Street, P.O. Box 40279, Jacksonville, FL 32203 · 904-549-4670

METABOLIC DISEASES
(See also Child Neurology, Metabolic Diseases)

Arthur Louis Beaudet · (General, Cystic Fibrosis, Urea Cycle Disorders) · Professor, Institute for Molecular Genetics, and Department of Pediatrics, Baylor College of Medicine · Texas Children's Hospital · Institute for Molecular Genetics, One Baylor Plaza, Houston, TX 77030 · 713-798-4795

Saul W. Brusilow · (Urea Cycle Disorders) · Professor of Pediatrics, Johns Hopkins University School of Medicine · Attending Staff, The Johns Hopkins Medical Institutions · 600 North Wolfe Street, Park 339, Baltimore, MD 21205 · 410-955-0885

Neil R. M. Buist · (Hereditary & Acquired) · Professor of Pediatrics and Molecular & Medical Genetics, Oregon Health Sciences University · Director, Metabolic Birth Defects Center and Pediatric Metabolic Laboratory, Oregon Health Sciences University · 3181 Southwest Sam Jackson Park Road, Portland, OR 97201-3098 · 503-494-8392

Stephen Cederbaum · (Genetics, Urea Cycle Disorders, Lactic Acidosis) · Professor of Pediatrics & Psychiatry, University of California, Los Angeles School of Medicine · University of California, Los Angeles Medical Center · Mental Retardation Research Center, 760 Westwood Plaza, Los Angeles, CA 90024 · 310-825-0402

Y. T. Chin · (Glycogen Storage Disease) · Associate Professor, Division of Pediatrics, Genetics and Metabolism, Duke University School of Medicine · Duke University Medical Center · Box 3028, DUMC, Durham, NC 27710 · 919-684-2036

Robert J. Desnick · (Genetics, Lysosomal Diseases) · Professor of Pediatrics & Genetics, Mt. Sinai School of Medicine · Chief, Division of Medical & Molecular Genetics, Mt. Sinai Medical Center · Fifth Avenue & 100th Street, Box 1203, New York, NY 10029-6574 · 212-241-6944

Louis J. Elsas II · (General, Medical Genetics) · Professor of Pediatrics, Emory University School of Medicine · Henrietta Egleston Hospital for Children; Emory University Affiliated Hospitals · 2040 Ridgewood Drive, Atlanta, GA 30322 · 404-727-5731

William Gahl · (Cystinosis) · Chief, Human Genetics Branch, National Institute of Child Health & Human Development, National Institutes of Health · Building 10, Room 9S242, Bethesda, MD 20892 · 301-496-6683

Stephen I. Goodman · (Organic Acidemias) · Professor of Pediatrics, and Head, Division of Genetics, University of Colorado School of Medicine · Director, B. F. Stolinsky Laboratories · 4200 East Ninth Avenue, Box C-233, Denver CO 80262 303-270-7301

Stephen G. Kahler · (General) · Assistant Professor of Pediatrics, Duke University School of Medicine · Duke University Medical Center · P.O. Box 3028, Durham, NC 27710 · 919-684-2036

Douglas S. Kerr · (Lactic Acidosis) · Associate Professor of Pediatrics, Biochemistry, & Nutrition, Case Western Reserve University School of Medicine · Director, Center for Inherited Disorders of Energy Metabolism, Rainbow Babies & Childrens Hospital · 2074 Abington Road, Cleveland, OH 44106 · 216-844-3661

Harvey L. Levy · (Amino Acid Disorders) · Associate Professor of Neurology, Harvard Medical School · Senior Associate in Medicine and Genetics, Children's Hospital · 300 Longwood Avenue, Gardener 818, Boston, MA 02115 · 617-735-6346

Edward R. B. McCabe · (Genetics) · Professor of Molecular Genetics & Pediatrics, and Director, R. J. Kleberg, Jr. Clinical Center, and Director, Baylor Mental Retardation Research Center, and Director, Baylor Child Health Research Center, Baylor College of Medicine · Texas Children's Hospital · Institute for Molecular Genetics, One Baylor Plaza, S-921, Houston, TX 77030 · 713-798-5820

William L. Nyhan · (Amino Acid Disorders) · Professor of Pediatrics, University of California at San Diego School of Medicine · Chief of the Biochemical Genetics Division of Pediatrics, University of California at San Diego Medical Center · 9500 Gilman Drive, Mail Code 0609A, La Jolla, CA 92093-0609 · 619-534-4150

William J. Rhead · (Fatty Acid Oxidation) · Professor of Pediatrics, The University of Iowa College of Medicine · Attending Staff, The University of Iowa Hospitals & Clinics · 200 Hawkins Drive, Room 2606 JCP, Iowa City, IA 52242 · 319-356-2674

Charles Stanley · (Disorders of Fatty Acid Oxidation) · Professor of Pediatrics, University of Pennsylvania School of Medicine · The Children's Hospital of Philadelphia · Division of Endocrine and Diabetes, 34th Street and Civic Center Boulevard, Philadelphia, PA 19104 · 215-590-3420

Jess G. Thoene · (Cystinosis) · Professor of Pediatrics and Associate Professor of Biological Chemistry, The University of Michigan Medical School · Attending Pediatrician, C. S. Mott Children's Hospital; The University of Michigan Medical Center · 109 Observatory Street, 2612SPH1, Ann Arbor, MI 48109-2029 · 313-763-3427

David Valle · (Genetics, Hereditary Eye Diseases) · Professor of Pediatrics, and Professor of Medicine, Johns Hopkins University School of Medicine · Attending Staff, The Johns Hopkins Medical Institutions · 725 North Wolfe Street, PCTB 802, Baltimore, MD 21205 · 410-955-4260

Barry Wolf · (Biotinidase) · Professor of Human Genetics and Pediatrics, Virginia Commonwealth University, Medical College of Virginia · Medical College of Virginia Hospital · 1101 East Marshall Street, Room 11003, Richmond, VA 23298-0033 · 804-786-9632

NEONATAL-PERINATAL MEDICINE
(See also Obstetrics & Gynecology, Maternal & Fetal Medicine; Addiction Medicine, Addicted Pregnant Women)

Henrietta Salvilla Bada · Professor of Pediatrics and Obstetrics & Gynecology, The University of Tennessee at Memphis, College of Medicine · Regional Medical Center at Memphis · Newborn Center, 853 Jefferson Avenue, Memphis, TN 38163 · 901-528-5950

Eduardo Bancalari · Professor of Pediatrics, and Professor of Obstetrics & Gynecology, and Director, Division of Neonatology, University of Miami School of Medicine · Chief, Newborn Service, University of Miami-Jackson Memorial Medical Center · Department of Pediatrics, (R131), P.O. Box 016960, Miami, FL 33101 · 305-585-6380

Charles R. Bauer · Professor of Pediatrics, Obstetrics & Gynecology, and Psychology, University of Miami School of Medicine · Associate Director, Division of Neonatology, and Director of Developmental Evaluation & Intervention Program, Jackson Memorial Medical Center; University of Miami Hospital & Clinics · Mailman Center for Child Development (D-820), 1601 Northwest 12th Avenue, P.O. Box 016960, Miami, FL 33101 · 305-547-5808

Elizabeth Ruth Brown · (Addicted Pregnant Women) · Associate Professor of Pediatrics, Boston University School of Medicine · Director of Neonatology, Boston City Hospital · 818 Harrison Avenue, Maternity 2, Boston, MA 02118 · 617-534-5461

George Cassady · Clinical Professor of Pediatrics, University of California, San Francisco School of Medicine · Chairman, Department of Pediatrics, California Pacific Medical Center · 3700 California Street, San Francisco, CA 94118 · 415-750-6171

Ira J. Chasnoff · (Addicted Pregnant Women) · President, National Association for Perinatal Addiction Research & Education, and Associate Professor of Pediatrics & Psychiatry, Northwestern University Medical School · Children's Memorial Hospital · 11 East Hubbard Street, Suite 200, Chicago, IL 60611 · 312-329-2512

Robert B. Cotton · Professor of Pediatrics, Vanderbilt University School of Medicine · Director, Division of Neonatology, and Chief of Nurseries, Vanderbilt University Medical Center · A-016 Medical Center North, Nashville, TN 37232-2370 · 615-322-2823

Avroy Arnold Fanaroff · Professor, Department of Pediatrics, Case Western Reserve University School of Medicine · Director, Division of Neonatology, Rainbow Babies & Childrens Hospital · 2074 Abington Road, Cleveland, OH 44106 · 216-844-3387

Loretta P. Finnegan · (Addicted Pregnant Women and Their Children) · Professor of Pediatrics, Psychiatry and Human Behavior, Jefferson Medical College of Thomas Jefferson University · Senior Advisor on Women's Issues, National Institute on Drug Abuse · 5600 Fishers Lane, Rockwell 2, Suite 615, Rockville, MD 20857 · 301-443-2158

Sheldon Bernarr Korones · Professor of Pediatrics & Obstetrics & Gynecology, The University of Tennessee, Memphis, College of Medicine · Regional Medical Center at Memphis · 853 Jefferson Avenue, Memphis, TN 38103 · 901-528-5950

James A. Lemons · The Hugh McK. Landon Professor of Pediatrics, Indiana University School of Medicine · Director, Section of Neonatal-Perinatal Medicine, Indiana University Medical Center · 702 Barnhill Drive, Room RK208, Indianapolis, IN 46202 · 317-274-4716

Jerold F. Lucey · Professor, Department of Pediatrics, University of Vermont School of Medicine · Chief, Newborn Services, Medical Center Hospital of Vermont · Pediatrics Editorial Office, McClure 718, 111 Colchester Avenue, Burlington, VT 05401 · 802-862-8778

M. Jeffrey Maisels · Clinical Professor of Pediatrics and Communicable Diseases, The University of Michigan Medical School · Chairman, Department of Pediatrics, William Beaumont Hospital · 3601 West Thirteen Mile Road, Royal Oak, MI 48073 · 313-551-0412

William Oh · Professor and Chairman of Pediatrics, Brown University School of Medicine · Pediatrician-in-Chief, Rhode Island Hospital; Women & Infants Hospital · 101 Dudley Street, Providence, RI 02905 · 401-274-5983

Enrique M. Ostrea · Professor of Pediatrics, Wayne State University Medical Center · Chief of Pediatrics, Hutzel Hospital · 4707 Saint Antonie Boulevard, Detroit, MI 48201 · 313-745-7231

Lu-Ann Papile · Professor of Pediatrics, and Professor of Obstetrics & Gynecology, The University of New Mexico School of Medicine · The University Hospital ·

Department of Pediatrics, ACC3 West, Albuquerque, NM 87131-5311 · 505-272-3967

Rosita Stephan Pildes · Professor and Interim Chairman, Department of Pediatrics, University of Health Sciences, The Chicago Medical School · Acting Chairman, Department of Pediatrics, and Chairman, Division of Neonatology, Cook County Children's Hospital · 700 South Wood, Third Floor, Chicago, IL 60612 · 312-633-6545

David K. Stevenson · Professor of Pediatrics and Chief, Division of Neonatal and Development Medicine, Stanford University School of Medicine · Director of Newborn Nurseries, Stanford University Hospital; Lucile Salter Packard Children's Hospital at Stanford · 750 Welch Road, Suite 315, Palo Alto, CA 94304 · 415-723-5711

PEDIATRIC ALLERGY & IMMUNOLOGY

Oscar L. Frick · (Allergy) · Professor of Pediatrics, University of California at San Francisco School of Medicine · Director, Allergy & Immunology Research & Training, University of California at San Francisco Medical Center · 505 Parnassus Avenue, Box 0546, San Francisco, CA 94143-0546 · 415-476-3148

Andrew B. Murray · (Asthma) · Professor of Pediatrics, The University of British Columbia · Head, Allergy Division, Children's Hospital · 4480 Oak Street, Room 1C32, Vancouver, British Columbia V6H 3V4 · 604-875-2345 x7103

Savita G. Pahwa · (Immunodeficiency) · Professor of Pediatrics, Cornell University Medical College · Chief, Division of Allergy/Immunology, Department of Pediatrics, North Shore University Hospital · Research Building, 350 Community Drive, Third Floor, Manhasset, NY 11030 · 516-562-4641

Robert H. Schwartz · (Asthma, Cow's Milk Allergy) · Professor of Pediatrics and Medicine, University of Rochester School of Medicine & Dentistry · Director of Pediatric Allergy, Strong Memorial Hospital, University of Rochester Medical Center · 919 Westfall Road, Rochester, NY 14618 · 716-442-0150

Jay E. Selcow · (Asthma) · Associate Clinical Professor, Department of Pediatrics, University of Connecticut School of Medicine · Senior Staff, Department of Pediatrics, Hartford Hospital · 836 Farmington Avenue, Suite 207, West Hartford, CT 06119 · 203-232-9911

Frances Estelle Reed Simons · Professor and Head, Section of Allergy & Clinical Immunology, and Deputy Chairman, Department of Pediatrics & Child Health, University of Manitoba School of Medicine · Children's Hospital of Winnipeg · Children's Hospital, 40 Sherbrook Street, Room AE101, Winnipeg, Manitoba R3A 1S1 · 204-787-2440

Ricardo U. Sorensen · (Immunodeficiency) · Professor of Pediatrics, Louisiana State University School of Medicine · Children's Hospital of New Orleans · 1542 Tulane Avenue, New Orleans, LA 70112 · 504-568-2578

Jerry A. Winkelstein · (Immunodeficiency) · Eudowood Professor of Pediatrics, Johns Hopkins University School of Medicine · The Johns Hopkins Medical Institutions · 600 North Wolfe Street, CMSC 1103, Baltimore, MD 21205 · 410-955-5883

Robert S. Zeiger · (Allergy) · Clinical Associate Professor of Pediatrics, University of California at San Diego School of Medicine · Chief of Allergy, Kaiser-Permanente Medical Center · 7060 Clairemont Mesa Boulevard, San Diego, CA 92111 619-268-5408

PEDIATRIC & ADOLESCENT GYNECOLOGY
(See also Obstetrics & Gynecology, Pediatric & Adolescent Gynecology)

S. Jean Emans · Associate Professor of Pediatrics, Harvard Medical School · Associate Chief, Division of Adolescent/Young Adult Medicine, Children's Hospital · 300 Longwood Avenue, Boston, MA 02115 · 617-735-6000

PEDIATRIC CARDIOLOGY

D. Woodrow Benson, Jr. · (General, Electrophysiology) · Professor of Pediatrics, Northwestern University Medical School · Head, Division of Cardiology, The Children's Memorial Hospital · The Children's Memorial Hospital, #21, 2300 Children's Plaza, Chicago, IL 60614 · 312-880-4367

Fredrick Z. Bierman · (Echocardiography) · Associate Professor of Pediatrics, Albert Einstein College of Medicine · Chief, Pediatric Cardiology, Long Island Jewish Medical Center, and Schneider Children's Hospital · New Hyde Park, NY 11042 · 718-470-7350

Edward B. Clark · (General) · Professor of Pediatrics, University of Rochester School of Medicine & Dentistry · Chief of Pediatric Cardiology, Strong Memorial Hospital, University of Rochester Medical Center · 601 Elmwood Avenue, Box 631, Rochester, NY 14642 · 716-275-4661

Macdonald Dick II · (Electrophysiology) · Professor of Pediatrics, The University of Michigan Medical School · Director of Pediatric Clinical Electrophysiology, C.S. Mott Children's Hospital, The University of Michigan Medical Center · 1500 East Medical Center Drive, F-1310, Box 0204, Ann Arbor, MI 48109-0204 · 313-936-7418

David J. Driscoll · Professor of Pediatrics, Mayo Medical School · Head, Section of Pediatric Cardiology, Mayo Clinic · 200 First Street SW, Rochester, MN 55905 507-284-3372

Ann Dunnigan · (Electrophysiology) · Associate Professor of Pediatrics, University of Minnesota School of Medicine · University of Minnesota Hospital & Clinics 420 Delaware Street SE, Box 94, Minneapolis, MN 55455 · 612-626-2755

David E. Fixler · (General) · Professor of Pediatrics, The University of Texas Southwestern Medical Center at Dallas · Director of Cardiology, Children's Medical Center of Dallas · 1935 Motor Street, Cardiology, Dallas, TX 75235 · 214-920-2333

Michael David Freed · (General) · Associate Professor of Pediatrics, Harvard Medical School · Chief, Inpatient Cardiovascular Service, Children's Hospital · 300 Longwood Avenue, Boston, MA 02115 · 617-735-6276

William F. Friedman · (General) · J. H. Nicholson Professor of Pediatrics (Cardiology) and Executive Chairman, Department of Pediatrics, University of California at Los Angeles School of Medicine · University of California at Los Angeles Medical Center · 10833 LeConte Avenue, Room 22-412, Los Angeles, CA 90024-1752 · 213-206-6327

Arthur Garson, Jr. · (General, Electrophysiology, Pacemakers) · Professor of Pediatrics and Medicine, Baylor College of Medicine · Chief of Pediatric Cardiology, Texas Children's Hospital · 6621 Fannin Street, Houston, TX 77030 · 713-770-5600

Henry Gelband · (Electrophysiology) · Professor of Pediatrics (Cardiology), and Professor of Pharmacology, University of Miami School of Medicine · Director, Pediatric Cardiology, University of Miami-Jackson Memorial Medical Center · 1611 Northwest 12th Avenue, P.O. Box 016960 (R-76), Miami, FL 33101 · 305-585-6659

Welton M. Gersony · (General) · Professor of Pediatrics, College of Physicians & Surgeons of Columbia University · Attending Pediatrician, and Director, Pediatric Cardiology, Columbia-Presbyterian Medical Center, Babies Hospital · 3959 Broadway, Room 102A, New York, NY 10032 · 212-305-8509

Ira H. Gessner · (General) · Eminent Scholar and Professor of Pediatrics, University of Florida College of Medicine · Shands Hospital at the University of Florida · Department of Pediatrics, University of Florida College of Medicine, P.O. Box 100296, Gainesville, FL 32610 · 904-392-6431

Paul C. Gillette · (Electrophysiology, Pacemakers) · Professor & Director of Pediatric Cardiology, and Professor of Surgery, Medical University of South Carolina · Director, Division of Pediatric Cardiology, Medical University of South Carolina Hospital · Children's Hospital, 171 Ashley Avenue, Charleston, SC 29425-0682 · 803-792-3287

Thomas P. Graham, Jr. · (General) · Professor of Pediatrics, Vanderbilt University School of Medicine · Director of Pediatric Cardiology, Vanderbilt University Medical Center · Medical Center North, 1161 Twenty-First Avenue South, Room P2217, Nashville, TN 37232 · 615- 322-7447

Howard P. Gutgesell · (Echocardiography) · Director, Pediatric Cardiology, University of Virginia School of Medicine · University of Virginia Health Sciences/ Children's Medical Center · Box 386, Charlottesville, VA 22908 · 804-924-2486

William E. Hellenbrand · (Interventional Catheterization) · Professor of Pediatrics & Diagnostic Imaging, Yale University School of Medicine · Yale-New Haven Hospital · 333 Cedar Street, New Haven, CT 06510 · 203-785-2022

Julien I. E. Hoffman · (General) · Professor of Pediatrics and Senior Staff Member, Cardiovascular Research Institute, University of California at San Francisco School of Medicine · University of California at San Francisco Medical Center; California Campus of California Pacific Medical Center · 505 Parnassus Avenue, Room HSE-1403, Box 0544, San Francisco, CA 94143 · 415-476-9313

Charles Kleinman · (Fetal Cardiology, Echocardiography) · Professor of Pediatrics, Yale University School of Medicine · Yale-New Haven Hospital · 333 Cedar Street, New Haven, CT 06510 · 203-785-2022

Ronald M. Lauer · (Preventive Cardiology) · Professor of Pediatrics and Preventive Medicine, and Director, Division of Pediatric Cardiology, The University of Iowa College of Medicine · The University of Iowa Hospitals & Clinics · Iowa City, IA 52242 · 319-356-2839

James E. Lock · (Interventional Catheterization) · Associate Professor of Pediatrics, Harvard Medical School · Chief, Clinical Cardiology, Children's Hospital · 300 Longwood Avenue, Boston, MA 02115 · 617-735-7313

Douglas D. Mair · (General) · Professor of Pediatrics, Mayo Medical School · Co-Director, Cardiac Catheterization Laboratory, Mayo Clinic · 200 First Street, SW, Rochester, MN 55905 · 507-284-3351

Gerard Robert Martin · (Fetal Cardiology) · Associate Professor of Pediatrics, The George Washington University School of Medicine · Director of Echocardiography, Children's National Medical Center · 111 Michigan Avenue NW, Washington, DC 20010 · 202-745-2090

Charles Edward Mullins · (Interventional Catheterization) · Professor of Clinical Pediatrics, Baylor College of Medicine · Director, Cardiac Catheterization Laboratory, and Associate Director of Pediatric Cardiology, Texas Children's Hospital 6621 Fannin Street, Houston, TX 77030 · 713-770-5901

Alexander S. Nadas · (General) · Senior Associate in Cardiology, and Professor of Pediatrics Emeritus, Harvard Medical School · Chief Emeritus in Cardiology, Children's Hospital · 300 Longwood Avenue, Hunnewell 2, Boston, MA 02115 · 617-735-8211

Jane W. Newburger · (Preventive Cardiology, Kawasaki Disease) · Associate Professor of Pediatrics, Harvard Medical School · Senior Associate in Cardiology, Children's Hospital · 300 Longwood Avenue, Boston, MA 02115 · 617-735-6276

Arthur S. Pickoff · (General) · Professor of Pediatrics and Director, Section of Cardiology, Tulane University School of Medicine · Tulane University Medical Center · 1415 Tulane Avenue, Room 4924, New Orleans, LA 70112-2699 · 504-588-5012

William W. Pinsky · (General) · Professor of Pediatrics, Wayne State University School of Medicine · Chief of Cardiology and Vice-Chairman, Department of Pediatrics, Children's Hospital of Michigan · 3901 Beaubien Boulevard, Detroit, MI 48201 · 313-745-5831

Samuel Beryl Ritter · (Echocardiography) · Associate Professor of Pediatrics & Radiology, Mt. Sinai School of Medicine · Associate Director of Pediatric Cardiology, and Chief, Non-invasive Cardiology, Mt. Sinai Medical Center · One Gustave L. Levy Place, Pediatric Cardiology, Box 1201, New York, NY 10029 · 212-241-8662

Albert P. Rocchini · (General, Interventional Catheterization) · Professor of Pediatrics, and Director of Pediatric Cardiology, The Rueben/Bentson Chair in Pediatric Cardiology, University of Minnesota School of Medicine · Variety Club Children's Hospital; University of Minnesota Hospital & Clinics · 420 Delaware Street SE, Box 94 UMHC, Minneapolis, MN 55455 · 612-626-2755

Amnon Rosenthal · (General) · Professor and Associate Chair, Department of Pediatrics, The University of Michigan Medical School · Director of Pediatric Cardiology, C.S. Mott Children's Hospital, The University of Michigan Medical Center · 1500 East Medical Center Drive, Mott F-1310, Ann Arbor, MI 48109 · 313-936-8993

Abraham M. Rudolph · (General, Fetal Physiology) · Professor of Pediatrics, and Professor of Obstetrics, Gynecology & Reproductive Sciences, University of California at San Francisco School of Medicine · Director of Pediatric Cardiology, and Senior Staff Member, Cardiovascular Research Institute, University of California at San Francisco Medical Center · 505 Parnassus Avenue, HSE1403, Box 0544, San Francisco, CA 94143 · 415-476-1373

David J. Sahn · (Echocardiography, Fetal Cardiac Diagnosis) · Professor of Pediatrics and Radiology, University of California, San Diego School of Medicine · Director of Pediatric Cardiology, University of California, San Diego Medical Center · 225 Dickinson Street, 8445, San Diego, CA 92103 · 619-543-3820

Stephen P. Sanders · (Echocardiography) · Senior Associate of Cardiology, and Director, Cardiac Noninvasive Laboratory, Department of Cardiology, Children's Hospital · 300 Longwood Avenue, Boston, MA 02115 · 617-735-7893

Norman H. Silverman · (Echocardiography) · Professor of Pediatrics and Radiology (Cardiology), University of California at San Francisco School of Medicine · Director, Pediatric Echocardiography Laboratory, University of California at San Francisco Medical Center · 505 Parnassus Avenue, Room M-342, San Francisco, CA 94143 · 415-476-5887

A. Rebecca Snider · (Echocardiography) · Professor of Pediatrics, The University of Michigan Medical School · C.S. Mott Children's Hospital, The University of Michigan Medical Center · 1500 East Medical Center Drive, Box 0204, Ann Arbor, MI 48109-0204 · 313-764-3718

Paul Stanger · (General, Interventional Catheterization) · Professor of Pediatrics (Cardiology), University of California, San Francisco School of Medicine · Director of Pediatric Cardiac Catheterization Laboratory, University of California, San Francisco Medical Center · Pediatric Cardiology Room 344C, Third and Parnassus, San Francisco, CA 94143-0110 · 415-476-1040

William Bryan Strong · (Preventive Cardiology) · Leon Henri Charbonnier Professor of Pediatrics, and Chief, Section of Pediatric Cardiology, Medical College of Georgia; Director, Georgia Institute for the Prevention of Human Disease & Accidents · 1120 Fifteenth Street, Room BA A800W, Augusta, GA 30912-3710 · 404-721-2336

Norman S. Talner · (Diagnostic Imaging) · Professor of Pediatrics, Yale University School of Medicine · Professor Pediatrics & Diagnostic Imaging, Yale-New Haven Hospital · 333 Cedar Street, New Haven, CT 06510 · 203-785-2022

Victoria L. Vetter · (Electrophysiology) · Associate Professor of Pediatrics, University of Pennsylvania School of Medicine · Director, Electrophysiology & Electrocardiography Laboratories, The Children's Hospital of Philadelphia · Division of Cardiology, 34th and Civic Center Boulevard, Philadelphia, PA 19104 · 215-590-3529

Roberta Gay Williams · (Echocardiography) · Professor of Pediatrics, University of California at Los Angeles School of Medicine · Chief, Division of Cardiology, University of California at Los Angeles Center for Health Sciences · Marion Davies Childrens Center, 10833 LeConte Avenue, B2-427, Los Angeles, CA 90024 · 310-825-5085

Grace S. Wolff · (Electrophysiology) · Professor of Pediatrics, University of Miami School of Medicine · Director of Pediatric Clinical Electrophysiology, University of Miami-Jackson Memorial Medical Center · 1611 Northwest 12th Avenue, Room 5043, P.O. Box 016960 (R-76), Miami, FL 33101 · 305-585-6681

J. R. Zuberbuhler · (General) · Professor of Pediatrics, University of Pittsburgh School of Medicine · Director, Division of Cardiology, Children's Hospital of Pittsburgh · One Children's Plaza, 3705 Fifth Avenue, Pittsburgh, PA 15213 · 412-692-5540

PEDIATRIC CRITICAL CARE

Robert K. Crone · Professor of Anesthesiology and Pediatrics, University of Washington School of Medicine · Director of Anesthesiology, Children's Hospital & Medical Center · 4800 Sand Point Way NE, Seattle, WA 98105 · 206-526-2052

J. Michael Dean · Associate Professor of Pediatrics, University of Utah School of Medicine · Director, Pediatric Intensive Care Unit, Primary Children's Medical Center · 100 North Medical Drive, Salt Lake City, UT 84113 · 801-588-3280

John J. Downes · Professor of Anesthesia & Pediatrics, University of Pennsylvania School of Medicine · Anesthesiologist-in-Chief, and Director, Department of Anesthesiology & Critical Care Medicine, The Children's Hospital of Philadelphia · 34th and Civic Center Boulevard, Suite 4330, Philadelphia PA 19104 · 215-590-1863

Alan I. Fields · Professor of Anesthesiology; and Associate Professor of Pediatrics, The George Washington University School of Medicine · Associate Director, Department of Critical Care Medicine, Children's National Medical Center · 111 Michigan Avenue, Washington, DC 20010 · 202-745-5107

Bradley P. Fuhrman · Professor of Pediatrics, State University of New York Health Science Center at Buffalo · Chief of Pediatric Critical Care, Children's Hospital of Buffalo · 219 Bryant Street, Buffalo, NY 14222 · 716-878-7442

Thomas P. Green · Professor of Pediatrics, University of Minnesota School of Medicine · Director, Pediatric Critical Care Medicine, University of Minnesota Hospital an&d Clinics · 420 Delaware Street SE, Box 737 UMHC, Minneapolis, MN 55455 · 612-626-2916

George Gregory · Professor, Department of Pediatrics & Anesthesia, University of California at San Francisco School of Medicine · University of California at San Francisco Medical Center · 521 Parnassus Avenue, San Francisco, CA 94143-0648 415-476-4887

Peter R. Holbrook · Professor of Anesthesiology, Child Health & Development, The George Washington University School of Medicine · Chairman, Department of Critical Care Medicine, Children's National Medical Center · 111 Michigan Avenue, NW, Washington, DC 20010-2970 · 202-745-2131

Larry S. Jefferson · Assistant Professor of Pediatrics, and Head, Critical Care Section, Baylor College of Medicine · Medical Director, Pediatric Intensive Care Unit, Texas Children's Hospital · 6621 Fannin Street, Suite 440, MC2-3450, Houston, TX 77030 · 713-770-6232

Patrick M. Kochanek · Associate Professor of Anesthesiology/Critical Care Medicine and Pediatrics, University of Pittsburgh School of Medicine · Associate Director of Pediatric Intensive Care Unit, Children's Hospital of Pittsburgh · 3705 Fifth Avenue, Room 6840, Pittsburgh, PA 15213 · 412-692-5164

Daniel L. Levin · Professor of Pediatrics, The University of Texas Southwestern Medical Center at Dallas · Medical Director, Pediatric Intensive Care, Children's Medical Center of Dallas · 1935 Motor Street, Dallas, TX 75235 · 214-920-2360

George Lister · Professor of Pediatrics and Anesthesiology, Yale University School of Medicine · Director, Pediatric Intensive Care Unit, Yale-New Haven Hospital 333 Cedar Street, New Haven, CT 06510 · 203-785-4651

P. Pearl O'Rourke · Associate Professor of Pediatrics and Anesthesiology, University of Washington School of Medicine · Director, Pediatric Intensive Care Unit, Children's Hospital & Medical Center · 4800 Sand Point Way NE, CH35, Seattle, WA 98105 · 206-526-2170

Murray M. Pollack · Professor of Anesthesiology & Pediatrics, The George Washington University School of Medicine · Associate Director of Critical Care, Children's National Medical Center · 111 Michigan Avenue NW, Washington, DC 20010 · 202-745-2131

Russell C. Raphaely · Professor of Anesthesia & Pediatrics, University of Pennsylvania School of Medicine · Chief, Division of Critical Care Medicine, and Medical Director, Pediatric Intensive Care Unit, The Children's Hospital of Philadelphia · 34th Street and Civic Center Boulevard, Philadelphia, PA 19104 · 215-590-1872

Mark C. Rogers · Distinguished Faculty Professor and Chairman, Department of Anesthesiology & Critical Care Medicine, and Dean for Clinical Practice, Johns Hopkins University School of Medicine · The Johns Hopkins Medical Institutions 600 North Wolfe Street, Blalock 1415, Baltimore, MD 21205 · 410-955-8408

Fernando Stein · Assistant Professor of Pediatrics, Baylor College of Medicine · Medical Director, Progressive Care Unit, and Deputy Director, Pediatric Intensive Care, Texas Children's Hospital · Critical Care & Surgical Facility, 6621 Fannin Street, Suite 440, MC 2-3450, Houston, TX 77030-2399 · 713-770-1403

Ann E. Thompson · Associate Professor of Anesthesiology/Critical Care Medicine and Pediatrics, University of Pittsburgh School of Medicine · Director, Pediatric ICU & Director Critical Care Medicine Training Program, Children's Hospital of Pittsburgh · 3705 Fifth Avenue, Room 6840, Pittsburgh, PA 15213 · 412-692-5164

Jerry J. Zimmerman · Associate Professor of Pediatrics, University of Wisconsin-Madison School of Medicine · Director, Pediatric Critical Care Medicine Research & Fellowship Programs, University of Wisconsin Hospital & Clinics; University of Wisconsin Children's Hospital · 600 Highland Avenue, Room H4-470, Madison, WI 53792-4108 · 608-263-8537

PEDIATRIC DERMATOLOGY
(See also Dermatology, Pediatric Dermatology)

Bernard Alan Cohen · Associate Professor of Pediatrics & Dermatology, Johns Hopkins University School of Medicine · Director, Pediatric Dermatology, The Johns Hopkins Medical Institutions · 600 North Wolfe Street, Baltimore, MD 21205 · 410-955-2049

Ilona Frieden · Assistant Clinical Professor of Pediatrics in Dermatology, University of California at San Francisco School of Medicine · University of California at San Francisco Medical Center · Department of Dermatology, 400 Parnassus, Third Floor, Box 0316, San Francisco, CA 94143-0316 · 415-476-4239

Ronald C. Hansen · Professor, The University of Arizona College of Medicine · The University of Arizona Health Sciences Center · Section of Dermatology, 1501 North Campbell, Tucson, AZ 85724 · 602-626-7783

Paul Joseph Honig · Professor of Pediatrics & Dermatology, University of Pennsylvania School of Medicine · Director, Pediatric Dermatology, The Children's Hospital of Philadelphia · Department of Dermatology, 34th and Civic Center Boulevard, Philadelphia, PA 19104 · 215-590-2169

Sidney Hurwitz · Clinical Professor of Pediatrics & Dermatology, Yale University School of Medicine · Yale-New Haven Hospital, Hospital of St. Raphael · 2 Church Street South, New Haven, CT 06519 · 203-776-0600

Alvin H. Jacobs · Professor Emeritus of Dermatology, Stanford University School of Medicine · Lucile Salter Packard Children's Hospital at Stanford · Edwards Building, R-144, 300 Pasteur Drive, Stanford, CA 94305 · 415-723-6101

Alfred T. Lane · Associate Professor of Dermatology and Pediatrics, Stanford University School of Medicine · Director of Pediatric Dermatology, Stanford University Hospital; Lucile Salter Packard Children's Hospital at Stanford · 300 Pasteur Drive, Edwards Building R-144, Stanford CA 94305-5334 · 415-725-7022

Moise L. Levy · Assistant Professor of Dermatology and Pediatrics, Baylor College of Medicine · Chief, Pediatric Dermatology, Texas Children's Hospital · 6621 Fannin Street, Houston, TX 77030 · 713-770-3720

Anne Lucky · (Acne) · Children's Hospital Medical Center · 7691 Five Mile Road, Cincinnati, OH 45230 · 513-559-4215, 232-3332, 791-6161

Susan B. Mallory · Associate Professor of Dermatology and Pediatrics, Washington University School of Medicine · Director of Pediatric Dermatology, St. Louis Children's Hospital · 400 South Kingshighway Boulevard, Room 8E6, St. Louis, MO 63110 · 314-454-2714

Joseph McGuire · (Psoriasis) · Carl Herzog Professor of Dermatology and Pediatrics, Stanford University School of Medicine · Stanford University Hospital; Lucile Salter Packard Children's Hospital at Stanford · 300 Pasteur Drive, Edwards Building, R114, Stanford, CA 94305 · 415-725-5272

Joseph G. Morelli · (Birthmarks, Laser Surgery) · Assistant Professor of Dermatology and Pediatrics, University of Colorado School of Medicine · University Hospital · 4200 East Ninth Avenue, Room B153, Denver, CO 80262 · 303-372-1111

Amy S. Paller · Associate Professor of Pediatrics and Dermatology, Northwestern University Medical School · Head, Division of Dermatology, The Children's Memorial Hospital · 2300 Children's Plaza, Box 107, Chicago, IL 60614 · 312-880-4698

Neil S. Prose · (AIDS, General) · Duke University School of Medicine · Duke University Medical Center · Box 3252, DUMC, Durham, NC 27710 · 919-684-5146

Lawrence Schachner · Professor of Dermatology and Pediatrics, University of Miami School of Medicine · Director, Division of Pediatric Dermatology, University of Miami-Jackson Memorial Medical Center · P.O. Box 016250 (R-250), Miami, FL 33101 · 305-547-6742

Lawrence M. Solomon · Professor of Dermatology, The University of Illinois College of Medicine at Chicago · The University of Illinois Hospital · Box 6998, Chicago, IL 60680 · 312-996-6966

Mary K. Spraker · Associate Professor of Dermatology and Pediatrics, Emory University School of Medicine · Chief of Dermatology, Henrietta Egleston Hospital for Children; Emory University Affiliated Hospitals · 1365 Clifton Road, NE, Atlanta, GA 30322 · 404-248-3336

Oon Tian Tan · (Pediatric Laser Surgery) · Associate Professor of Pathology, Boston University School of Medicine · Director, Laser Research Laboratory, Boston City Hospital · 29 Commonwealth Avenue, Suite 101, Boston, MA 02116 617-424-8335

Walter W. Tunnessen, Jr. · Professor, Department of Pediatrics, University of Pennsylvania School of Medicine · Associate Chairman for Medical Education, The Children's Hospital of Philadelphia · 34th Street and Civic Center Boulevard, Suite 2143, Philadelphia, PA 19104 · 215-590-2438

Samuel Weinberg · Clinical Professor of Dermatology, New York University School of Medicine · Attending Staff, Dermatology, New York University Medical Center · 2035 Lakeville Road, New Hyde Park, NY 11040 · 516-352-6151

William L. Weston · Professor and Chairman, Department of Dermatology; and Professor of Pediatrics, University of Colorado School of Medicine · University of Colorado Health Sciences Center · 4200 East Ninth Avenue, Box E-153, Denver, CO 80262 · 303-372-1111

Mary L. Williams · (Keratinizing Disorders) · Associate Professor of Dermatology and Pediatrics, University of California at San Francisco School of Medicine · University of California at San Francisco Medical Center; San Francisco Veterans Administration Medical Center · 400 Parnassus Avenue, San Francisco, CA 94143-0316 · 415-476-4239

PEDIATRIC ENDOCRINOLOGY

Val Abbassi · (Growth Disorders) · Professor of Pediatrics, Georgetown University School of Medicine · Georgetown University Children's Medical Center · Pasquerilla Health Care Center, Second Floor, 3800 Reservoir Road, NW, Washington, DC 20007 · 202-687-8881

Thomas Aceto, Jr. · (General, Growth) · Chairman Emeritus and Professor of Pediatrics, St. Louis University School of Medicine · Pediatrician-in-Chief, Emeritus, Cardinal Glennon Children's Hospital · 1465 South Grand Boulevard, St. Louis, MO 63104 · 314-577-5648

Gilbert Paul August · (General, Growth) · Professor of Pediatrics, The George Washington University School of Medicine · Acting Chairman, Department of Endocrinology, Children's National Medical Center · 111 Michigan Avenue NW, Washington, DC 20010 · 202-745-2122

Lester Baker · (Diabetes) · Professor of Pediatrics, University of Pennsylvania School of Medicine · Director, Division of Endocrinology/Diabetes, The Children's Hospital of Philadelphia · Division of Endocrinology, 34th and Civic Center Boulevard, Philadelphia, PA 19104 · 215-590-3172

Dorothy J. Becker · (Diabetes) · Professor of Pediatrics, Department of Pediatrics, University of Pittsburgh School of Medicine · Children's Hospital of Pittsburgh · One Children's Place, 3705 Fifth Avenue, Pittsburgh, PA 15213 · 412-692-5170

Dennis M. Bier · (Diabetes, Growth Hormone, Nutrition) · Professor of Pediatrics & Medicine, Washington University School of Medicine · Co-Director, Pediatric Endocrinology & Metabolism Division, St. Louis Children's Hospital · 400 South Kingshighway Boulevard, St. Louis, MO 63110 · 314-362-8190

Robert M. Blizzard · (General, Growth, Growth Hormone, Sexual Development) Professor of Pediatrics, University of Virginia School of Medicine · University of Virginia Health Sciences Center · Box 386, Charlottesville, VA 22908 · 804-924-2760

Jo Anne Brasel · (General, Nutrition) · Professor of Pediatrics and Medicine, University of California, Los Angeles · Program Director of Clinical Study Center, and Chief, Division of Pediatric Endocrinology, Harbor-UCLA Medical Center · 1000 West Carson Street, Torrance, CA 90509 · 310-533-2503

Ian M. Burr · (General, Diabetes) · Professor and Chairman, Department of Pediatrics, Vanderbilt University School of Medicine · Medical Director, Children's Hospital of Vanderbilt University · 1161 Twenty-Second Avenue South, Room AA-0216, Medical Center North, Nashville, TN 37232-2574 · 615-322-3377

H. Peter Chase · (Diabetes) · Professor of Pediatrics, and Clinical Director of Barbara Davis Center for Childhood Diabetes, University of Colorado School of Medicine · University of Colorado Health Science Center; The Children's Hospital; Denver General Hospital · 4200 East Ninth Avenue, Box 140, Denver, CO 80262 · 303-270-7451

Steven D. Chernausek · (General) · Associate Professor of Pediatrics, University of Cincinnati College of Medicine · Associate Director, Division of Endocrinology, Children's Hospital Medical Center · Elland and Bethesda Avenues, Cincinnati, OH 45229 · 513-559-4744

George Panagiotis Chrousos · (Pediatric Neuroendocrinology) · Professor of Pediatrics, Georgetown University School of Medicine · Chief, Pediatric Endocrinology Section, National Institute on Child Development, National Institutes of Health · 9000 Rockville Pike, Building 10, Room 10N262, Bethesda, MD 20892 301-496-4686

William L. Clarke · (Diabetes) · Professor of Pediatrics, University of Virginia School of Medicine · University of Virginia Health Sciences Center · Box 386, Charlottesville, VA 22908 · 804-924-5897

Eleanor Colle · (Diabetes) · Professor of Pediatrics, McGill University · Endocrinologist, Montreal Children's Hospital · 2300 Tupper Street, Room E316, Montreal, Quebec H3H 1P3 · 514-934-4315

Felix A. Conte · (General, Growth, Sexual Development) · Professor of Pediatrics, University of California at San Francisco School of Medicine · University of California at San Francisco Medical Center · 505 Parnassus Avenue, Box 0434, San Francisco, CA 94143-0434 · 415-476-1016

John D. Crawford · (General) · Professor Emeritus, Harvard Medical School · Massachusetts General Hospital · Department of Pediatric Endocrinology, Fruit Street, Boston, MA 02114 · 617-726-2909

A. Joseph D'Ercole · (Growth) · Professor of Pediatrics, University of North Carolina School of Medicine · University of North Carolina Hospitals · 509 Burnett-Womack Building, Manning Drive, Campus Box 7220, Chapel Hill, NC 27599-7220 · 919-966-4435

William Dahms · (Diabetes) · Case Western Reserve University School of Medicine · Rainbow Babies & Childrens Hospital · Pediatric Endocrinology, 2075 Abington Road, Room 790, Cleveland, OH 44106 · 216-844-3661

Denis Daneman · (Diabetes) · Associate Professor of Pediatrics, University of Toronto School of Medicine · Staff Endocrinologist, The Hospital for Sick Children · 555 University Avenue, Suite 5110, Toronto, Ontario M5G 1X8 · 416-598-6217

Raphael R. David · (General, Sexual Development) · Professor of Pediatrics, New York University School of Medicine · Director of Pediatric Endocrinology, New York University Medical Center · Department of Pediatrics, 550 First Avenue, New York, NY 10016 · 212-263-6462

Angelo M. DiGeorge · (General) · Professor of Pediatrics, Temple University School of Medicine · St. Christopher's Hospital for Children · Erie Avenue at Front Street, Philadelphia, PA 19134-1095 · 215-427-5173

Allan L. Drash · (Diabetes) · Professor of Pediatrics, University of Pittsburgh School of Medicine · Children's Hospital of Pittsburgh · One Children's Place, 3705 Fifth Avenue, Pittsburgh, PA 15213 · 412-692-5170

Stephen C. Duck · (Diabetes) · Associate Professor of Pediatrics, Section of Endocrinology & Metabolism, Medical College of Wisconsin · Children's Hospital of Wisconsin · 8701 Watertown Plank Road, Suite 3056, Milwaukee, WI 53226 · 414-266-4640

Donnell D. Etzwiler · (Diabetes) · Clinical Professor of Pediatrics, and Clinical Professor of Family Practice & Community Medicine, University of Minnesota School of Medicine · Methodist Hospital, St. Louis Park, MN · International Diabetes Center, 5000 West 39th Street, Minneapolis, MN 55416 · 612-927-3393

Thomas P. Foley, Jr. · (General, Thyroid) · Professor of Pediatrics, University of Pittsburgh School of Medicine · Director, Division of Endocrinology, Metabolism & Diabetes Mellitus, Children's Hospital of Pittsburgh · 3705 Fifth Avenue, Pittsburgh, PA 15213-2583 · 412-692-5170

S. Douglas Frasier · (Growth) · Professor of Pediatrics, University of California at Los Angeles School of Medicine · Chief of Pediatrics, Los Angeles County Olive View Medical Center · 14445 Olive View Drive, Sylmar, CA 91342 · 818-364-3233

Joseph M. Gertner · (Mineral Metabolism) · Professor of Pediatrics, and Program Director of Children's Clinical Research Center, Cornell University Medical College · The New York Hospital-Cornell Medical Center · 535 East 68th Streeet, Room N236, New York, NY 10021 · 212-746-3455

Fredda Ginsberg-Fellner · (Diabetes) · Professor of Pediatrics, Mt. Sinai School of Medicine · Chief, Pediatric Endocrinology & Metabolism, Mt. Sinai Medical Center · One Gustave L. Levy Place, Box 1198, New York, NY 10029 · 212-241-6936

Francis H. Glorieux · (Mineral Metabolism) · Professor, Departments of Pediatrics, Surgery and Human Genetics, McGill University · Director of Research, Shriners Hospital · 1529 Cedar Avenue, Montreal, Quebec H3G 1A6 · 514-849-7685

David E. Goldstein · (Diabetes) · Professor of Pediatrics, Medicine and Pathology, University of Missouri · Director, Division of Pediatric Endocrinology/Diabetes, University of Missouri Hospital & Clinics · Department of Child Health, One Hospital Drive, Columbia, MO 65212 · 314-882-6979

Melvin M. Grumbach · (General, Developmental Biology, Growth) · Edward B. Shaw Professor of Pediatrics and Emeritus Chairman, Department of Pediatrics, University of California, San Francisco School of Medicine · Attending Physician, University of California, San Francisco Medical Center · Department of Pediatrics, 505 Parnassus Avenue, San Francisco, CA 94143-0106 · 415-476-2244

Stuart Handwerger · (General, Growth) · Director of Endocrinology, Children's Hospital Medical Center · Elland and Bethesda Avenues, Cincinnati, OH 45229 513-559-4744

Morey W. Haymond · (Metabolic Diseases, Diabetes, Glucose Metabolism) · Professor and Vice-Chairman, Department of Pediatrics, University of Florida · Medical Director, Nemours Children's Clinic · 807 Nira Street, Jacksonville, FL 32207 · 904-390-3646

Raymond Hintz · (General, Growth) · Chief of Endocrinology and Professor of Pediatrics, Stanford University School of Medicine · Stanford University Hospital; Lucile Salter Packard Children's Hospital at Stanford · Room S-322, Stanford, CA 94305 · 415-723-5791

Weillington Hung · (General) · Professor of Pediatrics, Division of Pediatric Endocrinology & Metabolism, Georgetown University School of Medicine · Georgetown University Children's Medical Center · Pasquerilla Health Care Center, Second Floor, 3800 Reservoir Road, NW, Washington, DC 20007 · 202-687-8881

Selna L. Kaplan · (Growth, Sexual Development) · Professor of Pediatrics, University of California, San Francisco School of Medicine · University of California, San Francisco Medical Center · Box 0434, San Francisco, CA 94143 · 415-476-1016

Michael Steven Kappy · (Diabetes) · Clinical Professor, Department of Pediatrics, The University of Arizona College of Medicine · Medical Director, Children's Health Center of St. Joseph's Hospital & Medical Center · 350 West Thomas Road, Phoenix, AZ 85013 · 602-285-3699

Francine R. Kaufman · (Diabetes) · Associate Professor of Pediatrics, University of Southern California School of Medicine · Pediatric Endocrinologist, Children's Hospital of Los Angeles · 4650 Sunset Boulevard, Los Angeles, CA 90027 · 213-660-2450

Robert P. Kelch · (Pubertal Development, Sexual Development) · Professor and Chairman, Department of Pediatrics & Communicable Diseases, The University of Michigan Medical School · Physician-in-Chief, C.S. Mott Children's Hospital; The University of Michigan Medical Center · 1500 East Medical Center Drive, D-3202, Box 0718, Ann Arbor, MI 48109-0718 · 313-764-5173

L. Lyndon Key, Jr. · (Mineral Metabolism) · Associate Professor of Pediatrics, Medical University of South Carolina · Division Director, Pediatric Endocrinology, Medical University of South Carolina Hospital · Children's Hospital, 171 Ashley Avenue, Charleston, SC 29425 · 803-792-6807

John Lindsey Kirkland · (General, Growth) · Professor of Pediatrics, Baylor College of Medicine · Texas Children's Hospital · Pediatric Endocrinology, One Baylor Plaza, Houston TX 77030 · 713-798-4793

Georgeanna Klingensmith · (General Endocrinology, Growth Problems, Diabetes) · Associate Professor of Pediatrics, University of Colorado School of Medicine The Children's Hospital · 1056 East 19th Avenue, B265, Denver, CO 80218 · 303-861-6627

Stephen Henry LaFranchi · (General, Thyroid) · Professor of Pediatrics, and Head, Pediatric Residency Program, and Head, Pediatric Endocrinology, Oregon Health Sciences University · 3181 Southwest Sam Jackson Park Road, Portland, OR 97201 · 503-494-8194

Peter A. Lee · (Pubertal Development, Sexual Development) · Professor of Pediatrics, University of Pittsburgh School of Medicine · Director, Clinical Research Center, Children's Hospital of Pittsburgh · 3705 Fifth Avenue, Pittsburgh, PA 15213 · 412-692-5177

Lynne Lipton Levitsky · (Diabetes) · Associate Professor of Pediatrics, Harvard Medical School · Chief, Pediatric Endocrinology Unit, Massachusetts General Hospital · 15 Parkman Street, Wang Building, Ambulatory Care Center, Room 709, Boston, MA 02114 · 617-726-2909

Barbara M. Lippe · (Growth, Sexual Development, Turner Syndrome) · Professor of Pediatrics, University of California, Los Angeles School of Medicine · Chief, Division of Pediatric Endocrinology, University of California, Los Angeles Center for Health Sciences · University of California, Los Angeles Medical Center, 10833 LeConte Avenue, 22-315, Los Angeles, CA 90024-1752 · 310-825-6389

Margaret Hilda MacGillivray · (Growth) · Professor of Pediatrics, State University of New York Health Science Center at Buffalo · Chief, Division of Pediatric Endocrinology & Diabetes, Children's Hospital of Buffalo · 219 Bryant Street, Buffalo, NY 14222 · 716-878-7588

John I. Malone · (Diabetes) · Professor of Pediatrics, University South Florida College of Medicine · Tampa General Hospital; All Childrens Hospital (St. Petersburg, FL) · 12901 Bruce B. Downs Boulevard, Box 15, Tampa, FL 33612 · 813-974-4360

Claude J. Migeon · (Adrenal, Sex Differentiation) · Professor of Pediatrics, Johns Hopkins University School of Medicine · Director, Pediatric Endocrine Clinic & Laboratories, The Johns Hopkins Medical Institutions · 600 North Wolfe Street, CMSC 3-110, Baltimore, MD 21205 · 410-955-3533

Wayne V. Moore · (Growth) · Professor of Pediatrics, University of Kansas School of Medicine · Director, Section of Pediatric Endocrinology, University of Kansas Medical Center · 39th and Rainbow Boulevard, Kansas City, KS 66103 · 913-588-6326

Maria I. New · (Sexual Development, Adrenogenital Syndrome, Hypertension) · Professor and Chairman, Department of Pediatrics, Cornell University Medical College · Pediatrician-in-Chief, The New York Hospital-Cornell Medical Center 525 East 68th Street, Room N236, New York, NY 10021 · 212-746-3450

Songya Pang · (Adrenal, Adrenogenital Syndrome) · Professor of Pediatrics, The University of Illinois College of Medicine at Chicago · Chief, Pediatric Endocrinology, The University of Illinois Hospital; Michael Reese Hospital · 840 South Wood Street, MC856, Chicago, IL 60612 · 312-996-1795

Elsa P. Paulsen · (Diabetes) · Clinical Associate, Department of Pediatrics, University of Virginia School of Medicine · Martha Jefferson Hospital; University of Virginia Health Sciences Center · 316 Tenth Street NE, Charlottesville, VA 22902 804-293-8207, 293-7121

Leslie P. Plotnick · (Diabetes) · Associate Professor of Pediatrics, Pediatric Endocrine Division, Johns Hopkins University School of Medicine · Director, Pediatric Diabetes Clinic, The Johns Hopkins Medical Institutions · 600 North Wolfe Street, CMSC 3-110, Baltimore, MD 21205 · 410-955-6463

Edward O. Reiter · (Sexual Development, Growth Disorders) · Professor of Pediatrics, Tufts University School of Medicine · Chairman, Department of Pediatrics, Baystate Medical Center · 759 Chestnut Street, Springfield, MA 01199 · 413-784-5060

Alan D. Rogol · (Growth, Growth Hormone, Sexual Development) · Professor of Pediatrics & Pharmacology, and Chief, Division of Endocrinology & Metabolism, University of Virginia School of Medicine · University of Virginia Health Sciences Center · Building MR4, Room 3037, Charlottesville, VA 22908 · 804-924-5895

Allen W. Root · (General, Sexual Development, Growth, Mineral Metabolism, Pituitary) · Professor of Pediatrics and Biochemistry, University South Florida College of Medicine · Chief, Department of Pediatric Endocrinology, All Children's Hospital; Tampa General Hospital · Children's Hospital, 801 Sixth Street South, St. Petersburg, FL 33731 · 813-892-4237

Arlen L. Rosenbloom · (Diabetes) · Professor of Pediatrics, University of Florida College of Medicine · Chief, Division of Endocrinology, Shands Hospital at the University of Florida · 1600 Southwest Archer Road, Room HG518, P.O. Box 100296, Gainesville, FL 32610 · 904-392-2708

Ron G. Rosenfeld · (Growth, Growth Hormone, Sexual Development, Turner Syndrome) · Professor of Pediatric Endocrinology, Stanford University School of Medicine · Stanford University Hospital; Lucille Salter Packard Children's Hospital at Stanford · Room S-322, Stanford, CA 94305 · 415-723-5791

Robert L. Rosenfield · (Growth, Development) · Professor of Pediatrics and Medicine, The University of Chicago, Pritzker School of Medicine · Head, Section of Pediatric Endocrinology, University of Chicago Medical Center · 5841 South Maryland Avenue, Box 118, Chicago, IL 60637-1470 · 312-702-6432

Paul Saenger · (General, Sexual Development) · Professor of Pediatrics, Albert Einstein College of Medicine · Head, Division of Pediatric Endocrinology, Montefiore Medical Center · 111 East 210th Street, Bronx, NY 10467 · 212-920-4664

Julio V. Santiago · (Diabetes) · Professor of Pediatrics, Washington University School of Medicine · Director of Diabetes Research & Training Center, St. Louis Children's Hospital; Barnes Hospital · 400 South Kingshighway Boulevard, Room 1002, St. Louis, MO 63110 · 314-454-6046

Janet Silverstein · (Diabetes) · Professor of Pediatrics, University of Florida College of Medicine · Director, Diabetes Center, Shands Hospital at the University of Florida · 1600 Southwest Archer Road, Room HD517, P.O. Box 100296, Gainesville, FL 32610 · 904-392-2708

Juan F. Sotos · (General) · Professor, Department of Pediatrics, Ohio State University College of Medicine · Section Chief, Pediatric Endocrinology & Metabolism, Columbus Children's Hospital · 700 Children's Drive, Room C403, Columbus, OH 43205 · 614-461-2025

Mark A. Sperling · (Diabetes) · Professor & Chairman, Department of Pediatrics, University of Pittsburgh School of Medicine · Pediatrician-in-Chief, Children's Hospital of Pittsburgh · 3705 Fifth Avenue, Pittsburgh, PA 15213 · 412-692-5105

Dennis M. Styne · (Sexual Development and Puberty, Disorders of the Pituitary Gland) · Professor and Chair, Department of Pediatrics, University of California at Davis School of Medicine · Professor and Chair, Department of Pediatrics, University of California at Davis Medical Center · 2516 Stockton Boulevard, Sacramento, CA 95817 · 916-734-3745

William V. Tamborlane · (Diabetes) · Professor of Pediatrics, Yale University School of Medicine · Pediatric Endocrinologist, Yale-New Haven Hospital · 330 Cedar Street,LMP3103, New Haven, CT 06510-8064 · 203-785-4648

Louis E. Underwood · (Growth, Sexual Development) · Professor of Pediatrics and Chief, Division of Pediatric Endocrinology, University of North Carolina School of Medicine · University of North Carolina Hospitals · 509 Burnett-Womack Building, Manning Drive, Campus Box 7220, Chapel Hill, NC 27599-7220 · 919-966-4435

Judson J. Van Wyk · (General, Growth, Growth Factors) · Kenan Professor of Pediatrics, University of North Carolina School of Medicine · Attending Physician, North Carolina Children's Hospital · 509 Burnett-Womack Building, Manning Drive, Campus Box 7220, Chapel Hill, NC 27599-7220 · 919-966-4435

Samuel M. Wentworth · (Diabetes) · Methodist Hospital; Hendricks Community Hospital · 1300 East Main Street, Indianapolis, IN 46122 · 317-745-7128

Neil H. White · (Diabetes) · Associate Professor of Pediatrics, Washington University School of Medicine · St. Louis Children's Hospital · 400 South Kingshighway Boulevard, St. Louis, MO 63110 · 314-454-6051

Joseph Wolfsdorf · (Diabetes, Disorders of Carbohydrate Metabolism) · Assistant Professor of Pediatrics, Harvard Medical School · Chief of Pediatrics, Joslin Diabetes Center; Director, Diabetes Program, and Associate in Endocrinology, The Children's Hospital, Boston, New England Deaconess Hospital · One Joslin Place, Boston, MA 02215 · 617-732-2603

Donald Zimmerman · (General) · Associate Professor of Pediatrics, Mayo Medical School · Mayo Clinic · 200 First Street, SW, Rochester MN 55905 · 507-284-2511

PEDIATRIC GASTROENTEROLOGY

Daniel B. Caplan · (Cystic Fibrosis) · Professor of Pediatrics, and Director, Division of Gastroenterology, Cystic Fibrosis, & Nutrition, Emory University School of Medicine · Director, Division of Digestive Diseases, Egleston Hospital for Children · 2040 Ridgewood Drive NE, Atlanta, GA 30322 · 404-727-5728

Dennis L. Christie · Associate Professor of Pediatrics, University of Washington School of Medicine · Head, Division of Pediatric Gastroenterology, Children's Hospital & Medical Center · 4800 Sand Point Way NE, Seattle, WA 98105 · 206-526-2521

Fredric Daum · Associate Professor of Clinical Pediatrics, Cornell University Medical College · North Shore University Hospital · 300 Community Drive, New York, NY 10030 · 516-562-4642

George D. Ferry · (Inflammatory Bowel Disease) · Associate Professor of Clinical Pediatrics, Baylor College of Medicine · Chief, Gastroenterology Ambulatory Service, Texas Children's Hospital · 6621 Fannin Street, Houston, TX 77030 · 713-770-2940

Richard J. Grand · (Nutrition, Cystic Fibrosis, Inflammatory Bowel Disease, Wilson's Disease) · Professor of Pediatrics, Tufts University School of Medicine · Chief of Pediatric Gastroenterology and Nutrition, New England Medical Center Hospitals; The Boston Floating Hospital for Infants and Children · 750 Washington Street, Box 213, Boston, MA 02111 · 617-956-0130

Melvin B. Heyman · (Nutrition) · Associate Professor of Pediatrics, University of California at San Francisco School of Medicine · Chief of Pediatric Gastroenterology and Nutrition, University of California at San Francisco Medical Center · 505 Parnassus Avenue, Room M-680; Box 0136, San Francisco, CA 94143 · 415-476-5892

James P. Keating · Professor of Pediatrics, Washington University School of Medicine · Director, Pediatric Residency Program, St. Louis Children's Hospital · 400 South Kingshighway Boulevard, St. Louis, MO 63110 · 314-454-6006

Barbara S. Kirschner · Professor of Pediatrics and Medicine, University of Chicago, Pritzker School of Medicine · Wyler Children's Hospital · 5841 South Maryland Avenue, Box 107, Chicago, IL 60637-1470 · 312-702-6152

Alan M. Lake · Associate Professor of Pediatrics, Johns Hopkins University School of Medicine · The Johns Hopkins Medical Institutions · 10807 Falls Road, Suite 200, Lutherville, MD 21093 · 301-321-9393

John D. Lloyd-Still · (Cystic Fibrosis) · Professor of Pediatrics, Northwestern University Medical School · Head, Division of Gastroenterology, The Children's Memorial Hospital · 2300 Children's Plaza, Box 65, Chicago, IL 60614 · 312-880-4354

Claude C. Roy · (Cystic Fibrosis) · Professor and Chairman of Pediatrics, University of Montreal · St. Justine Hospital · 3175 Chemin St. Catherine Road, Montreal, Quebec H3T 1C5 · 514-345-4931

Arnold Silverman · (Liver Disease) · Professor of Pediatrics, University of Colorado School of Medicine · Director of Pediatrics, Denver General Hospital · 777 Bannock Street, Denver, CO 80204 · 303-893-7781

John B. Watkins · (Nutrition, Pediatric Liver Disease) · Professor of Pediatrics, Washington University School of Medicine · Director of Ambulatory Division, and Medical Director of Ambulatory Services, St. Louis Children's Hospital · 400 South Kingshighway Boulevard, St. Louis, MO 63110 · 314-454-6299

PEDIATRIC HEMATOLOGY-ONCOLOGY

W. Archie Bleyer · (Pediatric Neuroncology, Pediatric Leukemia, New Agent Trials) · Professor of Pediatrics, and Mosbacher Chair in Pediatrics, The University of Texas Medical School at Houston · Head, Division of Pediatrics, and Chairman, Department of Pediatrics, The University of Texas MD Anderson Cancer Center · 1515 Holcombe Boulevard, Houston, TX 77030 · 713-792-6603

George R. Buchanan · (Pediatric Leukemia) · Professor of Pediatrics, The University of Texas Southwestern Medical Center at Dallas · Director of Hematology-Oncology, Children's Medical Center of Dallas · 5323 Harry Hines Boulevard, Dallas, TX 75235 · 214-688-3388

James J. Casper · (Pediatric Bone Marrow Transplantation) · Professor of Pediatrics, Medical College of Wisconsin · Children's Hospital of Wisconsin · 8701 Watertown Plank Road, Milwaukee, WI 53226 · 414-266-4620

Peter F. Coccia · (Pediatric Leukemia, Pediatric Bone Marrow Transplantation) · Professor of Pediatrics, University of Nebraska College of Medicine · Director, Section of Pediatric Hematology-Oncology & Bone Marrow Transplantation, University of Nebraska Medical Center · 600 South 42nd Street, Omaha, NE 68198-2165 · 402-559-7257

Harvey J. Cohen · (Pediatric Leukemia) · Professor and Associate Chairman for Research & Development, Department of Pediatrics; Chief, Division of Pediatric Hematology-Oncology; Director, Strong Children's Research Center, University of Rochester School of Medicine and Dentistry · Strong Memorial Hospital, University of Rochester Medical Center · 601 Elmwood Drive, Box 777, Rochester, NY 14642 · 716-275-2981

William Miles Crist · (Pediatric Leukemia) · Professor, Department of Pediatrics, The University of Tennessee at Memphis, College of Medicine · Chairman, Department of Hematology-Oncology, St. Jude Children's Research Hospital · 332 North Lauderdale, Memphis, TN 38105 · 901-522-0524

George J. Dover · Professor of Pediatrics, Johns Hopkins University School of Medicine · Attending Staff, The Johns Hopkins Medical Institutions · 600 North Wolfe Street, Traylor 902, Baltimore, MD 21205 · 410-955-3886

Jonathan L. Finlay · (Pediatric Brain Tumors, Neurooncology) · Associate Professor of Pediatrics, Cornell University Medical College · Vice-Chairman, Department of Pediatrics, Memorial Sloan-Kettering Cancer Center · 1275 York Avenue, Room H1408, New York, NY 10021 · 212-639-7990

Arnold I. Freeman · (Pediatric Leukemia) · Professor of Pediatrics, University of Missouri at Kansas City School of Medicine · Chief, Department of Hematology-Oncology, The Children's Mercy Hospital · 2401 Gillham Road, Kansas City, MO 64108 · 816-234-3265

Henry S. Friedman · (Pediatric Brain Tumors, Neuroncology) · Professor of Pediatrics, Duke University School of Medicine · Duke University Medical Center Box 2916, DUMC, Durham, NC 27710 · 919-684-3401

Marc E. Horowitz · (Pediatric Brain Tumor, Neuro-oncology) · Senior Investigator, Pediatric Branch, National Cancer Institute, National Institutes of Health · 9000 Rockville Pike, Building 10, Room 13N240, Bethesda, MD 20892 · 301-496-5007

Nancy A. Kernan · (Pediatric Bone Marrow Transplantation) · Cornell University Medical College · Assistant Attending Pediatrician, and Assistant Chief of Bone Marrow Transplant Service, and Assistant Member, Memorial Sloan-Kettering Cancer Center · 1275 York Avenue, New York, NY 10021 · 212-639-7250

John H. Kersey · (Bone Marrow Transplantation) · Professor of Pediatrics, Laboratory Medicine and Pathology, University of Minnesota School of Medicine · Director, Bone Marrow Transplantation Program, University of Minnesota Hospital & Clinics · 420 Delaware Street, SE, Box 86, Minneapolis, MN 55455 · 612-625-4659

Joanne Kurtzberg · (Bone Marrow Transplantation) · Associate Professor of Pediatrics, and Assistant Professor of Pathology, Duke University School of Medicine · Director of Pediatric Bone Marrow Laboratory, Duke University Medical Center · P.O. Box 3350, Durham, NC 27710 · 919-684-8963

Beatrice C. Lampkin · (Leukemia) · Professor Emeritus, Department of Pediatric Hematology-Oncology, University of Cincinnati College of Medicine · Children's Hospital Medical Center · Elland and Bethesda Avenues, CHRF-2367, Cincinnati, OH 45229 · 513-559-4266

Brigid G. Leventhal · (Pediatric Leukemia, Hodgkin's Disease) · Associate Professor of Pediatrics, and Director, Clinical Research Administration, Johns Hopkins University School of Medicine · The Johns Hopkins Medical Institutions · Oncology Center, 550 North Broadway, Suite 1121, Baltimore, MD 21205 · 410-955-7224

Michael P. Link · (Pediatric Hodgkin's Disease, Non-Hodgkin's Lymphomas, Bone Tumors) · Professor of Pediatrics, Stanford University School of Medicine · Stanford University Hospital; Lucile Salter Packard Childrens Hospital at Stanford 725 Welch Road, Palo Alto, CA 94304 · 415-723-5535

Joseph Mirro, Jr. · (Pediatric Leukemia) · Professor of Pediatrics, University of Pittsburgh School of Medicine · Associate Director, Pittsburgh Cancer Institute; Chief, Division of Hematology-Oncology, Children's Hospital of Pittsburgh · 3705 Fifth Avenue, Pittsburgh, PA 15213 · 412-692-5947

Sharon Boehm Murphy · (Pediatric Leukemia; Pediatric Lymphoma Therapy, Hodgkin's Disease) · Professor of Pediatrics, Northwestern University Medical School · Chief, Division of Hematology/Oncology, The Children's Memorial Hospital · 2300 Children's Plaza, 30, Chicago, IL 60614 · 312-880-4584

Mark E. Nesbit · (Pediatric Leukemia) · Professor of Pediatrics, Therapeutic Radiology & Nursing, and Director, Section of Pediatric Hematology-Oncology, University of Minnesota School of Medicine · 420 Delaware Street, SE, Box 484, Minneapolis, MN 55455 · 612-626-2778

Richard J. O'Reilly · (Pediatric Bone Marrow Transplantation) · Professor of Pediatrics, Cornell University Medical College · Chairman, Department of Pediatrics, Memorial Sloan-Kettering Cancer Center · 1275 York Avenue, New York, NY 10021 · 212-639-2000

Lorrie Furman Odom · (Pediatric Leukemia) · Associate Professor, Department of Pediatrics, University of Colorado School of Medicine · Clinical Director, Hematology & Oncology, The Children's Hospital · 1056 East 19th Avenue, Box B-115, Denver, CO 80218 · 303-861-6750

Robertson Parkman · (Pediatric Bone Marrow Transplantation) · Professor of Pediatrics and Microbiology, University of Southern California School of Medicine Head, Division of Research Immunology/Bone Marrow Transplantation, Children's Hospital of Los Angeles · 4650 Sunset Boulevard,Box 62, Los Angeles, CA 90027 · 213-669-2546

Donald Pinkel · (Pediatric Leukemia) · Professor of Pediatrics, The University of Texas Medical School at Houston · Kana Chair in Pediatric Leukemia Research, The University of Texas MD Anderson Cancer Center · 1515 Holcombe Boulevard, Box 87, Houston, TX 77030 · 713-792-3326

David G. Poplack · (Pediatric Leukemia) · Head, Pharmacology & Experimental Therapeutics Section, Pediatric Branch, National Cancer Institute, National Institutes of Health · 9000 Rockville Pike, Building 10, Room 13N240, Bethesda, MD 20892 · 301-496-5008

Norma K. C. Ramsay · (Pediatric Bone Marrow Transplantation) · Professor of Pediatrics, University of Minnesota School of Medicine · Director, Pediatric Bone Marrow Transplantation, University of Minnesota Hospital & Clinics · 420 Delaware Street, SE, Box 366, Minneapolis, MN 55455 · 612-626-2778

Gregory H. Reaman · (Pediatric Leukemia) · Professor of Pediatrics, The George Washington University School of Medicine & Health Sciences · Chairman, Department of Hematology-Oncology, Children's National Medical Center · 111 Michigan Avenue NW, Washington, DC 20010 · 202-745-2147

Gaston K. Rivera · (Pediatric Leukemia) · Professor, Department of Pediatrics, The University of Tennessee at Memphis, College of Medicine · Member, Department of Hematology-Oncology, St. Jude Children's Research Hospital · 332 North Lauderdale, Memphis, TN 38105 · 901-531-2153

Stephen E. Sallan · (Pediatric Leukemia, Childhood Brain Tumors) · Professor of Pediatrics, Harvard Medical School · Clinical Director, Dana-Farber Cancer Institute; Children's Hospital · 44 Binney Street, Boston, MA 02115 · 617-732-3316

Jean E. Sanders · (Pediatric Bone Marrow Transplantation) · Professor of Pediatrics, University of Washington School of Medicine · Attending Staff, Fred Hutchinson Cancer Research Center · 1124 Columbia Street, E-100, Seattle, WA 98104 · 206-667-4348

Victor M. Santana · (Pediatric Leukemia, Neuroblastoma, Bone Marrow Transplantation) · Assistant Professor, Department of Pediatrics, University of Tennessee at Memphis · Assistant Member, Department of Hematology-Oncology, St. Jude Children's Research Hospital · 332 North Lauderdale, P.O. Box 318, Memphis, TN 38101-0318 · 901-522-0300

Molly Schwenn · (Pediatric Lymphoma [Non-Hodgkin's]) · Associate Professor of Pediatrics, University of Massachusetts Medical School · Clinical Director of Pediatric Hematology/Oncology, University of Massachusetts Medical Center · 55 Lake Avenue North, Worcester, MA 01655 · 508-856-4225

Michael Edward Trigg · (Pediatric Bone Marrow Transplantation) · Professor of Pediatrics, The University of Iowa College of Medicine · Director, Pediatric Bone Marrow Transplantation, The University of Iowa Hospitals & Clinics · 2524 John Colloton Pavilion, Iowa City, IA 52242 · 319-356-1608

Teresa J. Vietti · (Pediatric Cancer Chemotherapy) · Professor of Pediatrics and Pediatrics in Radiology, Washington University School of Medicine · Attending Pediatrician, and Consultant in Hematology & Oncology, St. Louis Children's Hospital, Shriners Hospital for Crippled Children, Barnes Hospitals · 400 South Kingshighway, Room 2 South 58, St. Louis, MO 63110 · 314-454-6228

Howard J. Weinstein · (Pediatric Leukemia, Pediatric Lymphoma [Non-Hodgkin's], Pediatric Bone Marrow Transplantation) · Associate Professor of Pediatrics, Harvard Medical School · Director, Division of Pediatric Bone Marrow Transplantation, Dana-Farber Cancer Institute; Children's Hospital · 44 Binney Street, Room 1842, Boston, MA 02115 · 617-732-3317

William G. Woods · (Pediatric Leukemia, Pediatric Bone Marrow Transplantation, Childhood Cancer Screening) · Professor of Pediatrics, University of Minnesota School of Medicine · University of Minnesota Hospital & Clinics · 420 Delaware Street, SE, Box 454, Minneapolis, MN 55455 · 612-626-2778

Andrew M. Yeager · (Pediatric Bone Marrow Transplantation) · Associate Professor of Oncology, Pediatrics and Neurology, Johns Hopkins University School of Medicine · Pediatrician-in-Charge, Johns Hopkins Bone Marrow Transplantation Program, The Johns Hopkins Medical Institutions · Johns Hopkins Oncology Center, 600 North Wolfe Street, Room 3-127, Baltimore, MD 21205 · 410-955-8783

PEDIATRIC INFECTIOUS DISEASE
(See also Infectious Disease, Pediatric Infectious Disease)

Warren A. Andiman · (Pediatric AIDS) · Associate Professor of Pediatrics, Laboratory Medicine, & Epidemiology, Yale University School of Medicine · Director, Pediatric AIDS Care Program, and Associate Director, Clinical Virology Laboratory, Yale-New Haven Hospital · 333 Cedar Street, Room 418, LSOG, New Haven, CT 06510 · 203-785-4730

Ann M. Arvin · (Herpes Virus Infections) · Professor of Pediatrics, Stanford University School of Medicine · Lucile Salter Packard Children's Hospital at Stanford 300 Pasteur Drive #A367, Stanford, CA 94305 · 415-723-5682

Carol Jane Baker · Professor of Pediatrics, Microbiology & Immunology, and Head, Section of Infectious Diseases, Department of Pediatrics, Baylor College of Medicine · Head, Section of Infectious Diseases, Texas Children's Hospital · Pediatric Infectious Disease, One Baylor Plaza, Houston, TX 77030 · 713-798-4790

Henry H. Balfour, Jr. · (Herpes Virus Infections) · Professor of Pediatrics, University of Minnesota School of Medicine · University of Minnesota Hospital & Clinics · 420 Delaware Street SE, Box 437, Minneapolis, MN 55455 · 612-626-5670

William Borkowsky · (Pediatric AIDS) · Associate Professor of Pediatrics, New York University School of Medicine · Director, Infectious Diseases & Immunology, New York University Medical Center, Bellevue Hospital · 550 First Avenue, Room Eight, North 16, New York, NY 10016 · 212-263-6426, 561-3612

Philip A. Brunell · Professor of Pediatrics, University of California at Los Angeles School of Medicine · Associate Director of Academic Affairs, Department of Pediatrics, and Chief, Pediatric Infectious Diseases, Cedars-Sinai Medical Center · 8700 Beverly Boulevard, Room 4316, Los Angeles, CA 90048 · 213-855-4471

Yvonne J. Bryson · (AIDS, Herpes Virus Infections, Sexually Transmitted Disease) · Professor of Pediatrics, University of California at Los Angeles School of Medicine · University of California at Los Angeles Medical Center · 10833 Le Conte Avenue, Room 22-442, Los Angeles, CA 90024-1752 · 310-825-5235

Edward M. Connor · (Pediatric AIDS, Immunodeficiency) · Associate Professor of Pediatrics, University of Medicine & Dentistry of New Jersey · Director, AIDS Clinical Trials Unit, University Hospital, and Children's Hospital · 185 South Orange Avenue, Newark, NJ 07103-2714 · 201-456-4300

Ralph D. Feigin · (Meningitis) · Distinguished Service Professor, and J. S. Abercrombie Professor of Pediatrics, and Chairman, Department of Pediatrics, Baylor College of Medicine · Physician-in-Chief, Texas Children's Hospital · 6621 Fannin Street, MC 1-3420, Houston, TX 77030 · 713-798-4780

Anne A. Gershon · (Herpes Virus Infections, Chicken Pox) · Director, Pediatric Infectious Diseases, College of Physicians & Surgeons of Columbia University · Columbia-Presbyterian Medical Center · 650 West 168th Street, BB4-427, New York, NY 10032 · 212-305-1556

Janet R. Gilsdorf · Associate Professor of Pediatrics, The University of Michigan Medical School · Director of Pediatric Infectious Diseases, The University of Michigan Medical Center · 1500 East Medical Center Drive, Box 0244, Ann Arbor, MI 48109-0244 · 313-763-2440

Caroline Breese Hall · Professor of Pediatrics and Medicine in Infectious Diseases, University of Rochester School of Medicine & Dentistry · Strong Memorial Hospital, University of Rochester Medical Center · 601 Elmwood Drive, Box 689, Rochester, NY 14642-8689 · 716-275-5242

Margaret C. Heagarty · (Pediatric AIDS) · Professor of Pediatrics, College of Physicians & Surgeons of Columbia University · Director of Pediatrics, Harlem Hospital Center · 506 Lennox Avenue, New York, NY 10037 · 212-491-1600

Walter Hughes · Professor of Pediatrics, The University of Tennessee at Memphis, College of Medicine · Chairman and Member, Department of Infectious Diseases, St. Jude Children's Research Hospital · 332 North Lauderdale, P.O. Box 318, Memphis, TN 38101-0318 · 901-522-0485

Richard F. Jacobs · (Tuberculosis) · Professor of Pediatrics, University of Arkansas for Medical Sciences · Chief, Pediatric Infectious Diseases, Arkansas Children's Hospital · 800 Marshall Street, Little Rock, AR 72202 · 501-320-1416

Samuel L. Katz · Wilburt C. Davison Professor of Pediatrics, Duke University School of Medicine · Duke University Medical Center · P.O. Box 2925—DUMC, Durham, NC 27710 · 919-684-3734

Jerome O. Klein · Professor of Pediatrics, Boston University School of Medicine Director, Division of Pediatric Infectious Diseases, Boston City Hospital · Maxwell Finland Laboratory for Infectious Diseases, 774 Albany Street, Room 509, Boston, MA 02118 · 617-534-5591

Keith Michael Krasinski · (Pediatric AIDS) · Associate Professor of Pediatrics, New York University School of Medicine · Associate Hospital Epidemiologist and Attending Physician, Bellevue Hospital Center; Attending Physician, New York University Medical Center · 550 First Avenue, Room Eight, North 16, New York, NY · 212-263-6427, 561-3612

Sarah S. Long · Professor of Pediatrics, Temple University School of Medicine · Chief, Section of Infectious Disease, St. Christopher's Hospital for Children · Erie Avenue at Front Street, Suite 1112, Philadelphia, PA 19134 · 215-427-5204

George McCracken · (Meningitis, Antibiotic Therapy) · The University of Texas Southwestern Medical Center at Dallas · Department of Pediatrics, 5323 Harry Hines Boulevard, Dallas TX 75235-9063 · 214-688-3439

Kenneth McIntosh · Professor of Pediatrics, Harvard Medical School · Chief, Infectious Diseases, Children's Hospital · 300 Longwood Avenue, Enders, Room 626, Boston, MA 02115 · 617-735-7622

Hermann A. Mendez · (Pediatric AIDS) · Associate Professor of Clinical Pediatrics, and Director, Brooklyn Pediatric AIDS Network, State University of New York Health Science Center at Brooklyn · 450 Clarkson Avenue, Box 49, Brooklyn, NY 11203 · 718-270-3825

John D. Nelson · (Meningitis, Antibiotic Pharmacology) · Professor of Pediatrics, and Chairman, Division of Infectious Disease, The University of Texas Southwestern Medical Center at Dallas · Parkland Memorial Hospital; Children's Medical Center of Dallas · 5323 Harry Hines Boulevard, Dallas, TX 75235-9063 · 214-688-3391

Stephen W. Nicholas · (Pediatric AIDS) · Assistant Professor of Pediatrics, College of Physicians & Surgeons of Columbia University · Assistant Attending, Pediatrics Medical Director, Incarnation Children's Center; Columbia Presbyterian Medical Center; Harlem Hospital Center · 142 Audubon Avenue, New York, NY 10032 · 212-928-2228

James M. Oleske · (Pediatric AIDS) · Francis-Xavier Bagnoud Professor of Pediatrics, University of Medicine & Dentistry of New Jersey · 185 South Orange Avenue, Newark, NJ 07103 · 201-456-5066

Wade P. Parks · (Pediatric AIDS) · The Pat & E. John Rosenwald Professor and Chairman of Pediatrics, New York University School of Medicine · Director of Pediatrics, Bellevue Hospital, and Tisch Hospital · 550 First Avenue, New York, NY 10016 · 212-263-7300

Georges Peter · Professor of Pediatrics, Brown University School of Medicine · Director, Division of Pediatric Infectious Diseases, Rhode Island Hospital · 593 Eddy Street, Providence, RI 02903 · 401-277-8360

Larry K. Pickering · David R. Park Professor of Pediatrics, Director of the Pediatric Infectious Diseases, and Vice-Chairman for Research, The University of Texas Medical School at Houston · Hermann Hospital · 6431 Fannin Street JFB 1.739, Houston, TX 77030 · 713-792-5330 x3114

Philip A. Pizzo · (Cancer & Infections, AIDS) · Professor of Pediatrics, Uniformed Services University of Health Sciences · Chief of Pediatrics and Head, Infectious Disease Section, National Cancer Institute, National Institutes of Health · 9000 Rockville Pike, Building 10, Room 13N240, Bethesda, MD 20892 301-496-4256

Paul G. Quie · Regents Professor, and Professor of Pediatrics, Microbiology and Laboratory Medicine Pathology and American Legion Memorial Heart Research Professor, University of Minnesota School of Medicine · University of Minnesota Hospital & Clinics · 420 Delaware Street Southeast,Box 483, UMHC, Minneapolis, MN 55455 · 612-624-5146

Gwendolyn B. Scott · (Pediatric AIDS) · Professor of Pediatrics, University of Miami School of Medicine · Director, Division of Pediatric Immunology & Infectious Diseases, University of Miami-Jackson Memorial Medical Center · 1550 Northwest 10th Avenue, Room 208, Miami, FL 33136 · 305-547-6676

John L. Sever · (Perinatal and Chronic Infections of the Nervous System, Pediatric AIDS) · Professor of Pediatrics, Obstetrics & Gynecology, and Microbiology & Immunology, The George Washington University School of Medicine · Chairman, Institutional Review Board, Children's National Medical Center · 111 Michigan Avenue NW, Washington, DC 20010 · 202-745-4132

Arnold L. Smith · (Cystic Fibrosis) · Professor of Pediatrics and Adjunct Professor of Microbiology, University of Washington School of Medicine · Chief, Division of Infectious Disease, Children's Hospital & Medical Center · 4800 Sand Point Way NE, Seattle, WA 98105 · 206-526-2116

Jeffrey R. Starke · (Tuberculosis) · Assistant Professor of Pediatrics, Baylor College of Medicine · Director, Children's Tuberculosis Clinic, Texas Children's Hospital; Ben Taub General Hospital · Department of Pediatrics, One Baylor Plaza, Houston, TX 77030 · 713-770-4330

Gregory A. Storch · (AIDS, Virology) · Associate Professor of Pediatrics and Medicine, Washington University School of Medicine · Director of Diagnostic Microbiology & Retrovirology, Department of Pediatrics, St. Louis Children's Hospital · 400 South Kingshighway Boulevard, St. Louis, MO 63110 · 314-454-6079

Richard J. Whitley · (Virology, Herpes Virus Infections, AIDS, Sexually Transmitted Disease) · Professor of Pediatrics, Microbiology and Medicine, and Scientist, Cancer Research & Training Center, and Associate Director, Center for AIDS Research, and Vice-Chairman, Department of Pediatrics, The University of Alabama School of Medicine · University Hospital; Children's Hospital · 1600 South Seventh Avenue, Suite 616, Birmingham, AL 35294 · 205-939-9594

Catherine M. Wilfert · (AIDS) · Professor of Pediatrics and Microbiology, Duke University School of Medicine · Chief of Pediatric Infectious Diseases, Duke University Medical Center · P.O. Box 2951, Durham, NC 27710 · 919-684-6610

Ram Yogev · (Pediatric AIDS) · Professor of Pediatrics, Northwestern University Medical School · Co-Director, Division of Infectious Disease, The Children's Memorial Hospital · 2300 Children's Plaza, Box 20, Chicago, IL 60614 · 312-880-3718

PEDIATRIC NEPHROLOGY

Raymond D. Adelman · (Hypertension) · Chairman, Department of Pediatrics, Eastern Virginia Medical School · Vice-President for Medical Affairs, and Physician-in-Chief, The Children's Hospital of the King's Daughters · 601 Children's Lane, Norfolk, VA 23510 · 804-628-7241

Steven Roy Alexander · (Dialysis, Kidney Transplantation) · Associate Professor of Pediatric Nephrology, The University of Texas Southwestern Medical Center at Dallas · Director, Dialysis, Kidney Transplantation, Children's Medical Center of Dallas · 5323 Harry Hines Boulevard, Dallas, TX 75235-9063 · 214-688-3438

Sharon P. Andreoli · (General) · Associate Professor of Pediatrics, Indiana University School of Medicine · James Whitcomb Riley Hospital for Children; Indiana University Medical Center · 702 Barnhill Drive, Room A583, Indianapolis, IN 46223 · 317-274-2563

Billy S. Arant, Jr. · (General, Reflux Nephropathy, Urinary Tract Infection, Problems of the Newborn Kidney) · Professor of Pediatrics, and Director, Division of Pediatric Nephrology, The University of Texas Southwestern Medical Center at Dallas · Director, Children's Kidney and Urology Center, Children's Medical Center of Dallas · 5323 Harry Hines Boulevard, Dallas, TX 75235-9063 · 214-688-3438

Gerald Stanley Arbus · (Dialysis, Kidney Transplantation) · Associate Professor of Pediatrics, University of Toronto School of Medicine · The Hospital for Sick Children · 555 University Avenue, Room 5123, Toronto, Ontario M5G 1X8 · 416-598-6288

J. Williamson Balfe · (Dialysis, Kidney Transplantation) · Professor of Pediatrics, University of Toronto School of Medicine · Clinical Director, Division of Nephrology, The Hospital for Sick Children · 555 University Avenue, Room 5109, Toronto, Ontario M5G 1X8 · 416-598-6289

H. Jorge Baluarte · (Dialysis, Kidney Transplantation) · Professor of Pediatrics, Temple University School of Medicine · Chief, Section of Nephrology, St. Christopher's Hospital for Children · Erie Avenue at Front Street, Suite 3301, Philadelphia, PA 19134 · 215-427-5190

L. Eileen Doyle Brewer · (General, Dialysis, Transplantation) · Associate Professor of Pediatrics, Baylor College of Medicine · Medical Director, Dialysis Unit & Renal Transplantation, Texas Children's Hospital · One Baylor Plaza, Renal Services, Houston, TX 77030 · 713-770-3800

Robert L. Chevalier · (General, Developmental Nephrology) · Professor & Vice-Chair, Department of Pediatrics, University of Virginia School of Medicine · University of Virginia Health Sciences Center · Department of Pediatrics, Box 386, Charlottesville, VA 22908 · 804-924-5093

Barbara R. Cole · (General, Polycystic Kidney Disease) · Associate Professor of Pediatrics, Washington University School of Medicine · Director, Division of Pediatric Nephrology, St. Louis Children's Hospital · 400 South Kingshighway Boulevard, St. Louis, MO 63110 · 314-454-6043

Susan B. Conley · (Dialysis, Kidney Transplantation) · Director of Pediatric Nephrology, California Pacific Medical Center · 2340 Clay Street, San Francisco, CA 94115 · 415-923-6565

Allison A. Eddy · (General) · Assistant Professor of Pediatrics, University of Toronto School of Medicine · Staff Nephrologist, The Hospital for Sick Children · 555 University Avenue, Toronto, Ontario M5G 1X8 · 416-598-6349

Demetrius Ellis · (Kidney Transplantation, Hypertension, Diabetic Nephropathy) · Professor of Pediatrics and Nephrology, and Director of Pediatric Nephrology, University of Pittsburgh School of Medicine · Children's Hospital of Pittsburgh · 3705 Fifth Avenue, Room 7457, Pittsburgh, PA 15213 · 412-692-5182

Robert Ettenger · (Kidney Transplantation) · Professor, Department of Pediatrics, Head, Division of Pediatric Nephrology and Vice-Chairman of Clinical Affairs, University of California at Los Angeles School of Medicine · A2-331 Marion Davies Children's Center, Los Angeles, CA 90024 · 213-206-6987

John W. Foreman · (General) · Professor of Pediatrics, Virginia Commonwealth University, Medical College of Virginia · Medical College of Virginia Hospital · 1101 East Marshall Street, Room 12-024, Box 498, MCV Station, Richmond, VA 23298 · 804-786-9608

Ira Greifer · (General) · Professor of Pediatrics, Director of Pediatrics and The Children's Kidney Center, Hospital of the Albert Einstein College of Medicine; Montefiore Medical Center · 1825 Eastchester Road, Bronx, NY 10461 · 212-904-2857

William E. Harmon · (Dialysis, Kidney Transplantation) · Harvard Medical School · Director, Pediatric Nephrology, Children's Hospital · 300 Longwood Avenue, Boston, MA 02115 · 617-735-6129

Diane Hebert · (Kidney Transplantation) · Assistant Professor of Pediatrics, Division of Nephrology, University of Toronto School of Medicine · Staff Nephrologist, and Director of the Renal Transplant Program, The Hospital for Sick Children · 555 University Avenue, Division of Nephrology, Room 5109, Elm Wing, Toronto, Ontario M5G 1X8 · 416-598-6287

Julie R. Ingelfinger · (Hypertension) · Associate Professor of Pediatrics, Harvard Medical School · Co-Chief, Pediatric Nephrology, Massachusetts General Hospital · 15 Parkman Street, Boston, MA 02114 · 617-726-2908

Bernard S. Kaplan · (Hemolytic Uremic Syndrome, Polycystic Kidney Disease) · Professor of Pediatrics & Medicine, University of Pennsylvania School of Medicine · Director of Nephrology, The Children's Hospital of Philadelphia · The Wood Building, 34th and Civic Center Boulevard, Philadelphia, PA 19104 · 215-590-2449

Edward C. Kohaut · (Dialysis, Kidney Transplantation) · Professor of Pediatrics, Division of Nephrology, University of Alabama at Birmingham · Children's Hospital of Alabama · 1600 Seventh Avenue South, Suite 735, Birmingham, AL 35233 205-934-3091

Craig B. Langman · (Stone Disease) · Associate Professor of Pediatrics, Northwestern University Medical School · Associate Chair for Research, Children's Memorial Hospital · 2300 Children's Plaza, Box 37, Chicago, IL 60614 · 312-880-4326

S. Michael Mauer · (Diabetic Kidney Disease) · Professor of Pediatrics, University of Minnesota School of Medicine · Department of Pediatrics, Box 491, 515 Delaware Street, SE, Minneapolis, MN 55455 · 612-626-2780

Paul T. McEnery · (Kidney Transplantation, General) · Professor of Pediatrics, University of Cincinnati College of Medicine · Director, ESRD Program, and Director, Quality Assessment & Improvement, Children's Hospital Medical Center · Elland and Bethesda Avenues, Fifth Floor CHRF, Cincinnati, OH 45229-2899 · 513-559-4531

Robert H. McLean · (General, Immunology) · Associate Professor of Pediatrics, Johns Hopkins University School of Medicine · Attending Staff, The Johns Hopkins Medical Institutions · 600 North Wolfe Street, Park 333, Baltimore, MD 21205 · 410-955-2467

Mark I. Mentser · Assistant Professor, Department of Pediatrics, Ohio State University College of Medicine · Chief, Section of Nephrology, Columbus Children's Hospital · 700 Children's Drive, Room 300, Columbus, OH 43205 · 614-461-2042

Thomas E. Nevins · (Dialysis, Kidney Transplantation) · Associate Professor of Pediatrics, University of Minnesota School of Medicine · University of Minnesota Hospital & Clinics · 515 Delaware Street, SE, Box 491 UMHC, Minneapolis, MN 55455 · 612-626-2922

Donald E. Potter · (Dialysis, Kidney Transplantation) · Clinical Professor of Pediatrics, University of California at San Francisco School of Medicine · University of California at San Francisco Medical Center · Children's Renal Center, 533 Parnassus Avenue, Room U-585, San Francisco, CA 94143-0748 · 415-476-2423

Edward Jerome Ruley · (General) · Professor of Pediatrics, The George Washington University School of Medicine · Chairman of Nephrology, Children's National Medical Center · 111 Michigan Avenue NW, Washington, DC 20010 · 202-745-5058

Isidro B. Salusky · (Dialysis) · Associate Professor of Pediatrics, University of California at Los Angeles School of Medicine · Director, Pediatric Dialysis Program, Division of Pediatric Nephrology, University of California at Los Angeles Medical Center · 10833 LeConte Avenue, A2-331 MDCC, Los Angeles, CA 90024-1752 · 213-206-6987

Aileen B. Sedman · (General) · Associate Professor of Pediatrics, The University of Michigan Medical School · C.S. Mott Children's Hospital, The University of Michigan Medical Center · 1521 Simpson Road East, Women's Building, Room L2602, Box 0297, Ann Arbor, MI 48109-0297 · 313-936-4210

Norman Siegel · (General, Acute Renal Failure, Electrolyte & Acid-Based Disorders) · Professor of Pediatrics & Medicine, and Vice Chairman, Department of Pediatrics, Yale University School of Medicine · Chief, Section of Nephrology, Department of Pediatrics, Yale-New Haven Hospital · 333 Cedar Street, New Haven, CT 06510 · 203-785-4643

Alan R. Sinaiko · (Hypertension) · Professor of Pediatrics, University of Minnesota School of Medicine · University of Minnesota Hospital & Clinics · 420 Delaware Street SE, Box 357, Minneapolis, MN 55455 · 612-625-8483

F. Bruder Stapleton · (General, Stone Disease) · Chairman of Pediatrics, State University of New York Health Science Center at Buffalo · Children's Hospital of Buffalo · 219 Bryant, Buffalo, NY 14222 · 716-878-7300

José Strauss · (AIDS and the Kidney) · Professor of Pediatrics, and Director of Division of Pediatric Nephrology, University of Miami School of Medicine · University of Miami-Jackson Memorial Medical Center · Division of Pediatric Nephrology, P.O. Box 016960 (R-131), Miami, FL 33101 · 305-585-6726

Amir Tejani · (Kidney Transplantation) · Professor of Pediatrics and Director, Renal Division, State University of New York Health Science Center at Brooklyn · 450 Clarkson Avenue, Box 49, Brooklyn, NY 11203 · 718-270-1913

Luther B. Travis · (Diabetes, Renal Disease) · William W. Glauser Professor of Pediatrics and Pediatric Nephrology, The University of Texas Medical Branch at Galveston · Director, Division of Nephrology & Diabetes, The Children's Hospital of University of Texas Medical Branch at Galveston · Ninth and Market Streets, Suite 221, Galveston, TX 77550 · 409-772-2538

Bradley A. Warady · (Dialysis, Kidney Transplantation) · Associate Professor of Pediatrics, University of Missouri at Kansas City School of Medicine · Medical Director, Dialysis and Transplantation, The Children's Mercy Hospital · 24th & Gillham Road, Kansas City, MO 64108 · 816-234-3010

Steven Joel Wassner · (General) · Professor & Vice-Chairman of Pediatrics, Pennsylvania State University · Directory, Pediatric Residency Program, and Chief, Division of Pediatric Nephrology & Pediatric Diabetes, The Milton S. Hershey Medical Center · 500 University Drive, Hershey, PA 17033 · 717-531-8521

PEDIATRIC PULMONOLOGY

Thomas F. Boat · (Cystic Fibrosis) · Professor and Chairman, Department of Pediatrics, University of North Carolina School of Medicine · University of North Carolina Hospitals · 509 Burnett-Womack Building, Manning Drive, Campus Box 7220, Chapel Hill, NC 27599-7220 · 919-966-4427

John G. Brooks · (General, Cystic Fibrosis, Sudden Infant Death Syndrome) · Professor of Pediatrics, University of Rochester School of Medicine & Dentistry · Director, Pediatric Pulmonology, Strong Memorial Hospital, University of Rochester Medical Center · Department of Pediatrics, Box 667, 601 Elmwood Avenue, Rochester, NY 14642 · 716-275-2464

Preston W. Campbell III · (Cystic Fibrosis) · Assistant Professor of Pediatrics, Vanderbilt University School of Medicine · 1161 Twenty-First Avenue South, Nashville, TN 37232 · 615-343-7617

Carl Frederick Doershuk · (Cystic Fibrosis) · Professor, Department of Pediatrics, Case Western Reserve University School of Medicine · Director, Pediatric Pulmonary Laboratory, University Hospitals of Cleveland; Rainbow Babies & Childrens Hospital · Cleveland, OH 44106 · 216-844-3267

Henry Lawrence Dorkin · (Cystic Fibrosis, General) · Associate Professor of Pediatrics, Tufts University School of Medicine · Chief, Pediatric Pulmonology and Allergy Division, and Director, Cystic Fibrosis Center, New England Medical Center · 750 Washington Street, Box 343, Boston, MA 02111 · 617-956-5085

Howard Eigen · (General, Cystic Fibrosis) · Professor of Pediatrics, Indiana University School of Medicine · Director, Section of Pulmonology & Critical Care, James Whitcomb Riley Hospital for Children · 702 Barnhill Drive, Room 2750, Indianapolis, IN 46202-5225 · 317-274-3434

Christopher G. Green · (General) · Associate Professor of Pediatrics, University of Wisconsin-Madison School of Medicine · University of Wisconsin Hospital & Clinics · 600 Highland Avenue, Madison, WI 53792-4108 · 608-263-8555

Gunyon Harrison · (Chronic Lung Disease, Cystic Fibrosis) · Professor of Pediatrics, Baylor College of Medicine · Texas Children's Hospital · One Baylor Plaza, Houston, TX 77030 · 713-770-3300

Ivan R. Harwood · (Cystic Fibrosis) · Professor of Pediatrics, University of California at San Diego School of Medicine · Chief, Pediatric Pulmonary Division, and Director, Cystic Fibrosis Center, University of California at San Diego Medical Center · 4130 Front Street, San Diego, CA 92103 · 619-294-6125

Bettina C. Hilman · (Cystic Fibrosis, Allergy) · Professor of Pediatrics, Louisiana State University School of Medicine · Louisiana State University Medical Center; Schumpert Medical Center · 1501 Kings Highway, 33932, Shreveport, LA 71130-3932 · 318-674-6094

Douglas S. Holsclaw, Jr. · (Cystic Fibrosis) · Professor of Pediatrics, Hahnemann University · Hahnemann Hospital · 230 North Broad Street, Philadelphia, PA 19102 · 215-448-7766

Allen Lapey · (Cystic Fibrosis, Allergy) · Clinical Assistant Professor of Pediatrics, Harvard Medical School · Associate Pediatrician, and Center Director, Center for Cystic Fibrosis Care & Research, and Director, Pediatric Allergy & Respiratory Disease, Massachusetts General Hospital · 15 Parkman Street, ACC Building, 709, Boston, MA 02114 · 617-726-8707

Gary L. Larsen · (Asthma) · Professor of Pediatrics, and Head, Section of Pediatric Pulmonary Medicine, University of Colorado School of Medicine · Senior Faculty Member, and Head, Division of Pulmonary Medicine, Department of Pediatrics, National Jewish Center for Immunology & Respiratory Medicine · 1400 Jackson Street, Denver, CO 80206 · 303-398-1617

Richard John Lemen · (General, Critical Care Medicine) · Professor of Pediatrics, The University of Arizona College of Medicine · The University of Arizona Health Sciences Center · Department of Pediatrics, 1501 North Campbell Avenue, Tucson, AZ 85724 · 602-626-5485

Gerald M. Loughlin · Associate Professor, Johns Hopkins University School of Medicine · Chief, Eudowood Division of Pediatric Respiratory Sciences, The Johns Hopkins Medical Institutions · 600 North Wolfe Street, Park Building, Room 316, Baltimore, MD 21205 · 410-955-2035

John T. McBride · (General) · Associate Professor of Pediatrics, University of Rochester School of Medicine & Dentistry · Director of Cystic Fibrosis Care, Strong Memorial Hospital, University of Rochester Medical Center · 601 Elmwood Avenue, Box 667, Rochester, NY 14642 · 716-275-2464

Robert B. Mellins · (General) · Professor of Pediatrics, College of Physicians & Surgeons of Columbia University · Attending Physician, and Director, Pediatric Pulmonary Division, Columbia-Presbyterian Medical Center · 630 West 168th Street, BHS1-101, New York, NY 10032 · 212-305-5122

Elaine H. Mischler · (Cystic Fibrosis) · Professor of Pediatrics, University of Wisconsin-Madison School of Medicine · Director, Pediatric Pulmonary/Cystic Fibrosis Center, University of Wisconsin Hospital & Clinics · 600 Highland Avenue, Madison, WI 53792-4108 · 608-263-8555

Shirley Murphy · (Asthma) · Professor of Pediatrics, The University of New Mexico School of Medicine · Director, Pediatric Pulmonary/Critical Care Division, The University Hospital · Ambulatory Care Center, 2211 Lomas Boulevard NE, Third Floor, Albuquerque, NM 87131 · 505-272-5551

David M. Orenstein · (General, Cystic Fibrosis) · Associate Professor of Pediatrics, University of Pittsburgh School of Medicine; Associate Professor of Instruction & Learning, School of Education, University of Pittsburgh · Director of Cystic Fibrosis & Pulmonology, Children's Hospital of Pittsburgh · 3705 Fifth Avenue, Floor 4A, Room 330, Pittsburgh, PA 15213 · 412-692-5630

Bonnie W. Ramsey · (Cystic Fibrosis) · Associate Professor, Department of Pediatrics, University of Washington School of Medicine · Director, Cystic Fibrosis, Children's Hospital & Medical Center, Seattle · P.O. Box C-5371, Seattle, WA 98105 · 206-526-2024

Gregory J. Redding · (General) · Associate Professor of Pediatrics, University of Washington School of Medicine · Head, Pediatric Pulmonary Medicine, Children's Hospital & Medical Center · 4800 Sand Point Way NE, Seattle, WA 98105 206-526-2174

Beryl J. Rosenstein · (Cystic Fibrosis) · Professor of Pediatrics, Johns Hopkins University School of Medicine · Attending Staff, The Johns Hopkins Medical Institutions · 600 North Wolfe Street, Park 315, Baltimore, MD 21205 · 410-955-2795

Daniel V. Schidlow · (Cystic Fibrosis) · Professor and Deputy Chairman, Department of Pediatrics, Temple University School of Medicine · Chief, Section of Pulmonology & Allergy, and Director, Pediatric Pulmonary & Cystic Fibrosis Center, St. Christopher's Hospital for Children · Erie Avenue at Front Street, Philadelphia, PA 19134-1095 · 215-427-5183

Robert C. Stern · (Cystic Fibrosis) · Professor, Department of Pediatrics, Case Western Reserve University School of Medicine · Rainbow Babies & Childrens Hospital · 2074 Abington Road, Cleveland, OH 44106 · 216-844-3267

Lynn M. Taussig · (Cystic Fibrosis, Pulmonary Function Testing) · Professor and Head, Department of Pediatrics, The University of Arizona College of Medicine The University of Arizona Health Sciences Center · 1501 North Campbell Avenue, Tucson, AZ 85724 · 602-626-6053

Michael A. Wall · (Cystic Fibrosis, General) · Professor of Pediatrics, Oregon Health Sciences University · Chief of Pediatrics, Pulmonary & Critical Care Division, and Director of Cystic Fibrosis Center, Oregon Health Sciences University 3181 Southwest Sam Jackson Park Road, Portland, OR 97201-3098 · 503-494-8023

Miles M. Weinberger · (Asthma, Allergy) · Professor of Pediatrics, The University of Iowa College of Medicine · Director, Pediatrics Allergy/Pulmonary Division, The University of Iowa Hospitals & Clinics · 650 Newton Road, Room 2449 2JCP, Iowa City, IA 52242 · 319-356-3485

Robert W. Wilmott · (Cystic Fibrosis, General) · Associate Professor, Division of Pediatric Pulmonology, University of Cincinnati College of Medicine · Director, Division of Pulmonary Medicine, Children's Hospital Medical Center · Division of Pulmonary Medicine, Elland and Bethesda Avenues, Cincinnati, OH 45229 · 513-559-6771

Glenna B. Winnie · (Cystic Fibrosis, Immunology) · Assistant Professor, Department of Pediatrics, Albany Medical College · Director, Pediatric Pulmonary & Cystic Fibrosis Center, Albany Medical Center · 22 New Scotland Avenue, Albany, NY 12208 · 518-432-1392

Robert E. Wood · (Cystic Fibrosis, Broncoscopy) · Professor of Pediatrics, and Chief, Division of Pediatric Pulmonary Medicine, University of North Carolina School of Medicine · University of North Carolina Hospitals; North Carolina Children's Hospital · 635 Burnett-Womack Building, Manning Drive, Campus Box 7220, Chapel Hill, NC 27599-7220 · 919-966-1001

PHYSICAL MEDICINE & REHABILITATION

ELECTROMYOGRAPHY
(See also Adult Neurology, Electromyography)

Randall Lee Braddom · Professor and Chairman, Department of Physical Medicine & Rehabilitation, Indiana University School of Medicine · Indiana University Medical Center; Community Hospital East · Hook Rehabilitation Associates, 1500 North Ritter Avenue, Room 3202, Indianapolis, IN 46219 · 317-355-5271

Murray E. Brandstater · Professor and Chairman, Department of Physical Medicine & Rehabilitation, Loma Linda University School of Medicine · Medical Director, Department of Physical Medicine & Rehabilitation, Loma Linda University Medical Center · 11234 Anderson Street, Room A-237, Loma Linda, CA 92354 · 714-824-4009

Joel Alan De Lisa · Professor and Chairman, Department of Physical Medicine and Rehabilitation, University of Medicine & Dentistry of New Jersey-New Jersey Medical School · Medical Director, Kessler Institute for Rehabilitation · 1199 Pleasant Valley Way, West Orange, NJ 07052 · 201-731-3600

Daniel Dumitru · Associate Professor and Deputy Chairman of Rehabilitation Medicine, The University of Texas Health Science Center at San Antonio · Medical Director, Brady Green Community Health Center; The University of Texas Clinic; The Audie L. Murphy Memorial Veterans Hospital; Warm Springs Rehabilitation Hospital · 7703 Floyd Curl Drive, San Antonio, TX 78284-7798 · 512-567-5347

Ernest W. Johnson · Professor, Department of Physical Medicine & Rehabilitation, and Associate Dean, External Affairs, Ohio State University College of Medicine · The Ohio State University Hospitals · 370 West Ninth Avenue, 235 Meiling Hall, Columbus, OH 43210 · 614-292-5671

James A. Leonard, Jr. · Clinical Assistant Professor, The University of Michigan Medical School · Associate Chairman, Department of Physical Medicine & Rehabilitation, The University of Michigan Medical Center · 1500 East Medical Center Drive, Ann Arbor, MI 48109-0042 · 313-936-7195

Ian C. MacLean · Associate Professor of Physical Medicine & Rehabilitation, Northwestern University Medical School · Rehabilitation Institute of Chicago · 448 East Ontario, Suite 420, Chicago, IL 60611 · 312-943-2475

John L. Melvin · (Disability Evaluation) · Professor and Deputy Chairman, Department of Physical Medicine & Rehabilitation, Temple University School of Medicine · Vice President of Medical Affairs, and Chairman, Department of Physical Medicine & Rehabilitation, Moss Rehabilitation Hospital, Albert Einstein Medical Center · 1200 West Tabor Road, Philadelphia, PA 19141-3099 · 215-456-9554

Walter C. Stolov · Professor and Chairman, Department of Rehabilitation Medicine, University of Washington School of Medicine · Medical Director, Rehabilitation Medicine, University of Washington Medical Center · Health Sciences Building, 1959 Northeast Pacific Street, BB-919, Seattle, WA 98195 · 206-543-3600

RHEUMATOLOGY

Jeanne E. Hicks · Assistant Professor of Medicine, George Washington University; Associate Professor of Rehabilitation, Georgetown University; Assistant Professor of Medicine, Uniformed Armed Services Institute · Deputy Chief, Department of Rehabilitation Medicine, National Institutes of Health · 9000 Rockville Pike, Building 10, Room 6S235, Bethesda, MD 20892 · 301-496-4733

Mary Jurisson · Instructor, Mayo Medical School · Mayo Clinic · 200 First Street, SW, RMH 3, Rochester, MN 55905 · 507-284-2511

John J. Nicholas · Professor of Physical Medicine & Rehabilitation, Rush Medical College · Chairman, Department of Physical Medicine & Rehabilitation, Rush-Presbyterian-St. Luke's Medical Center · 1653 West Congress Parkway, Chicago, IL 60612-3864 · 312-942-3675

PLASTIC SURGERY

AESTHETIC SURGERY

Bernard S. Alpert · (Breast Reconstruction, Muscle and Tissue Transplantation) Associate Clinical Professor of Surgery, Division of Plastic & Reconstructive Surgery, University of California at San Francisco School of Medicine · Chief, Division of Plastic Surgery, and Vice-Chief, Microsurgery Department, Davies Medical Center · San Francisco Institute of Plastic Surgery, Suite 150, San Francisco, CA 94114 · 415-565-6622

Eugene H. Courtiss · Associate Clinical Professor, Harvard Medical School · Newton-Wellesley Hospital · 2000 Washington Street, Suite 444, Newton Lower Falls, MA 02162 · 617-244-0990

Frederick M. Grazer · Clinical Professor of Surgery, Department of Plastic Surgery, Hershey School of Medicine; Associate Clinical Professor, Department of Plastic Surgery, University of California at Irvine School of Medicine · Hoag Memorial Hospital Presbyterian · 1101 Bayside Drive, Suite 100, Corona del Mar, CA 92625 · 714-644-5000

T. Roderick Hester, Jr. · (Breast Augmentation) · Associate Professor of Surgery, Plastic & Reconstructive, Emory University School of Medicine · Emory University Affiliated Hospitals · 1327 Clifton Road, Atlanta, GA 30322 · 404-248-3455

Stanley A. Klatsky · Assistant Professor of Plastic Surgery, Johns Hopkins University School of Medicine · Chief of Staff (1991-1993), and Chief, Division of Plastic & Reconstructive Surgery, Baltimore County General Hospital · 122 Slade Avenue, Suite 100, Baltimore, MD 21208 · 301-484-0400

G. Patrick Maxwell · Assistant Clinical Professor of Plastic Surgery, Vanderbilt University School of Medicine · Director, The Institute for Aesthetic and Reconstructive Surgery, Baptist Hospital · Nashville Plastic Surgery, Ltd., 2021 Church Street, Suite 806, Nashville, TN 37203 · 615-340-4500

John Q. Owsley, Jr. · Clinical Professor of Plastic Surgery, Division of Plastic Surgery, University of California at San Francisco School of Medicine · Davies Medical Center · 45 Castro Street, Suite 111, San Francisco, CA 94114 · 415-861-8040

Thomas D. Rees · Clinical Professor of Surgery, New York University Medical Center · Chairman, Department of Plastic Surgery, Manhattan Eye, Ear & Throat Hospital · 176 East 72nd Street, New York, NY 10021 · 212-535-1611

Harvey A. Zarem · Professor Emeritus, Department of Surgery, University of California at Los Angeles School of Medicine · St. John's Hospital & Health Center; Santa Monica Hospital · 1301 Twentieth Street, Suite 470, Santa Monica, CA 90404 · 310-315-0222

BODY CONTOURING

Lloyd N. Carlsen · (Buttock and Calf Implants) · Chief of Plastic Surgery, Scarborough General Hospital; Director of Plastic Surgery, Cosmetic Surgery Hospital in Woodbridge, Ontario · 2901 Lawrence Avenue East, Suite 408, Scarborough, Ontario M1P 2T3 · 416-269-7100

Eugene H. Courtiss · Associate Clinical Professor, Harvard Medical School · Newton-Wellesley Hospital · 2000 Washington Street, Suite 444, Newton Lower Falls, MA 02162 · 617-244-0990

Frederick M. Grazer · Clinical Professor of Surgery, Department of Plastic Surgery, Hershey School of Medicine; Associate Clinical Professor, Department of Plastic Surgery, University of California at Irvine School of Medicine · Hoag Memorial Hospital Presbyterian · 1101 Bayside Drive, Suite 100, Corona del Mar, CA 92625 · 714-644-5000

Ted E. Lockwood · Assistant Clinical Professor of Plastic Surgery, University of Missouri at Kansas City School of Medicine · Humana Hospital, Baptist Medical Center; St. Joseph Health Center · 10600 Quivira Road, Suite 470, Overland Park, KS 66215 · 913-894-1070

Gerald H. Pitman · Clinical Assistant Professor of Surgery, New York University School of Medicine · Attending Staff, Plastic Surgery, Manhattan Eye, Ear & Throat Hospital, University Hospital, and St. Luke's-Roosevelt Hospital Center 170 East 73rd Street, New York, NY 10021 · 212-517-2600

Bahman Teimourian · Clinical Professor of Plastic Surgery, Georgetown University School of Medicine · Former Chairman, Department of Surgery, Suburban Hospital · 8600 Old Georgetown Road, Bethesda, MD 20814 · 301-881-6363

BREAST SURGERY
(See also General Surgery, Breast Surgery)

Bernard S. Alpert · (Breast Reconstruction, Muscle and Tissue Transplantation) Associate Clinical Professor of Surgery, Division of Plastic & Reconstructive Surgery, University of California at San Francisco School of Medicine · Chief, Division of Plastic Surgery, and Vice-Chief, Microsurgery Department, Davies Medical Center · San Francisco Institute of Plastic Surgery, Suite 150, San Francisco, CA 94114 · 415-565-6622

Philip H. Beegle, Jr. · (Muscle and Tissue Transplantation, Breast Reconstruction) · Clinical Instructor, Emory University School of Medicine · Chief, Plastic Surgery, St. Joseph's Hospital · 975 Johnson Ferry Road NE, Suite 500, Atlanta, GA 30342 · 404-256-1311

John Bostwick III · (Breast Reconstruction) · Professor of Surgery, Division of Plastic Surgery, Emory University School of Medicine · Emory University Affiliated Hospitals; Crawford W. Long Memorial Hospital · 1365 Clifton Road, NE, Atlanta, GA 30322 · 404-248-3456

Lloyd N. Carlsen · (Aesthetic Breast Surgery) · Chief of Plastic Surgery, Scarborough General Hospital; Director of Plastic Surgery, Cosmetic Surgery Hospital in Woodbridge, Ontario · 2901 Lawrence Avenue East, Suite 408, Scarborough, Ontario M1P 2T3 · 416-269-7100

Benjamin E. Cohen · (Breast Reconstruction) · Academic Chief, and Director of Plastic Surgery Residency Program, St. Joseph Hospital · 1315 Calhoun Street, Suite 920, Houston, TX 77002 · 713-951-0400

I. Kelman Cohen · (Breast Reconstruction) · Professor of Surgery, Division of Plastic Surgery, Virginia Commonwealth University, Medical College of Virginia St. Mary's Hospital, Richmond Eye & Ear Hospital, St. Luke's Hospital, Henrico Doctors' Hospital · Division of Plastic Surgery, Richmond, VA 23298 · 804-786-9318

Lester Franklyn Elliott II · (Muscle and Tissue Transplantation, Breast Reconstruction) · Instructor, Emory University School of Medicine · Northside Hospital; Scottish Rite Children's Medical Center · 975 Johnson Ferry Road, Suite 500, Atlanta, GA 30342 · 404-256-1311

Jack Fisher · (Breast Reconstruction) · Assistant Clinical Professor of Plastic Surgery, Vanderbilt University School of Medicine · Baptist Hospital, The Institute for Aesthetic & Reconstructive Surgery · Nashville Plastic Surgery Clinic, 2021 Church Street, Suite 806, Nashville, TN 37203 · 615-340-4500

James C. Grotting · (Muscle and Tissue Transplantation, Breast Reconstruction) Associate Professor, The University of Alabama School of Medicine · The University of Alabama Hospital · 1813 Sixth Avenue South, Suite 524, Birmingham, AL 35294-3295 · 205-934-3312

Carl R. Hartrampf, Jr. · (Breast Reconstruction) · Clinical Professor, Emory University School of Medicine · St. Joseph's Hospital · 975 Johnson Ferry Road, NE, Suite 500, Atlanta, GA 30342 · 404-256-1311

T. Roderick Hester, Jr. · (Breast Augmentation) · Associate Professor of Surgery, Plastic & Reconstructive, Emory University School of Medicine · Emory University Affiliated Hospitals · 1327 Clifton Road, Atlanta, GA 30322 · 404-248-3455

David Lee Larson · (Breast Reconstruction) · Professor and Chairman, Department of Plastic & Reconstructive Surgery, Medical College of Wisconsin ·

Froedtert Memorial Lutheran Hospital · 9200 West Wisconsin Avenue, Milwaukee WI 53226 · 414-454-5445

John William Little III · (Breast Reconstruction) · Professor and Director, Division of Plastic Surgery, Georgetown University School of Medicine · Georgetown University Medical Center · 3800 Reservoir Road, Washington, DC 20007 · 202-687-8670

Stephen J. Mathes · (Breast Reconstruction) · Professor & Head of Plastic Surgery, University of California at San Francisco School of Medicine · University of California at San Francisco Medical Center · 350 Parnassus, Suite 509, San Francisco, CA 94143 · 415-476-3062

G. Patrick Maxwell · (Breast Reconstruction) · Assistant Clinical Professor of Plastic Surgery, Vanderbilt University School of Medicine · Director, The Institute for Aesthetic and Reconstructive Surgery, Baptist Hospital · Nashville Plastic Surgery, Ltd., 2021 Church Street, Suite 806, Nashville, TN 37203 · 615-340-4500

James W. May, Jr. · (Breast Reconstruction) · Clinical Associate Professor of Surgery, Harvard Medical School · Massachusetts General Hospital · Fruit Street, Ambulatory Care Unit, Floor 3A, Room 353, Boston, MA 02114 · 617-726-8220

John B. McCraw · (Breast Reconstruction) · Professor, Eastern Virginia Medical School · Norfolk General Hospital · 229 West Bute Street, 900 Wainwright Building, Norfolk, VA 23510 · 804-623-7072

Mary H. McGrath · (Breast Reconstruction) · Professor and Chief, Division of Plastic & Reconstructive Surgery, The George Washington University School of Medicine · The George Washington University Medical Center; Children's Hospital National Medical Center · 2150 Pennsylvania Avenue, Washington, DC 20037 · 202-994-8141

Walter R. Mullin · (Breast Reconstruction, Breast Reduction, Breast Augmentation) · Associate Professor of Plastic Surgery, University of Miami School of Medicine · University of Miami-Jackson Memorial Medical Center; Victoria Hospital; Miami Children's Hospital · 1444 Northwest 14th Avenue, Miami, FL 33125 · 305-325-1441

Foad Nahai · (Muscle and Tissue Transplantation, Breast Reconstruction) · Professor of Plastic Surgery, Emory University School of Medicine · Emory University Hospital · Emory University Clinic, 1365 Clifton Road NE, Atlanta, GA 30322 404-321-0111, 248-3793

James Joseph Ryan · (Breast Reconstruction) · Assistant Professor of Plastic Surgery, Johns Hopkins University School of Medicine · Chief of Plastic Surgery, Children's Hospital & Center for Reconstructive Surgery · 8415 Bellona Lane, Suite 201, Ruxton Towers, Baltimore, MD 21204 · 301-828-4577

Scott L. Spear · (Breast Reconstruction) · Professor of Surgery, Georgetown University School of Medicine · Georgetown University Medical Center · 3800 Reservoir Road NW, Washington, DC 20007 · 202-687-8751

William M. Swartz · (Muscle and Tissue Transplantation, Breast Reconstruction) Shadyside Hospital; Children's Hospital of Pittsburgh · 580 South Aiken Avenue, Suite 100, Pittsburgh, PA 15232 · 412-687-8810

John B. Tebbetts · (Aesthetic Breast Surgery) · Assistant Clinical Professor, The University of Texas Southwestern Medical Center at Dallas · Chief of Surgery, Mary Shiels Hospital · 2801 Lemon Avenue West, Suite 300, Dallas, TX 75204 · 214-220-2712

John E. Woods · (Breast Reconstruction) · Professor of Plastic Surgery, Mayo Medical School · Vice-Chairman, Department of Surgery, Mayo Clinic · 200 First Street, SW, Rochester, MN 55905 · 507-284-3252

CRANIOFACIAL SURGERY

Ian T. Jackson · Medical Director, Institute for Craniofacial Plastic and Reconstructive Surgery, Providence Hospital · 22250 Providence Drive, Suite 703, Southfield, MI 48075 · 313-424-5800

Henry K. Kawamoto · Clinical Professor of Plastic Surgery, University of California at Los Angeles School of Medicine · 1301 Twentieth Street, Suite 460, Santa Monica, CA 90404 · 213-829-0391

Paul N. Manson · (Trauma, Congenital Deformities) · Chairman, Division of Plastic Surgery, Johns Hopkins University School of Medicine · Chairman, Plastic Surgery, The Johns Hopkins Medical Institutions · 600 North Wolfe Street, Baltimore, MD 21205 · 410-955-6897

Jeffrey L. Marsh · Professor of Plastic & Reconstructive Surgery; and Associate Professor of Surgery in Pediatrics (Plastic & Reconstructive), Washington University School of Medicine · Medical Director of the Cleft Palate & Craniofacial Deformities Institute, and Director of Pediatric Plastic Surgery, St. Louis Children's Hospital · 400 South Kingshighway Boulevard, St. Louis, MO 63110 · 314-454-6020

Joseph G. McCarthy · Lawrence D. Bell Professor of Plastic Surgery, New York University School of Medicine · New York University Medical Center · 550 First Avenue, Department of IRPS, New York, NY 10016 · 212-628-4420

Louis Morales, Jr. · Associate Clinical Professor of Surgery, University of Utah School of Medicine · Associate Director of the Intermountain Cranial Facial Center, and Director, Plastic & Craniofacial Fellowship, Primary Children's Medical Center · 100 North Medical Drive, Suite 3600, Salt Lake City, UT 84113 · 801-588-3630

Ian R. Munro · Director, Humana Craniofacial Institute, Humana Hospital · 7777 Forest Lane, Suite C-700, Dallas, TX 75230 · 214-788-6464

Douglas K. Ousterhout · Clinical Professor of Plastic Surgery, University of California San Francisco, School of Medicine · St. Francis Memorial Hospital · Davies Medical Center, 45 Castro Street, Suite 150, San Francisco, CA 94114 · 415-565-6525

Jeffrey C. Posnick · Assistant Professor, Department of Surgery, Faculty of Medicine, and Assistant Professor, Faculty of Dentistry, University of Toronto School of Medicine · Medical Director, Craniofacial Program, The Hospital for Sick Children · 555 University Avenue, Toronto, Ontario M5G 1X8 · 416-598-6197

Kenneth Everett Salyer · (Cleft Lip and Palate Surgery) · Director & Founding Chairman, Humana Craniofacial Institute; Founding Chairman, Humana Advanced Surgical Institute (HASI); and, Humana Hospital · Medical City Dallas, 7777 Forest Lane, Suite C-717, Dallas, TX 75230 · 214-788-6555

Linton A. Whitaker · Professor of Surgery, University of Pennsylvania School of Medicine · Chief of Plastic Surgery, and Director of the Center for Human Appearance, Hospital of the University of Pennsylvania · 3400 Spruce Street, 10 Penn Tower, Philadelphia, PA 19104 · 215-662-2048

S. Anthony Wolfe · Clinical Professor of Plastic & Reconstructive Surgery, University of Miami School of Medicine · Chief of Plastic Surgery, Victoria Hospital; Miami Children's Hospital · 1444 Northwest 14th Avenue, Miami, FL 33125 · 305-325-1441

FACIAL AESTHETIC SURGERY

Sherrell Jerome Aston · (Facelift) · Associate Professor, Department of Plastic Surgery & Reconstructive Surgery, New York University School of Medicine · New York University Medical Center · 278 Park Avenue, New York, NY 10021 212-249-6000

Daniel C. Baker III · (Nasal Reconstruction, Facial Paralysis Reconstruction) · Associate Professor of Plastic Surgery, New York University Medical School; Institute of Reconstructive Plastic Surgery · Attending Surgeon, Manhattan Eye, Ear & Throat Hospital; Attending Surgeon, New York University Medical Center 630 Park Avenue, New York, NY 10021 · 212-734-9695

Thomas J. Baker, Jr. · Assistant Clinical Professor of Surgery, University of Miami School of Medicine · Senior Attending Physician, Mercy Hospital, and Cedars of Lebanon Hospital · Plastic Surgery Associates, 1501 South Miami Avenue, Miami, FL 33129 · 305-854-2424

Lloyd N. Carlsen · Chief of Plastic Surgery, Scarborough General Hospital; Director of Plastic Surgery, Cosmetic Surgery Hospital in Woodbridge, Ontario · 2901 Lawrence Avenue East, Suite 408, Scarborough, Ontario M1P 2T3 · 416-269-7100

James Howard Carraway · (Eyelid Surgery) · Professor, University of Eastern Virginia · Norfolk Medical Center Hospitals · 400 Gresham Drive, 508 Medical Tower, Norfolk, VA 23507 · 804-623-3749

Bruce F. Connell · Clinical Professor of Surgery (Plastic), University of California at Irvine School of Medicine; President, Canadian Society for Aesthetic (Cosmetic) Plastic Surgery · University of California at Irvine Medical Center · 2200 East Fruit Street, Suite 101, Santa Ana, CA 92701 · 714-972-0666

Rollin K. Daniel · (Rhinoplasty) · Clinical Professor of Plastic Surgery, University of California at Irvine School of Medicine · Hoag Memorial Hospital Presbyterian; Irvine Medical Center · 1441 Avocado Avenue, Suite 308, Newport Beach, CA 92660 · 714-721-0494

Jack A. Friedland · (Correction of Congenital Cleft Lip, Palate, and Craniofacial Deformities) · Attending Plastic Surgeon, Phoenix Plastic Surgery Fellowship Program, and Mayo Clinic Plastic Surgery Residency Training Program · Chief, Department of Plastic Surgery, Children's Rehabilitatiive Services; St. Joseph's Hospital & Medical Center · 101 East Coronado Road, Phoenix, AZ 85004-1556 602-257-8480

Howard L. Gordon · Plastic Surgery Associates, 1501 South Miami Avenue, Miami, FL 33129 · 305-854-2424

Gilbert P. Gradinger · Associate Clinical Professor of Surgery, Stanford University School of Medicine; Assistant Clinical Professor of Surgery, University of California at San Francisco School of Medicine · Chief of the Plastic & Reconstructive Surgery Section, Peninsula Hospital · 1750 ElCamino Real, Suite 405, Burlingame, CA 94010 · 415-692-0467

Jack Pershing Gunter · (Rhinoplasty) · Clinical Professor in Plastic Surgery and Otolaryngology, University of Texas Southwestern Medical Center · Past Chairman, Department of Plastic Surgery, Presbyterian Hospital of Dallas; Parkland Hospital of Dallas · 8315 Walnut Hill Lane, Suite 125, Dallas, TX 75231 · 214-369-8123

Sam T. Hamra · (Facelift) · Clinical Assistant Professor, The University of Texas Southwestern Medical Center at Dallas · Mary Shiels Hospital; Baylor Medical Center · 3707 Gaston Avenue, Suite 810, Dallas, TX 75246 · 214-823-9381

Bernard L. Kaye · Clinical Professor of Plastic Surgery, University of Florida · Baptist Medical Center · 820 Prudential Drive, Suite 702, Jacksonville, FL 32207 904-396-2816

Stanley A. Klatsky · (Eyelid Surgery) · Assistant Professor of Plastic Surgery, Johns Hopkins University School of Medicine · Chief of Staff (1991-1993), and Chief, Division of Plastic & Reconstructive Surgery, Baltimore County General Hospital · 122 Slade Avenue, Suite 100, Baltimore, MD 21208 · 301-484-0400

Vasilios Lambros · (Facelifts, Brow Lifts) · Clinical Instructor, University of California at Irvine School of Medicine · Western Medical Center · 2200 East Fruit Street, Suite 102, Santa Ana, CA 92701 · 714-972-0666

Peter McKinney · Professor of Clinical Surgery (Plastic), Northwestern University Medical School · Active Attending Staff, Northwestern Memorial Hospital · 707 North Fairbanks Court, Suite 1207, Chicago, IL 60611 · 312-266-0300

John Q. Owsley, Jr. · (Eyelid, Facelift) · Clinical Professor of Plastic Surgery, Division of Plastic Surgery, University of California at San Francisco School of Medicine · Davies Medical Center · 45 Castro Street, Suite 111, San Francisco, CA 94114 · 415-861-8040

George C. Peck, Sr. · (Rhinoplasty) · Hackensack Hospital · 1200 Route 46, Clifton, NJ 07013 · 201-471-3906

Rex A. Peterson · Director and Founder, Phoenix Plastic Surgery Residency Program · 2525 East Arizona Biltmore Circle, Phoenix, AZ 85106-2192 · 602-955-6777

Gerald H. Pitman · Clinical Assistant Professor of Surgery, New York University School of Medicine · Attending Staff, Plastic Surgery, Manhattan Eye, Ear & Throat Hospital, University Hospital, and St. Luke's-Roosevelt Hospital Center 170 East 73rd Street, New York, NY 10021 · 212-517-2600

Thomas D. Rees · Clinical Professor of Surgery, New York University Medical Center · Chairman, Department of Plastic Surgery, Manhattan Eye, Ear & Throat Hospital · 176 East 72nd Street, New York, NY 10021 · 212-535-1611

Bruno Ristow · Chief, Division of Plastic & Reconstructive Surgery, California Pacific Medical Center · 2100 Webster Street, Suite 502, San Francisco, CA 94115 415-923-3003

Jack H. Sheen · (Rhinoplasty) · Clinical Professor of Surgery, Section of Plastic & Reconstructive Surgery, University of Southern California; Associate Clinical Professor of Surgery, Division of Plastic Surgery, University of California at Los Angeles School of Medicine · 9201 Sunset Boulevard, Suite 814, Los Angeles, CA 90069 · 213-274-6603

John B. Tebbetts · (Rhinoplasty) · Assistant Clinical Professor, The University of Texas Southwestern Medical Center at Dallas · Chief of Surgery, Mary Shiels Hospital · 2801 Lemon Avenue West, Suite 300, Dallas, TX 75204 · 214-220-2712

John E. Williams · Clinical Faculty, University of California at Los Angeles School of Medicine · Medical Director, Aesthetica Surgical Center · 5757 Wilshire Boulevard, Los Angeles, CA 90036 · 213-935-3644

HEAD & NECK SURGERY
(See also Otolaryngology, Head & Neck Surgery)

Stephan Ariyan · Yale University School of Medicine · Yale-New Haven Hospital 40 Temple Street, New Haven, CT 06510 · 203-787-9888

John J. Coleman · Professor of Surgery, and Director, Plastic Surgery Department, Indiana University School of Medicine · Indiana University Medical Center 545 Barnhill Drive, Emerson Hall, Room 236, Indianapolis, IN 46202-5124 · 317-274-8106

Ian T. Jackson · Medical Director, Institute for Craniofacial Plastic and Reconstructive Surgery, Providence Hospital · 22250 Providence Drive, Suite 703, Southfield, MI 48075 · 313-424-5800

David Lee Larson · Professor and Chairman, Department of Plastic & Reconstructive Surgery, Medical College of Wisconsin · Froedtert Memorial Lutheran Hospital · 9200 West Wisconsin Avenue, Milwaukee WI 53226 · 414-454-5445

John E. Woods · Professor of Plastic Surgery, Mayo Medical School · Vice-Chairman, Department of Surgery, Mayo Clinic · 200 First Street, SW, Rochester, MN 55905 · 507-284-3252

LASER SURGERY & BIRTHMARKS
(See also Dermatology, Laser Surgery)

Bruce M. Achauer · Associate Adjunct Professor of Surgery, University of California at Irvine School of Medicine · Director, Burn Center, and Director, Plastic Surgery Division at Beckman Laser Institute, University of California at Irvine Medical Center · 705 West LaVeta Avenue, Suite 115, Orange, CA 92668; Effective 9-1-92: 1140 West LaVeta Avenue, 8th Floor, Orange, CA 92668 · 714-997-3330

David B. Apfelberg · Assistant Clinical Professor of Plastic Surgery, Stanford University Medical Center · Atherton Plastic Surgery Center; Stanford University Hospital · 3351 El Camino Real, Atherton, CA 94027 · 415-363-0300

Richard O. Gregory · Clinical Instructor, University of Central Florida · Chairman of Plastic Surgery, Florida Hospital; Orlando Regional Medical Center; Winter Park Memorial Hospital · Center for Plastic and Reconstructive Surgery, 2501 North Orange Avenue, Suite 310, Orlando, FL 32804 · 407-898-1436

Joel M. Noe · Clinical Assistant Professor of Plastic & Reconstructive Surgery, Harvard Medical School · Beth Israel Hospital · 575 Boylston Street, Newton Center, MA 02159 · 617-630-9400

MAXILLOFACIAL SURGERY

Joseph S. Gruss · (Trauma) · Professor of Surgery, Division of Plastic Surgery, University of Washington School of Medicine · Chief, Plastic Surgery, Childrens Hospital & Medical Center; Attending Staff, Harborview Medical Center · 4800 Sand Point Way, NE, Seattle, WA 98105; 325 Ninth Avenue (ZA-16), Seattle, WA 98104 · 206-223-3209, 527-3990

Henry K. Kawamoto · Clinical Professor of Plastic Surgery, University of California at Los Angeles School of Medicine · 1301 Twentieth Street, Suite 460, Santa Monica, CA 90404 · 213-829-0391

Edward Andrew Luce · (Trauma) · Professor of Surgery, University of Kentucky College of Medicine · Chief of Plastic Surgery, University of Kentucky Medical Center · 800 Rose Street, C233, Lexington, KY 40536 · 606-233-5887

Paul N. Manson · (Trauma, Congenital Deformities) · Chairman, Division of Plastic Surgery, Johns Hopkins University School of Medicine · Chairman, Plastic Surgery, The Johns Hopkins Medical Institutions · 600 North Wolfe Street, Baltimore, MD 21205 · 410-955-6897

Joseph G. McCarthy · Lawrence D. Bell Professor of Plastic Surgery, New York University School of Medicine · New York University Medical Center · 550 First Avenue, Department of IRPS, New York, NY 10016 · 212-628-4420

Louis Morales, Jr. · Associate Clinical Professor of Surgery, University of Utah School of Medicine · Associate Director of the Intermountain Cranial Facial Center, and Director, Plastic & Craniofacial Fellowship, Primary Children's Medical Center · 100 North Medical Drive, Suite 3600, Salt Lake City, UT 84113 · 801-588-3630

Ian R. Munro · Director, Humana Craniofacial Institute, Humana Hospital · 7777 Forest Lane, Suite C-700, Dallas, TX 75230 · 214-788-6464

Jeffrey C. Posnick · Assistant Professor, Department of Surgery, Faculty of Medicine, and Assistant Professor, Faculty of Dentistry, University of Toronto School of Medicine · Medical Director, Craniofacial Program, The Hospital for Sick Children · 555 University Avenue, Toronto, Ontario M5G 1X8 · 416-598-6197

S. Anthony Wolfe · Clinical Professor of Plastic & Reconstructive Surgery, University of Miami School of Medicine · Chief of Plastic Surgery, Victoria Hospital; Miami Children's Hospital · 1444 Northwest 14th Avenue, Miami, FL 33125 · 305-325-1441

MICROSURGERY
(See also Hand Surgery, Microsurgery)

Bernard S. Alpert · (Breast Reconstruction, Muscle and Tissue Transplantation) Associate Clinical Professor of Surgery, Division of Plastic & Reconstructive Surgery, University of California at San Francisco School of Medicine · Chief, Division of Plastic Surgery, and Vice-Chief, Microsurgery Department, Davies Medical Center · San Francisco Institute of Plastic Surgery, Suite 150, San Francisco, CA 94114 · 415-565-6622

Philip H. Beegle, Jr. · (Muscle and Tissue Transplantation, Breast Reconstruction) · Clinical Instructor, Emory University School of Medicine · Chief, Plastic Surgery, St. Joseph's Hospital · 975 Johnson Ferry Road NE, Suite 500, Atlanta, GA 30342 · 404-256-1311

Lester Franklyn Elliott II · (Muscle and Tissue Transplantation, Breast Reconstruction) · Instructor, Emory University School of Medicine · Northside Hospital; Scottish Rite Children's Medical Center · 975 Johnson Ferry Road, Suite 500, Atlanta, GA 30342 · 404-256-1311

James C. Grotting · (Muscle and Tissue Transplantation, Breast Reconstruction) Associate Professor, The University of Alabama School of Medicine · The University of Alabama Hospital · 1813 Sixth Avenue South, Suite 524, Birmingham, AL 35294-3295 · 205-934-3312

James W. May, Jr. · (Breast Reconstruction) · Clinical Associate Professor of Surgery, Harvard Medical School · Massachusetts General Hospital · Fruit Street, Ambulatory Care Unit, Floor 3A, Room 353, Boston, MA 02114 · 617-726-8220

William M. Swartz · (Muscle and Tissue Transplantation, Breast Reconstruction) Shadyside Hospital; Children's Hospital of Pittsburgh · 580 South Aiken Avenue, Suite 100, Pittsburgh, PA 15232 · 412-687-8810

OCULOPLASTIC & ORBITAL SURGERY
(See also Ophthalmology, Oculoplastic & Orbital Surgery)

Glenn W. Jelks · Associate Professor of Ophthalmology and Plastic Surgery, New York University Medical Center · Manhattan Eye, Ear & Throat Hospital; New York Eye & Ear Infirmary; Valley Hospital, Ridgewood, NJ · 830 Park Avenue, New York, NY 10021 · 212-988-3303

PEDIATRIC PLASTIC SURGERY

Michael John Boyajian · Assistant Professor of Plastic Surgery, The George Washington University School of Medicine · Chairman, Department of Plastic Surgery, Children's National Medical Center · 111 Michigan Avenue NW, Washington, DC 20010 · 202-745-2157

Jeffrey L. Marsh · (Cleft Lip and Palate Surgery) · Professor of Plastic & Reconstructive Surgery; and Associate Professor of Surgery in Pediatrics (Plastic & Reconstructive), Washington University School of Medicine · Medical Director of the Cleft Palate & Craniofacial Deformities Institute, and Director of Pediatric Plastic Surgery, St. Louis Children's Hospital · 400 South Kingshighway Boulevard, St. Louis, MO 63110 · 314-454-6020

John B. Mulliken · (Craniofacial Surgery, Vascular Anomalies) · Associate Professor of Surgery, Harvard Medical School · Associate in Surgery, Children's Hospital 300 Longwood Avenue, Boston, MA 02115 · 617-735-7686

John F. Reinisch · Chairman, Division of Plastic Surgery, and Associate Professor of Surgery, University of Southern California School of Medicine · Head, Division of Plastic Surgery, Children's Hospital of Los Angeles · Mail Stop 96, 4650 Sunset Boulevard, Los Angeles, CA 90027 · 213-669-4544

PERIPHERAL NERVE SURGERY
(See also Hand Surgery, Peripheral Nerve Surgery; Neurological Surgery, Peripheral Nerve Surgery; Orthopaedic Surgery, Peripheral Nerve Surgery)

A. Lee Dellon · Associate Professor of Plastic Surgery, and Associate Professor of Neurosurgery, Johns Hopkins University School of Medicine · The Johns Hopkins Medical Institutions; Children's Hospital & Center for Reconstructive Surgery · 3901 Greenspring Avenue, Suite 104, Baltimore, MD 21211 · 301-225-0300

Michael E. Jabaley · Clinical Professor of Plastic & Orthopaedic Surgery, University of Mississippi · University of Mississippi Medical Center; St. Dominic Hospital; River Oaks Hospital · 971 Lakeland Drive, Suite 515, Jackson, MS 39216 · 601-981-2525

Susan E. Mackinnon · (Thoracic Outlet Disorders, Brachial Plexus Surgery, Facial Palsy) · Professor of Surgery, Division of Plastic Surgery, Washington University School of Medicine · Director, Peripheral Nerve Surgical Center, Barnes Hospital · One Barnes Hospital Plaza, 17424 East Pavilion, St. Louis, MO 63110 314-362-4587

Allen L. Van Beek · Clinical Associate Professor of Surgery, University of Minnesota School of Medicine · North Memorial Medical Center; Fairview South Dale Hospital; Abbott Northwestern Hospital; Minneapolis Children's Medical Center · 7373 France Avenue South, Suite 510, Minneapolis, MN 55435 · 612-588-0593, 830-1028

H. Bruce Williams · Professor of Surgery, and Director, Division of Plastic & Reconstructive Surgery, McGill University · Director, Division of Plastic & Reconstructive Surgery, Montreal General Hospital; Montreal Children's Hospital · 1650 Cedar Avenue, Suite 646, Montreal, Quebec H3G 1A4 · 514-933-7730

RECONSTRUCTIVE SURGERY
(See also Hand Surgery, Reconstructive Surgery; Orthopaedic Surgery, Reconstructive Surgery)

Bruce M. Achauer · (Burn Reconstruction) · Associate Adjunct Professor of Surgery, University of California at Irvine School of Medicine · Director, Burn Center, and Director, Plastic Surgery Division at Beckman Laser Institute, University of California at Irvine Medical Center · 705 West LaVeta Avenue, Suite 115, Orange, CA 92668; Effective 9-1-92: 1140 West LaVeta Avenue, 8th Floor, Orange, CA 92668 · 714-997-3330

Bernard S. Alpert · (Breast Reconstruction, Muscle and Tissue Transplantation) Associate Clinical Professor of Surgery, Division of Plastic & Reconstructive Surgery, University of California at San Francisco School of Medicine · Chief, Division of Plastic Surgery, and Vice-Chief, Microsurgery Department, Davies Medical Center · San Francisco Institute of Plastic Surgery, Suite 150, San Francisco, CA 94114 · 415-565-6622

Phillip G. Arnold · (Chest Wall Reconstruction) · Professor of Plastic Surgery, Mayo Medical School · Mayo Clinic · 200 First Street, SW, Rochester, MN 55905 507-284-3214

Fritz E. Barton, Jr. · (Facial Reconstruction Surgery, Cosmetic) · Professor, Department of Plastic Surgery, The University of Texas Southwestern Medical Center at Dallas · Baylor University Medical Center · Wadley Tower, 3600 Gaston Avenue, Suite 751, Dallas, TX 75246 · 214-827-0925

Paul William Black · (Cleft Lip and Palate Surgery) · President, Atlanta Plastic Surgery · 975 Johnson Ferry Road, NE, Suite 500, Atlanta GA 30342 · 404-256-1311

Burton D. Brent · (Ear Reconstruction, Microtia, Congenital Atresia) · Associate Clinical Professor of Plastic Surgery, Stanford University School of Medicine · El Camino Hospital · 2995 Woodside Road, Suite 300, Woodside, CA 94062 · 415-851-5300

Harry J. Buncke · Clinical Professor of Surgery, University of California at San Francisco School of Medicine · Director, Neurosurgical Division, Davies Medical Center; Peninsula-Mills Hospitals · Davies Medical Center, M.O.B. Annex Suite 140, 45 Castro Street, San Francisco, CA 94114 · 415-342-8989

Gary C. Burget · (Nasal Reconstruction) · Clinical Associate, Section of Plastic & Reconstruction Surgery, Department of Surgery, University of Chicago, Pritzker School of Medicine · St. Joseph's Hospital · 2913 North Commonwealth Avenue, Suite 400, Chicago, IL 60657 · 312-880-0062

John J. Coleman · Professor of Surgery, and Director, Plastic Surgery Department, Indiana University School of Medicine · Indiana University Medical Center 545 Barnhill Drive, Emerson Hall, Room 236, Indianapolis, IN 46202-5124 · 317-274-8106

Loren H. Engrav · (Burn Reconstruction) · Professor of Plastic Surgery, University of Washington School of Medicine · Chief, Division of Plastic Surgery, Harborview Medical Center · 325 Ninth Avenue (ZA-16), Seattle, WA 98104 · 206-223-3209

Elof Eriksson · Professor and Chairman, Division of Plastic Surgery, Harvard Medical School · Brigham & Women's Hospital · 75 Francis Street, Boston, MA 02115 · 617-732-5500

Joel J. Feldman · (Facial Burn Reconstruction) · Teaching Consultant, Harvard Medical School · Mt. Auburn Hospital · Doctors' Office Building, 300 Mt. Auburn Street, Suite 304, Cambridge, MA 02238 · 617-661-5998

Robert M. Goldwyn · Clinical Professor of Surgery, Harvard Medical School · Head, Division of Plastic Surgery, Beth Israel Hospital · 1101 Beacon Street, Brookline, MA 02146 · 617-232-7523

Frederick R. Heckler · Clinical Associate Professor of Surgery, University of Pittsburgh School of Medicine · Chief, Division of Plastic & Reconstructive Surgery, Allegheny General Hospital · Division of Plastic Surgery, 320 East North Avenue, Pittsburgh, PA 15212 · 412-359-4352

Malcolm A. Lesavoy · Associate Professor, Division of Plastic Surgery, University of California at Los Angeles School of Medicine · Chief of Plastic & Reconstructive Surgery, Harbor-UCLA Medical Center · 1000 West Carson, Torrance, CA 90509 · 310-825-1647

Jeffrey L. Marsh · (Cleft Lip and Palate Surgery) · Professor of Plastic & Reconstructive Surgery; and Associate Professor of Surgery in Pediatrics (Plastic & Reconstructive), Washington University School of Medicine · Medical Director of the Cleft Palate & Craniofacial Deformities Institute, and Director of Pediatric Plastic Surgery, St. Louis Children's Hospital · 400 South Kingshighway Boulevard, St. Louis, MO 63110 · 314-454-6020

John B. McCraw · (Breast Reconstruction) · Professor, Eastern Virginia Medical School · Norfolk General Hospital · 229 West Bute Street, 900 Wainwright Building, Norfolk, VA 23510 · 804-623-7072

D. Ralph Millard, Jr. · (Cleft Lip and Palate Surgery, Rhinoplasty) · The Light Millard Professor of Plastic Surgery, and Chief, Division of Plastic Surgery, University of Miami School of Medicine · University of Miami-Jackson Memorial Medical Center; Miami Children's Hospital · 1444 Northwest 14th Avenue, Miami, FL 33125 · 305-325-1441

Foad Nahai · (Muscle and Tissue Transplantation, Breast Reconstruction) · Professor of Plastic Surgery, Emory University School of Medicine · Emory University Hospital · Emory University Clinic, 1365 Clifton Road NE, Atlanta, GA 30322 404-321-0111, 248-3793

Henry W. Neale · (Burn Reconstruction) · Director, Division of Plastic Reconstructive & Hand Surgery, University of Cincinnati College of Medicine · Director, Division of Plastic, Reconstructive & Hand Surgery, Shriners Burn Center, Children's Hospital Medical Center · 231 Bethesda Avenue, ML 558, Cincinnati, OH 45267-0558 · 513-558-4363

Martin C. Robson · (Burn Reconstruction) · Professor and Chief, Division of Plastic Surgery, The University of Texas Medical Branch at Galveston · Director, Surgical Services, Shriners Burns Institute · 610 Texas Avenue, Galveston, TX 77550 · 409-772-1255

Kenneth Everett Salyer · (Cleft Lip and Palate Surgery) · Director & Founding Chairman, Humana Craniofacial Institute; Founding Chairman, Humana Advanced Surgical Institute (HASI); and, Humana Hospital · Medical City Dallas, 7777 Forest Lane, Suite C-717, Dallas, TX 75230 · 214-788-6555

Alan E. Seyfer · (Chest Wall Reconstruction, Rheumatoid Arthritis) · Professor of Surgery, and Head of Plastic Surgery, Oregon Health Sciences University · 3181 Southwest Sam Jackson Park Road, L352A, Portland, OR 97201-3098 · 503-494-7824

David John Smith, Jr. · (Burn Reconstruction) · Associate Professor of Surgery, and Section Head, Plastic & Reconstructive Surgery, The University of Michigan Medical School · The University of Michigan Medical Center · 1500 East Medical Center Drive, Taubman Center, Room 2130, Ann Arbor, MI 48109-0340 · 313-936-8925

Luis Oswaldo Vasconez · Professor and Chief, Division of Plastic Surgery, The University of Alabama School of Medicine · The University of Alabama Hospital 1813 Sixth Avenue South (MEB-524), Birmingham, AL 35294-3295 · 205-934-3245

Harvey A. Zarem · Professor Emeritus, Department of Surgery, University of California at Los Angeles School of Medicine · St. John's Hospital & Health Center; Santa Monica Hospital · 1301 Twentieth Street, Suite 470, Santa Monica, CA 90404 · 310-315-0222

WOUND HEALING
(See also Dermatology, Wound Healing; Plastic Surgery, Wound Healing)

I. Kelman Cohen · Professor of Surgery, Division of Plastic Surgery, Virginia Commonwealth University, Medical College of Virginia · St. Mary's Hospital, Richmond Eye & Ear Hospital, St. Luke's Hospital, Henrico Doctors' Hospital · Division of Plastic Surgery, Richmond, VA 23298 · 804-786-9318

Elof Eriksson · Professor and Chairman, Division of Plastic Surgery, Harvard Medical School · Brigham & Women's Hospital · 75 Francis Street, Boston, MA 02115 · 617-732-5500

Thomas Anthony Mustoe · Professor of Surgery, Northwestern University Medical School · Chief, Division of Plastic & Reconstructive Surgery, Northwestern Memorial Hospital · 707 North Fairbanks Court, Suite 811, Chicago, IL 60611 · 312-908-5585

Martin C. Robson · The Truman G. Blocke, Jr. Professor of Surgery, The University of Texas Medical Branch at Galveston · Chief, Division of Plastic Surgery, The John Sealy Hospital · The McCullough Building, 301 University Boulevard, Room 6.130, Galveston, TX 77550 · 409-772-1255

PSYCHIATRY

ADDICTION MEDICINE
(See also Addiction Medicine, p. 1)

Jack David Blaine · Chief, Treatment Research Branch, Division of Clinical Research, National Institute on Drug Abuse, National Institutes of Health · 5600 Fishers Lane, Room 10 A30, Rockville, MD 20857 · 301-443-4060

Sheila Bierman Blume · (Alcoholism) · Clinical Professor of Psychiatry, State University of New York Health Science Center at Stony Brook · Medical Director, Alcoholism, Chemical Dependency and Compulsive Gambling Programs, South Oaks Hospital, Amityville, NY · 284 Greene Avenue, Sayville, NY 11782 · 516-264-4000 x5017

John Nelson Chappel · Professor, Department of Psychiatry & Behavioral Sciences, University of Nevada School of Medicine · Medical Director, Alcohol & Drug Programs, Truckee Meadows Hospital · Manville Medical Building, 354, Reno, NV 89557-0046 · 702-784-4917

Domenic A. Ciraulo · (Benzodiazepines,Addiction to Prescribed Drugs, Alcoholism) · Associate Professor of Psychiatry, Tufts University School of Medicine · Chief, Psychiatry Service, Department of Veterans Affairs Outpatient Clinic · 251 Causeway Street, Boston, MA 02114 · 617-248-1047

Thomas J. Crowley · Professor of Psychiatry, University of Colorado School of Medicine · University of Colorado Health Sciences Center; Colorado Psychiatric Hospital · 4200 East Ninth Avenue, Box C-268-35, Denver, CO 80262 · 303-270-7573

Robert Louis Dupont, Jr. · (Benzodiazepines) · Clinical Professor of Psychiatry, Georgetown University School of Medicine · President, Institute for Behavior & Health, Inc. · 6191 Executive Boulevard, Rockville, MD 20852 · 301-231-9010

Richard J. Frances · Vice-Chairman, Department of Psychiatry, and Director, Residency Training, and Professor of Clinical Psychiatry, University of Medicine & Dentistry of New Jersey · University Hospital · 144 East End Avenue, New York, NY 10028 · 212-996-7420

William A. Frosch · (Consultation) · Professor and Interim Chairman, Department of Psychiatry, Cornell University Medical College · Interim Psychiatrist-in-Chief, The New York Hospital-Cornell Medical Center · 525 East 68th Street, New York, NY 10021 · 212-746-3667

Marc Galanter · (Alcoholism) · Professor of Psychiatry, New York University School of Medicine · Director of the Division of Alcoholism and Drug Abuse, New York University Medical Center · 285 Central Park West, New York, NY 10024 · 212-877-4093

Donald M. Gallant · Professor Emeritus of Psychiatry, Tulane University School of Medicine · Tulane University Medical Center · 1415 Tulane Avenue, New Orleans, LA 70112 · 504-588-5687

Jerome Herbert Jaffe · Associate Director, Office for Treatment Improvement, Alcohol, Drug Abuse & Mental Health Administration · Clinical Professor of Psychiatry, University of Connecticut Medical Center · 5515 Security Lane, Rockwall II Building, 10th Floor, Rockville, MD 20852 · 301-443-6549

Edward R. Kaufman · (Substance Abuse in Families) · Professor of Psychiatry, University of California at Irvine School of Medicine · Director, University Substance Abuse Service, University of California at Irvine Medical Center; Capistrano by the Sea Hospital · 15615 Alton Parkway, Irvine, CA 92718 · 714-727-4333

Edward J. Khantzian · (Psychotherapy) · Associate Clinical Professor of Psychiatry, Harvard Medical School · Principal Psychiatrist for Substance Abuse Disorders, Cambridge Hospital; Associate Medical Director, Danvers State Hospital · 10-12 Phoenix Road, Haverhill, MA 01832 · 508-372-0240

Thomas R. Kosten · (Medical Treatment of Drug Abusers) · Associate Professor of Psychiatry, Yale University School of Medicine · Acting Co-director, Substance Abuse Treatment Unit, Yale-New Haven Hospital · 27 Sylvan Avenue, New Haven, CT 06519 · 203-782-2221

Walter Ling · (Medical Treatment of Drug Abusers) · Clinical Associate Professor of Psychiatry, Department of Psychiatry and Biobehavioral Sciences, University of California at Los Angeles School of Medicine · CPC Westwood Hospital; Pine Grove Hospital; University of California at Los Angeles Neuropsychiatric Institute 8447 Wilshire Boulevard, Suite 409, Beverly Hills, CA 90211 · 213-655-3258

Joyce H. Lowinson · (Drug Abuse) · Clinical Professor of Psychiatry, and Executive Director, Division of Substance Abuse, Albert Einstein College of Medicine 1300 Morris Park Avenue, Bronx, NY 10461 · 212-409-1916

Roger E. Meyer · (Alcoholism, Drug Abuse) · Physicians Health Services Professor & Chair, Department of Psychiatry, and Executive Dean, School of Medicine, University of Connecticut School of Medicine · John Dempsey Hospital · Department of Psychiatry, 10 Talcott Notch Road, East Wing, Farmington, CT 06032-1806 · 203-679-6732

Sheldon I. Miller · Chairman and Lizzie Gilman Professor, Northwestern University Medical School · Director, Institute of Psychiatry, Northwestern Memorial Hospital · 303 East Superior, Suite 561, Chicago, IL 60611 · 312-908-2323

Robert B. Millman · (Drug Abuse, Alcoholism) · Saul P. Steinberg Distinguished Professor of Psychiatry & Public Health, Cornell University Medical College · Project Director of Adolescent Development Program, and Director of Alcohol & Substance Abuse Services, Payne Whitney Clinic; Medical Director of Employee Assistance Program Consortium, The Employee Development Center, and Midtown Center for Treatment & Research, The New York Hospital-Cornell Medical Center · 411 East 69th Street, Room 305, New York, NY 10021 · 212-746-1248

Steven M. Mirin · Associate Professor of Psychiatry, Harvard Medical School · General Director/Psychiatrist in Chief, McLean Hospital · 115 Mill Street, Belmont, MA 02178 · 617-855-3615

Charles P. O'Brien · (Medical Treatment of Drug Abusers) · Professor and Vice Chairman, Department of Psychiatry, University of Pennsylvania School of Medicine · Chief of Psychiatry, Veterans Affairs Medical Center, Philadelphia; Hospital of the University of Pennsylvania · Treatment Research Center, 3900 Chestnut Street, Philadelphia, PA 19104-6178 · 215-222-3200 x132

Joseph A. Pursch · Attending Staff, College Hospital · 3151 Airway Avenue, Suite C-1, Costa Mesa, CA 92626 · 714-545-7114

Richard Boyce Resnick · Clinical Associate Professor, Department of Psychiatry, New York University School of Medicine · Attending Staff, Bellevue Hospital · Center for Psychiatry & Family Therapy, 43 West 94th Street, New York, NY 10025 · 212-662-1899

Bruce J. Rounsaville · (Drug Abuse) · Associate Professor of Psychiatry, Yale University School of Medicine · Director, Psycho-social Research, Substance Abuse Treatment Unit, Connecticut Mental Health Center · 27 Sylvan Avenue, New Haven, CT 06519 · 203-785-0705

Marc Alan Schuckit · (Alcoholism) · Professor of Psychiatry, University of California, San Diego School of Medicine · Director, Alcohol Research Center, San Diego Veterans Affairs Medical Center · 3350 La Jolla Village Drive, San Diego, CA 92161 · 619-552-8585 x7978

Anne Maxwell Seiden · (Addicted Pregnant Women) · Associate Professor of Psychiatry & Public Health, The University of Illinois College of Medicine at Chicago · Chairman, Department of Psychiatry, Cook County Hospital · 1825 West Harrison Street, 214 B-Building, Chicago, IL 60612 · 312-633-8902

Edward C. Senay · Professor of Psychiatry, University of Chicago, Pritzker School of Medicine · University of Chicago Medical Center · 5841 South Maryland Avenue, Box 411, Chicago, IL 60637 · 312-702-6185, 219-787-9126

Peter J. Steinglass · (Susbtance Abuse in Families) · Professor of Psychiatry & Behavioral Science, and Director, Center for Family Research, The George Washington University School of Medicine · 2300 "Eye" Street NW, Washington, DC 20037 · 202-994-2624

Roger Dale Walker · (Alcoholism) · Professor and Director, Division of Addictions & Social/Cultural Psychiatry, University of Washington School of Medicine · Chief, Addictions Treatment Center, Seattle Veterans Affairs Medical Center · 1660 South Columbian Way, ATC-116, Seattle, WA 98108 · 206-764-2782

Roger D. Weiss · Associate Professor of Psychiatry, Harvard Medical School · Clinical Director, Alcohol & Drug Abuse Program, McLean Hospital · 115 Mill Street, Belmont, MA 02178 · 617-855-2242

George E. Woody · (Medical Treatment of Drug Abusers) · Clinical Professor of Psychiatry, University of Pennsylvania School of Medicine · Chief, Substance Abuse Treatment Unit, Veterans Affairs Medical Center, Philadelphia · Department of Veteran Affairs, University and Woodland Avenues, Building Seven, Philadelphia, PA 19104 · 215-823-5809

AFFECTIVE DISORDERS

Hagop S. Akiskal · (Depression, Bipolar Disorder) · Professor of Psychiatry and Pharmacology, University of Tennessee, Memphis · Senior Science Advisor on Affective & Related Disorders, National Institute of Mental Health · 5600 Fishers Lane, Room 10C 24, Rockville, MD 20857 · 301-443-1636

James C. Ballenger · (Anxiety Disorders) · Professor and Chairman, Department of Psychiatry, and Director, Institute of Psychiatry, Medical University of South Carolina · 171 Ashley Avenue, Charleston, SC 29425 · 803-792-4037

Bernard J. Carroll · Professor of Psychiatry, Duke University School of Medicine Clinical Director, Geriatric Psychiatry Institute, John Umstead Hospital · Butner, NC 27509-1626 · 919-575-7923

Dennis S. Charney · Professor, Department of Psychiatry, Yale University School of Medicine · Chief, Psychiatry Service, West Haven Veterans Affairs Medical Center · 950 Campbell Avenue, West Haven, CT 06516 · 203-937-3837

Paula J. Clayton · Professor and Head, Department of Psychiatry, University of Minnesota Medical School · University of Minnesota Hospital & Clinic · Box 77 UMHC,420 Delaware Street, SE, Minneapolis, MN 55455 · 612-626-3853

J. Raymond DePaulo, Jr. · (Manic Depression) · Associate Professor of Psychiatry, Johns Hopkins University School of Medicine · The Johns Hopkins Medical Institutions · Meyer 3-181, Baltimore, MD 21205-2104 · 410-955-3246

Steven L. Dubovsky · Professor of Psychiatry and Medicine and Vice-Chairman, Department of Psychiatry, University of Colorado School of Medicine · University of Colorado Health Sciences Center · 4200 East Ninth Avenue, Box C-260, Denver, CO 80262 · 303-270-8481

David L. Dunner · Professor, Department of Psychiatry, University of Washington School of Medicine · Director, Outpatient Psychiatry, and Co-Director, Center for Anxiety & Depression, and Vice-Chairman for Clinical Services, University of Washington Medical Center · 4225 Roosevelt Way NE, Suite 306, Seattle, WA 98105 · 206-543-6768

Jan Fawcett · Professor and Chairman, Department of Psychiatry, Rush Medical College · Rush-Presbyterian-St. Luke's Medical Center · 1720 West Polk, Chicago, IL 60612 · 312-942-5372

John P. Feighner · Associate Clinical Professor of Psychiatry, University of California at San Diego School of Medicine · Director, Research, Feighner Research Institute, San Diego · 1101 Devonshire Drive, Suite E, Encinitas, CA 92024 · 619-753-1234

Alan J. Gelenberg · Professor and Head, Department of Psychiatry, The University of Arizona College of Medicine · The University of Arizona Health Sciences Center · 1501 North Campbell Avenue, Tucson, AZ 85724 · 602-626-6336

Robert H. Gerner · (Anxiety Disorders) · Associate Research Professor of Psychiatry, University of California at Los Angeles School of Medicine · Chief, Affective Disorders Unit and Director, Center for Mood Disorders, Veterans Affairs Hospital · Center for Mood Disorders, 1990 South Bundy, Suite 790, Los Angeles, CA 90025 · 213-207-8448

Elliot Sheldon Gershon · Chief of Clinical Neurogenetics Branch, National Institute of Mental Health, National Institutes of Health · 9000 Rockville Pike, Building 10, Room 3N218, Bethesda, MD 20892 · 301-496-3465

Alexander H. Glassman · (Depression, Cigarette Smoking Cessation) · Professor of Clinical Psychiatry, College of Physicians & Surgeons of Columbia University Chief, Department of Clinical Psychopharmacology, New York State Psychiatric Institute; Columbia-Presbyterian Medical Center · 722 West 168th Street, Box 116, New York, NY 10032 · 212-960-5750

Frederick K. Goodwin · Administrator, Alcohol, Drug Abuse & Mental Health Administration · Parklawn Building, 5600 Fishers Lane, Room 12-105; Rockville, MD 20857 · 301-443-4797

Jack M. Gorman · (Anxiety, Panic) · Professor of Clinical Psychiatry, College of Physicians & Surgeons of Columbia University · Attending Psychiatrist, Columbia- Presbyterian Medical Center · 722 West 168th Street, New York, NY 10032 212-799-5202

Robert M. A. Hirschfeld · (Depression) · Professor and Chairman, Department of Psychiatry & Behavioral Sciences, The University of Texas Medical Branch at Galveston · Galveston, TX 77550 · 409-772-3901

Lewis L. Judd · (Medication of Manic Depression Illness) · Mary Gilman Marston Professor of Psychiatry; and Chairman, Department of Psychiatry, University of California, San Diego, School of Medicine · University of California, San Diego Medical Center · Basic Science Building, La Jolla, CA 92093 · 619-534-3684

Martin B. Keller · (Bipolar Depression) · Professor and Chairman, Department of Psychiatry & Human Behavior, Brown University School of Medicine · Executive Psychiatrist and Chief, Butler Hospital · 345 Blackstone Boulevard, Room 204, Providence, RI 02906 · 401-455-6430

Donald F. Klein · (Anxiety) · Professor of Psychiatry, College of Physicians & Surgeons of Columbia University · Attending Psychiatrist, Columbia-Presbyterian Medical Center · 722 West 168th Street, Box 22, New York, NY 10032 · 212-960-2307

David J. Kupfer · (Depression) · Professor and Chairman, Department of Psychiatry, University of Pittsburgh School of Medicine · Western Psychiatric Institute and Clinic, University of Pittsburgh Medical Center · 3811 O'Hara Street, Pittsburgh, PA 15213-2593 · 412-624-2353

Michael R. Liebowitz · (Anxiety) · Professor of Clinical Psychiatry, College of Physicians & Surgeons of Columbia University · Director, Anxiety Disorder Clinic, New York State Psychiatric Institute · 722 West 168th Street, Box 120, New York, NY 10032 · 212-960-2366

Barnett Samuel Meyers · Associate Professor of Clinical Psychiatry, Cornell University Medical College · The New York Hospital-Cornell Medical Center, Westchester Division · 21 Bloomingdale Road, White Plains, NY 10605 · 914-997-5721

J. Craig Nelson · Professor of Psychiatry, Yale University School of Medicine · Director, Psychiatric Inpatient Service, Yale-New Haven Hospital · 20 York Street, MU-10-704, New Haven, CT 06504 · 203-785-2157

Charles B. Nemeroff · (Manic Depression) · Professor and Chairman, Department of Psychiatry, Emory University School of Medicine · 1701 Uppergate Drive, Atlanta, GA 30322 · 404-727-5881

Russell Noyes, Jr. · (Anxiety) · Professor of Psychiatry, The University of Iowa College of Medicine · The University of Iowa Hospitals & Clinics · 500 Newton Road, Iowa City, IA 52242 · 319-353-3898

Robert Morton Post · Chief, Biological Psychiatry Branch, National Institute of Mental Health · 9000 Rockville Pike, Building 10, Room 3N212, Bethesda, MD 20892 · 301-496-4805

Arthur J. Prange, Jr. · Boshamer Professor of Psychiatry, and Director, NIMH Clinical Research Center Chapel Hill, University of North Carolina School of Medicine · University of North Carolina Hospitals · 101 Manning Drive, Campus Box 7160, Chapel Hill, NC 27599-7160 · 919-966-1489

Frederic M. Quitkin · Professor of Clinical Psychiatry, College of Physicians & Surgeons of Columbia University · Director, Depression Evaluation Service, New York State Psychiatric Institute · 722 West 168th Street, Box 12, New York, NY 10032 · 212-960-5784, 516-484-0013

Victor I. Reus · (Affective Disorders Related to Brain Injury) · Professor, Department of Psychiatry, University of California at San Francisco School of Medicine Professor and Medical Director, Langley Porter Neuropsychiatric Institute · 401 Parnassus Avenue, San Francisco, CA 94143-0984 · 415-476-7478

Robert G. Robinson · (Affective Disorders Related to Brain Injury, Strokes) · Professor and Head of Psychiatry, The University of Iowa College of Medicine · The University of Iowa Hospitals & Clinics · 500 Newton Road, Room 1-289 MEB, Iowa City, IA 52242 · 319-356-4658

Gerald F. Rosenbaum · Chief of Psychopharmacology & Behavioral Therapy, Massachusetts General Hospital · 15 Parkman Street, WACC815, Boston, MA 02114 · 617-726-3488

Peter P. Roy-Byrne · (Anxiety) · Professor of Psychiatry, University of Washington School of Medicine · Director, Anxiety Disorders Program, University of Washington Medical Center · 1959 Northeast Pacific Street, RP-10, Seattle, WA 98195 · 206-543-3924

A. John Rush · Betty Jo Hay Distinguished Chair in Mental Health, and Professor of Psychiatry, The University of Texas Southwestern Medical Center at Dallas · Parkland Memorial Hospital · 5323 Harry Hines Boulevard, Dallas, TX 75235 · 214-688-8768

Alan F. Schatzberg · Kenneth T. Norris, Jr. Professor and Chairman, Department of Psychiatry & Behavioral Sciences, Stanford University School of Medicine · Chief of Psychiatry, Stanford University Hospital · Panama Street, Psychiatry Building, TD114, Stanford, CA 94305-5490 · 415-723-6811

David V. Sheehan · (Anxiety, Panic) · Professor of Psychology, University of South Florida College of Arts & Sciences; Professor of Psychiatry, and Director of the Office of Research, Department of Psychiatry & Behavioral Medicine, University of South Florida College of Medicine · Director of Clinical Research, University of South Florida Psychiatry Center · University of South Florida Psychiatry Center, 3515 East Fletcher Avenue, Tampa, FL 33613 · 813-974-3344

Peter E. Stokes · (Affective Disorders Related to Brain Injury) · Professor of Medicine & Psychiatry, Cornell University Medical College · Chief, Department of Psychobiology, The New York Hospital-Cornell Medical Center · Payne Whitney Clinic, 525 East 68th Street, New York, NY 10021 · 212-746-3819

Michael E. Thase · Associate Professor of Psychiatry, University of Pittsburgh School of Medicine · Medical and Research Director, Mood Disorders Module, Western Psychiatric Institute & Clinic, University of Pittsburgh Medical Center · 3811 O'Hara Street, Suite E-824, Pittsburgh, PA 15213 · 412-624-0752

Thomas Whitley Uhde · (Anxiety) · Clinical Professor, Department of Psychiatry, Uniformed Services University of the Health Sciences School of Medicine · Chief, Anxiety & Affective Disorders, National Institute of Mental Health, National Institutes of Health · Section on Anxiety & Affective Disorders, 9000 Rockville Pike, Room 3-S 239, Bethesda, MD 20892 · 301-496-6825

Paul H. Wender · (Attention Deficit Disorder, Pediatric Hyperactivity, Adult Hyperactivity · Distinguished Professor of Psychiatry, University of Utah School of Medicine · Director of Psychiatric Resources, University of Utah Health Sciences Center · 50 North Medical Drive, Salt Lake City, UT 84132 · 801-581-8075

Peter C. Whybrow · (Neuroendocrinology) · Professor and Chairman, Department of Psychiatry, University of Pennsylvania School of Medicine · Psychiatrist-in-Chief, Hospital of the University of Pennsylvania · 305 Blockley Hall, 418 Service Drive, Philadelphia, PA 19104 · 215-662-2818

George Winokur · The Paul W. Penningroth Professor of Psychiatry, The University of Iowa College of Medicine · The University of Iowa Hospitals & Clinics Medical Education Building, 500 Newton Road, Iowa City, IA 52242 · 319-353-4551

AUTISM

Magda Campbell · Professor of Psychiatry, New York University School of Medicine · Director, Division of Child & Adolescent Psychiatry, Bellevue Hospital · 550 First Avenue, 21S15, New York, NY 10016 · 212-263-6206

Donald J. Cohen · Director of the Child Study Center, and Irving B. Harris Professor of Child Psychiatry, Pediatrics & Psychology, Yale University School of Medicine · Chairman of the Department of Child Psychiatry, Yale-New Haven Hospital · P.O. Box 3333, 230 South Frontage Road, Room I-267, Sterling Hall of Medicine, New Haven, CT 06510 · 203-785-5759

Susan E. Folstein · Professor of Psychiatry (Joint Appointment in Medicine and Pediatrics), and Director of Psychiatric Genetics, and Director of Child & Adolescent Psychiatry, Johns Hopkins University School of Medicine · The Johns Hopkins Medical Institutions · Johns Hopkins Hospital, 600 North Wolfe Street, Meyer 2-181, Baltimore, MD 21205 · 410-955-2320

Edward R. Ritvo · (Family-Related Problems) · Professor of Psychiatry, University of California at Los Angeles School of Medicine · University of California at Los Angeles Neuropsychiatric Institute · 760 Westwood Plaza, Los Angeles, CA 90024 · 310-825-0220

Fred R. Volkmar · Harris Associate Professor of Child Psychiatry, Pediatrics and Psychiatry, Yale University School of Medicine · Attending Physician, Yale-New Haven Hospital · 230 South Frontage Road, New Haven, CT 06510 · 203-785-2510

BEHAVIORAL DISORDERS

Eric Douglas Caine · Professor of Psychiatry & Neurology, and Associate Chairman for Academic Affairs, University of Rochester School of Medicine & Dentistry, Department of Psychiatry · Strong Memorial Hospital, University of Rochester Medical Center · 300 Crittenden Boulevard, Rochester, NY 14642 · 716-275-3574

Susan E. Folstein · (Huntington's Disease) · Professor of Psychiatry (Joint Appointment in Medicine and Pediatrics), and Director of Psychiatric Genetics, and Director of Child & Adolescent Psychiatry, Johns Hopkins University School of Medicine · The Johns Hopkins Medical Institutions · Johns Hopkins Hospital, 600 North Wolfe Street, Meyer 2-181, Baltimore, MD 21205 · 410-955-2320

Paul R. McHugh · Director and Psychiatrist-in-Chief, Department of Psychiatry, Johns Hopkins University School of Medicine · Henry Phipps Professor of Psychiatry, The Johns Hopkins Medical Institutions · Meyer Building, 600 North Wolfe Street, Room 4113, Baltimore, MD 21205 · 410-955-3130

Gary J. Tucker · (Neuropsychiatric Disorders) · Professor and Chairman, Department of Psychiatry & Behavioral Sciences, University of Washington School of Medicine · University of Washington Medical Center · 1959 Northeast Pacific Street, RP-10, Seattle, WA 98195 · 206-543-3750

CHILD ABUSE
(See also Pediatrics, Abused Children)

Elissa P. Benedek · (Children and the Law) · Clinical Professor of Psychiatry, The University of Michigan Medical School · Director, Research & Training, Center for Forensic Psychiatry · 3607 Chatham Way, Ann Arbor, MI 48105 · 313-429-2531 x290

Arthur H. Green · (Adult & Child Psychoanalysis) · Clinical Professor of Psychiatry, College of Physicians & Surgeons of Columbia University · Columbia-Presbyterian Medical Center · 350 Central Park West, New York, NY 10025 · 212-678-4338

Diane H. Schetky · (Children and the Law, Abuse and Neglect) · Associate Clinical Professor, Department of Psychiatry, University of Vermont School of Medicine · Penobscot Bay Hospital · P.O. Box 429, Rockport, ME 04856 · 207-236-6588

CHILD PSYCHIATRY

Thomas F. Anders · (Sleep) · Head, Division of Child Psychiatry, Brown University School of Medicine · Executive Director, Bradley Hospital, East Providence · 18 Halsey Street, Providence, RI 02906 · 401-831-2339

Elwyn James Anthony · (Vulnerability and Invulnerabilty) · The George Washington University School of Medicine · Director, Chestnut Lodge Hospital · 500 West Montgomery Avenue, Rockville, MD 20850 · 301-424-8300

Myron L. Belfer · Professor of Psychiatry, Harvard Medical School · 643 Huntington Avenue, Boston, MA 02115 · 617-432-2114

Elissa P. Benedek · (Children and the Law) · Clinical Professor of Psychiatry, The University of Michigan Medical School · Director, Research & Training, Center for Forensic Psychiatry · 3607 Chatham Way, Ann Arbor, MI 48105 · 313-429-2531 x290

Joseph Biederman · Associate Professor of Psychiatry, Harvard Medical School · Director, Pediatric Psychopharmacology Unit, Massachusetts General Hospital · Child Psychiatry Department, 15 Parkman Street, Boston, MA 02114 · 617-726-2724

Hector Ramon Bird · (Child Psychoanalysis) · Professor of Clinical Psychiatry, College of Physicians & Surgeons of Columbia University · Deputy Director, Department of Child Psychiatry, Columbia-Presbyterian Medical Center · 722 West 168th Street, New York, NY 10032 · 212-874-5311

David A. Brent · Associate Professor of Child & Adolescent Psychiatry, University of Pittsburgh, Western Psychiatric Institute & Clinic (WPIC) · Chief, Division of Child and Adolescent Psychiatry, and Director, Services for Teens at Risk (STAR-Center), Western Psychiatric Institute & Clinic, University of Pittsburgh Medical Center · 3811 O'Hara Street, Pittsburgh, PA 15213 · 412-624-5172

Dexter Means Bullard, Jr. · (Hospitalized Children) · Medical Director, Chestnut Lodge Hospital · 500 West Montgomery Avenue, Rockville, MD 20850 · 301-424-8300

Justin David Call · Chief of Child & Adolescent Psychiatry, Director of Training in Child Psychiatry, and Professor of Psychiatry and Pediatrics, University of California, Irvine School of Medicine · University of California, Irvine Medical Center · 101 The City Drive, Building 53, Room 303, Orange, CA 92668 · 714-634-6023

Magda Campbell · Professor of Psychiatry, New York University School of Medicine · Director, Division of Child & Adolescent Psychiatry, Bellevue Hospital · 550 First Avenue, 21S15, New York, NY 10016 · 212-263-6206

Dennis P. Cantwell · (Hyperactivity, Learning Disabilities, Attention Deficit Disorder) · The Joseph Campbell Professor of Child Psychiatry, and Head, Child Psychiatry Training Program, University of California at Los Angeles School of Medicine · University of California at Los Angeles Neuropsychiatric Institute · 760 Westwood Plaza, Los Angeles, CA 90024 · 310-825-0506

Gabrielle A. Carlson · Professor of Child Psychiatry & Psychiatry, State University of New York Health Science Center at Stony Brook · SUNY at Stony Brook Hospital · Eight Schooners Cove, East Setauket, NY 11733 · 516-632-8840

Donald J. Cohen · (Learning Disabilities, Tic Disorders) · Director of the Child Study Center, and Irving B. Harris Professor of Child Psychiatry, Pediatrics & Psychology, Yale University School of Medicine · Chairman of the Department of Child Psychiatry, Yale-New Haven Hospital · P.O. Box 3333, 230 South Frontage Road, Room I-267, Sterling Hall of Medicine, New Haven, CT 06510 · 203-785-5759

Calvin A. Colarusso · Clinical Professor of Psychiatry, University of California at San Diego School of Medicine · Children's Hospital & Health Center; University of California at San Diego Medical Center · 1020 Prospect Street, Suite 415A, La Jolla, CA 92037 · 619-454-2473

James Egan · Clinical Professor, Psychiatry, The George Washington University School of Medicine · Senior Attending Physician, Children's National Medical Center · 35 Wisconsin Circle, Chevy Chase, MD 20815 · 301-913-5953

Glen R. Elliott · Associate Professor and Director, Child & Adolescent Psychiatry, University of California at San Francisco School of Medicine · Langley Porter Neuropsychiatric Institute · 401 Parnassus Avenue, Box F, San Francisco, CA 94143-0984 · 415-476-7162

Richard O. Gode · Division Head, Child, Adolescent & Family Psychiatry, Virginia Mason Medical Center · 1100 Olive Way, Metro Park Building, West Tower, 10th Floor, Seattle, WA 98101 · 206-625-7404

Arthur H. Green · (Child Psychoanalysis) · Clinical Professor of Psychiatry, College of Physicians & Surgeons of Columbia University · Columbia-Presbyterian Medical Center · 350 Central Park West, New York, NY 10025 · 212-678-4338

Laurence L. Greenhill · (Hyperactivity, Pediatric Psychoses) · Associate Professor of Clinical Psychiatry, College of Physicians & Surgeons of Columbia University · Director, Disruptive Behavior Clinic, New York State Psychiatric Institute · 722 West 168th Street, 905 North, New York, NY 10032 · 212-960-2340

Gregory J. Heimarck · Associate Professor of Clinical Psychiatry, College of Physicians & Surgeons of Columbia University · Columbia-Presbyterian Medical Center · 63 East 80th Street, New York, NY 10021 · 212-288-4304

Stephen Paul Herman · (Child Custody) · Associate Professor of Psychiatry, Yale Child Study Center, Yale University School of Medicine · Attending Psychiatist, The New York Hospital-Cornell Medical Center; Norwalk Hospital, Norwalk,

CT · 436 Danbury Road, Wilton, CT 06897; 123 West 79th Street, Suite 201, New York, NY 10024 · 203-761-9902, 212-721-3274

David B. Herzog · (Pediatrics) · Associate Professor of Psychiatry, Harvard Medical School · Director, Eating Disorders Unit, and Chief, Consult/Liaison Service, Massachusetts General Hospital · Eating Disorders Unit, ACC 725, 15 Parkman Street, Boston, MA 02114 · 617-726-2724

Joseph J. Jankowski · (Consultation) · Assistant Professor of Psychiatry and Pediatrics, Tufts University School of Medicine · Director, Child Psychiatry Consult Liaison and Emergency Services, New England Medical Center · 750 Washington Street, Box 39, Boston, MA 02111 · 617-956-5328

Michael Jellinek · Assistant Professor of Psychiatry (Pediatric), Harvard Medical School · Chief, Child Psychiatry Service, Massachusetts General Hospital · Child Psychiatry Unit, Massachusetts General Hospital, 15 Parkman Street, Boston, MA 02114 · 617-726-2711

Charles R. Keith · (Violent Children) · Associate Professor, Division of Child Psychiatry, Duke University School of Medicine · Assistant Clinical Director, and Training Director, Division of Child Psychiatry, Durham Community Guidance Clinic · Trent and Elba Streets, Durham, NC 27705 · 919-286-4456

John Fredric Kelley · Associate Medical Director, The St. Joseph's/Parkside Center for Behavioral Medicine · 600 Eighteenth Street, Suite 501, Parkersburg, WV 26101 · 304-424-4670

Paulina Kernberg · (Child Psychoanalysis) · Associate Professor of Psychiatry, Cornell University Medical College · Director of Child & Adolescent Psychiatry, The New York Hospital-Cornell Medical Center, Westchester Division · 21 Bloomingdale Road, White Plains, NY 10605 · 914-997-5951

Clarice J. Kestenbaum · (Psychoanalysis) · Clinical Professor of Psychiatry, and Director of Training, Division of Child & Adolescent Psychiatry, College of Physicians & Surgeons of Columbia University · Columbia-Presbyterian Medical Center · 722 West 168th Street, New York, NY 10032 · 212-873-1020

Robert A. King · (Adolescent Psychiatry) · Assistant Professor of Child Psychiatry, Yale University School of Medicine · Yale-New Haven Hospital · Yale Child Study Center, 230 South Frontage Road, New Haven, CT 06510 · 203-785-5880

Gilbert Wallace Kliman · Director, Preventive Psychiatric Service, St. Mary's Hospital & Medical Center · 450 Stanyan Street, San Francisco, CA 94115 · 415-750-4838

William Michael Klykylo · (Consultation, Interface with Medical Illnesses) · Director, Child & Adolescent Psychiatry, Wright State University School of Medicine · Good Samaritan Hospital; Dartmouth Hospital · P.O. Box 927, Dayton, OH 45435 · 513-276-8325

James F. Leckman · (Tourette's Syndrome, Genetic Aspects of Child Psychiatry) Neison Harris Professor of Child Psychiatry & Pediatrics, Yale University School of Medicine · Yale-New Haven Medical Center · 230 South Frontage Road, New Haven, CT 06510 · 203-785-2511

Dorothy Otnow Lewis · (Juvenile Deliquency) · Professor, Department of Psychiatry, New York University School of Medicine; Clinical Professor, Yale University Child Study Center · Attending Physican, New York University-Bellevue Medical Center, Tisch Hospital; Yale-New Haven Hospital · New Bellevue 21S25, 550 First Avenue, New York, NY 10016 · 212-263-6208

Melvin Lewis · Professor of Pediatrics and Psychiatry, Yale University School of Medicine · Director of Medical Studies, Yale University Child Study Center · 230 South Frontage Road, New Haven, CT 06510-8009 · 203-785-2546

Eugene J. Mahon · (Child Psychoanalysis) · Assistant Clinical Professor of Psychiatry, College of Physicians & Surgeons of Columbia University · Adult Analyst & Child Psychoanalyst, Columbia Psychoanalytic Center for Training & Research Six East 96th Street, New York, NY 10128 · 212-831-1414

Charles Mangham, Sr. · (Child Psychoanalysis) · Clinical Professor, University of Washington; Training Analyst & Supervising Child Analyst, Seattle Institute for Psychoanalysis · Northwest Psychoanalytic Hospital · 4033 East Madison Street, Seattle, WA 98112 · 206-323-1706

Richard E. Mattison · Blanche F. Ittleson Associate Professor of Child Psychiatry, Washington University School of Medicine · Director, Division of Child Psychiatry, Department of Psychiatry, Barnes Hospital; St. Louis Children's Hospital · 4940 Audubon Avenue, St. Louis, MO 63110 · 314-454-2303

Ake Erik Mattsson · (Liaison) · Clinical Professor of Psychiatry, University of Virginia School of Medicine · Blue Ridge Hospital; University of Virginia Health Sciences Center · 6E East Blue Ridge Hospital, Charlottesville, VA 22901 · 804-924-8787

John F. McDermott, Jr. · Professor and Chairman, Department of Psychiatry, John A. Burns School of Medicine, University of Hawaii · 1356 Lusitana Street, Fourth Floor, Honolulu, HI 96813 · 808-548-3420

William Martin McMahon · (Tourette's Syndrome, Movement Disorders) · Associate Professor, University of Utah School of Medicine · 100 North Medical Drive, Salt Lake City UT 84113-1100 · 801-581-3936

Cynthia Roberta Pfeffer · (Adolescent Psychiatry) · Professor of Psychiatry, Cornell University Medical College · Chief, Child-Psychiatry In-Patient Unit, The New York Hospital-Cornell Medical Center, Westchester Division · 21 Bloomingdale Road, White Plains, NY 10605 · 212-722-6856, 914-997-5849

Betty Pfefferbaum · Professor, Department of Psychiatry & Behavioral Sciences, The University of Oklahoma College of Medicine · Children's Hospital of Oklahoma · 1200 South Pickard Avenue, Norman, OK 73072 · 405-325-1000

Irving Philips · (Children and the Law, Psychotic Children, Mental Retardation) Professor of Psychiatry, University of California at San Francisco School of Medicine · Director, Child & Adolescent Psychiatry, Langley Porter Neuropsychiatric Institute · 401 Parnassus Avenue, Box F0984, San Francisco, CA 94143 · 415-476-7160

Judith L. Rapoport · (Obsessive Compulsive Disorder, Pediatric Psychopharmacology, Attention Deficit Disorder) · Clinical Professor of Psychiatry and Pediatrics, The George Washington University School of Medicine · Chief, Child Psychiatry Branch, National Institute of Mental Health, National Institutes of Health Child Psychiatry Branch, NIMH, Bethesda, MD 20892 · 301-496-6081

George M. Realmuto · Associate Professor, University of Minnesota School of Medicine · Medical Director, Autism Clinic & Research Center, University of Minnesota Hospital & Clinics · Harvard Street at East River Road, Box 95 UMHC, Minneapolis, MN 55455 · 612-626-6577

Robert Jay Reichler · Professor of Child Psychiatry, University of Washington School of Medicine · Children's Hospital & Medical Center · 4800 Sand Point Way NE, Seattle, WA 98105 · 206-368-4949

Edward R. Ritvo · (Family-Related Problems) · Professor of Psychiatry, University of California at Los Angeles School of Medicine · University of California at Los Angeles Neuropsychiatric Institute · 760 Westwood Plaza, Los Angeles, CA 90024 · 310-825-0220

Samuel Ritvo · (Child Psychoanalysis) · Clinical Professor, Yale University School of Medicine · 230 South Frontage Road, P.O. Box 3333, New Haven CT 06510 203-785-2513

Michael B. Rothenberg · Professor of Psychiatry & Pediatrics, University of Washington School of Medicine · Children's Hospital & Medical Center · 4800 Sand Point Way NE, P.O. Box C-5371, Seattle, WA 98105 · 206-221-2774

Richard M. Sarles · Clinical Professor of Psychiatry & Pediatrics, University of Maryland School of Medicine · Director, Division of Child & Adolescent Psychiatry, Sheppard Pratt Hospital · 6501 North Charles Street, Towson, MD 21204 · 301-938-3000

Diane H. Schetky · (Children and the Law, Abuse and Neglect) · Associate Clinical Professor, Department of Psychiatry, University of Vermont School of Medicine · Penobscot Bay Hospital · P.O. Box 429, Rockport, ME 04856 · 207-236-6588

John E. Schowalter · (Adolescent Psychiatry) · Albert J. Solnit Professor of Child Psychiatry & Pediatrics, Yale University School of Medicine · Professor of Pediatrics and Psychiatry, Yale University Child Study Center · 333 Cedar Street, P.O. Box 3333, New Haven, CT 06510 · 203-785-2516

Calvin F. Settlage · Clinical Professor of Psychiatry, University of California, San Francisco School of Medicine · Training & Supervising Analyst in Adult & Child Analysis, San Francisco Psychoanalytic Institute · 10 Crecienta Lane, Sausalito, CA 94965 · 415-332-2226

David Shaffer · (Diagnosis) · Irving Philips Professor of Child Psychiatry, and Professor of Psychiatry and Pediatrics, and Director, Division of Child & Adolescent Psychiatry, College of Physicians & Surgeons of Columbia University · New York State Psychiatric Institute · 722 West 168th Street, Box 78, New York, NY 10032 · 212-960-2548

Theodore Shapiro · (Development Disorders) · Professor of Psychiatry, and Professor of Psychiatry in Pediatrics, and Director, Child & Adolescent Psychiatry, Cornell University Medical College · The New York Hospital-Cornell Medical Center · 525 East 68th Street, New York, NY 10021 · 212-746-3926

Albert J. Solnit · (Child Psychoanalysis) · Sterling Professor of Pediatrics & Psychiatry, and Senior Research Scientist, Yale University School of Medicine; Commissioner of Department of Mental Health for State of Connecticut · Yale-New Haven Hospital · 333 Cedar Street, P.O. Box 3333, New Haven, CT 06510 203-785-2518

Ludwik Szymanski · (Mental Retardation) · Assistant Professor of Psychiatry, Harvard Medical School · Director of Psychiatry for the Developmental Evaluation Center, Children's Hospital · 300 Longwood Avenue; Fegan 10, Boston, MA 02115 · 617-735-6501

Peter E. Tanguay · (Childhood Psychoses) · Professor of Child & Adolescent Psychiatry, University of California at Los Angeles School of Medicine · Acting Chief, Division of Child & Adolescent Psychiatry, Neuropsychiatric Hospital, University of California at Los Angeles Medical Center · 760 Westwood Plaza, Los Angeles, CA 90024 · 310-825-0028

Lenore C. Terr · (Severe Trauma) · Clinical Professor of Psychiatry, University of California, San Francisco School of Medicine · Langley Porter Neuropsychiatric Institute · 450 Sutter Street, San Francisco CA 94108 · 415-433-7800

Dianne W. Trumbull · Assistant Professor, Department of Behavioral Medicine & Psychiatry, West Virginia University School of Medicine · West Virginia University Health Sciences Center; Chestnut Ridge Hospital · 930 Chestnut Ridge Road, Morgantown, WV 26505 · 304-293-2411

Luke Y. Tsai · Associate Professor of Psychiatry and Pediatrics, The University of Michigan Medical School · Chief, Child and Adolescent Psychiatric Hospital, The University of Michigan Medical Center · 1500 East Medical Center Drive, Room TC3896, Ann Arbor, MI 48109-0390 · 313-764-5357

Fred R. Volkmar · Harris Associate Professor of Child Psychiatry, Pediatrics and Psychiatry, Yale University School of Medicine · Attending Physician, Yale-New Haven Hospital · 230 South Frontage Road, New Haven, CT 06510 · 203-785-2510

Paul H. Wender · (Attention Deficit Disorder, Pediatric Hyperactivity) · Distinguished Professor of Psychiatry, University of Utah School of Medicine · Director of Psychiatric Resources, University of Utah Health Sciences Center · 50 North Medical Drive, Salt Lake City, UT 84132 · 801-581-8075

Jerry M. Wiener · (Diagnosis and Consultation) · Professor and Chairman, Department of Psychiatry, The George Washington University School of Medicine · George Washington University Medical Center · 2150 Pennsylvania Avenue, NW, Washington, DC 20037 · 202-994-4081

Alayne Yates · (Children & the Law) · Professor of Psychiatry & Pediatrics, The University of Arizona College of Medicine · Chief, Child Psychiatry, The University of Arizona Health Sciences Center · 1501 North Campbell Avenue, Tucson, AZ 85724 · 602-626-6473

DISSOCIATIVE DISORDER

Bennett G. Braun · (Multiple Personality Disorder) · Clinical Associate Professor, The University of Illinois at Chicago College of Medicine; Assistant Professor, Rush Medical College · Medical Director, Dissociative Disorders Program & Inpatient Unit, Rush North Shore Medical Center · 9701 North Knox #103, Skokie, IL 60676 · 312-372-1447

Philip M. Coons · Associate Professor of Psychiatry, Indiana University School of Medicine · Larue D. Carter Memorial Hospital · 1315 West 10th Street, Indianapolis, IN 46202 · 317-634-8401

George K. Ganaway · Clinical Assistant Professor of Psychiatry, Emory University, and Morehouse Schools of Medicine · Program Director, Ridgeview Center for Dissociative Disorders, Ridgeview Institute, Smyrna · Hardeman Square, 5064 Roswell Road NE, Suite D-201, Atlanta, GA 30342 · 404-252-4525

Nancy Louise Hornstein · Assistant Clinical Professor of Psychiatry, University of California at Los Angeles School of Medicine · Unit Director, Children's Inpatient Psychiatric Unit, Neuropsychiatric Hospital, University of California at Los Angeles Medical Center · 921 Westwood Boulevard, Suite 227, Los Angeles, CA 90024 · 213-824-5760

Richard P. Kluft · (Multiple Personality Disorder) · Clinical Professor of Psychiatry, Temple University School of Medicine · Director of Dissociative Disorders Program, The Institute of Pennsylvania Hospital · 111 North 49th Street, Philadelphia, PA 19139 · 215-471-2484

Richard J. Loewenstein · (Multiple Personality Disorder) · Assistant Clinical Professor, University of Maryland School of Medicine · Senior Psychiatrist and Director, Dissociative Disorders Program, Sheppard Pratt Hospital · 6501 North Charles Street, P.O. Box 6815, Baltimore, MD 21285-6815 · 410-938-3000

Stephen S. Marmer · 11980 San Vincente Boulevard, Suite 710, Los Angeles, CA 90049 · 213-820-4330, 820-5773

Frank W. Putnam · (Multiple Personality Disorder) · Senior Clinical Investigator, Department of Psychiatry, George Washington University; Senior Clinical Investigator, Department of Child & Adolescent Psychiatry, Georgetown University; Senior Clinical Investigator, Department of Child Psychiatry, Children's Hospital National Medical Center · National Institute of Mental Health, National Institutes of Health · 9000 Rockville Pike, Building 15K, Bethesda, MD 20892 · 301-496-4406

Colin A. Ross · (Multlple Personality Disorder) · Director, Dissociative Disorders Unit, Charter Hospital of Dallas · 6800 Preston Road, Plano, TX 75024 · 214-618-3939

David Spiegel · (Hypnosis, Multiple Personality Disorders) · Professor of Psychiatry & Behavioral Sciences, Stanford University School of Medicine · Attending Psychiatrist, Stanford University Hospital · TD-114, Stanford, CA 94305 · 415-723-6421

Walter C. Young · (Multiple Personality Disorder) · Medical Director, National Center for the Treatment of Dissociative Disorders · 1290 South Potomac, Aurora, CO 80012 · 303-888-6559, 800-441-6921

EATING DISORDERS
(See also Eating Disorders, p. 73)

Arnold E. Andersen · (Anorexia Nervosa, Bulimia Nervosa) · Professor, Department of Psychiatry, The University of Iowa College of Medicine · The University of Iowa Hospitals & Clinics · 500 Newton Road, Iowa City, IA 52242 · 319-356-1354

Regina Klaere Casper · (Depression) · Professor of Psychiatry and Committee on Human Nutrition, The University of Chicago, Pritzker School of Medicine · Director, Biological Psychiatry, The University of Chicago Hospitals · Department of Psychiatry, 5841 S. Maryland Avenue, Chicago, IL 60637-1470 · 312-702-5844

Paul Earl Garfinkel · Professor and Vice-Chairman, Department of Psychiatry, University of Toronto School of Medicine · Psychiatrist-in-Chief, The Toronto Hospital · 101 College Street, East Wing, Eighth Floor, Toronto, Ontario M5G 1L7 · 416-928-0920, 340-3044

Harry Edward Gwirtsman · Chief, Somatic Treatment Disorders Program of the Mood, Anxiety, & Personality Disorders Research Branch, National Institute of Mental Health, Alcohol, Drub Abuse, and Mental Health Administration · Parklawn Building, Room 10C-24, Rockville, MD 20857 · 301-443-1636

Katherine A. Halmi · Professor of Psychiatry, and Director, Anorexia Nervosa & Bulimia Program, Cornell University Medical College · The New York Hospital-Cornell Medical Center, Westchester Division · 21 Bloomingdale Road, White Plains, NY 10605 · 914-997-5875

David B. Herzog · (Pediatrics) · Associate Professor of Psychiatry, Harvard Medical School · Director, Eating Disorders Unit, and Chief, Consult/Liaison Service, Massachusetts General Hospital · Eating Disorders Unit, ACC 725, 15 Parkman Street, Boston, MA 02114 · 617-726-2724

James I. Hudson · Associate Professor of Psychiatry, Harvard Medical School · Chief of the Clinical Neurophysiology Laboratory, McLean Hospital · 115 Mill Street, Belmont, MA 02178 · 617-855-2911

Jack L. Katz · Professor of Clinical Psychiatry, Cornell University Medical College Chairman, Department of Psychiatry, North Shore University Hospital · 400 Community Drive, Manhasset, NY 11030 · 516-562-3065

James E. Mitchell · Professor of Psychiatry, University of Minnesota School of Medicine · Director, Division of Adult Psychiatry, University of Minnesota Hospital & Clinics · Mayo Building, 420 Delaware Street, SE, Box 393 UMHC, Minneapolis, MN 55455 · 612-626-3633

Pauline S. Powers · (Obesity) · Professor of Psychiatry & Behavioral Medicine, and Director of the Eating Disorders Clinic, University South Florida College of Medicine · Director of Psychosomatic Medicine Unit, University of South Florida, Psychiatry Center · 3515 East Fletcher Avenue, Tampa, FL 33613 · 813-972-7073

Albert J. Stunkard · (Obesity) · Professor of Psychiatry, University of Pennsylvania School of Medicine · Psychiatrist, Hospital of the University of Pennsylvania 133 South 36th Street, Suite 507, Philadelphia, PA 19104-3246 · 215-898-7314

B. Timothy Walsh · Professor of Clinical Psychiatry, College of Physicians & Surgeons of Columbia University · Director, Eating Disorders Clinic, New York State Psychiatric Institute; Columbia-Presbyterian Medical Center · 722 West 168th Street, Box 98, New York, NY 10032 · 212-960-5752

Joel Yager · Professor and Associate Chair for Education, Department of Psychiatry and Biobehavioral Sciences, University of California at Los Angeles School of Medicine · Director of Residency Education, University of California at Los Angeles Neuropsychiatric Institute · 760 Westwood Plaza, Los Angeles, CA 90024 310-825-0018

FORENSIC PSYCHIATRY

Paul S. Appelbaum · A. F. Zeleznik Professor of Psychiatry, University of Massachusetts Medical School · Director, Law and Psychiatry Program, University of Massachusetts Medical Center · 55 Lake Avenue North, Worcester, MA 01655 · 508-856-3983

Elissa P. Benedek · (Children and the Law) · Clinical Professor of Psychiatry, The University of Michigan Medical School · Director, Research & Training, Center for Forensic Psychiatry · 3607 Chatham Way, Ann Arbor, MI 48105 · 313-429-2531 x290

Joseph D. Bloom · Professor and Chairman, Department of Psychiatry, Oregon Health Sciences University · University Hospital · 3181 Southwest Sam Jackson Park Road, Portland, OR 97201-3098 · 503-494-8144

James L. Cavanaugh · Professor of Psychiatry, Rush Medical College · Rush-Presbyterian-St. Luke's Medical Center · 1725 West Harrison Street, Suite 303, Chicago, IL 60612 · 312-829-1463

J. Richard Ciccone · Professor of Psychiatry, and Director, Psychiatry Law Program, University of Rochester School of Medicine & Dentistry · Strong Memorial Hospital, University of Rochester Medical Center · 300 Crittenden Boulevard, Rochester, NY 14642 · 716-275-4986

Park E. Dietz · Clinical Professor of Psychiatry and Biobehavioral Sciences, University of California at Los Angeles School of Medicine · 537 Newport Center Drive, Newport Beach, CA 92660 · 714-760-0422

Seymour L. Halleck · Professor of Psychiatry, University of North Carolina School of Medicine · Chapel Hill, NC 27514 · 919-966-4447

Abraham L. Halpern · Clinical Professor, Department of Psychiatry, New York Medical College · Director of Psychiatry, United Hospital Medical Center · 720 The Parkway, Mamaroneck, NY 10543-4299 · 914-698-2136

Kathleen May Quinn · (Child Sexual Abuse, Children and the Law) · Assistant Professor of Psychiatry, Case Western Reserve University School of Medicine · Staff Psychiatrist, Cleveland Metropolitan General Hospital · 3395 Scranton Road, Cleveland, OH 44109 · 216-459-3745

Jonas Ralph Rappeport · Clinical Professor of Psychiatry, University of Maryland School of Medicine; Adjunct Professor of Law, University of Maryland School of Law; Associate Professor of Psychiatry, Johns Hopkins University School of Medicine · University of Maryland Medical Center; The Johns Hopkins Medical Institutions; Sheppard Pratt Hospital · Professional Arts Building, 101 West Read Street, Suite 323, Baltimore, MD 21201 · 301-837-7888

Phillip J. Resnick · Professor of Psychiatry, Case Western Reserve University School of Medicine · Director, Forensic Psychiatry, University Hospitals of Cleveland · 2040 Abington Road, Cleveland, OH 44106 · 216-844-3415

Loren H. Roth · (Ethics and Psychiatry and Medicine) · Professor and Vice-Chairman, Department of Psychiatry, and Director, Law & Psychiatry Program, University of Pittsburgh School of Medicine · Chief, Clinical Services, Western Psychiatric Institute & Clinic, University of Pittsburgh Medical Center · 3811 O'Hara Street, Room E820, Pittsburgh, PA 15213 · 412-624-2161

Robert Leslie Sadoff · Clinical Professor of Psychiatry, and Director of the Center for Studies in Social-Legal Psychiatry, University of Pennsylvania School of Medicine · Consultant in Forensic Psychiatry, Philadelphia Psychiatric Center; Albert Einstein University Hospital · Suite 326, The Benjamin Fox Pavilion, Jenkintown, PA 19046 · 215-887-6144

Alan A. Stone · The Touroff-Glueck Professor of Law & Medicine, the Faculty of Law and the Faculty of Medicine, Harvard Law School · Harvard Law School, 1545 Massachusetts Avenue, Cambridge, MA 02138 · 617-495-3124

Howard V. Zonana · Associate Professor of Psychiatry, Yale University School of Medicine · Yale-New Haven Hospital · 34 Park Street, New Haven, CT 06519 · 203-789-7421

GENERAL PSYCHIATRY

Kenneth Z. Altshuler · (Psychtherapy, Geriatrics, Early Profound Deafness) · Stanton Sharp Professor and Chairman, Department of Psychiatry, The University of Texas Southwestern Medical Center at Dallas · Chief of Service, Parkland Memorial Hospital, and Zale-Lipshy University Hospital; Consulting Physician, Presbyterian Hospital, and Children's Hospital · 5325 Harry Hines Boulevard, F5 400, Dallas TX 75235 · 214-688-3300

Boris M. Astrachan · Professor and Head, Department of Psychiatry, The University of Illinois College of Medicine at Chicago · The University of Illinois Hospital · P.O. Box 6998, Chicago, IL 60680 · 312-996-3580

Dennis S. Charney · Professor, Department of Psychiatry, Yale University School of Medicine · Chief, Psychiatry Service, West Haven Veterans Affairs Medical Center · 950 Campbell Avenue, West Haven, CT 06516 · 203-937-3837

Jonathan O. Cole · Professor of Psychiatry, Harvard Medical School · Program Director, Affective Disorders Program, McLean Hospital · 115 Mill Street, Belmont, MA 02178 · 617-855-2900

Jonathan R. T. Davidson · Associate Professor of Psychiatry, Duke University School of Medicine · Director, Psychiatry Outpatient Programs and Anxiety Disorders Program, Duke University Medical Center · P.O. Box 3812, Durham, NC 27710 · 919-684-2880

Shervert H. Frazier, Jr. · Psychiatrist-in-Chief Emeritus, and Director, Post-Graduate & Continuing Medical Education, McLean Hospital · 115 Mill Street, Belmont, MA 02178 · 617-855-3245

William Jay Gershell · (Psychopharmacology) · Assistant Clinical Professor, Department of Psychiatry, Mt. Sinai School of Medicine · Assistant Attending, Mt. Sinai Medical Center · 40 East 89th Street, Apartment 10E, New York NY 10028 212-534-2400

Robert M. A. Hirschfeld · (Depression) · Professor and Chairman, Department of Psychiatry & Behavioral Sciences, The University of Texas Medical Branch at Galveston · Galveston, TX 77550 · 409-772-3901

John R. Lion · Clinical Professor of Psychiatry, University of Maryland School of Medicine · Sheppard Pratt Hospital · 328 East Quadrangle, 5100 Falls Road, Baltimore, MD 21210 · 301-433-6333

Gordon L. Moore · Associate Professor, Mayo Medical School · Chair, Department of Psychiatry & Psychology, Mayo Clinic · 200 First Street, SW, Rochester, MN 55905 · 507-284-2933

Samuel W. Perry III · Professor of Clinical Psychiatry, Cornell University Medical College · The New York Hospital-Cornell Medical Center · 525 East 68th Street, Payne Whitney Clinic, New York NY 10021 · 212-746-3918

Arnold Rothstein · 320 Central Park West, Suite 3A, New York, NY 10025 · 212-496-6209

Alan F. Schatzberg · Kenneth T. Norris, Jr. Professor and Chairman, Department of Psychiatry & Behavioral Sciences, Stanford University School of Medicine · Chief of Psychiatry, Stanford University Hospital · Panama Street, Psychiatry Building, TD114, Stanford, CA 94305-5490 · 415-723-6811

Alan A. Stone · The Touroff-Glueck Professor of Law & Medicine, the Faculty of Law and the Faculty of Medicine, Harvard Law School · Harvard Law School, 1545 Massachusetts Avenue, Cambridge, MA 02138 · 617-495-3124

John Andrew Talbott · Professor and Chairman of Psychiatry, University of Maryland School of Medicine · Director, Institute of Psychiatry & Human Behavior, Baltimore; Maryland Medical Systems; Walter P. Carter Center; Baltimore Veterans Affairs Medical Center · 645 West Redwood Street, Baltimore, MD 21201 · 410-328-6735

Paul H. Wender · (Attention Deficit Disorder, Pediatric Hyperactivity, Adult Hyperactivity · Distinguished Professor of Psychiatry, University of Utah School of Medicine · Director of Psychiatric Resources, University of Utah Health Sciences Center · 50 North Medical Drive, Salt Lake City, UT 84132 · 801-581-8075

GERIATRIC PSYCHIATRY

F. M. Baker · (Cross-Cultural and Transcultural Psychiatry) · Associate Professor of Psychiatry, University of Maryland School of Medicine · Consulting Scientist, Mental Disorders of the Aging Research Branch, National Institute of Mental Health; Consulting Scientist, Division of Geriatrics, National Institute on Aging, National Institutes of Health; Institute of Psychiatry & Human Behavior · 645 West Redwood Street, Baltimore, MD 21201-1549 · 301-328-2431

David G. Bienenfeld · Vice Chair, Department of Psychiatry, and Director of Residency Training Program, Wright State University School of Medicine · Good Samaritan Hospital · P.O. Box 927, Dayton, OH 45401-0927 · 513-276-8329

Nathan Billig · Professor of Psychiatry, Georgetown University School of Medicine · Georgetown University Medical Center · Kober Cogan Building, Room 619, 3800 Reservoir Road, NW, Washington, DC 20007 · 202-687-8770, 687-8537

Dan G. Blazer · (Depression in Late Life) · Duke University School of Medicine Duke University Medical Center · P.O. Box 3215, Durham, NC 27710 · 919-684-4128

Soo Borson · Associate Professor of Psychiatry, University of Washington School of Medicine · University of Washington Hospital · RP-10, Seattle, WA 98195 · 206-543-3996

Robert N. Butler · Brookdale Professor of Geriatrics & Adult Development, Mt. Sinai School of Medicine · Chairman, Department of Geriatrics, Mt. Sinai Medical Center · One Gustave L. Levy Place, Box 1070, New York, NY 10029 · 212-241-4633

Eric Douglas Caine · Professor of Psychiatry & Neurology, and Associate Chairman for Academic Affairs, University of Rochester School of Medicine & Dentistry, Department of Psychiatry · Strong Memorial Hospital, University of Rochester Medical Center · 300 Crittenden Boulevard, Rochester, NY 14642 · 716-275-3574

Gene D. Cohen · Acting Director, National Institute on Aging, National Institutes of Health · Clinical Professor, Department of Psychiatry, Georgetown University Medical Center · 9000 Rockville Pike, Building 31, Room 2C02, Bethesda, MD 20892 · 301-496-9265

Christopher C. Colenda · Associate Professor of Psychiatry & Behavioral Medicine, and Associate in Public Health Sciences, The Bowman Gray School of Medicine of Wake Forest University · North Carolina Baptist Hospital · Medical Center Boulevard, Winston-Salem, NC 27157-1087 · 919-748-6992

Maurice William Dysken · (Clinical Psychopharmacology) · Professor of Psychiatry, University of Minnesota School of Medicine · Psychopharmacologist, GRECC Program, Minneapolis Veterans Affairs Medical Center · One Veterans Drive, Minneapolis, MN 55417 · 612-725-2000 x3308

M. Robin Eastwood · (Epidemiology) · Professor of Psychiatry & Preventive Medicine & Biostatistics, University of Toronto School of Medicine · Head, Neuroepidemiology Research Unit, The Clarke Institute of Psychiatry · 250 College Street, Toronto, Ontario M5T 1R8 · 416-979-6841

Carl Eisdorfer · Professor and Chairman of Psychiatry, and Director, Center on Aging & Adult Development, University of Miami School of Medicine · Chairman, Mental Health Services, University of Miami-Jackson Memorial Medical Center · P.O. Box 016960 (D-28), Miami, FL 33101 · 305-545-6319

Sanford I. Finkel · Associate Professor of Psychiatry, Northwestern University Medical School · Director, Gero-psychiatric Services, Northwestern Memorial Hospital · 259 East Erie Street, Room 448, Chicago, IL 60611 · 312-908-9481

Barry S. Fogel · Associate Professor of Psychiatry, Brown University School of Medicine · Rhode Island Hospital · 593 Eddy Street, Jane Brown 5, Providence, RI 02903 · 401-277-5228

David G. Folks · Geropsychiatry Research Professor; and Professor of Psychiatry, The University of Alabama at Birmingham · The University of Alabama Hospital N275 Jefferson Tower, 619 South 19th Street, Birmingham, AL 35294-6912 · 205-934-6054

Marshal F. Folstein · Eugene Meyer III Professor of Psychiatry and Medicine, Johns Hopkins University School of Medicine · The Johns Hopkins Medical Institutions · Osler Building, 600 North Wolfe Street, Room 320, Baltimore, MD 21205 · 410-955-3347

Jeffrey Robert Foster · Assistant Professor of Clinical Psychiatry, New York University School of Medicine · New York University Medical Center · 155 East 29th Street, Suite 5-D, New York, NY 10016 · 212-686-9668

Charles Milton Gaitz · Clinical Professor, Department of Psychiatry, Baylor College of Medicine · Medical Director of Geropsychiatry, Bellaire Hospital · 6550 Mapleridge, Suite 208, Houston, TX 77081 · 713-669-4138

Marion Zucker Goldstein · Clinical Associate Professor of Psychiatry, State University of New York at Buffalo School of Medicine & Biomedical Sciences · Director, Division of Geriatric Psychiatry, Erie County Medical Center · 462 Grider Street, Buffalo, NY 14215-3098 · 716-898-3630

Gary L. Gottlieb · Associate Chairman, Department of Psychiatry, University of Pennsylvania School of Medicine · Director, Section of Geriatric Psychiatry, Hospital of the University of Pennsylvania · 3615 Chestnut Street, Philadelphia, PA 19104 · 215-662-2824

James Allen Greene · Clinical Associate Professor, The University of Tennessee College of Medicine · Center for Health & Creative Aging, 9330 Park West Boulevard, Knoxville, TN 37923 · 615-694-0076

George T. Grossberg · Professor of Psychiatry, St. Louis University School of Medicine · Director, Division of Geriatric Psychiatry, St. Louis University Medical Center · 1221 South Grand Boulevard, St. Louis, MO 63104 · 314-577-8726

Bennett S. Gurian · Associate Professor of Psychiatry, Harvard Medical School · Director of Geropsychiatry, Massachusetts Mental Health Center · Positive Aging Services, 74 Fenwood Road, Boston, MA 02115 · 617-734-1300

Donald Peter Hay · (Electroconvulsive Therapy) · Associate Professor of Psychiatry, and Director, Division of Geriatric Psychiatry, Medical College of Wisconsin; Associate Clinical Professor of Psychiatry, University of Wisconsin Medical School Chief, Older Adult Service, St. Mary's Hill Hospital · 2350 North Lake Drive, Milwaukee, WI 53211 · 414-271-5555

Lissy F. Jarvik · (Alzheimers) · Professor of Psychiatry, University of California at Los Angeles School of Medicine · Chief of the Section on Neuropsychogeriatrics, University of California at Los Angeles Neuropsychiatric Institute · 760 Westwood Plaza, Los Angeles, CA 90024-1759 · 310-825-3885

Dilip V. Jeste · Professor, Department of Psychiatry and Neuroscience, University of California at San Diego School of Medicine · Chief, Psychiatry Service, VA Medical Center · 3350 La Jolla Village Drive (V116A), San Deigo, CA 92161 · 619-534-4020

Ira R. Katz · Professor of Psychiatry and Director, Division of Geriatric Psychiatry, Medical College of Pennsylvania · 3200 Henry Avenue, EPPI, Philadelphia PA 19129 · 215-842-4376

Gary J. Kennedy · Director of Geriatric Psychiatry, Albert Einstein College of Medicine · Montefiore Medical Center; Bronx Psychiatric Center · 111 East 210th Street, Bronx, NY 10467 · 212-920-4236

Lawrence W. Lazarus · Assistant Professor of Psychiatry, Rush Medical College Attending Psychiatrist, Rush-Presbyterian-St. Luke's Medical Center · 1653 North Congress Parkway, Chicago IL 60612 · 312-236-2482

Andrew F. Leuchter · (Neuro-Psychology, EEG) · Assistant Professor of Psychiatry, University of California at Los Angeles School of Medicine · Co-Director, Geriatric Inpatient Service, and Director, Clinical Electrophysiology Laboratory, University of California, Los Angeles Neuropsychiatric Hospital, University of California at Los Angeles Geriatric Psychiatry Service · Neuropsychiatric Institute, 760 Westwood Plaza, Los Angeles, CA 90024 · 310-825-0207

Jonathan D. Lieff · Associate Clinical Professor of Psychiatry, Boston University School of Medicine · Chief of Psychiatry, Hahnemann Hospital; American Geriatric Service · 22 Carlton Street, Brookline, MA 02146 · 617-739-9067

Benjamin Liptzin · Professor and Deputy Chair of Psychiatry, Tufts University School of Medicine · Chairman, Department of Psychiatry, Baystate Medical Center · Department of Psychiatry, Springfield, MA 01199 · 413-784-4235

Gabe J. Maletta · Associate Chief of Staff and Associate Professor of Psychiatry, Department of Geriatrics & Extended Care, University of Minnesota School of Medicine · Minnesota Veterans Affairs Medical Center · One Veterans' Drive, Minneapolis, MN 55417 · 612-725-2051

Richard Alan Margolin · (Neuro-radiology) · Assistant Professor of Psychiatry & Radiology, Vanderbilt University School of Medicine · Vanderbilt University Medical Center · The Vanderbilt Clinic, 22nd Avenue South, Room 3945, Nashville, TN 37232-5646 · 615-322-0325

Barnett Samuel Meyers · Associate Professor of Clinical Psychiatry, Cornell University Medical College · The New York Hospital-Cornell Medical Center, Westchester Division · 21 Bloomingdale Road, White Plains, NY 10605 · 914-997-5721

Gary Stuart Moak · Assistant Professor of Psychiatry, University of Massachusetts Medical School · Medical Director of Geriatric Medical Psychiatry Unit, Clinton Hospital · 201 Highland Street, Clinton, MA 01510 · 508-365-4531

Edwin J. Olsen · University of Miami School of Medicine; Mount Sinai Medical Center, Miami Beach, FL · Vice Chairman, Department of Psychiatry, University of Miami School of Medicine; Chairman, Mount Sinai Medical Center, Miami Beach, FL; University of Miami-Jackson Memorial Medical Center · 4300 Alton Road, Main #204, Miami Beach, FL 33140 · 305-647-2194

George H. Pollock · (Psychosomatic Medicine) · Ruth & Evelyn Dunbar Distinguished Professor of Psychiatry & Behavioral Sciences, Northwestern University Medical School · Senior Attending Staff Member, Northwestern Memorial Hospital · 303 East Superior Street, Room 544, Chicago, IL 60611 · 312-908-6828

Peter Vincent Rabins · (Alzheimers) · Associate Professor of Psychiatry & Behavioral Sciences, Johns Hopkins University School of Medicine · The Johns Hopkins Medical Institutions · 600 North Wolfe Street, Baltimore, MD 21205 · 410-955-6736

Murray A. Raskind · Professor and Vice-Chairman for Research, Department of Psychiatry & Behavioral Sciences, University of Washington School of Medicine · Seattle Veterans Affairs Medical Center; University of Washington Medical Center 1660 South Columbian Way, Seattle, WA 98108 · 206-764-2308

Burton V. Reifler · Professor and Chairman, Department of Psychiatry & Behavioral Medicine, The Bowman Gray School of Medicine of Wake Forest University North Carolina Baptist Hospital · Medical Center Boulevard, Winston-Salem, NC 27157-1087 · 919-748-4552

Barry Reisberg · (Alzheimers) · Professor of Psychiatry, New York University School of Medicine · New York University Medical Center · The Aging and Dementia Research Center, Millhauser Laboratory, 550 First Avenue, Room HN314, New York, NY 10016 · 212-263-8550

Charles F. Reynolds III · Professor of Psychiatry & Neurology, University of Pittsburgh School of Medicine · Western Psychiatric Institute & Clinic, University of Pittsburgh Medical Center · 3811 O'Hara Street, Room E-1135, Pittsburgh, PA 15213 · 412-624-2246

Joseph E. V. Rubin · Maine Medical Center · 121 Middle Street, Portland, ME 04101 · 207-772-8634

Joel Sadavoy · Associate Professor of Psychiatry, University of Toronto School of Medicine · Senior Consultant, and Director, Geriatric Psychiatry Services, Mount Sinai Hospital · 600 University Avenue, Suite 941A, Toronto, Ontario M5G 1X5 416-586-5262

Kenneth M. Sakauye · Associate Professor of Clinical Psychiatry, Louisiana State University School of Medicine in New Orleans · Chief of Geriatric Psychiatry Service, Touro Infirmary · 1401 Fourcher Street, New Orleans, LA 70115 · 504-568-6001

Andrew Satlin · Instructor, Department of Psychiatry, Harvard Medical School · McLean Hospital · 115 Mill Street, Belmont, MA 02178 · 617-855-3183

Charles A. Shamoian · (Psychopharmacology) · Professor of Clinical Psychiatry, Cornell University Medical College · Director, Acute Treatment Services, The New York Hospital-Cornell Medical Center, Westchester Division · 21 Bloomingdale Road, White Plains, NY 10605 · 914-997-5841

Kimberly A. Sherrill · Assistant Professor of Psychiatry & Behavioral Medicine, The Bowman Gray School of Medicine of Wake Forest University · North Carolina Baptist Hospital · Medical Center Boulevard, Winston-Salem, NC 27157-1087 919-748-6028

Alan P. Siegal · Assistant Professor of Psychiatry, Yale University School of Medicine · Hospital of St. Raphael, and Yale-New Haven Hospital · 60 Washington Avenue, Suite 304, Hamden, CT 06518 · 203-288-0414

Gary W. Small · Associate Professor of Psychiatry, University of California at Los Angeles School of Medicine · Director, Geriatric Consultation Liaison Services, University of California at Los Angeles Neuropsychiatric Hospital; Chief, Geriatric Psychiatry, Veterans Affairs Medical Center, West Los Angeles · Neuropsychiatric Institute, 760 Westwood Plaza, Room 37-432, Los Angeles, CA 90024 · 310-825-0291

Elliott M. Stein · Clinical Assistant Professor, University of Miami School of Medicine · Cedars-Lebanon Medical Center · 1680 Michigan Avenue, Suite 1010, Miami Beach, FL 33139 · 305-534-3636

Alan Stoudemire · (Consultation-Liaison Psychiatry) · Professor of Psychiatry, Emory University School of Medicine · Director, Medical Psychiatry Unit, Emory University Hospital · Emory Central Clinic, 1365 Clifton Road, NE, Section of Psychiatry, Atlanta, GA 30322 · 404-248-3969

Hugo Van Dooren · Clinical Professor, University of Washington School of Medicine · Medical Director, Mental Health Unit, Puget Sound Hospital · 2314 North 31st Street, Unit #1, Tacoma, WA 98403 · 206-627-8448

Richard C. Veith · Professor of Psychiatry & Behavioral Sciences, University of Washington School of Medicine · Director, Geriatric Research Education & Clinical Center, Seattle Veterans Affairs Medical Center · 1660 South Columbian Way, Seattle, WA 98108 · 206-764-2308

Myron F. Weiner · Professor and Vice Chairman, Department of Psychiatry, The University of Texas Southwestern Medical Center at Dallas · Zale-Lipshy University Hospital · 5323 Harry Hines Boulevard, Department of Psychiatry, F5.400, Dallas, TX 75235-9070 · 214-688-3400

Jerome A. Yesavage · Professor of Psychiatry, Stanford University School of Medicine · Stanford University Hospital; Veterans Administration Hospital · Room TD114, Stanford University School of Medicine, Stanford, CA 94305 · 415-852-3287

HEADACHE
(See also Adult Neurology, Headache)

Fred D. Sheftell · Clinical Assistant Professor, Department of Psychiatry, New York Medical College · Director, New England Center for Headache; Associate Medical Director, Headache Inpatient Unit, Greenwich Hospital · New England Center for Headache, 778 Long Ridge Road, Stamford, CT 06906 · 203-968-1799

Bernard Swerdlow · Clinical Assistant Professor, University of Central Florida · Winter Park Memorial Hospital · 1925 Mitzell Avenue, Suite 100, Winter Park, FL 32792 · 407-628-2905

MENTAL RETARDATION/MENTAL HEALTH: DUAL DIAGNOSIS

Henry F. Crabbe · (Diagnosis & treatment of mental disorders in individuals with developmental disabilities and/or mental retardation) · Psychiatric Medicine Center, 501 Ocean Avenue, New London, CT 06320 · 203-442-6364

Frank Menolascino · (Autism, Diagnosis & treatment of mental disorders in individuals with developmental disabilities and/or mental retardation) · Professor and Chairperson, Combined Creighton-Nebraska Department of Psychiatry, University of Nebraska College of Medicine, and Creighton University School of Medicine · University of Nebraska Medical Center; St. Joseph Center for Mental Health · 600 South 42nd Street, Omaha, NE 68198-5575 · 402-559-5100

Stephen L. Ruedrich · (Diagnosis & treatment of mental disorders in individuals with developmental disabilities and/or mental retardation) · Associate Professor, Department of Psychiatry, Case Western Reserve University School of Medicine Interim Director, Office of Education, MetroHealth Medical Center · 3395 Scranton Road, Cleveland, OH 44109 · 216-459-5287

Robert Sovner · (Diagnosis & treatment of mental disorders in individuals with developmental disabilities and/or mental retardation) · Coordinator, Neuropsychiatric/Developmental Disabilities Service, Harvard Community Health Plan · 26 City Hall Mall, Medford, MA 02155 · 617-381-5463

Steven A. Weisblatt · (Diagnosis & treatment of mental disorders in individuals with developmental disabilities and/or mental retardation) · Assistant Professor of Clinical Psychiatry, Albert Einstein College of Medicine · Weiler Hospital of the Albert Einstein College of Medicine · 1825 Eastchester Road, Suite 2 South 56, Bronx, NY 10461-2373 · 212-405-0494

NEUROPSYCHIATRY
(See also Adult Neurology, Neuropsychiatry)

Eric Douglas Caine · Professor of Psychiatry & Neurology, and Associate Chairman for Academic Affairs, University of Rochester School of Medicine & Dentistry, Department of Psychiatry · Strong Memorial Hospital, University of Rochester Medical Center · 300 Crittenden Boulevard, Rochester, NY 14642 · 716-275-3574

Barry S. Fogel · Associate Professor of Psychiatry, Brown University School of Medicine · Rhode Island Hospital · 593 Eddy Street, Jane Brown 5, Providence, RI 02903 · 401-277-5228

Susan E. Folstein · (Huntington's Disease) · Professor of Psychiatry (Joint Appointment in Medicine and Pediatrics), and Director of Psychiatric Genetics, and Director of Child & Adolescent Psychiatry, Johns Hopkins University School of

Medicine · The Johns Hopkins Medical Institutions · Johns Hopkins Hospital, 600 North Wolfe Street, Meyer 2-181, Baltimore, MD 21205 · 410-955-2320

Robert E. Hales · Clinical Professor of Psychiatry, University of California at San Francisco School of Medicine · Chairman, Department of Psychiatry, California Pacific Medical Center · 2340 Clay Street, Seventh Floor, San Francisco, CA 94115 · 415-923-3624

Thomas W. McAllister · Associate Professor of Clinical Psychiatry, Dartmouth Medical School · Director of Section of Neuropsychiatry, Dartmouth-Hitchcock Medical Center; New Hampshire Hospital · New Hampshire Hospital, Section of Neuropsychiatry, 105 Pleasant Street, Concord, NH 03301-3861 · 603-271-5203

Paul R. McHugh · (Huntington's Disease) · Director and Psychiatrist-in-Chief, Department of Psychiatry, Johns Hopkins University School of Medicine · Henry Phipps Professor of Psychiatry, The Johns Hopkins Medical Institutions · Meyer Building, 600 North Wolfe Street, Room 4113, Baltimore, MD 21205 · 410-955-3130

Vernon M. Neppe · Associate Professor of Psychiatry, and Director, Division of Neuropsychiatry, University of Washington School of Medicine · Attending Physician, University of Washington Medical Center; Harborview Medical Center · Department of Psychiatry ZA99, Harborview Medical Center, Seattle, WA 98104-2499 · 206-223-3425

Trevor R. P. Price · Professor of Psychiatry and Medicine, and Chairman, Department of Psychiatry, Medical College of Pennsylvania-Allegheny Campus · Allegheny General Hospital; Allegheny Neuropsychiatric Institute · 320 East North Avenue, 14th Floor, South Tower, Pittsburgh, PA 15212 · 412-359-5050

Robert G. Robinson · (Affective Disorders Related to Brain Injury, Strokes) · Professor and Head of Psychiatry, The University of Iowa College of Medicine · The University of Iowa Hospitals & Clinics · 500 Newton Road, Room 1-289 MEB, Iowa City, IA 52242 · 319-356-4658

Randolph B. Schiffer · Associate Professor of Neurology & Psychiatry, University of Rochester School of Medicine & Dentistry · Strong Memorial Hospital, University of Rochester Medical Center · 601 Elmwood Avenue, Box 605, Rochester, NY 14642 · 716-275-3301

Jonathan M. Silver · Assistant Professor of Clinical Psychiatry, College of Physicians & Surgeons of Columbia University · Director, Neuropsychiatry, Columbia-Presbyterian Medical Center · Allen Pavilion, 5141 Broadway, New York, NY 10034 · 212-932-4165, 799-7620

Michael Alan Taylor · Professor and Chairman, Department of Psychiatry & Behavioral Sciences, University of Health Sciences/The Chicago Medical School 3333 Green Bay Road, North Chicago, IL 60064-3095 · 312-578-3330

Paula T. Trzepacz · Associate Professor of Psychiatry, University of Pittsburgh School of Medicine · Western Psychiatric Institute & Clinic, University of Pittsburgh Medical Center · 3811 O'Hara Street, Pittsburgh, PA 15213 · 412-624-0701

Gary J. Tucker · (Neuropsychiatric Disorders) · Professor and Chairman, Department of Psychiatry & Behavioral Sciences, University of Washington School of Medicine · University of Washington Medical Center · 1959 Northeast Pacific Street, RP-10, Seattle, WA 98195 · 206-543-3750

Daniel R. Weinberger · Chief, Clinical Brain Disorders Branch, National Institute of Mental Health, National Institutes of Health · Neuroscience Center, 2700 Martin Luther King, Jr., Avenue, SE, Room 500, Washington DC 20032 · 202-373-6228

Stuart C. Yudofsky · (Aggressive Disorders) · Professor and Chairman, Department of Psychiatry, University of Chicago, Pritzker School of Medicine · University of Chicago Medical Center · 5841 South Maryland Avenue, Box 411, Chicago, IL 60637-1470 · 312-702-6192

PERSONALITY DISORDER

Philip R. Slavney · Associate Professor of Psychiatry & Behavioral Science, and Director, Research Education, and Attending Physician, Johns Hopkins Medical Institutions · 600 North Wolfe Street, Baltimore, MD 21205 · 410-955-6767

POST-TRAUMATIC STRESS DISORDERS

Bennett G. Braun · Clinical Associate Professor, The University of Illinois at Chicago College of Medicine; Assistant Professor, Rush Medical College · Medical Director, Dissociative Disorders Program & Inpatient Unit, Rush North Shore Medical Center · 9701 North Knox #103, Skokie, IL 60676 · 312-372-1447

Bessel A. van der Kolk · Lecturer, Department of Psychiatry, Harvard Medical School · Director, Trauma Clinic, Massachusetts General Hospital · 16 Braddock Park, Boston, MA 02116 · 617-247-3918

PSYCHOANALYSIS

Sander M. Abend · Training Analyst, New York Psychoanalytic Institute · 1040 Park Avenue, New York, NY 10028 · 212-860-0680

Steven L. Ablon · (Adult & Child Psychoanalysis) · Assistant Professor of Psychiatry, Harvard Medical School · Massachusetts General Hospital · 62 Chestnut Hill Road, Chestnut Hill, MA 02167 · 617-734-3279

Samuel Abrams · (Adult & Child Psychoanalysis) · Clinical Professor of Psychiatry, New York University School of Medicine · 25 East 83rd Street, Suite 2D, New York, NY 10028 · 212-628-1071

Carl P. Adatto · (Adult & Child Psychoanalysis) · Clinical Professor Emeritus, Louisiana State University School of Medicine · Training & Supervising Analyst, Emeritus, New Orleans Psychoanalytic Institute · 6205 Garfield Street, New Orleans, LA 70118 · 504-895-3681

George H. Allison · Clinical Professor of Psychiatry, University of Washington School of Medicine · 2271 Northeast 51st Street, Seattle, WA 98105 · 206-522-8553

Kenneth Z. Altshuler · (Psychtherapy, Geriatrics, Early Profound Deafness) · Stanton Sharp Professor and Chairman, Department of Psychiatry, The University of Texas Southwestern Medical Center at Dallas · Chief of Service, Parkland Memorial Hospital, and Zale-Lipshy University Hospital; Consulting Physician, Presbyterian Hospital, and Children's Hospital · 5325 Harry Hines Boulevard, F5 400, Dallas TX 75235 · 214-688-3300

Elwyn James Anthony · (Vulnerability and Invulnerabilty) · The George Washington University School of Medicine · Director, Chestnut Lodge Hospital · 500 West Montgomery Avenue, Rockville, MD 20850 · 301-424-8300

Jacob A. Arlow · 120 East 36th Street, New York, NY 10016 · 212-684-2871

Gerald J. Aronson · Assistant Professor of Clinical Psychiatry, University of California at Los Angeles School of Medicine · Training Analyst, Los Angeles Psychoanalytic Institute · 11980 San Vicente Boulevard, Suite 902, Los Angeles, CA 90049 · 213-826-7701

Roy N. Aruffo · (Adult & Child Psychoanalysis) · 5300 San Jacinto, Suite 105, Houston TX 77004 · 713-523-9389

Harold Philip Blum · Clinical Professor of Psychiatry, New York University · Long Island Jewish Hospital · 23 The Hemlocks, Roslyn, NY 11576 · 516-621-6850

Dale Boesky · Clinical Associate Professor of Psychiatry, Wayne State University School of Medicine · 755 West Big Beaver Road, Suite 510, Troy, MI 48084 · 313-362-0966

John Iverson Boswell, Jr. · Associate Professor of Psychiatry, University of North Carolina School of Medicine · Director, Eating Disorder Clinic; and Director, University of North Carolina-Duke Psychoanalytic Education Program, University of North Carolina Hospitals · Wing C, Campus Box 7160, Chapel Hill, NC 27599-7160 · 919-966-3379

Charles Brenner · Clinical Professor of Psychiatry, State University of New York Health Science Center at Brooklyn · 1040 Park Avenue, New York, NY 10028 · 212-722-0428

Justin David Call · Chief of Child & Adolescent Psychiatry, Director of Training in Child Psychiatry, and Professor of Psychiatry and Pediatrics, University of California, Irvine School of Medicine · University of California, Irvine Medical Center · 101 The City Drive, Building 53, Room 303, Orange, CA 92668 · 714-634-6023

C. Glenn Cambor · Training & Supervising Analyst, Houston Galveston Psychoanalytic Institute · 5300 San Jacinto, Suite 110, Houston, TX 77004 · 713-522-3986

Pietro Castelnuovo-Tedesco · James G. Blakemore Professor of Psychiatry, Vanderbilt University School of Medicine · Vanderbilt University Medical Center AA2206 Medical Center North, Nashville, TN 37232 · 615-322-6608

Judith Fingert Chused · (Adult, Adolescent, & Child Psychoanalysis) · Clinical Professor of Psychiatry and Pediatrics, The George Washington University School of Medicine · Supervising & Training Analyst, Washington Psychoanalytic Institute, Children's National Medical Center; George Washington University Medical Center · 1805 Randolph Street, NW, Washington, DC 20011 · 202-726-9273, 723-7896

Calvin A. Colarusso · Clinical Professor of Psychiatry, University of California at San Diego School of Medicine · Children's Hospital & Health Center; University of California at San Diego Medical Center · 1020 Prospect Street, Suite 415A, La Jolla, CA 92037 · 619-454-2473

Alan Bruce Cooper · Hermann Hospital; Harris County Psychiatric Hospital · P.O. Box 1628, La Porte, TX 77571-1628 · 713-792-4865

Arnold M. Cooper · Professor of Psychiatry, Cornell University Medical College Attending Psychiatrist, The New York Hospital-Cornell Medical Center · 525 East 68th Street, New York, NY 10021 · 212-746-3678

Homer C. Curtis · Clinical Professor of Psychiatry, Hahnemann University · Training & Supervising Analyst, Philadelphia Association of Psychoanalysis · 111 North 49th Street, Philadelphia, PA 19139 · 215-471-2468, 476-7115

Carl L. Davis · Clinical Professor of Psychiatry, Louisiana State University School of Medicine · Touro Infirmary · 3412 Prytania Street, New Orleans, LA 70115 · 504-895-8328

Paul A. Dewald · (Psychotherapy) · Clinical Professor of Psychiatry, St. Louis University School of Medicine · Training & Supervising Analyst, St. Louis Psychoanalytic Institute · 4524 Forest Park Avenue, St. Louis, MO 63108 · 314-367-5817

Scott Dowling · (Child & Adolescent Psychoanalysis) · Associate Clinical Professor of Psychiatry, Case Western Reserve University School of Medicine · University Hospitals of Cleveland · 11328 Euclid Avenue, Cleveland, OH 44106 · 216-229-3366

Roger Eddy · Clinical Professor, Department of Psychiatry, University of Washington School of Medicine · Hillclimb Court, 1425 Western, Suite 202, Seattle, WA 98101 · 206-623-3488

Newell Fischer · (Adult & Child Psychoanalysis) · Clinical Professor of Psychiatry, University of Pennsylvania School of Medicine · Institute of the Pennsylvania Hospital · 111 North 49th Street, Philadelphia, PA 19139 · 215-471-2386

John A. Fowler · Professor Emeritus, Department of Psychiatry, Duke University School of Medicine · Duke University Medical Center · 2721 Spencer Street, Durham NC 27705 · 919-489-5339

Alvin R. Frank · Professor of Clinical Psychiatry, St. Louis University School of Medicine · The Jewish Hospital of St. Louis · 7751 Carondelet Street, St. Louis, MO 63105-3316 · 314-721-8344

David A. Freedman · Professor, Department of Psychiatry, and Associate Professor, Department of Neurology, Baylor College of Medicine · The Methodist Hospital · 6560 Fannin Street, Suite 832, Houston, TX 77030 · 713-798-4877

Henry J. Friedman · Associate Clinical Professor of Psychiatry, Harvard University School of Medicine · Cambridge Hospital · Six Garden Terrace, Cambridge, MA 02138 · 617-876-4610

William A. Frosch · (Consultation) · Professor and Interim Chairman, Department of Psychiatry, Cornell University Medical College · Interim Psychiatrist-in-Chief, The New York Hospital-Cornell Medical Center · 525 East 68th Street, New York, NY 10021 · 212-746-3667

Robert Milton Galatzer-Levy · (Adult & Child Psychoanalysis) · Lecturer, University of Chicago; Institute for Psychoanalysis · 180 North Michigan, Chicago, IL 60601 · 312-236-0245

M. Robert Gardner · 97 Avon Hill Street, Cambridge, MA 02140 · 617-547-9135

Herbert Stockton Gaskill · Professor Emeritus, Department of Psychiatry, University of Colorado School of Medicine · 4900 Cherry Creek Drive South, Denver, CO 80222 · 303-758-2058

John E. Gedo · Chicago Institute for Psychoanalysis · 680 North Lake Shore Drive, Chicago, IL 60611 · 312-944-6485

Robert M. Gilliland · Professor of Clinical Psychiatry, Baylor College of Medicine 2201 West Holcombe Boulevard, Suite 320, Houston, TX 77030 · 713-664-7281

Jules Glenn · (Adult & Child Psychoanalysis) · Clinical Professor of Psychiatry, New York University Medical Center · Eight Preston Road, Great Neck, NY 11023 · 516-482-6302

Arnold I. Goldberg · Professor of Psychiatry, Rush-Presbyterian-St. Luke's Medical Center · Director, Institute for Psychoanalysis · 180 North Michigan, Chicago, IL 60601 · 312-726-6300

Marianne R. Goldberger · (Adult & Child Psychoanalysis) · Clinical Assistant Professor of Psychiatry, Cornell University Medical College, and New York University Medical Center · Training & Supervising Analyst, Psychoanalytic Institute of New York at the NYU Medical Center; The New York Hospital-Cornell Medical Center · 1130 Park Avenue, New York, NY 10128 · 212-534-3070, 543-6655

Stanley Goodman · Training Analyst, San Francisco Psychoanalytic Institute · 3021 Telegraph Avenue, Berkeley, CA 94705 · 415-848-1871

Paul Gray · Faculty: Supervising Analyst, Baltimore-Washington Institute for Psychoanalysis · 3315 Wisconsin Avenue, NW, Suite 803, Washington, DC · 202-244-0333

Arthur H. Green · (Adult & Child Psychoanalysis) · Clinical Professor of Psychiatry, College of Physicians & Surgeons of Columbia University · Columbia-Presbyterian Medical Center · 350 Central Park West, New York, NY 10025 · 212-678-4338

Richard M. Greenberg · Clinical Professor of Psychiatry, University of California at San Francisco School of Medicine · 2340 Sutter Street, Suite 303, San Francisco, CA 94115 · 415-389-0729

Daniel Peter Greenson · Associate Clinical Professor of Psychiatry, University of California at San Francisco School of Medicine · Assistant Chief, Department of Psychiatry, Mt. Zion Hospital & Medical Center · 2486 Shattuck Avenue, Berkeley, CA 94704 · 415-549-0218

Alexander Grinstein · Clinical Professor of Psychiatry, Wayne State University School of Medicine · Training & Supervising Psychoanalyst, Michigan Psychoanalytic Institute, Southfield · 31510 Bellvine Trail, Birmingham, MI 48010 · 313-646-1060

Cornelis Heijn, Jr. · Clinical Professor, Department of Psychiatry, and Director, Medical Student Education, Tufts University School of Medicine · New England Medical Center · 750 Washington Street, Box 1007, Boston, MA 02111 · 617-956-5774

John Hitchcock · Clinical Associate Professor of Psychiatry, University of Pittsburgh School of Medicine · 3708 Fifth Avenue, Suite 408, Pittsburgh, PA 15213 412-681-8772

Samuel Hoch · 2345 California Street, San Francisco, CA 94115 · 415-922-0500

John S. Howie · 3129 Essex Circle, Raleigh, NC 27608 · 919-782-0616

David Michael Hurst · Clinical Associate Professor of Psychiatry, University of Colorado School of Medicine · Training & Supervising Analyst, Denver Institute of Psychoanalysis · 601 Emerson Street, Denver, CO 80218 · 303-832-5024

Peggy B. Hutson · Clinical Professor of Psychiatry, University of Miami School of Medicine · University of Miami Hospital & Clinics · 3170 Munroe Drive, Miami, FL 33133 · 305-854-6349

Jacob G. Jacobson · Clinical Professor of Psychiatry, University of Colorado, Department of Psychiatry; Training and Supervising Analyst, Denver Institute for Psychoanalysis, 1636 Sixteenth Street, Boulder, CO 80302 · 303-443-1337

John S. Kafka · Clinical Professor, Department of Psychiatry, The George Washington University School of Medicine · George Washington University Medical Center · 5323 Connecticut Avenue, NW, Washington, DC 20015 · 202-362-0087, 301-652-8226

Lila Joyce Kalinich · Associate Clinical Professor of Psychiatry, College of Physicians & Surgeons of Columbia University; Training & Supervising Analyst, Columbia University Psychoanalytic Center for Training & Research · Columbia-Presbyterian Medical Center · 300 Central Park West, Suite 1-K, New York, NY 10024 · 212-769-4000

Alex H. Kaplan · Clinical Professor of Psychiatry, Washington University School of Medicine · Attending Physician, Barnes Hospital; The Jewish Hospital of St. Louis · 4524 Forest Park, St. Louis, MO 63108 · 314-367-6243

Joseph G. Kepecs · Professor Emeritus, Department of Psychiatry, University of Wisconsin-Madison School of Medicine · University of Wisconsin Hospital & Clinics · Clinical Science Center, 600 Highland Avenue, Madison, WI 53792 · 608-263-6080

Otto F. Kernberg · Professor of Psychiatry, Cornell University Medical College · Associate Chairman & Medical Director, The New York Hospital-Cornell Medical Center, Westchester Division · 21 Bloomingdale Road, White Plains, NY 10605 · 914-997-5714

Paulina Kernberg · (Adult & Child Psychoanalysis) · Associate Professor of Psychiatry, Cornell University Medical College · Director of Child & Adolescent Psychiatry, The New York Hospital-Cornell Medical Center, Westchester Division · 21 Bloomingdale Road, White Plains, NY 10605 · 914-997-5951

Edward H. Knight · Emeritus Clinical Professor, Department of Psychiatry, Louisiana State University School of Medicine · 1303 Antoinine Street, New Orleans, LA 70115 · 504-895-5381

George P. Kochis · (Adult & Child Psychoanalysis) · Clinical Associate Professor of Psychiatry, Baylor College of Medicine, and The University of Texas Medical Branch at Houston · Doctors Hospital, Conroe; Cypress Creek Hospital, Houston 2201 West Holcombe Boulevard, Suite 320, Houston, TX 77030 · 713-661-4225

Selma Kramer · (Adult & Child Psychoanalysis) · Professor of Psychiatry, Thomas Jefferson University School of Medicine; Training Analyst, Philadelphia Psychoanalytic Institute · Thomas Jefferson University Hospital · 3902 Netherfield Road, Philadelphia, PA 19129 · 215-849-7272

Anton O. Kris · Training & Supervising Analyst, The Boston Psychoanalytic Society & Institute · 37 Philbrick Road, Brookline, MA 02146 · 617-734-7972

Maimon Leavitt · 1800 Fairburn Avenue, Los Angeles, CA 90025 · 213-475-1811

Roy K. Lilleskov · (Adult & Child Psychoanalysis) · Clinical Professor of Psychiatry, New York University Medical Center · 55 East 87th Street, New York, NY 10128 · 212-876-0405

James Welton Lomax II · Director, Psychiatric Residency Program, Baylor College of Medicine · Baylor University Medical Center · One Baylor Plaza, Houston, TX 77030 · 713-798-4878

Roger A. MacKinnon · Professor of Clinical Psychiatry, College of Physicians & Surgeons of Columbia University; Director, Columbia University Psychoanalytic Center for Training & Research · Attending Psychiatrist, Columbia-Presbyterian Medical Center · 11 East 87th Street, New York, NY 10028 · 212-289-0511

John Adams MacLeod · Professor Emeritus of Psychiatry, Department of Psychiatry, University of Cincinnati, College of Medicine · The Christ Hospital · 3001 Highland Avenue, Cincinnati, OH 45219 · 513-961-8830

Eugene J. Mahon · (Child Psychoanalysis) · Assistant Clinical Professor of Psychiatry, College of Physicians & Surgeons of Columbia University · Adult Analyst & Child Psychoanalyst, Columbia Psychoanalytic Center for Training & Research Six East 96th Street, New York, NY 10128 · 212-831-1414

Charles Mangham, Sr. · (Child Psychoanalysis) · Clinical Professor, University of Washington; Training Analyst & Supervising Child Analyst, Seattle Institute for Psychoanalysis · Northwest Psychoanalytic Hospital · 4033 East Madison Street, Seattle, WA 98112 · 206-323-1706

Marvin O. Margolis · (Adult & Child Psychoanalysis) · Associate Professor of Psychiatry, Wayne State University School of Medicine · Training & Supervising Psychoanalyst, Michigan Psychoanalytic Institute, Southfield · 31425 Baffin Drive, Franklin, MI 48025 · 313-626-6466

James T. McLaughlin · Clinical Associate Professor, Emeritus, University of Pittsburgh School of Medicine · Training & Supervising Analyst, Pittsburgh Psychoanalytic Institute · 820 Devonshire Street, Pittsburgh, PA 15213 · 412-621-4159

Robert D. Mehlman · Assistant Clinical Professor of Psychiatry, Harvard Medical School; Training & Supervising Analyst, Boston Psychoanalytic Society & Institute · Brigham & Women's Hospital; Faulkner Hospital; Massachusetts Mental Health Center · 20 Netherlands Road, Brookline, MA 02146 · 617-232-0073

Jon Keith Meyer · Professor of Psychoanalysis, and Director, Division of Psychoanalysis, Medical College of Wisconsin · Columbia-Presbyterian Medical Center; Milwaukee Psychiatric Hospital · 2321 East Stratford Court, Milwaukee, WI 53211 · 414-963-2431

Robert Weigel Meyers · Clinical Professor of Psychiatry, St. Louis University School of Medicine · Director, & Training & Supervising Analyst, St. Louis Psychoanalytic Institute, St. Louis University Medical Center · 4524 Forest Park Boulevard, St. Louis, MO 63108 · 314-367-8424

Robert Michels · Professor and Chairman, Department of Psychiatry, Cornell University Medical College · 525 East 68th Street, New York NY 10021 · 212-746-3770

Paul G. Myerson · 25 Larch Road, Waban, MA 02168 · 617- 527-0324

Calvern E. Narcisi · (Adult & Child Psychoanalysis) · Assistant Clinical Professor of Psychiatry, University of Colorado School of Medicine · 4900 Cherry Creek South Drive, Denver, CO 80222 · 303-691-0941

Stanley Stuart Needell · Clinical Associate Professor of Psychiatry, University of Miami School of Medicine · 2699 Bayshore Drive,Suite 900-A, Miami, FL 33133 305-858-3535

Robert A. Nemiroff · Clinical Professor of Psychiatry, and Director, Research & Training, University of California at San Diego School of Medicine · Training & Supervising Analyst, San Diego Psychoanalytic Institute, University Hospital; Veterans Affairs Medical Center · 2803 Inverness Drive, La Jolla, CA 92037 · 619-459-0111

Peter B. Neubauer · (Adult & Child Psychoanalysis) · Clinical Professor of Psychiatry, New York University Medical Center · 33 East 70th Street, New York, NY 10021 · 212-288-2348

Kenneth M. Newman · Training and Supervising Analyst, Chicago Psychoanalytic Institute · Michael Reese Hospital · 180 North Michigan Avenue, Chicago, IL 60601 · 312-263-6172

William C. Offenkrantz · Director, Psychotherapy Training, Maricopa Medical Center · El Dorado Square, 6623 North Scottsdale Road, Scottsdale, AZ 85253 · 602-998-1928

Shelley Orgel · Clinical Professor of Psychiatry, The Psychoanalytic Institute, Department of Psychiatry, New York University College of Medicine, New York University Medical Center · 245 East 87th Street, New York, NY 10128 · 212-427-7163

Anna Ornstein · Professor of Child Psychiatry, University of Cincinnati College of Medicine · University of Cincinnati Hospital · 4177 Rose Hill Avenue, Cincinnati, OH 45267-0539 · 513-558-5841

Paul H. Ornstein · Professor of Psychiatry, University of Cincinnati College of Medicine · University of Cincinnati Hospital · 4177 Rose Hill Avenue, Cincinnati, OH 45229 · 513-558-5900

Thomas L. Pappadis · Clinical Assistant Professor of Psychiatry, University of Chicago, Pritzker School of Medicine · Michael Reese Hospital · 180 North Michigan Avenue, Chicago, IL 60601 · 312-372-3373

H. Gunther Perdigao · (Adult & Child Psychoanalysis) · Training & Supervising Analyst, New Orleans Psychoanalytic Institute · Supervising Child Analyst, New Orleans Psychoanalytic Society · 1424 Amelia Street, New Orleans, LA 70115-3618 · 504-895-7841

David Peretz · (Thanatology) · Assistant Clinical Professor of Psychiatry, College of Physicians & Surgeons of Columbia University; Teaching Faculty, Columbia University Psychoanalytic Center for Training & Research · 300 Central Park West, New York, NY 10024 · 212-873-7860

Ethel S. Person · Professor of Clinical Psychiatry, College of Physicians & Surgeons of Columbia University · Columbia-Presbyterian Medical Center · 135 Central Park West, New York, NY 10023 · 212-873-2700

Warren S. Poland · 5225 Connecticut Avenue, NW, Washington, DC 20015 · 202-362-4522

George H. Pollock · (Psychosomatic Medicine) · Ruth & Evelyn Dunbar Distinguished Professor of Psychiatry & Behavioral Sciences, Northwestern University Medical School · Senior Attending Staff Member, Northwestern Memorial Hospital · 303 East Superior Street, Room 544, Chicago, IL 60611 · 312-908-6828

Sydney Lawrence Pomer · (Adult & Adolescent Psychoanalysis) · Clinical Professor of Psychiatry, University of Southern California School of Medicine · Training Analyst, Southern California Psychoanalytic Institute, Los Angeles County-University of Southern California Medical Center; Cedars-Sinai Medical Center · 10444 Santa Monica Boulevard, Los Angeles, CA 90025 · 310-279-1131

Robert Cooley Prall · (Adult & Child Psychoanalysis) · Consultant in Psychiatry, Child Guidance Center · Consultant in Child Psychiatry, Austin State Hospital, Child Unit · 5750 Balcones Drive, Suite 101B, Austin, TX 78731 · 512-453-3323

Naomi Ragins · (Child & Adolescent Psychoanalysis) · Clinical Associate Professor of Child Psychiatry, University of Pittsburgh School of Medicine · Training & Supervising Analyst, Adult & Child Psychoanalysis, Pittsburgh Psychoanalytic Institute; Volunteer Staff, Western Psychiatric Institute & Clinic, Cathedral Mansions, 4716 Ellsworth Avenue, Suite 118-119, Pittsburgh, PA 15213 · 412-621-9992

Leo Rangell · Clinical Professor of Psychiatry, University of California at Los Angeles School of Medicine · Westwood Hospital · 456 North Carmelina Avenue, Los Angeles, CA 90049 · 213-472-5311

Owen Dennis Renik · Associate Clinical Professor of Psychiatry, University of California at San Francisco School of Medicine · 244 Myrtle Street, San Francisco, CA 94109 · 415-673-9692

Samuel Ritvo · (Child Psychoanalysis) · Clinical Professor, Yale University School of Medicine · 230 South Frontage Road, P.O. Box 3333, New Haven CT 06510 203-785-2513

Ana-Maria Rizzuto · Training & Supervising Analyst, Psychoanalytic Institute of New England, East · 75 Gardner Road, Brookline, MA 02146-4523 · 617-232-5363

James Robinson · (Adult & Child Psychoanalysis) · 320 Westcott, Suite 103, Houston, TX 77007 · 713-524-2959

F. Robert Rodman · (Adult & Child Psychoanalysis) · University of California at Los Angeles School of Medicine · 450 North Bedford, Suite 211, Beverly Hills, CA 90210 · 213-275-4662

Arthur Louis Rosenbaum · (Adult & Child Psychoanalysis) · Assistant Clinical Professor, Department of Psychiatry, Case Western Reserve University School of Medicine · University Hospitals of Cleveland · 2680 Fairmount Boulevard, Cleveland Heights, OH 44106 · 216-321-2376

Allan D. Rosenblatt · Clinical Professor of Psychiatry, University of California at San Diego School of Medicine · Training & Supervising Analyst, San Diego Psychoanalytic Institute · 3252 Holiday Court, Suite 205, La Jolla, CA 92037 · 619-453-6108

Arnold Morton Rothstein · 320 Central Park West, Suite 3A, New York, NY 10025 · 212-496-6209

Ralph Emerson Roughton, Jr. · Clinical Professor of Psychiatry, Emory University School of Medicine · Director, Emory University Psychoanalytic Institute · 1175 Peachtree Street NE, Suite 412, Atlanta, GA 30361 · 404-892-7561

David Morton Sachs · Clinical Professor of Child & Adult Psychiatry, Hahnemann University · Hahnemann Hospital · 255 South 17th Street, Philadelphia, PA 19103 · 215-735-1116

Judith S. Schachter · (Adult & Child Psychoanalysis) · Director, and Training & Supervising Analyst, Pittsburgh Psychoanalytic Institute · 401 Shady Avenue, Suite B202, Pittsburgh, PA 15206 · 412-661-6096

Melvin A. Scharfman · (Adult & Child Psychoanalysis) · Clinical Professor of Psychiatry, New York University Medical Center, Bellevue Medical Center · 89 Bayview Avenue, Great Neck, NY 10021 · 516-466-8155

Evelyne Albrecht Schwaber · Training & Supervising Analyst, Psychoanalytic Institute of New England East · Faculty, Boston Psychoanalytic Society & Institute · Four Welland Road, Brookline, MA 02146 · 617-232-3088

Lawrence H. Schwartz · Clinical Professor, Department of Psychiatry & Behavioral Science, University of Washington School of Medicine · Swedish Hospital Medical Center · 1120 Cherry, Suite 240, Seattle, WA 98104 · 206-624-0296

Lester Schwartz · 322 Central Park West, New York, NY 10025 · 212-864-8055

I. Gene Schwarz · Associate Clinical Professor, Department of Psychiatry, University of Colorado School of Medicine · Director, Denver Institute for Psychoanalysis; Colorado General Hospital · 4200 East Ninth Avenue, Box C255-64, Denver, CO 80262 · 303-270-7776,758-3155

Calvin F. Settlage · Clinical Professor of Psychiatry, University of California, San Francisco School of Medicine · Training & Supervising Analyst in Adult & Child Analysis, San Francisco Psychoanalytic Institute · 10 Crecienta Lane, Sausalito, CA 94965 · 415-332-2226

Louis B. Shapiro · 180 North Michigan, Chicago, IL 60601 · 312-726-6300

Leonard L. Shengold · Training Analyst, New York University Analytic Institute 1199 Park Avenue, Apartment 1C, New York, NY 10128 · 212-369-3011

Moisy Shopper · (Adult, Adolescent & Child Psychoanalysis) · Clinical Professor of Child Psychiatry & Pediatrics, St. Louis University School of Medicine · Cardinal Glennon Children's Hospital · 4524 Forest Park, St. Louis, MO 63108 · 314-361-4646

Lorraine D. Siggins · (College Psychiatry) · Psychiatrist-in-Chief, Mental Hygiene, Division of the Yale Health Services, Yale University School of Medicine · Yale-New Haven Hospital · Division of Mental Hygiene, 17 Hillhouse Avenue, New Haven, CT 06520 · 203-432-0306

Austin Silber · Clinical Professor of Psychiatry, New York University School of Medicine · Former Director, and Training & Supervising Psychoanalyst, Psychoanalytic Institute, Department of Psychiatry, New York University Medical Center · 1199 Park Avenue, New York, NY 10128 · 212-369-7851

Martin A. Silverman · (Adult & Child Psychoanalysis) · Clinical Professor of Psychiatry, New York University Medical Center; Training & Supervising Analyst, The Psychoanalytic Institute · The New York University Medical Center · 551 Ridgewood Road, Maplewood, NJ 07040 · 201-762-1387

Richard C. Simons · Professor of Psychiatry, University of Colorado School of Medicine · University of Colorado Health Sciences Center · 4200 East Ninth Avenue, Box C-249-44, Denver, CO 80262 · 303-270-7393

Albert J. Solnit · (Adult & Child Psychoanalysis) · Sterling Professor of Pediatrics & Psychiatry, and Senior Research Scientist, Yale University School of Medicine; Commissioner of Department of Mental Health for State of Connecticut · Yale-New Haven Hospital · 333 Cedar Street, P.O. Box 3333, New Haven, CT 06510 203-785-2518

Rebecca Z. Solomon · Clinical Professor of Psychiatry, University of Connecticut School of Medicine · Hartford Hospital · 85 Seymour Street, Hartford, CT 06106 203-247-2123

Vann Spruiell · Clinical Professor of Psychiatry, Tulane University School of Medicine · Touro Infirmary · P.O. Box 56270, Metairie, LA 70055 · 504-837-3606

Brandt F. Steele · Professor Emeritus of Psychiatry, University of Colorado School of Medicine · Training & Supervising Analyst, Denver Psychoanalytic Institute · 4200 East Ninth Avenue, C270-50, Denver, CO 80262 · 303-270-7378

Leo Stone · Instructor, New York Psychoanalysis Institute · One Gracie Terrace, New York, NY 10028 · 212-288-3209

James Lampton Titchener · Professor Emeritus, University of Cincinnati, College of Medicine · University of Cincinnati Hospital · Logan Hall, 3259 Elland Avenue, Cincinnati, OH 45267-0539 · 513-558-5838

Paul H. Tolpin · Senior Attending Psychiatrist, Michael Reese Hospital · 180 North Michigan Avenue, Chicago, IL 60601 · 312-236-2371

Robert L. Tyson · (Psychotherapy, also child) · Professor of Psychiatry, Department of Psychiatry, University of California at San Diego School of Medicine; Training and Supervising Analyst (Adult and Child), San Diego Psychoanalytic Society and Institute · 3252 Holiday Court, La Jolla, CA 92037 · 619-452-0733

Arthur F. Valenstein · Clinical Professor Emeritus, Department of Psychiatry, Harvard Medical School · 140 Foster Street, Cambridge, MA 02138 · 617-547-6152

Vamik D. Volkan · Professor of Psychiatry, University of Virginia School of Medicine · Medical Director, University of Virginia Blue Ridge Hospital; University of Virginia Health Sciences Center · Blue Ridge Hospital, Charlottesville, VA 22901 804-924-9001

Samuel Wagonfeld · (Adult & Child Psychoanalysis) · Assistant Clinical Professor, University of Colorado School of Medicine · 240 St. Paul Street, Denver, CO 80206 · 303-321-3275

Robert S. Wallerstein · Professor Emeritus, University of California, San Francisco School of Medicine · 655 Redwood Highway, Suite 261, Mill Valley, CA 94941 · 415-389-9323

Edward M. Weinshel · Clinical Professor of Psychiatry, University of California at San Francisco School of Medicine · Mt. Zion Hospital & Medical Center · 2625 Scott Street, San Francisco, CA 94123 · 415-567-1238

Samuel Weiss · (Adult & Child Psychoanalysis) · Clinical Associate Professor, The University of Illinois College of Medicine at Chicago · Training & Supervising Analyst, Chicago Institute of Psychoanalysis · 500 North Michigan Avenue, Chicago, IL 60611 · 312-527-4541

David S. Werman · (Psychotherapy) · Professor of Psychiatry, Duke University School of Medicine · Duke University Medical Center · Box 3812, DUMC, Durham, NC 27710 · 919-684-6605

Ernest Simon Wolf · Assistant Professor of Psychiatry, Northwestern University Medical School · 180 North Michigan Avenue, Chicago, IL 60601 · 312-236-4582

Anna K. Wolff · McLean Hospital · 115 Mill Street, Belmont, MA 02178 · 617-855-2868

Edwin C. Wood · Professor of Clinical Psychiatry, Baylor College of Medicine · Training & Supervising Analyst, Houston Galveston Psychoanalytic Institute · 5300 San Jacinto, Suite 150, Houston, TX 77004-6886 · 713-524-8566

Alan Barry Zients · (Adult & Child Psychoanalysis) · Assistant Clinical Professor, Child Psychiatry & Child Development, The George Washington University School of Medicine · Training, Supervising & Teaching Analyst, Baltimore—Washington Institute of Psychoanalysis, Baltimore · 5410 Connecticut Avenue, NW, Washington, DC 20015 · 202-362-2336

PSYCHOPHARMACOLOGY

Ross J. Baldessarini · (Psychopharmacology of Psychotic Disorders) · Professor of Psychiatry & in Neuroscience, Harvard Medical School · Director, Laboratories for Psychiatric Research & Psychotic Disorders Program, Mailman Research Center, McLean Hospital · Mailman Research Center, 115 Mill Street, Belmont, MA 02178 · 617-855-3203

James C. Ballenger · (Anxiety Disorders) · Professor and Chairman, Department of Psychiatry, and Director, Institute of Psychiatry, Medical University of South Carolina · 171 Ashley Avenue, Charleston, SC 29425 · 803-792-4037

Joseph Biederman · Associate Professor of Psychiatry, Harvard Medical School · Director, Pediatric Psychopharmacology Unit, Massachusetts General Hospital · Child Psychiatry Department, 15 Parkman Street, Boston, MA 02114 · 617-726-2724

Bernard J. Carroll · Professor of Psychiatry, Duke University School of Medicine · Clinical Director, Geriatric Psychiatry Institute, John Umstead Hospital · Butner, NC 27509-1626 · 919-575-7923

Jesse O. Cavenar, Jr. · Professor of Psychiatry, Duke University School of Medicine · Division Chief for Outpatient Services, Duke University Medical Center · P.O. Box 3837, Durham, NC 27710 · 919-286-6933

Dennis S. Charney · Professor, Department of Psychiatry, Yale University School of Medicine · Chief, Psychiatry Service, West Haven Veterans Affairs Medical Center · 950 Campbell Avenue, West Haven, CT 06516 · 203-937-3837

Paula J. Clayton · Professor and Head, Department of Psychiatry, University of Minnesota Medical School · University of Minnesota Hospital & Clinic · Box 77 UMHC, 420 Delaware Street, SE, Minneapolis, MN 55455 · 612-626-3853

Jonathan O. Cole · Professor of Psychiatry, Harvard Medical School · Program Director, Affective Disorders Program, McLean Hospital · 115 Mill Street, Belmont, MA 02178 · 617-855-2900

Jonathan R. T. Davidson · Associate Professor of Psychiatry, Duke University School of Medicine · Director, Psychiatry Outpatient Programs and Anxiety Disorders Program, Duke University Medical Center · P.O. Box 3812, Durham, NC 27710 · 919-684-2880

David L. Dunner · Professor, Department of Psychiatry, University of Washington School of Medicine · Director, Outpatient Psychiatry, and Co-Director, Center for Anxiety & Depression, and Vice-Chairman for Clinical Services, University of Washington Medical Center · 4225 Roosevelt Way NE, Suite 306, Seattle, WA 98105 · 206-543-6768

Burr S. Eichelman · (Pharmacology of Violence) · Professor & Chairman, Department of Psychiatry, Temple University School of Medicine · Temple University Hospital · 3401 North Broad, Philadelphia, PA 19140 · 215-221-3364

Jan Fawcett · Professor and Chairman, Department of Psychiatry, Rush Medical College · Rush-Presbyterian-St. Luke's Medical Center · 1720 West Polk, Chicago, IL 60612 · 312-942-5372

Alexander H. Glassman · (Depression, Cigarette Smoking Cessation) · Professor of Clinical Psychiatry, College of Physicians & Surgeons of Columbia University Chief, Department of Clinical Psychopharmacology, New York State Psychiatric Institute; Columbia-Presbyterian Medical Center · 722 West 168th Street, Box 116, New York, NY 10032 · 212-960-5750

Jack M. Gorman · (Anxiety, Panic) · Professor of Clinical Psychiatry, College of Physicians & Surgeons of Columbia University · Attending Psychiatrist, Columbia- Presbyterian Medical Center · 722 West 168th Street, New York, NY 10032 212-799-5202

Laurence L. Greenhill · (Hyperactivity, Pediatric Psychoses) · Associate Professor of Clinical Psychiatry, College of Physicians & Surgeons of Columbia University Director, Disruptive Behavior Clinic, New York State Psychiatric Institute · 722 West 168th Street, 905 North, New York, NY 10032 · 212-960-2340

Samuel B. Guze · Spencer T. Olin Professor of Psychiatry, Washington University School of Medicine · Psychiatrist and Assistant Physician, Department of Internal Medicine, Barnes Hospital · 4940 Audubon Avenue, St. Louis, MO 63110 · 314-362-7772

Jeffrey L. Houpt · (Consultation-Liaison Psychiatry) · Dean of School of Medicine, Emory University School of Medicine · 1440 Clifton Road NE, Atlanta, GA 30322 · 404-727-5630

Donald F. Klein · (Anxiety) · Professor of Psychiatry, College of Physicians & Surgeons of Columbia University · Attending Psychiatrist, Columbia-Presbyterian Medical Center · 722 West 168th Street, Box 22, New York, NY 10032 · 212-960-2307

David J. Kupfer · (Depression) · Professor and Chairman, Department of Psychiatry, University of Pittsburgh School of Medicine · Western Psychiatric Institute and Clinic, University of Pittsburgh Medical Center · 3811 O'Hara Street, Pittsburgh, PA 15213-2593 · 412-624-2353

Michael R. Liebowitz · (Anxiety) · Professor of Clinical Psychiatry, College of Physicians & Surgeons of Columbia University · Director, Anxiety Disorder Clinic, New York State Psychiatric Institute · 722 West 168th Street, Box 120, New York, NY 10032 · 212-960-2366

J. Craig Nelson · Professor of Psychiatry, Yale University School of Medicine · Director, Psychiatric Inpatient Service, Yale-New Haven Hospital · 20 York Street, MU-10-704, New Haven, CT 06504 · 203-785-2157

Charles B. Nemeroff · (Manic Depression) · Professor and Chairman, Department of Psychiatry, Emory University School of Medicine · 1701 Uppergate Drive, Atlanta, GA 30322 · 404-727-5881

Robert Morton Post · Chief, Biological Psychiatry Branch, National Institute of Mental Health · 9000 Rockville Pike, Building 10, Room 3N212, Bethesda, MD 20892 · 301-496-4805

Frederic M. Quitkin · Professor of Clinical Psychiatry, College of Physicians & Surgeons of Columbia University · Director, Depression Evaluation Service, New York State Psychiatric Institute · 722 West 168th Street, Box 12, New York, NY 10032 · 212-960-5784, 516-484-0013

Judith L. Rapoport · (Obsessive Compulsive Disorder, Pediatric Psychopharmacology, Attention Deficit Disorder) · Clinical Professor of Psychiatry and Pediatrics, The George Washington University School of Medicine · Chief, Child Psychiatry Branch, National Institute of Mental Health, National Institutes of Health Child Psychiatry Branch, NIMH, Bethesda, MD 20892 · 301-496-6081

Gerald F. Rosenbaum · Chief of Psychopharmacology & Behavioral Therapy, Massachusetts General Hospital · 15 Parkman Street, WACC815, Boston, MA 02114 · 617-726-3488

A. John Rush · Betty Jo Hay Distinguished Chair in Mental Health, and Professor of Psychiatry, The University of Texas Southwestern Medical Center at Dallas · Parkland Memorial Hospital · 5323 Harry Hines Boulevard, Dallas, TX 75235 · 214-688-8768

Carl Salzman · Associate Professor of Psychiatry, Harvard Medical School · Director of Psychopharmacology, Massachusetts Mental Health Center · 74 Fenwood Road, Boston, MA 02115 · 617-232-1113

Alan F. Schatzberg · Kenneth T. Norris, Jr. Professor and Chairman, Department of Psychiatry & Behavioral Sciences, Stanford University School of Medicine · Chief of Psychiatry, Stanford University Hospital · Panama Street, Psychiatry Building, TD114, Stanford, CA 94305-5490 · 415-723-6811

Richard I. Shader · (Antianxiety Agents and Antidepressants) · Chairman, Department of Pharmacology and Experimental Therapeutics, Tufts University School of Medicine · Chief, Division of Clinical Pharmacology, New England Medical Center Hospitals · 136 Harrison Avenue, M and V Building, Room 308, Boston, MA 02111 · 617-956-6897

David V. Sheehan · Professor of Psychology, University of South Florida College of Social & Behavioral Sciences; Professor of Psychiatry, and Director of the Office of Research, Department of Psychiatry & Behavioral Medicine, University of

South Florida College of Medicine · Director of Clinical Research, Univerisity of South Florida Psychiatry Center · Univerisity of South Florida Psychiatry Center, 3500 East Fletcher Avenue, Suite 321, Tampa, FL 33613 · 813-974-3344

Gary J. Tucker · (Neuropsychiatric Disorders) · Professor and Chairman, Department of Psychiatry & Behavioral Sciences, University of Washington School of Medicine · University of Washington Medical Center · 1959 Northeast Pacific Street, RP-10, Seattle, WA 98195 · 206-543-3750

Thomas Whitley Uhde · (Anxiety) · Clinical Professor, Department of Psychiatry, Uniformed Services University of the Health Sciences School of Medicine · Chief, Anxiety & Affective Disorders, National Institute of Mental Health, National Institutes of Health · Section on Anxiety & Affective Disorders, 9000 Rockville Pike, Room 3-S 239, Bethesda, MD 20892 · 301-496-6825

Paul H. Wender · (Attention Deficit Disorder, Pediatric Hyperactivity, Adult Hyperactivity) · Distinguished Professor of Psychiatry, University of Utah School of Medicine · Director of Psychiatric Resources, University of Utah Health Sciences Center · 50 North Medical Drive, Salt Lake City, UT 84132 · 801-581-8075

Joel Yager · Professor and Associate Chair for Education, Department of Psychiatry and Biobehavioral Sciences, University of California at Los Angeles School of Medicine · Director of Residency Education, University of California at Los Angeles Neuropsychiatric Institute · 760 Westwood Plaza, Los Angeles, CA 90024 · 310-825-0018

Stuart C. Yudofsky · (Aggressive Disorders) · Professor and Chairman, Department of Psychiatry, University of Chicago, Pritzker School of Medicine · University of Chicago Medical Center · 5841 South Maryland Avenue, Box 411, Chicago, IL 60637-1470 · 312-702-6192

SCHIZOPHRENIA

Nancy C. Andreasen · Professor of Psychiatry, The University of Iowa College of Medicine · Director, Mental Health Clinical Research Center, The University of Iowa Hospitals & Clinics · 200 Hawkins Drive, Iowa City, IA 52242 · 319-356-1616

Magda Campbell · (Diagnosis, Childhood Schizophrenia) · Professor of Psychiatry, New York University School of Medicine · Director, Division of Child & Adolescent Psychiatry, Bellevue Hospital · 550 First Avenue, 21S15, New York, NY 10016 · 212-263-6206

William T. Carpenter, Jr. · (Etiology of Schizophrenia, Treatment of Schizophrenia) · Professor of Psychiatry & Pharmacology, University of Maryland School of Medicine · Director, Maryland Psychiatric Research Center · Box 21247, Baltimore, MD 21228 · 301-455-7101

John G. Gunderson · Associate Professor of Psychiatry, Harvard Medical School Director, Psychotherapy & Psychosocial Research, McLean Hospital · Belmont, MA 02178 · 617-855-2293

Marvin Ira Herz · (Treatment and Rehabilitation of Schizophrenia) · Professor of Psychiatry, University of Rochester School of Medicine & Dentistry · Director, Longterm Program, and Director, Mental Health Services Research, Strong Memorial Hospital, University of Rochester Medical Center · 300 Crittenden Boulevard, Rochester, NY 14642 · 716-275-2716

Barry Jones · Director, Schizophrenia Program, University of Ottawa School of Medicine · Royal Ottawa Hospital · 1145 Carling, Ottawa, Ontario K1Z 7K4 · 613-724-6502

Samuel J. Keith · (Rehabilitation of Schizophrenia) · Clinical Professor of Psychiatry, Georgetown University School of Medicine · Acting Deputy Director, and Acting Director, Division of Applied & Services Research, National Institute of Mental Health, National Institutes of Health · 5600 Fishers Lane, Room 1799, Rockville, MD 20857 · 301-443-3673

H. Richard Lamb · (Rehabilitation of Schizophrenia) · Professor of Psychiatry, University of Southern California School of Medicine · The Los Angeles County + University of Southern California Medical Center · 1934 Hospital Place, Los Angeles, CA 90033 · 213-226-5618

Anthony F. Lehman · (Rehabilitation of Schizophrenia) · Associate Professor of Psychiatry, University of Maryland School of Medicine · 645 West Redwood Street, Baltimore, MD 21201 · 301-328-8667

Robert Paul Liberman · (Rehabilitation of Schizophrenia) · Professor of Psychiatry, University of California at Los Angeles School of Medicine · Chief of Rehabilitation Medicine, and Director, Clinical Research Center for Schizophrenia & Psychiatric Rehabilitation (Brentwood Division); Director, Clinical Research Unit, Camarillo-UCLA Research Center; Camarillo State Hospital; Veterans Affairs Medical Center, West Los Angeles; UCLA Center for the Health Sciences, and UCLA Neuropsychiatric Institute & Hospital · Rehabilitation Service (B117), Wilshire and Sawtelle Boulevards, Los Angeles, CA 90073 · 213-824-6620

William R. McFarlane · (Treatment and Rehabilitation of Schizophrenia) · Associate Clinical Professor of Psychiatry, College of Physicians & Surgeons of Columbia University · Director, Biosocial Treatment Research Division, New York

State Psychiatric Institute · 722 West 168th Street, Box 117, New York, NY 10032
212-960-2554

Thomas H. McGlashan · (Rehabilitation of Schizophrenia) · Executive Director, The Yale Psychiatric Institute; Psychiatrist-in-Chief, Yale University School of Medicine · P.O. Box 12A, Yale Station, New Haven, CT 06520 · 203-785-7849

Leonard I. Stein · (Rehabilitation of Schizophrenia) · Professor of Psychiatry, University of Wisconsin-Madison School of Medicine · Director of Research & Training, Mental Health Center of Dane County, Inc.; University of Wisconsin Hospital & Clinics · 600 Highland Avenue, Room B6-240, Madison, WI 53792 · 608-263-6064

John S. Strauss · (Rehabilitation of Schizophrenia) · Professor of Psychiatry, Yale University School of Medicine · Yale-New Haven Hospital · Connecticut Mental Health Center, 34 Park Street, Room 160, New Haven, CT 06519 · 203-789-7417

Kenneth Terkelsen · (Rehabilitation of Schizophrenia) · Associate Professor of Clinical Psychiatry, Cornell University Medical College · Director, Adult Day Treatment Program, The New York Hospital-Cornell Medical Center, Westchester Division · 21 Bloomingdale Road, White Plains, NY 10605 · 914-997-5930

SCHIZOPHRENIA/PSYCHOPHARMACOLOGY

Malcolm B. Bowers, Jr. · (Psychopharmacology of Schizophrenia, Rehabilitation of Schizophrenia) · Professor of Psychiatry and Associate Chairman for Clinical Services, Yale University School of Medicine · Attending Psychiatrist, Yale-New Haven Hospital · New Haven, CT 06510 · 203-785-2121

Alan Francis Breier · (Psychopharmacology of Schizophrenia) · Research Associate Professor, Department of Psychiatry, and Chief, Outpatient Department, Maryland Psychiatric Research Center, University of Maryland School of Medicine · P.O. Box 21247, Baltimore, MD 21228 · 301-455-7871

John M. Davis · (Psychopharmacology of Schizophrenia) · Gilman Professor of Psychiatry & Experimental Medicine, The University of Illinois College of Medicine at Chicago · Director of Research, Illinois State Psychiatric Institute · 1153 N. Lavergne Avenue, Chicago, IL 60659 · 312-854-6550

William M. Glazer · (Psychopharmacology of Schizophrenia) · Associate Clinical Professor of Psychiatry, Yale University School of Medicine · Yale-New Haven Hospital · Connecticut Mental Health Center, 34 Park Street, Room 269, New Haven, CT 06519 · 203-789-6985

John Michael Kane · (Psychopharmacology of Schizophrenia) · Professor of Psychiatry, Albert Einstein College of Medicine · Chairman, Department of Psychiatry, Hillside Hospital, Division of Long Island Jewish Medical Center · 75-59 Two Hundred Sixty-Third Street, Glen Oaks, NY 11004 · 718-470-8141

Joel Edward Kleinman · (Psychopharmacology of Schizophrenia) · Associate Clinical Professor of Psychiatry and Neurology, The George Washington University School of Medicine · Deputy Chief, Clinical Brain Disorders Branch, and Chief of Neuropathology Section, National Institute of Mental Health, National Institutes of Health · 5415 Connecticut Avenue, NW, Suite L30, Washington, DC 20015 · 202-363-2718

Stephen R. Marder · (Psychopharmacology of Schizophrenia) · Professor of Psychiatry, University of California at Los Angeles School of Medicine · Associate Chief of Psychiatry for Special Programs, West Los Angeles Veterans Affairs Medical Center, Brentwood Division · 11301 Wilshire Boulevard, Building 210, Los Angeles, CA 90073 · 213-824-6715

Herbert Yale Meltzer · (Psychopharmacology of Schizophrenia) · Douglas D. Bond Professor of Psychiatry, and Vice-Chairman for Research, Department of Psychiatry, Case Western Reserve University School of Medicine · University Hospitals of Cleveland · 2040 Abington Road, Cleveland, OH 44106 · 312-844-8750

David Pickar · (Psychopharmacology of Schizophrenia) · Clinical Professor of Psychiatry, Uniformed Services University of Health Sciences · Chief, Experimental Therapeutics Branch, National Institute of Mental Health, National Institutes of Health · 9000 Rockville Pike, Building 10, Room 4N214, Bethesda, MD 20892 · 301-496-6295

Charles S. Schulz · (Psychopharmacology of Schizophrenia and other Serious Mental Disorders) · Chairman, Department of Psychiatry, Case Western Reserve University School of Medicine · Director, Department of Psychiatry, University Hospitals of Cleveland · 2074 Abington Road, Cleveland OH 44106 · 216-844-3883

George M. Simpson · (Psychopharmacology of Schizophrenia) · Professor & Director, Clinical Psychopharmacology, Medical College of Pennsylvania · Consultant, Haverford State Hospital; Professor of Psychiatry, Medical College of Pennsylvania · 3200 Henry Avenue, Philadelphia, PA 19129 · 215-842-4390

Carol A. Tamminga · (Psychopharmacology of Schizophrenia) · Professor of Psychiatry, University of Maryland School of Medicine · Chief, Inpatient Program, Maryland Psychiatric Research Center · P.O. Box 21247, Baltimore, MD 21228 · 301-455-7915, 455-7695

Joe P. Tupin · (Psychopharmacology of Schizophrenia) · Professor of Psychiatry, University of California, Davis School of Medicine · Medical Director, University of California, Davis Medical Center · 2315 Stockton Boulevard, Sacramento, CA 95817 · 916-734-2777

Theodore Van Putten · (Psychopharmacology of Schizophrenia) · Professor of Psychiatry, University of California at Los Angeles School of Medicine · Head of Research, Veterans Affairs Hospital · 11301 Wilshire Boulevard, Ward 210-C, Los Angeles, CA 90073 · 213-824-4422

Daniel R. Weinberger · (Psychopharmacology of Schizophrenia) · Chief, Clinical Brain Disorders Branch, National Institute of Mental Health, National Institutes of Health · Neuroscience Center, 2700 Martin Luther King, Jr., Avenue, SE, Room 500, Washington DC 20032 · 202-373-6228

Richard Jed Wyatt · (Psychopharmacology of Schizophrenia) · Chief, Neuropsychiatry Branch, National Institute of Mental Health · St. Elizabeth's Hospital · Neuroscience Center, WAW Building, 2700 Martin Luther King, Jr. Avenue, SE, Room 536, Washington, DC 20032 · 202-373-6233

SEXUAL ABUSE

Elissa P. Benedek · (Children and the Law) · Clinical Professor of Psychiatry, The University of Michigan Medical School · Director, Research & Training, Center for Forensic Psychiatry · 3607 Chatham Way, Ann Arbor, MI 48105 · 313-429-2531 x290

Jean Patricia Goodwin · Professor of Psychiatry, Medical College of Wisconsin · Milwaukee County Mental Health Complex; Milwaukee Psychiatric Hospital · 9455 Watertown Plank Road, Milwaukee, WI 53226 · 414-257-4886

Arthur H. Green · (Adult & Child Psychoanalysis) · Clinical Professor of Psychiatry, College of Physicians & Surgeons of Columbia University · Columbia-Presbyterian Medical Center · 350 Central Park West, New York, NY 10025 · 212-678-4338

Domeena C. Renshaw · (Sexual Dysfunction Treatment, Sex Education) · Professor of Psychiatry, Loyola Stritch School of Medicine · Loyola University Medical Center · 2160 South First Avenue, Maywood, IL 60153 · 708-216-3752

SUICIDOLOGY

David A. Brent · Associate Professor of Child & Adolescent Psychiatry, University of Pittsburgh, Western Psychiatric Institute & Clinic (WPIC) · Chief, Division of Child and Adolescent Psychiatry, and Director, Services for Teens at Risk (STAR-

Center), Western Psychiatric Institute & Clinic, University of Pittsburgh Medical Center · 3811 O'Hara Street, Pittsburgh, PA 15213 · 412-624-5172

Bruce Leonard Danto · 100 East Valencia Drive, Suite 208, Fullerton, CA 92635 714-992-5111

Jan Fawcett · Professor and Chairman, Department of Psychiatry, Rush Medical College · Rush-Presbyterian-St. Luke's Medical Center · 1720 West Polk, Chicago, IL 60612 · 312-942-5372

Herbert M. Hendin · Professor of Psychiatry, New York Medical College · Director, American Suicide Association · 1045 Park Avenue, New York, NY 10028 · 212-348-4035

Robert M. Littman · Associate Professor of Psychiatry, University of California at San Diego School of Medicine · University of California at San Diego Medical Center; Mercy Hospital · 3914 Third Avenue, San Diego, CA 92103 · 619-291-4808

Jerome A. Motto · Professor of Psychiatry Emeritus, University of California, San Francisco School of Medicine · University of California, San Francisco Medical Center · 401 Parnassus Avenue, Room LPPI-379, San Francisco, CA 94143 · 415-476-1485

Cynthia Roberta Pfeffer · (Adolescent Psychiatry) · Professor of Psychiatry, Cornell University Medical College · Chief, Child-Psychiatry In-Patient Unit, The New York Hospital-Cornell Medical Center, Westchester Division · 21 Bloomingdale Road, White Plains, NY 10605 · 212-722-6856, 914-997-5849

Charles Lambert Rich · Professor of Psychiatry, State University of New York Health Science Center at Stony Brook · SUNY at Stony Brook Hospital · Health Science Center 510-020, Stonybrook, NY 11794 · 516-444-2990

Alec Roy · Professor of Psychiatry, Albert Einstein College of Medicine · Director of Affective Services, Hillside Hospital · 75-59 Two Hundred Sixty-Third Street, P.O. Box 38, Glen Oaks, NY 11004 · 718-470-8075

David Shaffer · (Diagnosis) · Irving Philips Professor of Child Psychiatry, and Professor of Psychiatry and Pediatrics, and Director, Division of Child & Adolescent Psychiatry, College of Physicians & Surgeons of Columbia University · New York State Psychiatric Institute · 722 West 168th Street, Box 78, New York, NY 10032 · 212-960-2548

Andrew Edmund Slaby · Clinical Professor of Psychiatry, New York University School of Medicine · Psychiatrist-in-Chief, Regent Hospital · 425 East 61st Street, New York, NY 10021 · 212-935-3400

Bryan L. Tanney · Associate Professor of Psychiatry, University of Calgary · Calgary General Hospital · 841 Center Avenue East, Room M7-024, Calgary, Alberta T2E 0A1 · 403-268-9894

VIOLENCE

David M. Bear · Professor of Psychiatry, University of Massachusetts Medical School · Chairman, Department of Psychiatry, Medical Center of Central Massachusetts · 119 Belmont Street, Worcester, MA 01605 · 508-793-6228

Magda Campbell · Professor of Psychiatry, New York University School of Medicine · Director, Division of Child & Adolescent Psychiatry, Bellevue Hospital · 550 First Avenue, 21S15, New York, NY 10016 · 212-263-6206

Bruce Leonard Danto · 100 East Valencia Drive, Suite 208, Fullerton, CA 92635 714-992-5111

Park E. Dietz · Clinical Professor of Psychiatry and Biobehavioral Sciences, University of California at Los Angeles School of Medicine · 537 Newport Center Drive, Newport Beach, CA 92660 · 714-760-0422

William R. Dubin · Professor, Department of Psychiatry, Temple University School of Medicine · Deputy Medical Director, Philadelphia Psychiatric Center · 4200 Monument Road, Philadelphia, PA 19131 · 215-581-3771

Burr S. Eichelman · (Pharmacology of Violence) · Professor & Chairman, Department of Psychiatry, Temple University School of Medicine · Temple University Hospital · 3401 North Broad, Philadelphia, PA 19140 · 215-221-3364

Frank R. Ervin · (Brain Disorders, Behavioral Genetics) · Professor, Department of Psychiatry & Center for Human Genetics, McGill University · Medical Scientist, Royal Victoria Hospital · 1033 Pine Avenue West, Room 409, Montreal, Quebec H3A 1A1 · 514-842-0340

Charles R. Keith · (Violent Children) · Associate Professor, Division of Child Psychiatry, Duke University School of Medicine · Assistant Clinical Director, and Training Director, Division of Child Psychiatry, Durham Community Guidance Clinic · Trent and Elba Streets, Durham, NC 27705 · 919-286-4456

Dorothy Otnow Lewis · (Juvenile Deliquency) · Professor, Department of Psychiatry, New York University School of Medicine; Clinical Professor, Yale University Child Study Center · Attending Physican, New York University-Bellevue Medical Center, Tisch Hospital; Yale-New Haven Hospital · New Bellevue 21S25, 550 First Avenue, New York, NY 10016 · 212-263-6208

John R. Lion · Clinical Professor of Psychiatry, University of Maryland School of Medicine · Sheppard Pratt Hospital · 328 East Quadrangle, 5100 Falls Road, Baltimore, MD 21210 · 301-433-6333

Richard Thomas Rada · President and CEO, College Health Enterprises · One Pacific Plaza, 7711 Center Avenue, Suite 300, Huntington Beach, CA 92647 · 714-891-5000

Loren H. Roth · (Ethics and Psychiatry and Medicine) · Professor and Vice-Chairman, Department of Psychiatry, and Director, Law & Psychiatry Program, University of Pittsburgh School of Medicine · Chief, Clinical Services, Western Psychiatric Institute & Clinic, University of Pittsburgh Medical Center · 3811 O'Hara Street, Room E820, Pittsburgh, PA 15213 · 412-624-2161

Robert Leslie Sadoff · Clinical Professor of Psychiatry, and Director of the Center for Studies in Social-Legal Psychiatry, University of Pennsylvania School of Medicine · Consultant in Forensic Psychiatry, Philadelphia Psychiatric Center; Albert Einstein University Hospital · Suite 326, The Benjamin Fox Pavilion, Jenkintown, PA 19046 · 215-887-6144

Jonathan M. Silver · Assistant Professor of Clinical Psychiatry, College of Physicians & Surgeons of Columbia University · Director, Neuropsychiatry, Columbia-Presbyterian Medical Center · Allen Pavilion, 5141 Broadway, New York, NY 10034 · 212-932-4165, 799-7620

Kenneth Tardiff · Professor of Psychiatry, Cornell University Medical College · Associate Medical Director, The New York Hospital-Cornell Medical Center · Payne Whitney Clinic, 525 East 68th Street, New York, NY 10021 · 212-746-3730

Joe P. Tupin · Professor of Psychiatry, University of California, Davis School of Medicine · Medical Director, University of California, Davis Medical Center · 2315 Stockton Boulevard, Sacramento, CA 95817 · 916-734-2777

PULMONARY & CRITICAL CARE MEDICINE

AIDS
(See also Infectious Disease, AIDS; Medical Oncology & Hematology, AIDS)

Jeffrey Glassroth · Marquardt Professor of Medicine, and Vice-Chairman, Department of Medicine, Northwestern University Medical School · Chief, Medical Service, Northwestern Memorial Hospital · 250 East Superior Street, Room 296, Chicago, IL 60611 · 312-908-2118

Philip Hopewell · Professor of Medicine, University of California at San Francisco School of Medicine · Chief, Chest Service, San Francisco General Hospital · 1001 Potrero Avenue, Chest Service, Room 5K1, San Francisco, CA 94110 · 415-648-5010

Diane E. Stover · Professor of Medicine, Cornell University Medical College · Chief of Pulmonary Service, and Head, Division of General Medicine, Department of Medicine, Memorial Sloan-Kettering Cancer Center · 1275 York Avenue, New York, NY 10021 · 212-639-8380

Jeanne M. Wallace · Associate Professor of Medicine, University of California at Los Angeles School of Medicine · Director of Diagnostic Procedures, Olive View Medical Center · 14445 Olive View Drive, Sylmar, CA 91342 · 818-364-3205

ASTHMA
(See also Allergy & Immunology, Adult and Pediatric; Pediatrics, Pediatric Allergy & Immunology, Asthma; Pediatric Pulmonology, Asthma)

Jeffrey Drazen · Parker B. Francis Professor of Medicine, Harvard Medical School Chief, Combined Program in Pulmonary/Critical Care Medicine, Beth Israel Hospital and Brigham and Women's Hospital; Director, Ina Sue Perlmutter Laboratory, Children's Hospital · Combined Program in Pulmonary/Critical Care Medicine, c/o Program Office, Brigham and Women's Hospital, 75 Francis Street, Boston, MA 02115 · 617-732-7420

Frederick E. Hargreave · Professor of Medicine, McMaster University · Active Staff, Firestone Regional Chest & Allergy Unit, St. Joseph's Hospital · 50 Charlton Avenue East, Hamilton, Ontario L8N 4A6 · 416-521-6000

Leonard D. Hudson · Professor of Medicine, Division of Pulmonary & Critical Care Medicine, and Head, Division of Pulmonary & Critical Care Medicine, University of Washington School of Medicine · Chief, Division of Pulmonary & Critical Care Medicine, Harborview Medical Center · 325 Ninth Avenue (ZA-62), Seattle, WA 98104-2499 · 206-223-3533

Roland H. Ingram · Professor of Medicine, Emory University School of Medicine Chief of Medicine, Crawford W. Long Hospital of Emory University · 550 Peachtree Street, NE, Atlanta, GA 30365 · 404-892-4411

Richard E. Kanner · Associate Professor of Medicine, University of Utah School of Medicine · University of Utah Health Sciences Center · 50 North Medical Drive, Salt Lake City, UT 84132 · 801-581-7806

E. R. McFadden, Jr. · Argyl J. Beams Professor of Medicine, Case Western Reserve University School of Medicine · Division Chief, Airway Disease Center, University Hospitals of Cleveland · 2074 Abington Road, Cleveland, OH 44106 · 216-844-8668

Thomas L. Petty · Professor of Medicine, University of Colorado School of Medicine · Director of Academic & Research Affairs, Presbyterian-St. Luke's Medical Center · 1719 East 19th Avenue, Denver, CO 80218 · 303-839-6740

Susan K. Pingleton · (Chronic Obstructive Pulmonary Disease, Nutrition) · Professor of Medicine, University of Kansas School of Medicine · Interim Director, Pulmonary Division, University of Kansas Medical Center · 4030 Sudler Building, 39th and Rainbow Boulevard, Kansas City, KS 66160-7381 · 913-588-6045

Herbert Y. Reynolds · Professor and Chairman, Department of Medicine, Pennsylvania State University · The Milton S. Hershey Medical Center · 500 University Drive, P.O. Box 850, Hershey, PA 17033 · 717-531-5016

Robert M. Rogers · (Emphysema) · Professor of Medicine and Anesthesiology, University of Pittsburgh School of Medicine · Chief of Pulmonary/Critical Care Medicine Division, University of Pittsburgh Medical Center · 440 Scaife Hall, Pittsburgh, PA 15261 · 412-648-9340

Dean Sheppard · Associate Professor of Medicine, University of California at San Francisco School of Medicine · Director, Lung Biology Center · UCSF 0854, San Francisco, CA 94143 · 415-821-5959

Gordon L. Snider · Maurice B. Strauss Professor of Medicine, Boston University School of Medicine; Tufts University School of Medicine · Chief of Medicine, Boston Veterans Affairs Medical Center · Medical Service (111), 150 South Huntington Avenue, Boston, MA 02130 · 617-739-3405

Adam Wanner · Professor of Medicine, University of Miami School of Medicine Chief, Pulmonary Division, Mt. Sinai Medical Center · Blum Building, Fourth Floor, 4300 Alton Road, Miami, FL 33140 · 305-674-2610

M. Henry Williams · Professor of Medicine, Albert Einstein College of Medicine Director, Chest Service, Bronx Municipal Hospital Center · Van Etten Hospital, Pelham Parkway and Eastchester Road, Room 3A4, Bronx, NY 10461 · 212-430-2182

BRONCHOESOPHEGOLOGY

Denis A. Cortese · Professor of Medicine, Mayo Medical School · Mayo Clinic · 200 First Street, SW, Rochester, MN 55905 · 507-284-2158

James H. Harrell · Professor of Medicine, University of California at San Diego School of Medicine · Chief, Pulmonary Care Unit, University of California at San Diego Medical Center · 225 Dickinson Street, Suite 157, San Diego, CA 92103 · 619-543-5840

Udaya B. S. Prakash · (Rare and Uncommon Lung Diseases) · Professor of Medicine, Mayo Medical School · Consultant in Thoracic Diseases and Internal Medicine, Mayo Clinic · 200 First Street, SW, Rochester, MN 55905 · 507-284-4162

David R. Sanderson · Professor of Medicine, Mayo Medical School; Chairman, Department of Internal Medicine, and Vice-Chairman, Board of Governors, Mayo Clinic-Scottsdale; Mayo Graduate School of Medicine · Scottsdale Memorial-North · 13400 East Shea Boulevard, Scottsdale, AZ 85259 · 602-391-8265

CYSTIC FIBROSIS
(See also Allergy & Immunology, Pediatric; Pediatrics, Gastroenterology; Pediatrics, Pediatric Pulmonology)

Michael Ray Knowles · Associate Professor of Medicine, University of North Carolina School of Medicine · University of North Carolina Hospitals · 209 Boulder Bluff, Chapel Hill, NC 27516 · 919-966-2531

James R. Yankaskas · Assistant Professor of Medicine, University of North Carolina School of Medicine · University of North Carolina Hospitals · 724 Burnett-Womack Building, Manning Drive, Campus Box 7020, Chapel Hill, NC 27599-7020 · 919-966-1077

GENERAL PULMONARY & CRITICAL CARE MEDICINE

Arnold Aberman · Professor and Chairman of Medicine, University of Toronto School of Medicine · Physician-in-Chief, The Toronto Hospital · 585 University Avenue, Suite BW1-628, Toronto, Ontario M5G 2C4 · 416-978-6430

Richard K. Albert · Professor of Medicine, University of Washington School of Medicine · Section Head, Pulmonary & Critical Care Medicine, University of Washington Medical Center · Health Sciences Building, BB-1253, Mail Stop RM-12, Seattle, WA 98195 · 206-543-3166

Roger C. Bone · Professor of Medicine, and Ralph C. Brown, M.D. Professor, Department of Internal Medicine, and Acting Dean, Rush Medical College · Chairman, Department of Internal Medicine, Rush-Presbyterian-St. Luke's Medical Center · 1653 West Congress Parkway, Suite 301 Jones, Chicago, IL 60612 · 312-942-5269

Dick D. Briggs, Jr. · Eminent Scholar Chair in Pulmonary Diseases, and Professor and Vice-Chairman, Department of Medicine, and Director of Pulmonary & Critical Care Medicine, and President, Health Services Foundation, The University of Alabama School of Medicine · The University of Alabama Hospital · 215 THT, 1900 University Boulevard, Birmingham, AL 35294 · 205-934-5400

Nausherwan K. Burki · Professor of Medicine, University of Kentucky College of Medicine · Chief, Division of Pulmonary & Critical Care Medicine, University of Kentucky Medical Center · 800 Rose Street, MN578, Lexington, KY 40536 · 606-233-5045

David R. Dantzker · Professor of Medicine, Albert Einstein College of Medicine · Chairman, Department of Medicine, Long Island Jewish Medical Center · New Hyde Park, NY 11042 · 718-470-7270

James E. Fish · Professor of Medicine, and Acting Chairman, Department of Medicine, Jefferson Medical College of Thomas Jefferson University · Director, Division of Pulmonary Medicine & Critical Care, Thomas Jefferson University Hospital · 1025 Walnut Street, Room 821, Philadelphia, PA 19107 · 215-955-6946

William J. Fulkerson · Associate Professor of Medicine, Duke University School of Medicine · Director, Medical Intensive Care Unit, and Chief, Critical Care Medicine, Duke University Medical Center · P.O. Box 3121, Durham, NC 27710 919-681-5850

Ronald B. George · Professor of Medicine, and Chief, Section of Pulmonary & Critical Care Medicine, Louisiana State University School of Medicine · Louisiana State University Medical Center · 1501 Kings Highway, Shreveport, LA 71130 · 318-674-5920

Philip M. Gold · Professor of Medicine, Loma Linda University School of Medicine · Chief of Pulmonary & Intensive Care Medicine Section, Loma Linda University Medical Center · 11234 Anderson Street, Loma Linda, CA 92354 · 714-824-4489

Thomas Morgan Hyers · Professor of Medicine, St. Louis University School of Medicine · Director, Division of Pulmonology & Pulmonary Occupational Medicine, St. Louis University Medical Center · 3635 Vista at Grand Boulevard, P.O. Box 15250, St. Louis, MO 63110-0250 · 314-577-8000

Steven Jenkenson · Professor of Medicine, The University of Texas at San Antonio · Chief, Pulmonary Section, Audie L. Murphy Memorial Veterans Hospital Pulmonary Division, 7703 Floyd Curl Drive, San Antonio, TX 78284 · 512-567-1904

Mark A. Kelley · Vice Dean for Clinical Affairs, University of Pennsylvania School of Medicine · Hospital of the University of Pennsylvania · 34th Street and Civic Center Boulevard, 21 Penn Tower, Philadelphia, PA 19104 · 215-662-7277

Richard W. Light · Associate Chief-of-Staff for Research & Development, Long Beach Veterans Affairs Hospital · (151) 5901 East Seventh Street, Long Beach, CA 90822 · 213-494-5816

John M. Luce · Associate Professor of Medicine and Anesthesia, University of California at San Francisco School of Medicine · Associate Director, Medical and Surgical Intensive Care Unit, San Francisco General Hospital · The Chest Service, Room 5K1 San Francisco General Hospital, San Francisco, CA 94110 · 415-821-8289

Joseph P. Lynch III · Associate Professor of Internal Medicine, Division of Pulmonary & Critical Care Medicine, The University of Michigan Medical School · Medical Director of Pulmonary Outpatient Services & Bronchoscopy Suite, The University of Michigan Medical Center · 3916 Taubman Center, 1500 East Medical Center Drive, Box 0360, Ann Arbor, MI 48109-0360 · 313-936-5040

Neil MacIntyre · Associate Professor of Medicine, Duke University School of Medicine · Medical Director, Respiratory Care Services, Duke University Medical Center · 400 Irwin Road, Box 3911, Durham, NC 27710 · 919-681-2720

John J. Marini · Professor of Medicine, University of Minnesota School of Medicine · Director, Pulmonary & Critical Care Medicine, St. Paul-Ramsey Medical Center · 640 Jackson Street, St. Paul, MN 55101 · 612-221-3135

Michael Anthony Matthay · Associate Professor of Medicine and Anesthesia, and Associate Director, Intensive Care Unit, and Associate, Cardiovascular Research Institute, University of California at San Francisco School of Medicine · University of California at San Francisco Medical Center · 513 Parnassus Avenue, San Francisco, CA 94143 · 415-476-1116

Richard A. Matthay · Professor and Associate Chairman, Department of Medicine, Yale University School of Medicine · Yale-New Haven Hospital · 333 Cedar Street, P. O. Box 3333, New Haven, CT 06510 · 203-785-4196

Melvin L. Morganroth · Clinical Associate Professor of Medicine, University of Oregon · The Thoracic Clinic, and Providence Medicine Center · 507 Northeast 47th Avenue, Portland, OR 97213 · 503-238-7220

Alan Morris · (Research) · Professor of Medicine, University of Utah · Director of Research, Pulmonary Division, LDS Hospital · Eighth Avenue and C Street, Salt Lake City, UT 84143 · 801-321-1100

Michael S. Niederman · Associate Professor of Medicine, State University of New York Health Science Center at Stony Brook · Director, Medical Intensive Care Unit, Winthrop University Hospital · 222 Station Plaza North, Suite 400, Mineola, NY 11501 · 516-663-2005

James R. Patterson · The Thoracic Clinic · 507 Northeast 47th Avenue, Portland, OR 97213 · 503-238-7220

Alan K. Pierce · Professor of Medicine, The University of Texas Southwestern Medical Center at Dallas · Medical Director, Parkland Memorial Hospital · 5323 Harry Hines Boulevard, Dallas, TX 75235-9034 · 214-688-3429

David J. Pierson · Medical Director, Department of Respiratory Care, Harborview Medical Center · 325 Ninth Avenue (ZA-62), Seattle, WA 98104 · 206-223-8022

Stuart F. Quan · (Sleep Disorders) · Associate Professor of Internal Medicine & Anesthesiology, The University of Arizona College of Medicine · Chief, Pulmonary & Critical Care Medicine Section, and Director, Sleep Disorders Center, The University of Arizona Health Sciences Center · 1501 North Campbell Avenue, Tucson, AZ 85724 · 602-626-6115

Thomas Raffin · Chief, Division of Pulmonary & Critical Care Medicine, and Co-director, Stanford University Center for Biomedical Ethics; Medical Director, Department of Respiratory Therapy, Stanford University School of Medicine · Stanford University Hospital · Department of Medicine, Room H3149, SUMC, Stanford, CA 94305-5236 · 415-723-6381

Stephen I. Rennard · Professor of Internal Medicine, University of Nebraska College of Medicine · University of Nebraska Medical Center · 600 South 42nd Street, Omaha, NE 68198-2465 · 402-559-7313

Edward C. Rosenow III · Arthur M. & Gladys D. Gray Professor of Medicine, Mayo Medical School · Chairman, Division of Thoracic Diseases, Mayo Clinic · 200 First Street, SW, Rochester MN 55905 · 507-284-2964

James A. Russell · Head, Program of Critical Care Medicine and Associate Professor of Medicine, The University of British Columbia · Director, Intensive Care Unit, St. Paul's Hospital · 1081 Burrard Street, Vancouver, British Columbia V6Z 1Y6 · 604-682-2344 x2265

Steven Alan Sahn · Professor of Medicine and Director, Pulmonary & Critical Care Medicine, Medical University of South Carolina · Co-Director, Medical Intensive Care Unit, Medical University of South Carolina Hospital · 171 Ashley Avenue, Charleston, SC 29425 · 803-792-3161

Deborah Shure · Associate Professor of Medicine, University of California at San Diego School of Medicine · San Diego Veterans Administration Medical Center · 3350 La Jolla Village Drive, San Diego, CA 92161 · 619-552-8585 x3541

James P. Smith · Clinical Professor of Medicine, Cornell University Medical College · Attending Physican, Pulmonary Disease, The New York Hospital-Cornell Medical Center · 170 East 77th Street, New York, NY 10021 · 212-879-2180

James K. Stoller · Head, Section of Respiratory Therapy, Department of Pulmonary Disease, The Cleveland Clinic Foundation · One Clinic Center, 9500 Euclid Avenue, Cleveland, OH 44195-5001 · 216-444-1960

Warren R. Summer · Howard Buechner Professor, and Section Chief, Department of Pulmonary & Critical Care Medicine, Louisiana State University School of Medicine · Hotel Dieu Hospital; Charity Hospital of New Orleans · 1901 Perdido Street, Room 3205, New Orleans, LA 70112 · 504-568-4634

John G. Weg · Professor of Internal Medicine, The University of Michigan Medical School · Physician, Division of Pulmonary & Critical Care Medicine, and Director of Respiratory Therapy, The University of Michigan Medical Center · 1500 East Medical Center Drive, B1H245 UH/0024, Ann Arbor, MI 48109-0024 · 313-936-5245

Dorothy A. White · Associate Professor, Cornell University Medical College · Attending Physician, The Pulmonary Service, Memorial Sloan-Kettering Cancer Center · 1275 York Avenue, New York, NY 10021 · 212-639-8022

Herbert P. Wiedemann · Chairman, Department of Pulmonary & Critical Care Medicine, The Cleveland Clinic Foundation · One Clinic Center, 9500 Euclid Avenue, Cleveland, OH 44195-5038 · 216-444-8335

LUNG INFECTIONS
(See also Infectious Disease, Respiratory Infections)

John Burrell Bass, Jr. · (Tuberculosis) · Professor of Medicine, University of South Alabama · University of South Alabama Medical Center · 2451 Fillingim Street, Mobile, AL 36617 · 205-471-7888

Jeffrey Glassroth · (Tuberculosis) · Marquardt Professor of Medicine, and Vice-Chairman, Department of Medicine, Northwestern University Medical School · Chief, Medical Service, Northwestern Memorial Hospital · 250 East Superior Street, Room 296, Chicago, IL 60611 · 312-908-2118

Philip Hopewell · (Tuberculosis) · Professor of Medicine, University of California at San Francisco School of Medicine · Chief, Chest Service, San Francisco General Hospital · 1001 Potrero Avenue, Chest Service, Room 5K1, San Francisco, CA 94110 · 415-648-5010

Michael D. Iseman · (Tuberculosis) · Professor of Medicine, University of Colorado School of Medicine · Chief, Clinical Mycobacteriology, Division of Infectious Diseases, National Jewish Center for Immunology & Respiratory Medicine 1400 Jackson Street, Room J-205, Denver, CO 80206 · 303-398-1279

Edward A. Nardell · (Tuberculosis) · Assistant Professor of Medicine, Harvard Medical School · Chief of Pulmonary Medicine, Cambridge Hospital · 1493 Cambridge Street, Cambridge MA 02139 · 617-498-1029

Lee Brodersohn Reichman · (Tuberculosis) · Professor of Medicine, University of Medicine & Dentistry of New Jersey · Director of Pulmonary Division, University Hospital · 150 Bergen Street, Pulmonary Laboratory, I 354, Newark, NJ 08002 · 201-456-6111

Gisela F. Schecter · (Tuberculosis) · Assistant Clinical Professor of Medicine, University of California at San Francisco School of Medicine · Director, City & County of San Francisco Department of Public Health, Division of TB Control, San Francisco General Hospital · 1001 Potrero Avenue, San Francisco, CA 94110 415-821-8524

Gordon L. Snider · (Bronchitis, Emphysema) · Maurice B. Strauss Professor of Medicine, Boston University School of Medicine; Tufts University School of Medicine · Chief of Medicine, Boston Veterans Affairs Medical Center · Medical Service (111), 150 South Huntington Avenue, Boston, MA 02130 · 617-739-3405

PULMONARY DISEASE

A. Jay Block · (Sleep Apnea) · Professor of Medicine & Anesthesiology, and Chief, Pulmonary Division, University of Florida College of Medicine · Shands Hospital at the University of Florida; Gainesville Veterans Affairs Medical Center Health Center, P.O. Box 10025, Gainesville, FL 32610 · 904-392-2666

Norma M.T. Wang Braun · (Emphysema, Obstructive Diseases of the Airways) · Associate Professor of Clinical Medicine, College of Physicians & Surgeons of Columbia University · Associate Attending, Department of Medicine, Pulmonary Division, St. Luke's Roosevelt Hospital Center; Consultant, Helen Hayes Rehabilitation Hospital · 1090 Amsterdam Avenue, Room 408, New York, NY 10025 · 212-523-3655

Antonino Catanzaro · (Fungal Diseases of the Lung, Mycobacterial Diseases) · Associate Professor of Medicine, University of California at San Diego School of Medicine · University of California at San Diego Medical Center · 225 Dickinson Street, Mail Code 8374, San Diego, CA 92103 · 619-543-5550

Leonard D. Hudson · (Emphysema) · Professor of Medicine, Division of Pulmonary & Critical Care Medicine, and Head, Division of Pulmonary & Critical Care Medicine, University of Washington School of Medicine · Chief, Division of Pulmonary & Critical Care Medicine, Harborview Medical Center · 325 Ninth Avenue (ZA-62), Seattle, WA 98104-2499 · 206-223-3533

Richard E. Kanner · (Emphysema) · Associate Professor of Medicine, University of Utah School of Medicine · University of Utah Health Sciences Center · 50 North Medical Drive, Salt Lake City, UT 84132 · 801-581-7806

Talmadge E. King, Jr. · (Interstitial Lung Disease) · Professor of Medicine, University of Colorado School of Medicine · Chairman of Clinical Affairs, National Jewish Center for Immunology & Respiratory Medicine · 1400 Jackson Street, Denver, CO 80206 · 303-398-1333

Kenneth Moser · (Pulmonary Embolism) · Professor of Medicine, University of California at San Diego School of Medicine · Director, Pulmonary & Critical Care Division, University of California at San Diego Medical Center · 225 Dickinson Street, San Diego, CA 92103 · 619-543-5970

John F. Murray · (Physiology) · Professor of Medicine, University of California at San Francisco School of Medicine · San Francisco General Hospital · 1001 Potrero Avenue, Room 5K1, San Francisco, CA 94110 · 415-476-2916

Thomas L. Petty · (Emphysema) · Professor of Medicine, University of Colorado School of Medicine · Director of Academic & Research Affairs, Presbyterian-St. Luke's Medical Center · 1719 East 19th Avenue, Denver, CO 80218 · 303-839-6740

Susan K. Pingleton · (Chronic Obstructive Pulmonary Disease, Nutrition) · Professor of Medicine, University of Kansas School of Medicine · Interim Director, Pulmonary Division, University of Kansas Medical Center · 4030 Sudler Building, 39th and Rainbow Boulevard, Kansas City, KS 66160-7381 · 913-588-6045

Herbert Y. Reynolds · (Interstitial Lung Disease) · Professor and Chairman, Department of Medicine, Pennsylvania State University · The Milton S. Hershey Medical Center · 500 University Drive, P.O. Box 850, Hershey, PA 17033 · 717-531-5016

Robert M. Rogers · (Emphysema) · Professor of Medicine and Anesthesiology, University of Pittsburgh School of Medicine · Chief of Pulmonary/Critical Care Medicine Division, University of Pittsburgh Medical Center · 440 Scaife Hall, Pittsburgh, PA 15261 · 412-648-9340

Marvin I. Schwarz · (Interstitial Lung Disease) · Professor of Medicine, University of Colorado School of Medicine · Head, Division of Pulmonary Sciences, University of Colorado Health Sciences Center · 4200 East Ninth Avenue, Box C272, Denver, CO 80262 · 303-270-7047

Om P. Sharma · (Interstitial Lung Disease, Sarcoidosis) · Professor of Medicine, University of Southern California School of Medicine · The Los Angeles County + University of Southern California Medical Center · 1200 North State Street, Room 11900, Los Angeles, CA 90033 · 213-226-7923

Gordon L. Snider · (Bronchitis, Emphysema) · Maurice B. Strauss Professor of Medicine, Boston University School of Medicine; Tufts University School of Medicine · Chief of Medicine, Boston Veterans Affairs Medical Center · Medical Service (111), 150 South Huntington Avenue, Boston, MA 02130 · 617-739-3405

David P. White · (Sleep Apnea) · Associate Professor of Medicine, University of Colorado Health Sciences Center · Director, Sleep Laboratory, Denver Department of Veterans Affairs Medical Center, National Jewish Center/University of Colorado Sleep Center · Respiratory Care 111A, 1055 Clermont Street, Denver, CO 80220 · 303-393-2869

Richard Winterbauer · (Interstitial Lung Disease) · Head, Section of Pulmonary & Critical Care Medicine, Virginia Mason Medical Center · 1100 Ninth Avenue, Seattle, WA 98111 · 206-223-6687

Clifford W. Zwillich · (Sleep Apnea) · Professor of Medicine, Chief Pulmonary/ Critical Care Medicine, The Pennsylvania State University, College of Medicine The Milton S. Hershey Medical Center · 500 University Drive, Room C7521, Hershey, PA 17033 · 717-531-6525

RADIATION ONCOLOGY

BRACHYTHERAPY

Karen King-Wah Fu · Professor of Radiation Oncology, University of California at San Francisco School of Medicine · University of California at San Francisco Medical Center · 505 Parnassus Avenue, San Francisco, CA 94143-0226 · 415-476-4815

Don R. Goffinet · Stanford University School of Medicine · Stanford University Hospital · 300 Pasteur Drive,Room M-121, Palo Alto, CA 94305-5302 · 415-723-5714

Louis Benjamin Harrison · Associate Professor of Radiation Oncology, Cornell University Medical College · Chief, Brachytherapy Service, and Associate Attending Radiation Oncologist, Memorial Sloan-Kettering Cancer Center · 1275 York Avenue, New York, NY 10021 · 212-639-7637

Basil S. Hilaris · Professor and Chairman of Radiation Medicine, New York Medical College · Director, Department of Radiation Medicine, Westchester County Medical Center · Department of Radiation Medicine, Valhalla, NY 10595 914-285-8560

Alvaro A. Martinez · Chairman, Radiation Oncology, William Beaumont Hospital 3601 West Thirteen Mile Road, Royal Oak, MI 48073 · 313-551-7058

J. Frank Wilson · Professor and Chairman, Department of Radiation Oncology, Medical College of Wisconsin · President, Medical Staff, Milwaukee County Medical Complex, Froedtert Memorial Lutheran Hospital, West Allis Memorial Hospital · 8700 West Wisconsin Avenue, Milwaukee, WI 53226 · 414-257-5636

BRAIN CANCER
(See Adult Neurology, Neuro-oncology; Child Neurology, Neuro-oncology; Medical Oncology & Hematology, Brain Cancer)

David A. Larson · Associate Professor and Vice-Chairman, Department of Radiation Oncology, and Director of Medical Education, University of California at San Francisco School of Medicine · University of California at San Francisco Medical Center · 505 Parnassus Avenue, Room L-75, San Francisco, CA 94143 · 415-476-4815

Steven A. Leibel · Vice-Chairman & Clinical Director, Department of Radiation Oncology, Memorial Sloan-Kettering Cancer Center · 1275 York Avenue, 208H, New York, NY 10021 · 212-639-6800

Jay S. Loeffler · Assistant Professor of Radiation Therapy, Harvard Medical School · Co-Director of Stereotactic Radiosurgery, Joint Center for Radiation Therapy · 75 Francis Street, Boston, MA 02115 · 617-732-6310

Theodore Locke Phillips · Professor and Chairman of Radiation Oncology, University of California at San Francisco School of Medicine · University of California at San Francisco Medical Center · 505 Parnassus Avenue, Room L-08, Box 0226, San Francisco, CA 94143 · 415-476-4815

BREAST CANCER
(See also Medical Oncology, Breast Cancer; Medical Oncology & Hematology, Breast Cancer; Surgical Oncology, Breast Cancer)

John M. Bedwinek · Medical Director of Radiation Oncology, St. Joseph's Hospital · 525 Couch Avenue, Kirkwood, MO 63122 · 314-966-1650

Luther W. Brady · Professor and Chairman, Department of Radiation Oncology & Nuclear Medicine, Hahnemann University · Hahnemann Hospital · 230 North Broad Street, Mail Stop 200, Philadelphia, PA 19102-1192 · 215-448-8419

R. M. Clark · Professor of Radiation Oncology, University of Toronto Faculty of Medicine · Senior Staff, Ontario Cancer Institute, Princess Margaret Hospital · 500 Sherbourne Street, Toronto, Ontario M4X 1K9 · 416-924-0671 x5152

Barbara Fowble · Professor of Radiation Oncology, University of Pennsylvania School of Medicine · Hospital of the University of Pennsylvania · Department of Radiation Oncology, 3400 Spruce Street, Philadelphia, PA 19104 · 215-662-3075

Robert L. Goodman · Henry K. Pancoast Professor and Chairman of Radiation Oncology, University of Pennsylvania School of Medicine · Hospital of the University of Pennsylvania · US Health Care, 980 Jolly Road, Blue Bell, PA 19422 · 215-283-6514

Francine E. Halberg · University of California, San Francisco · Marin General Hospital · Department of Radiation Therapy, P.O. Box 8010, San Rafael, CA 94912-8010 · 415-925-7326

Jay R. Harris · Professor of Radiation Oncology, and Clinical & Educational Director, Joint Center for Radiation Therapy, Harvard Medical School · Clinical & Educational Director, Beth Israel Hospital; Dana-Farber Cancer Institute · Joint Center for Radiation Therapy, 50 Binney Street, Boston, MA 02115 · 617-432-1889

Seymour Levitt · Professor and Head, Department of Therapeutic Radiology-Radiation Oncology, University of Minnesota School of Medicine · Clinical Chief, Department of Therapeutic Radiology-Radiation Oncology, University of Minnesota Hospital & Clinics · Harvard Street at East River Road, Box 436, Minneapolis, MN 55455 · 612-626-3000

Allen S. Lichter · Professor and Chair, Department of Radiation Oncology, The University of Michigan Medical School · The University of Michigan Medical Center · 1500 East Medical Center Drive, B-2C502, Box 0010, Ann Arbor, MI 48109-0010 · 313-936-4000

Beryl McCormick · Associate Professor of Radiation Oncology in Medicine, Cornell University Medical College · Associate Attending Radiation Oncologist, Memorial Sloan-Kettering Cancer Center · 1275 York Avenue, New York, NY 10021 212-639-6828

Marsha Diane McNeese · Associate Professor of Radiology, The University of Texas · The University of Texas MD Anderson Cancer Center · 1515 Holcombe Boulevard, Box 97, Houston, TX 77030 · 713-792-3400

Nancy P. Mendenhall · Associate Professor of Radiation Oncology, University of Florida College of Medicine · Shands Cancer Center · 2000 Southwest Archer Road, Gainesville, FL 32610-0385 · 904-395-0287

Carlos A. Perez · Professor of Radiology, Washington University School of Medicine · Director, Radiation Oncology Center, Mallinckrodt Institute of Radiology 510 South Kings Highway, St. Louis, MO 63110 · 314-362-8542

Leonard R. Prosnitz · Professor of Radiation Oncology, Duke University School of Medicine · Duke University Medical Center · Box 3085, DUMC, Durham, NC 27710 · 919-684-3805

Abram Recht · Assistant Professor of Radiation Oncology, Harvard Medical School · Deputy Chief, Department of Radiation Oncology, Beth Israel Hospital 330 Brookline Avenue, FNB25, Boston, MA 02215 · 617-735-2345

Lawrence J. Solin · Associate Professor of Radiation Oncology, University of Pennsylvania School of Medicine · The Fox Chase Cancer Center · Department of Radiation Oncology, 7701 Burholme Avenue, Philadelphia, PA 19111 · 215-728-2908

Leonard M. Toonkel · Associate Professor of Radiology, University of Miami School of Medicine · Chairman, Department of Radiation Oncology, Mt. Sinai Medical Center, Comprehensive Cancer Center · Blum Building, 4300 Alton Road, Miami, FL 33140 · 305-535-3400

GASTROENTEROLOGIC CANCER
(See also Gastroenterology, Gastroenterologic Cancer; Surgical Oncology, Gastroenterologic Cancer)

Bernard J. Cummings · Chairman, Department of Radiation Oncology, University of Toronto Faculty of Medicine · Chief, Department of Radiation Oncology, Ontario Cancer Institute; Princess Margaret Hospital · 500 Sherbourne Street, Toronto, Ontario M4X 1K9 · 416-924-0671

Leonard L. Gunderson · Professor of Oncology, Mayo Medical School · Chairman of Radiation Oncology, Mayo Clinic · 200 First Street, SW, Rochester, MN 55905 507-284-2949

Joel E. Tepper · Professor of Radiation Oncology, University of North Carolina School of Medicine · Chair, Department of Radiation Oncology, University of North Carolina Hospitals · UNC School of Medicine, Campus Box 7512, Chapel Hill, NC 27599-7512 · 919-966-7700

Richard Whittington · Assistant Professor of Radiation Oncology, University of Pennsylvania · Hospital of the University of Pennsylvania · 3400 Spruce Street, 2 Donner, Philadelphia, PA 19104 · 215-662-6515

Christopher G. Willett · Assistant Professor of Radiation Oncology, Harvard Medical School · Assistant Radiation Oncologist, Department of Radiation Oncology, Massachusetts General Hospital · 100 Blossom Street, Boston, MA 02114 617-726-6826

GENERAL RADIATION ONCOLOGY

C. Norman Coleman · Professor and Chairman, Joint Center for Radiation Therapy, and Alvan T. & Viola D. Fuller—American Cancer Society Professor, Harvard Medical School · Beth Israel Hospital; Brigham & Women's Hospital; Dana Farber Cancer Institute; New England Deaconess Hospital; The Children's Hospital; Framingham Union Hospital · Joint Center for Radiation Therapy, 50 Binney Street, Boston, MA 02115 · 617-432-1889

Anatoly Dritschilo · Professor and Chairman, Department of Radiation Medicine, Georgetown University School of Medicine · Director, Radiation Oncology, Georgetown University Medical Center · Bles Building, Lower Level, 3800 Reservoir Road, NW, Washington, DC 20007 · 202-687-2144

John D. Earle · Professor of Oncology, Mayo Medical School · Mayo Clinic · 200 Second Street, SW, Rochester, MN 55905 · 507-284-2511

Thomas W. Griffin · Professor and Chairman, Department of Radiation Oncology, University of Washington School of Medicine · Director, University Cancer Center, University of Washington Medical Center · 1959 Northeast Pacific Street, RC-08, Seattle, WA 98195 · 206-548-4110

Anthony E. Howes · Assistant Professor of Radiation Therapy, Harvard Medical School · Medical Director, Radiation Therapy, Brigham & Women's Hospital · 75 Francis Street, Boston, MA 02115 · 617-732-6310

David H. Hussey · Professor of Radiology, The University of Iowa College of Medicine · Director, Division of Radiation Oncology, The University of Iowa Hospitals & Clinics · Newton Road, Room W189Z-GH, Iowa City, IA 52242-1059 319-356-2699

Timothy J. Kinsella · Professor and Chairman, Department of Human Oncology, University of Wisconsin-Madison School of Medicine · University of Wisconsin Hospital & Clinics · 600 Highland Avenue, Room K4/312, Madison, WI 53792 · 608-263-5009

Peter M. Mauch · Associate Professor of Therapeutic Radiology, Harvard Medical School · Brigham & Women's Hospital, Dana-Farber Cancer Institute, Beth Israel Hospital, New England Deaconess, Children's Hospital · Joint Center for Radiation Therapy, 50 Binney Street, Boston, MA 02115 · 617-732-6310

Robert G. Parker · Professor and Chairman, Department of Radiation Oncology, University of California, Los Angeles School of Medicine · University of California, Los Angeles Center for the Health Sciences · 200 UCLA Medical Plaza, Suite B-265, Los Angeles, CA 90024-6951 · 310-825-9304

David A. Pistenmaa · Chairman, Department of Radiation Oncology, Fairfax Hospital · 3300 Gallows Road, Falls Church, VA 22046 · 703-698-3731

Robert H. Sagerman · Professor and Director of Radiology, State University of New York Health Science Center at Syracuse · 750 Adams Street, Syracuse, NY 13210 · 315-464-5276

James G. Schwade · Professor and Chairman of Radiation Oncology, University of Miami School of Medicine, and Bascom Palmer Eye Institute · Associate Director, Clinical Research Program, The Sylvester Cancer Center, Jackson Memorial Medical Center · 1611 Northwest 12th Avenue, D-31, Miami, FL 33136 · 305-585-6673

Robert Stewart · Professor and Director, Department of Radiation Oncology, University of Utah School of Medicine · University of Utah Health Sciences Center · 50 North Medical Drive, Salt Lake City, UT 84132 · 801-581-8793

Herman D. Suit · Andres Soriano Professor of Radiation Oncology, Harvard Medical School · Chief, Department of Radiation Oncology, Massachusetts General Hospital · Department of Radiation Oncology, Boston, MA 02114 · 617-726-8150

Joel E. Tepper · Professor of Radiation Oncology, University of North Carolina School of Medicine · Chair, Department of Radiation Oncology, University of North Carolina Hospitals · UNC School of Medicine, Campus Box 7512, Chapel Hill, NC 27599-7512 · 919-966-7700

Ralph R. Weichselbaum · Harold H. Hines, Jr. Professor and Chairman of Radiation & Cellular Oncology, University of Chicago, Pritzker School of Medicine University of Chicago Medical Center · 5841 South Maryland Avenue, Box 442, Chicago, IL 60637-1470 · 312-702-6819

GENITO-URINARY CANCER
(See also Medical Oncology & Hematology, Genito-Urinary Cancer)

Malcolm A. Bagshaw · (Prostate Cancer) · Professor and Chairman, Department of Radiation Oncology, Stanford University School of Medicine · Stanford University Hospital · 300 Pasteur Drive, Stanford, CA 94305 · 415-723-5510

Zvi Y. Fuks · (Prostate Cancer) · Chairman, Department of Radiation Oncology, Memorial Sloan-Kettering Cancer Center · 1275 York Avenue, New York, NY 10021 · 212-639-5868

Mary K. Gospodarowicz · Associate Professor, Department of Radiology, University of Toronto School of Medicine · Radiation Oncologist, Princess Margaret Hospital · 500 Sherbourne Street, Room 251, Toronto, Ontario M4X 1K9 · 416-924-0671

Gerald Eugene Hanks · (Prostate Cancer) · Professor of Radiation Oncology, University of Pennsylvania School of Medicine · Chairman, Department of Radiation Oncology, The Fox Chase Cancer Center · 7701 Burholme Avenue, Philadelphia, PA 19111 · 215-728-2940

Allen S. Lichter · (Prostate Cancer) · Professor and Chair, Department of Radiation Oncology, The University of Michigan Medical School · The University of Michigan Medical Center · 1500 East Medical Center Drive, B-2C502, Box 0010, Ann Arbor, MI 48109-0010 · 313-936-4000

James T. Parsons · Associate Professor of Radiation Oncology, University of Florida College of Medicine · Shands Hospital at the University of Florida · 1600 Southwest Archer Road, Room HG518, P.O. Box 100385 JHMHC, Gainesville, FL 32610 · 904-392-5397

Carlos A. Perez · Professor of Radiology, Washington University School of Medicine · Director, Radiation Oncology Center, Mallinckrodt Institute of Radiology 510 South Kings Highway, St. Louis, MO 63110 · 314-362-8542

Arthur T. Porter · Professor and Chairman, Department of Radiation Oncology, Wayne State University School of Medicine · Chief, Department of Radiation Oncology, Harper Hospital · 3990 John R, Detroit, MI 48201 · 313-745-2101

William U. Shipley · (Bladder Cancer) · Professor of Radiation Oncology, Harvard Medical School · Radiation Therapist and Associate Director, Massachusetts General Hospital Cancer Center · Cox-3, Boston, MA 02114 · 617-726-8146

GYNECOLOGIC CANCER

Hywel Madoc-Jones · Professor and Chairman, Department of Radiation Oncology, Tufts University School of Medicine · New England Medical Center · 750 Washington Street, Box 359, Boston, MA 02111 · 617-956-6161

Carlos A. Perez · Professor of Radiology, Washington University School of Medicine · Director, Radiation Oncology Center, Mallinckrodt Institute of Radiology 510 South Kings Highway, St. Louis, MO 63110 · 314-362-8542

Theodore Locke Phillips · Professor and Chairman of Radiation Oncology, University of California at San Francisco School of Medicine · University of California at San Francisco Medical Center · 505 Parnassus Avenue, Room L-08, Box 0226, San Francisco, CA 94143 · 415-476-4815

Marvin Rotman · (Bladder Cancer, Infusion Chemotherapy) · Professor and Chairman, Department of Radiation Oncology, State University Of New York Health Science Center at Brooklyn · Director, Radiation Oncology, Long Island Colege Hospital · 450 Clarkson Avenue, Box 1211, Brooklyn, NY 11203 · 718-270-2181

HEAD & NECK CANCER
(See also Medical Oncology & Hematology, Head & Neck Cancer)

Karen King-Wah Fu · Professor of Radiation Oncology, University of California at San Francisco School of Medicine · University of California at San Francisco Medical Center · 505 Parnassus Avenue, San Francisco, CA 94143-0226 · 415-476-4815

Don R. Goffinet · Stanford University School of Medicine · Stanford University Hospital · 300 Pasteur Drive, Room M-121, Palo Alto, CA 94305-5302 · 415-723-5714

George E. Laramore · Professor of Radiation Oncology, and Clinical Director, Fast Neutron Radiotherapy Therapy Project, University of Washington School of Medicine · 1959 Northeast Pacific Street, RC-08, Seattle, WA 98195 · 206-548-4120

Robert Dery Lindberg · Professor of Radiation Oncology, University of Louisville School of Medicine · Chairman, Department of Radiation Oncology, James Graham Brown Cancer Center · 529 South Jackson Street, Louisville, KY 40292 · 502-588-7171

William M. Mendenhall · (Laryngeal Cancer, Management of Neck Cancer) · Associate Professor of Radiation Oncology, University of Florida College of Medicine · Shands Hospital at the University of Florida · 2000 Southwest Archer Road, Box 100385, Gainesville, FL 32610 · 904-395-0287

Rodney Reiff Million · Professor and Chairman, Department of Radiation Oncology, University of Florida College of Medicine · Shands Hospital at the University of Florida · 2000 Southwest Archer Road, Gainesville, FL 32610-0385 · 904-395-0287

James T. Parsons · Associate Professor of Radiation Oncology, University of Florida College of Medicine · Shands Hospital at the University of Florida · 1600 Southwest Archer Road, Room HG518, P.O. Box 100385 JHMHC, Gainesville, FL 32610 · 904-392-5397

Lester J. Peters · Professor of Radiotherapy, The University of Texas MD Anderson Cancer Center · Head, Division of Radiotherapy, and Chairman, Department of Radiotherapy, The University of Texas MD Anderson Cancer Center · 1515 Holcombe Boulevard, Box 97, Houston, TX 77030 · 713-792-3411

Theodore Locke Phillips · Professor and Chairman of Radiation Oncology, University of California at San Francisco School of Medicine · University of California at San Francisco Medical Center · 505 Parnassus Avenue, Room L-08, Box 0226, San Francisco, CA 94143 · 415-476-4815

C. C. Wang · Professor of Radiation Oncology, Harvard Medical School · Clinical Chief, Department of Radiation Oncology, Massachusetts General Hospital · Department of Radiation Oncology, Boston, MA 02114 · 617-726-8150

HODGKINS DISEASE

Seymour Levitt · Professor and Head, Department of Therapeutic Radiology-Radiation Oncology, University of Minnesota School of Medicine · Clinical Chief, Department of Therapeutic Radiology-Radiation Oncology, University of Minnesota Hospital & Clinics · Harvard Street at East River Road, Box 436, Minneapolis, MN 55455 · 612-626-3000

HYPOTHERMIA

Frederic A. Gibbs · Professor and Chief, Department of Radiation Oncology, University of Utah School of Medicine · University of Utah Health Sciences Center · 50 North Medical Drive, Salt Lake City, UT 84132 · 801-581-2396

LUNG CANCER
(See also Medical Oncology & Hematology, Lung Cancer; Medical Oncology, Lung Cancer)

Noah C. Choi · Associate Professor, Department of Radiation Oncology, Harvard Medical School · Associate Radiation Oncologist, Massachusetts General Hospital; Chief, Division of Radiation Therapy, Department of Radiology, Mt. Auburn Hospital; Massachusetts General Hospital · Fruit Street, Department of Radiation Oncology, Boston, MA 02114 · 617-726-8146

James D. Cox · Professor of Radiotherapy, The University of Texas Medical School at Houston · Vice President for Patient Care, and Physician-in-Chief, The University of Texas MD Anderson Cancer Center · 1515 Holcombe Boulevard, Box 43, Houston, TX 77030 · 713-792-7475

Eli Glatstein · Professor of Radiology, Uniformed Services University of Health Sciences · Chief, Radiation Oncology Branch, National Cancer Institute, National Institutes of Health · 9000 Rockville Pike, Building 10, Room B3B69, Bethesda, MD 20892 · 301-496-5457

Allen S. Lichter · Professor and Chair, Department of Radiation Oncology, The University of Michigan Medical School · The University of Michigan Medical Center · 1500 East Medical Center Drive, B-2C502, Box 0010, Ann Arbor, MI 48109-0010 · 313-936-4000

Carlos A. Perez · Professor of Radiology, Washington University School of Medicine · Director, Radiation Oncology Center, Mallinckrodt Institute of Radiology 510 South Kings Highway, St. Louis, MO 63110 · 314-362-8542

Andrew T. Turrisi · Associate Professor and Associate Chairman, Department of Radiation Oncology, The University of Michigan Medical School · Director of Clinical Programs, The University of Michigan Medical Center · 1500 East Medical Center Drive, Room B-2C490, Box 0010, Ann Arbor, MI 48109-0010 · 313-936-9338

LYMPHOMAS

Robert L. Goodman · Henry K. Pancoast Professor and Chairman of Radiation Oncology, University of Pennsylvania School of Medicine · Hospital of the University of Pennsylvania · US Health Care, 980 Jolly Road, Blue Bell, PA 19422 · 215-283-6514

Mary K. Gospodarowicz · Associate Professor, Department of Radiology, University of Toronto School of Medicine · Radiation Oncologist, Princess Margaret Hospital · 500 Sherbourne Street, Room 251, Toronto, Ontario M4X 1K9 · 416-924-0671

Richard T. Hoppe · Professor of Radiation Oncology, Stanford University School of Medicine · Stanford University Hospital · 300 Pasteur Drive,Room A-091, Stanford, CA 94305 · 415-723-5338

Peter M. Mauch · Associate Professor of Therapeutic Radiology, Harvard Medical School · Brigham & Women's Hospital, Dana-Farber Cancer Institute, Beth Israel Hospital, New England Deaconess, Children's Hospital · Joint Center for Radiation Therapy, 50 Binney Street, Boston, MA 02115 · 617-732-6310

Leonard R. Prosnitz · Professor of Radiation Oncology, Duke University School of Medicine · Duke University Medical Center · Box 3085, DUMC, Durham, NC 27710 · 919-684-3805

PARTICLE BEAM RADIATION

Joseph Castro · Professor of Radiation Oncology, University of California Medical Center, San Francisco · Faculty Senior Physician, Department of Radiation Oncology, University of California, Lawrence Berkeley Laboratory · Building 55, Room 106, Berkeley, CA 94720 · 510-486-6325

James M. Slater · Professor and Chairman, Department of Radiation Medicine, Loma Linda University School of Medicine · Loma Linda University Medical Center · 11234 Anderson Street, Loma Linda, CA 92354 · 714-824-4378

Herman D. Suit · Andres Soriano Professor of Radiation Oncology, Harvard Medical School · Chief, Department of Radiation Oncology, Massachusetts General Hospital · Department of Radiation Oncology, Boston, MA 02114 · 617-726-8150

PEDIATRIC RADIATION ONCOLOGY

J. Robert Cassady · Professor of Radiation Oncology, The University of Arizona College of Medicine · Head, Department of Radiation Oncology, The University of Arizona Health Sciences Center · 1501 North Campbell Avenue, Tucson, AZ 85724 · 602-626-6724

Sarah S. Donaldson · (Lymphomas, Hodgkin's Disease) · Professor of Radiation Oncology, Stanford University School of Medicine · Stanford University Hospital; Lucile Salter Packard Children's Hospital at Stanford · 300 Pasteur Drive, Room A-083, Stanford, CA 94305 · 415-723-6195

Carolyn R. Freeman · (Brain Tumors, Neuro-oncology) · Professor and Rosenbloom Chairman, Department of Oncology, Division of Radiation Oncology, McGill University · Director of Radiation Oncology, Montreal General Hospital · 1650 Cedar Avenue, Room 5700, Montreal, Quebec H3G 1A4 · 514-934-8040

Christopher Fryer · Clinical Professor of Pediatrics, The University of British Columbia · Head, Developmental Radio Therapy, and Head, Department of Pediatric Oncology, British Columbia Cancer Agency · 600 West 10th Avenue, Vancouver, British Columbia V5Z 4V6 · 604-877-6000

Larry E. Kun · (Brain Cancer, Neuro-oncology) · Professor of Radiology and Pediatrics, and Chairman, Section of Radiation Oncology, The University of Tennessee at Memphis, College of Medicine · Chairman, Department of Radiation Oncology, St. Jude Children's Research Hospital · 332 North Lauderdale, Memphis, TN 38105 · 901-522-0596

Robert B. Marcus, Jr. · (Bone and Soft Tissue Sarcomas) · Professor of Radiation Oncology and Pediatrics, University of Florida College of Medicine · Shands Cancer Center · 2000 Southwest Archer Road, Room 1204, P.O. Box 100385, Gainesville, FL 32610 · 904-395-0287

Nancy J. Tarbell · (Lymphomas, Medulloblastoma, Leukemia, Bone Marrow Transplantation) · Division Chief of Radiation Oncology, Children's Hospital · 300 Longwood Avenue, Boston, MA 02115 · 617-735-8399

William M. Wara · (Brain Tumors, Neuro-oncology) · Professor and Executive Vice-Chair, Department of Radiation Oncology, University of California at San Francisco School of Medicine · University of California at San Francisco Medical Center · 505 Parnassus Avenue, Room L75, San Francisco, CA 94143 · 415-476-4815

Moody D. Wharam · Associate Professor of Oncology and Radiological Sciences, Johns Hopkins University School of Medicine · Acting Director, Department of Radiation Oncology, The Johns Hopkins Medical Institutions · 600 North Wolfe Street, Oncology Center, B1-170I, Baltimore, MD 21205 · 410-955-7312

RADIOSURGERY

David A. Larson · Associate Professor and Vice-Chairman, Department of Radiation Oncology, and Director of Medical Education, University of California at San Francisco School of Medicine · University of California at San Francisco Medical Center · 505 Parnassus Avenue, Room L-75, San Francisco, CA 94143 · 415-476-4815

SARCOMAS

Robert Dery Lindberg · Professor of Radiation Oncology, University of Louisville School of Medicine · Chairman, Department of Radiation Oncology, James Graham Brown Cancer Center · 529 South Jackson Street, Louisville, KY 40292 · 502-588-7171

James T. Parsons · Associate Professor of Radiation Oncology, University of Florida College of Medicine · Shands Hospital at the University of Florida · 1600 Southwest Archer Road, Room HG518, P.O. Box 100385 JHMHC, Gainesville, FL 32610 · 904-392-5397

SKIN CANCER

Peter Fitzpatrick · Physician-in-Chief, Cancer Treatment & Research Foundation of Nova Scotia · 5820 University Avenue, Halifax, Nova Scotia B3H 1V7 · 902-428-4209

SKIN CANCER SURGERY & RECONSTRUCTION

Arthur H. Gladstein · Professor of Clinical Dermatology, New York University School of Medicine · New York University Medical Center, Skin & Cancer · 566 First Avenue, New York, NY 10016 · 212-263-5247

RADIOLOGY

CARDIOVASCULAR DISEASE

Leon Axel · Professor of Radiology, University of Pennsylvania School of Medicine · Hospital of the University of Pennsylvania · Pendergrass Diagnostic Research Laboratory, 308 Stemmler Hall, 36th and Hamilton Walk, Philadelphia, PA 19104-6086 · 215-662-6225

Robert J. Herfkens · Associate Professor of Radiology, Stanford University School of Medicine · Stanford University Hospital · 300 Pasteur Drive, Stanford, CA 94305 · 415-723-4733

Charles B. Higgins · Professor of Radiology, University of California at San Francisco School of Medicine · Chief, Magnetic Resonance Imaging Section, University of California at San Francisco Medical Center · 505 Parnassus Avenue, Room L-308, San Francisco, CA 94143-0628 · 415-476-4742

Justin D. Pearlman · Assistant Professor of Medicine, with joint appointment at MIT, Harvard Medical School · Director of NMR Computing & Technology, Massachusetts General Hospital · Cardiac Group, Bulfinch Four, MSH, Boston, MA 02114 · 617-726-1707

Elias A. Zerhouni · (Computed Tomography) · Associate Professor of Radiology, Johns Hopkins University School of Medicine · Medical Director of MRI and Thoracic Imaging, The Johns Hopkins Medical Institutions · Radiology Department, 600 North Wolfe Street, Baltimore, MD 21205 · 410-955-4062

CHEST

John Austin · Professor of Clinical Radiology, College of Physicians & Surgeons of Columbia University · Columbia-Presbyterian Medical Center · 177 Fort Washington, Milstein 3, Room 124B, New York, NY 10032 · 212-305-2639

Gordon Gamsu · Professor of Radiology and Medicine, University of California at San Francisco School of Medicine · Director of Thoracic Imaging, University of California at San Francisco Medical Center · 505 Parnassus Avenue, Room M-396, San Francisco, CA 94143 · 415-476-1451

Gary M. Glazer · Professor and Chairman, Department of Radiology, Stanford University School of Medicine · Stanford University Hospital · 300 Pasteur Drive, Stanford, CA 94305-5105 · 415-723-7863

J. David Godwin · Professor of Radiology, University of Washington School of Medicine · Director, Chest Radiology, University of Washington Medical Center 1959 Northeast Pacific Street, SB-05, Seattle, WA 98195 · 206-543-3320

Lawrence R. Goodman · Professor of Radiology, Medical College of Wisconsin · Milwaukee County Medical Complex · 8700 West Wisconsin Avenue, Milwaukee, WI 53226 · 414-257-6130

E. Robert Heitzman · Distinguished Service Professor, Department of Radiology, State University of New York Health Science Center at Syracuse · 750 East Adams Street, Syracuse, NY 13210 · 315-464-7407

Herman I. Libshitz · The University of Texas MD Anderson Cancer Center · 1515 Holcombe Boulevard, Houston, TX 77030 · 713-792-2121

Theresa C. McLoud · Associate Professor of Radiology, Harvard Medical School Chief of Thoracic Radiology, Massachusetts General Hospital · Ellison Building, Room 234, 32 Fruit Street, Boston, MA 02114 · 617-724-4255

Nestor L. Müller · Associate Professor and Program Director of Residency Training Program, Department of Radiology, The University of British Columbia · Deputy Chief of Radiology, Vancouver General Hospital · 855 West 12th Avenue, Vancouver, British Columbia V5Z 1M9 · 604-875-4355

David P. Naidich · Professor of Radiology, New York University Medical Center Attending Physician, Tisch Hospital, and Bellevue Hospital · Department of Radiology, 27th Street and First Avenue, New York, NY 10016 · 212-263-5229

Robert D. Pugatch · Associate Professor of Radiology, Harvard Medical School · Co-Director of Thoracic Radiology, Brigham & Women's Hospital · 75 Francis Street, Boston, MA 02115 · 617-732-5500

Stuart S. Sagel · (Computed Body Tomography) · Professor of Radiology, Washington University School of Medicine, Mallinckrodt Institute of Radiology · Attending Staff, Barnes Hospital · 510 South Kingshighway Boulevard, St. Louis, MO 63110 · 314-362-2927

Stanley S. Seigelman · Professor of Radiology, and Advisor of Academic Affairs, Johns Hopkins University School of Medicine · The Johns Hopkins Medical Institutions · Radiology Building, 600 North Wolfe Street, Baltimore, MD 21205 301-327-0124

Frederick P. Stitik · Professor of Radiology, Eastern Virginia Medical School · Chairman, Radiology, Virginia Beach General Hospital · 1060 First Colonial Road, Virginia Beach, VA 23454 · 804-496-6177, 889-5422

W. Richard Webb · Professor of Radiology, University of California at San Francisco School of Medicine · University of California at San Francisco Medical Center · 505 Parnassus Avenue, Room M-396, San Francisco, CA 94143-0628 · 415-476-5926

MAGNETIC RESONANCE IMAGING
(See also Adult Neurology, Magnetic Resonance Imaging; Cardiovascular Disease, Magnetic Resonance Imaging)

Leon Axel · Professor of Radiology, University of Pennsylvania School of Medicine · Hospital of the University of Pennsylvania · Pendergrass Diagnostic Research Laboratory, 308 Stemmler Hall, 36th and Hamilton Walk, Philadelphia, PA 19104-6086 · 215-662-6225

Robert J. Herfkens · Associate Professor of Radiology, Stanford University School of Medicine · Stanford University Hospital · 300 Pasteur Drive, Stanford, CA 94305 · 415-723-4733

Charles B. Higgins · Professor of Radiology, University of California at San Francisco School of Medicine · Chief, Magnetic Resonance Imaging Section, University of California at San Francisco Medical Center · 505 Parnassus Avenue, Room L-308, San Francisco, CA 94143-0628 · 415-476-4742

Elias A. Zerhouni · (Computed Tomography) · Associate Professor of Radiology, Johns Hopkins University School of Medicine · Medical Director of MRI and Thoracic Imaging, The Johns Hopkins Medical Institutions · Radiology Department, 600 North Wolfe Street, Baltimore, MD 21205 · 410-955-4062

NEURORADIOLOGY

Alex Berenstein · (Interventional) · Professor of Radiology, New York University School of Medicine · New York University Medical Center · 560 First Avenue, Room 390, New York, NY 10016 · 212-263-6325

Nick R. Bryan · (Diagnostic) · Professor of Radiology, Neurosurgery & Otolaryngology, Johns Hopkins University School of Medicine · Director, Department of Neuroradiology, The Johns Hopkins Medical Institutions · 600 North Wolfe Street, Meyer 8-140, Baltimore, MD 21205 · 410-955-2685

Robert I. Grossman · (Diagnostic) · Professor of Radiology, University of Pennsylvania School of Medicine · Section Chief of Neuroradiology, Hospital of the University of Pennsylvania · 3400 Spruce Street, Ground Floor, Founder's Building, Philadelphia, PA 19104 · 215-662-6865

Van V. Halbach · (Interventional) · Associate Professor of Radiology and Neurological Surgery, University of California at San Francisco School of Medicine · University of California at San Francisco Medical Center · 505 Parnassus Avenue, Room L-352, San Francisco, CA 94143 · 415-476-5262

Grant B. Hieshima · (Interventional) · Professor of Radiology and Neurological Surgery, University of California at San Francisco School of Medicine · Director of Interventional Neuroradiology, University of California at San Francisco Medical Center · 505 Parnassus Avenue, Room L-352, San Francisco, CA 94143 · 415-476-5262

Sadek K. Hilal · (Diagnostic, Interventional) · Professor of Radiology, College of Physicians & Surgeons of Columbia University · Director of Neuroradiology, Columbia-Presbyterian Medical Center · Department of Radiology, Neurological Institute, 710 West 168th Street, New York, NY 10032 · 212-305-5118

Michael T. Modic · (Magnetic Resonance Imaging/Spinal Imaging) · Chairman, Division of Radiology, The Cleveland Clinic Foundation · One Clinic Center, 9500 Euclid Avenue, Cleveland, OH 44195 · 216-444-9308

David Norman · (Diagnostic) · Professor of Radiology, University of California at San Francisco School of Medicine · Chief, Neuroradiology, University of California at San Francisco Medical Center · 505 Parnassus Avenue, Room L-371, San Francisco, CA 94143 · 415-476-6553

Robert M. Quencer · (Diagnostic) · Professor of Radiology, Neurological Surgery and Ophthalmology, University of Miami School of Medicine · University of Miami-Jackson Memorial Medical Center · 1115 Northwest 14th Avenue, Miami, FL 33136 · 305-548-4701

Fernando Vinuela · (Interventional) · Professor of Radiology, University of California at Los Angeles School of Medicine · Director, Endovascular Therapy Service, University of California at Los Angeles Center for the Health Sciences · 10833 LeConte Avenue, Room BL 1211, Los Angeles, CA 90024-1721 · 310-825-6576

Robert A. Zimmerman · (Diagnostic) · Professor of Radiology, University of Pennsylvania School of Medicine · Chief, Pediatric Neuroradiology, The Children's Hospital of Philadelphia · 34th and Civic Center Boulevard, Philadelphia PA 19104 · 215-590-2569

RHEUMATOLOGY

FIBROMYALGIA

Robert M. Bennett · Professor of Medicine, Oregon Health Sciences University Director, Division of Arthritis & Rheumatic Diseases, Oregon Health Sciences University · 3181 Southwest Sam Jackson Park Road, Portland, OR 97201 · 503-494-8963

Don Lee Goldenberg · Professor of Medicine, Tufts University School of Medicine · Chief of Rheumatology, Newton-Wellesley Hospital · 2014 Washington Street, Newton, MA 02162 · 617-527-7485

Glenn A. McCain · Professor of Medicine, The University of Western Ontario · Consultant in Rheumatology, University Hospital · 339 Windermere Road, London, Ontario N6A 5A5 · 519-663-3491

Hugh A. Smythe · Professor of Medicine, University of Toronto School of Medicine · Chief, Division of Rheumatology, Wellesley Hospital · 160 Wellesley Street East, Suite 647, Toronto, Ontario M4Y 1J3 · 416-926-7627

Frederick Wolfe · Clinical Professor of Medicine, University of Kansas School of Medicine · St. Francis Regional Medical Center · Arthritis Center, 1035 North Emporia, Suite 230, Wichita, KS 67214 · 316-263-2125

GENERAL RHEUMATOLOGY

Larry G. Anderson · Clinical Associate Professor of Medicine, University of Vermont School of Medicine · Maine Medical Center; Mercy Hospital · Rheumatology Associates, 51 Sewall Street, Portland, ME 04102 · 207-774-5761

Andrew R. Baldassare · Associate Clinical Professor of Internal Medicine, St. Louis University School of Medicine · DePaul Health Center; St. John's Mercy Medical Center; St. Joseph's Hospital (St. Charles) · 522 North New Ballas, Suite 240, St. Louis, MO 63141 · 314-567-5100

Gene V. Ball · Professor of Medicine, The University of Alabama School of Medicine · The University of Alabama Hospital · 625 Medical Education Building, 1813 Sixth Avenue South, Birmingham, AL 35294-3296 · 205-934-4703

Gerson Charles Bernhard · Clinical Professor of Medicine, Stanford University Medical School · Medical Director, The Arthritis Center at Mills-Peninsula Hospital · 100 South San Mateo Drive, San Mateo, CA 94401 · 415-696-4753

Neal S. Birnbaum · Associate Clinical Professor of Medicine, University of California at San Francisco · Chief of Staff, and Chief of Rheumatology, California Pacific Medical Center · 2100 Webster Street, Suite 112, San Francisco, CA 94115 · 415-923-3060

Sidney R. Block · Head, Rheumatology Department, Eastern Maine Medical Center · 275 Union Street, Bangor, ME 04401 · 207-945-9442

Rodney Bluestone · 436 North Bedford , Suite 303, Beverly Hills, CA 90210 · 213-657-2222

Kenneth D. Brandt · Professor of Medicine, Head, Rheumatology Division, Director, Multipurpose Arthritis & Musculoskeletal Disease Center, and Director, Specialized Center of Research in Osteoarthritis, Indiana University School of Medicine · Indiana University Medical Center · 541 Clinical Drive, Room 492, Indianapolis IN 46202-5103 · 317-274-4225

Walter G. Briney · Clinical Professor of Medicine, Rheumatology Division, University of Colorado School of Medicine · Chairman, Rheumatology Division, Rose Medical Center · Denver Arthritis Clinic, 4545 East Ninth Avenue, Suite 510, Denver, CO 80220 · 303-394-2828

Andrew Chubick · Clinical Assistant Professor, Department of Internal Medicine, The University of Texas Southwestern Medical Center at Dallas · Chief of Rheumatology, Baylor University Medical Center · 712 North Washington Avenue, Suite 200, Dallas, TX 75246 · 214-823-6503

Doyt LaDean Conn · Professor of Medicine, Mayo Medical School · Mayo Clinic 200 First Street, SW, Rochester, MN 55905 · 507-284-2002

Joseph David Croft, Jr. · Clinical Professor of Medicine, Department of Rheumatology, Georgetown University School of Medicine · Georgetown University Medical Center · 5530 Wisconsin Avenue, Suite 730, Chevy Chase, MD 20815 · 301-656-9030

John G. Curd · Head, Division of Rheumatology, and Vice Chairman, Department of Medicine, Scripps Clinic & Research Foundation · 10666 North Torrey Pines Road, La Jolla, CA 92037 · 619-554-8819

John S. Davis · Professor of Medicine and Head, Division of Rheumatology, and Trolinger Professor of Rheumatology, University of Virginia School of Medicine · University of Virginia Health Sciences Center · Box 412, Charlottesville, VA 22908 804-924-5213

Robert A. Gatter · (Fibromyalgia, Crystal Induced Arthritis, Lyme Disease) · Associate Clinical Professor of Medicine, University of Pennsylvania School of Medicine · Chief of Rheumatology, Abington Memorial Hospital · Regency Park Towers, 1003 Easton Road, Suite 104, Willow Grove, PA 19090 · 215-657-6776

Bernard F. Germain · Professor of Medicine and Director, Division of Rheumatology, Department of Internal Medicine, University of South Florida College of Medicine · Chief, Rheumatology Section, Medical Service, James A. Haley Veterans Hospital; Medical Director, Arthritis Care & Treatment Center, Tampa General Hospital; Staff Physician, H. Lee Moffitt Cancer Center & Research

Institute, and Shriners Hospital for Crippled Children · 12901 Bruce B. Downs Boulevard, Box 19, Tampa, FL 33612 · 813-974-2681

William W. Ginsburg · Associate Professor, Mayo Medical School · Mayo Clinic Jacksonville · 4500 San Pablo Road, Jacksonville, FL 32224 · 904-223-2062

J. Timothy Harrington · Professor, University of Wisconsin-Madison School of Medicine · Meriter Park Hospital · 20 South Park Street, Suite 505, Madison, WI 53715 · 608-282-8330

Louis A. Healey · Head, Division of Rheumatology, Virginia Mason Medical Center · 1100 Ninth Avenue (X-6RHE), Seattle, WA 98101 · 206-223-6823

Kahler P. Hench · Senior Consultant in Rheumatology, Scripps Clinic & Research Foundation · 10666 North Torrey Pines Road, La Jolla, CA 92037 · 619-554-8637

John Settle Johnson · Associate Professor of Clinical Medicine, Vanderbilt University School of Medicine · Midstate Baptist Hospital · Plaza II, Suite 100, 2021 Church Street, Nashville, TN 37203 · 615-340-4611

Robert Katz · Associate Professor of Medicine, Rush Medical College · Rush-Presbyterian-St. Luke's Medical Center · 1725 West Harrison Street, Suite 1039, Chicago, IL 60612 · 312-226-8228

Warren A. Katz · Clinical Professor of Medicine, University of Pennsylvania School of Medicine · Chairman, Department of Medicine, and Chief, Division of Rheumatology, Presbyterian Medical Center of Philadelphia; Moss Rehabilitation Hospital · 39th & Market Streets, Department of Medicine, Suite W285, Philadelphia, PA 19104 · 215-662-9292

Franklin Kozin · Scripps Clinic Medical Group · 10666 North Torrey Pines Road, La Jolla, CA 92037 · 619-554-8818

Joel M. Kremer · Professor of Medicine, Albany Medical College · Albany Medical Center · 47 New Scotland Avenue, Albany, NY 12208 · 518-445-5212

Robert W. Lightfoot, Jr. · Professor of Medicine, University of Kentucky College of Medicine · Director, Division of Rheumatology, University of Kentucky Medical Center · 800 Rose Street, MN614, Lexington, KY 40536-0084 · 606-233-6700

Daniel J. McCarty · Will and Cava Ross Professor of Medicine, Medical College of Wisconsin; Director, Arthritis Institute · Milwaukee County Medical Complex; Froedert Memorial Lutheran Hospital; St. Francis Hospital · 8700 West Wisconsin Avenue, Milwaukee, WI 53226 · 414-257-5946

David H. Neustadt · Clinical Professor of Medicine, University of Louisville School of Medicine · Jewish Hospital · 328 Medical Towers South, Louisville, KY 40202 · 502-585-4163

Harold A. Paulus · Professor of Medicine, University of California, Los Angeles School of Medicine · University of California, Los Angeles Medical Center · 1000 Veteran Avenue, 32-47, Los Angeles, CA 90024-1670 · 310-825-6439

Paulding Phelps · Clinical Professor of Medicine, University of Vermont School of Medicine · Maine Medical Center; Mercy Hospital; Westbrook Community Hospital · Rheumatology Associates, 51 Sewall Street, Portland, ME 04102 · 207-774-5761

Robert S. Pinals · Professor of Medicine, Robert Wood Johnson Medical School Chairman, Department of Medicine, Medical Center at Princeton · 253 Witherspoon Street, Princeton, NJ 08540 · 609-497-4301

Theodore Pincus · Professor of Medicine & Microbiology, Vanderbilt University School of Medicine, Division of Rheumatology and Immunology · T-3219 Medical Center North, Nashville, TN 37232 · 615-322-4746

Richard Mitchell Pope · Professor of Medicine, Northwestern University Medical School · Chief, Division of Arthritis & Connective Tissue Diseases, Northwestern Memorial Hospital · 222 East Superior, Chicago, IL 60611 · 312-908-8628

Mark Ruderman · Associate Clinical Professor, Department of Medicine, University of Connecticut School of Medicine · Senior, Department of Medicine, and Chief, Section of Rheumatology, Hartford Hospital · 85 Seymour Street, Hartford, CT 06106 · 203-246-4260

H. Ralph Schumacher, Jr. · Professor of Medicine, and Acting Chief of the Rheumatology Section, University of Pennsylvania School of Medicine · Director, Arthritis Immunology, Philadelphia VA Medical Center; Acting Chief of Rheumatology, Hospital of the University of Pennsylvania · 570 Maloney Building, 3400 Spruce Street, Philadelphia, PA 19104 · 215-662-2454, 823-5800 x6460

John S. Sergent · Professor Department of Medicine, Vanderbilt University School of Medicine · Chief of Medicine, St. Thomas Hospital · 4220 Harding Road, P.O. Box 380, Nashville, TN 37202 · 615-386-6609

Mary Betty Stevens · Professor of Medicine, Johns Hopkins University School of Medicine · Good Samaritan Hospital · Russell Morgan Building, 5601 Loch Raven Boulevard, Suite 507, Baltimore, MD 21239 · 301-323-2200

Elizabeth A. Tindall · Clinical Assistant Professor, Department of Medicine, Division of Arthritis and Rheumatic Diseases, Oregon Health Sciences University · Director of Rheumatology, Portland Adventist Medical Center · 10123 Southeast Market Street, Portland, OR 97216 · 503-255-5828

Arthur Lawrence Weaver · Clinical Associate Professor of Medicine, University of Nebraska College of Medicine · Attending Staff, Bryan Memorial Hospital · Arthritis Center of Nebraska, 2121 South 56th Street, Lincoln, NE 68506 · 402-489-0333

Michael Eliot Weinblatt · Associate Professor of Medicine, Harvard Medical School · Vice Chairman of Clinical Affairs, Department of Rheumatology & Immunology, Brigham & Women's Hospital · 75 Francis Street, Boston, MA 02115 · 617-732-5331

Michael H. Weisman · Professor of Medicine, University of California, San Diego School of Medicine · University of California, San Diego Medical Center · 225 Dickinson Street, Mail Code 8418, San Diego, CA 92103-8418 · 619-543-5635

Robert F. Willkens · Clinical Professor of Medicine/Rheumatology, University of Washington School of Medicine · Chief of Rheumatology, Harborview Medical Center · 325 Ninth Avenue (ZA-94), Seattle, WA 98104; Madison Street Internists, 1229 Madison Street, Suite 860, Seattle, WA 98104 · 206-223-3156, 386-6860

Kenneth Ray Wilske · Virginia Mason Medical Center · 1100 Ninth Avenue (X-6RHE), Seattle, WA 98111 · 206-223-6824

Robert A. Yood · Assistant Professor of Medicine, University of Massachusetts Medical School · Director of Rheumatology, St. Vincent's Hospital · Fallon Clinic, 135 Gold Star Boulevard, Worcester, MA 01606 · 508-856-9596

GOUT

Daniel J. McCarty · Will & Cava Ross Professor of Medicine, Medical College of Wisconsin; Director, Arthritis Institute · Milwaukee County Medical Complex; Froedert Memorial Lutheran Hospital; St. Francis Hospital · 8700 West Wisconsin Avenue, Milwaukee, WI 53226 · 414-257-5946

INFECTIOUS ARTHRITIS

Don Lee Goldenberg · Professor of Medicine, Tufts University School of Medicine · Chief of Rheumatology, Newton-Wellesley Hospital · 2014 Washington Street, Newton, MA 02162 · 617-527-7485

LUPUS

Bevra Hannahs Hahn · Professor of Medicine, University of California at Los Angeles School of Medicine · Chief of Rheumatology, University of California at Los Angeles Center for the Health Sciences · 10833 LeConte Avenue, Los Angeles, CA 90024-7991 · 310-825-7991

OSTEOARTHRITIS

Roy D. Altman · Professor of Medicine, University of Miami School of Medicine Chief, Arthritis Section, Miami Veterans Affairs Medical Center · 1201 Northwest 16th Street, Room D-1009, Miami, FL 33125 · 305-547-5735

Kenneth D. Brandt · Professor of Medicine, Head, Rheumatology Division, Director, Multipurpose Arthritis & Musculoskeletal Disease Center, and Director, Specialized Center of Research in Osteoarthritis, Indiana University School of Medicine · Indiana University Medical Center · 541 Clinical Drive, Room 492, Indianapolis IN 46202-5103 · 317-274-4225

David S. Howell · Professor of Medicine, University of Miami School of Medicine Chief, Arthritis Division, University of Miami Affiliated Hospitals; Medical Investigator, Miami Veterans Administration Medical Center · 1201 Northwest 16th Street, P.O. Box 016960, Miami, FL 33101 · 305-547-6325

Roland W. Moskowitz · Professor of Medicine, Case Western Reserve University School of Medicine · Director, Division of Rheumatic Diseases, University Hospitals of Cleveland · 2074 Abington Road, Cleveland, OH 44106 · 216-844-3168

OSTEOPOROSIS

Stephen M. Krane · Persis, Cyrus & Marlow B. Harrison Professor of Medicine, Harvard Medical School · Physician-in-Chief of the Arthritis Unit, Massachusetts General Hospital · 32 Fruit Street, Boston, MA 02114 · 617-726-2870

PAGET'S DISEASE
(See also Endocrinology & Metabolism, Paget's Disease)

Roy D. Altman · Professor of Medicine, University of Miami School of Medicine Chief, Arthritis Section, Miami Veterans Affairs Medical Center · 1201 Northwest 16th Street, Room D-1009, Miami, FL 33125 · 305-547-5735

REHABILITATION
(See also Physical Medicine and Rehabilitation, Rheumatology)

Joseph J. Biundo · Professor of Medicine, Louisiana State University School of Medicine · Chief, Section of Physical Medicine & Rehabilitation, Louisiana State University Medical Center · 1542 Tulane Avenue, Suite 602, New Orleans, LA 70112 · 504-568-2173

Naomi Lynn Gerber · Professor of Medicine, Georgetown University School of Medicine · Chief, Department Rehabilitation Medicine, National Institutes of Health · 9000 Rockville Pike, Building 10, Room 6S235, Bethesda, MD 20892 · 301-496-4733

Jeanne E. Hicks · Assistant Professor of Medicine, George Washington University; Associate Professor of Rehabilitation, Georgetown University; Assistant Professor of Medicine, Uniformed Armed Services Institute · Deputy Chief, Department of Rehabilitation Medicine, National Institutes of Health · 9000 Rockville Pike, Building 10, Room 6S235, Bethesda, MD 20892 · 301-496-4733

Mary Jurisson · Instructor, Mayo Medical School · Mayo Clinic · 200 First Street, SW, RMH 3, Rochester, MN 55905 · 507-284-2511

John J. Nicholas · Professor of Physical Medicine & Rehabilitation, Rush Medical College · Chairman, Department of Physical Medicine & Rehabilitation, Rush-Presbyterian-St. Luke's Medical Center · 1653 West Congress Parkway, Chicago, IL 60612-3864 · 312-942-3675

Robert L. Swezey · Clinical Professor of Medicine, University of California at Los Angeles School of Medicine · Medical Director, Arthritis & Back Pain Center, St. John's Hospital & Health Center · 1328 Sixteenth Street, Santa Monica, CA 90404 213-394-1113

RHEUMATIC FEVER

Richard Mitchell Pope · Professor of Medicine, Northwestern University Medical School · Chief, Division of Arthritis & Connective Tissue Diseases, Northwestern Memorial Hospital · 222 East Superior, Chicago, IL 60611 · 312-908-8628

RHEUMATOID ARTHRITIS

Neal S. Birnbaum · Associate Clinical Professor of Medicine, University of California at San Francisco · Chief of Staff, and Chief of Rheumatology, California Pacific Medical Center · 2100 Webster Street, Suite 112, San Francisco, CA 94115 415-923-3060

Joseph David Croft, Jr. · Clinical Professor of Medicine, Department of Rheumatology, Georgetown University School of Medicine · Georgetown University Medical Center · 5530 Wisconsin Avenue, Suite 730, Chevy Chase, MD 20815 · 301-656-9030

Louis A. Healey · Head, Division of Rheumatology, Virginia Mason Medical Center · 1100 Ninth Avenue (X-6RHE), Seattle, WA 98101 · 206-223-6823

Herbert Kaplan · Clinical Professor of Medicine, University of Colorado Health Sciences Center · Rose Medical Center · Denver Arthritis Clinic, P.C., 4545 East Ninth Avenue, Suite 510, Denver, CO 80220 · 303-394-2828

Michael Eliot Weinblatt · Associate Professor of Medicine, Harvard Medical School · Vice Chairman of Clinical Affairs, Department of Rheumatology & Immunology, Brigham & Women's Hospital · 75 Francis Street, Boston, MA 02115 617-732-5331

Kenneth Ray Wilske · Virginia Mason Medical Center · 1100 Ninth Avenue (X-6RHE), Seattle, WA 98111 · 206-223-6824

Frederick Wolfe · Clinical Professor of Medicine, University of Kansas School of Medicine · St. Francis Regional Medical Center · Arthritis Center, 1035 North Emporia, Suite 230, Wichita, KS 67214 · 316-263-2125

SCLERODERMA

Roy D. Altman · Professor of Medicine, University of Miami School of Medicine Chief, Arthritis Section, Miami Veterans Affairs Medical Center · 1201 Northwest 16th Street, Room D-1009, Miami, FL 33125 · 305-547-5735

Phillip J. Clements · Professor of Rheumatology, University of California at Los Angeles School of Medicine · University of California at Los Angeles Medical Center; Wadsworth West Los Angeles Veterans Administration Hospital · 1000 Veteran Avenue, Room 32-47, Los Angeles, CA 90024-1670 · 310-825-7704

Sergio A. Jimenez · Professor of Medicine, Biochemistry & Molecular Biology, Jefferson Medical College of Thomas Jefferson University · Director, Rheumatology Research, and Director, Scleroderma Center, Thomas Jefferson University Hospital · Bluemle Life Sciences Building, 233 South 10th Street, Room 509, Philadelphia, PA 19107 · 215-955-5042

E. Carwile LeRoy · Professor of Medicine, Medical University of South Carolina 171 Ashley Avenue, Charleston, SC 29425-2229 · 803-792-4152

Thomas A. Medsger, Jr. · Professor of Medicine, University of Pittsburgh School of Medicine · Chief, Division of Rheumatology & Clinical Immunology, Presbyterian University Hospital; Professor of Medicine, Montefiore University Hospital 985 Scaife Hall, Pittsburgh, PA 15261 · 412-648-9698

James Richard Seibold · Associate Professor of Medicine, Robert Wood Johnson Medical School-University of Medicine & Dentistry of New Jersey · Director of Clinical Research Center, Robert Wood Johnson University Hospital · One Robert Wood Johnson Place, CN-19, New Brunswick, NJ 08903-0019 · 908-828-3000

UVEITIS
(See also Ophthalmology, Uveitis)

James T. Rosenbaum · Professor of Medicine, Ophthalmology and Cell Biology, Oregon Health Sciences University · Oregon Health Sciences University · 3181 Southwest Sam Jackson Park Road, Portland, OR 97201 · 503-494-5023

VASCULITIS
(See also Infectious Disease, Vasculitis)

Gene G. Hunder · Professor of Medicine, and Chairman, Division of Rheumatology, Mayo Medical School · Mayo Clinic · 200 First Street, SW, Rochester, MN 55905 · 507-284-2060

Robert W. Lightfoot, Jr. · Professor of Medicine, University of Kentucky College of Medicine · Director, Division of Rheumatology, University of Kentucky Medical Center · 800 Rose Street, MN614, Lexington, KY 40536-0084 · 606-233-6700

SURGICAL ONCOLOGY

BREAST CANCER
(See also Medical Oncology, Breast Cancer; Medical Oncology &
Hematology, Breast Cancer; Radiation Oncology, Breast Cancer)

Kirby I. Bland · Professor and Associate Chairman, Department of Surgery, University of Florida College of Medicine · Shands Hospital at the University of Florida · 1600 Southwest Archer Road, Room 6186, P.O. Box 100286, Gainesville, FL 32610 · 904-395-0630

Edward M. Copeland III · The Edward R. Woodward Professor and Chairman, Department of Surgery, University of Florida College of Medicine · Chief of Surgery, Shands Hospital at the University of Florida · 1600 Southwest Archer Road, Room 6172, P.O. Box 100286, Gainesville, FL 32610-0286 · 904-395-0630

William L. Donegan · Professor of Surgery, Medical College of Wisconsin · Chairman of Surgery, Sinai Samaritan Medical Center · 950 North 12th Street, P.O. Box 342, Milwaukee, WI 53201 · 414-283-6809

Armando E. Giuliano · Clinical Professor of Surgery, University of California, Los Angeles Medical Center · Chief of Surgical Oncology, St. John's Hospital & Health Center, John Wayne Institute · 1328 Twenty-Second Street, Three West, Santa Monica, CA 90404 · 213-829-8089

William H. Goodson III · Professor of Surgery, University of California, San Francisco School of Medicine · Professor-in-Residence, University of California, San Francisco Medical Center · 400 Parnassus Avenue, Room A-680, Box 0338, San Francisco, CA 94143 · 415-476-1161

Alfred S. Ketcham · Professor of Surgery, and The Sylvester Professor of Oncology, and Chief, Division of Oncology, University of Miami School of Medicine · Chief, Division of Oncology, Jackson Memorial Medical Center; University of Miami Hospital & Clinics; The Sylvester Comprehensive Cancer Center · Department of Surgery (310T), P.O. Box 016310, Miami, FL 33101 · 305-547-6364

David W. Kinne · Memorial Sloan-Kettering Cancer Center · 1275 York Avenue, New York, NY 10021 · 212-639-7962

Richard G. Margolese · Herbert Black Professor of Surgical Oncology, Department of Surgery, and Chairman, Division of Clinical Oncology, Department of Oncology, McGill University · Surgeon and Director, Department of Oncology, Jewish General Hospital · 3755 Cote St. Catherine Road, Suite E177, Montreal, Quebec H3T 1E2 · 514-342-3504

Michael P. Moore · Professor of Surgery, Cornell University Medical College · Assistant Attending Physician, Memorial Sloan-Kettering Cancer Center · 1275 York Avenue, New York, NY 10021 · 212-639-8261

Monica Morrow · Associate Professor of Surgery, University of Chicago, Pritzker School of Medicine · University of Chicago Medical Center · 5841 South Maryland Avenue, Box 402, Chicago, IL 60637-1470 · 312-702-0921

Michael P. Osborne · Professor of Surgery, Cornell University Medical College · Director of the Strang Cancer Prevention Center in Manhattan; Chief of The Breast Service, The New York Hospital-Cornell Medical Center · 428 East 72nd Street, Suite 600, New York, NY 10021 · 212-794-6085

Jeanne A. Petrek · Assistant Professor of Surgery, Cornell University Medical College · Assistant Attending Surgeon, Breast Service, Memorial Sloan-Kettering Cancer Center · 1275 York Avenue, New York, NY 10021 · 212-639-2000

Gordon F. Schwartz · Professor of Surgery, Jefferson Medical College of Thomas Jefferson University · Consulting Surgeon, Pennsylvania Hospital; Consulting Surgeon, Bryn Mawr Hospital; Attending Surgeon, Thomas Jefferson University Hospital · 1015 Chestnut Street, Suite 510, Philadelphia, PA 19107 · 215-627-8487

Thomas J. Smith · Associate Professor of Surgery, Tufts University School of Medicine · Chief, Division of Surgical Oncology, and Director, Surgical Education Program, New England Medical Center · 750 Washington Street, Box 28, Boston, MA 02111 · 617-956-6093

David P. Winchester · Associate Professor of Clinical Surgery, Northwestern University Medical School · Chief, Division of General Surgery, Evanston Hospital · 2500 Ridge, Suite 310, Evanston, IL 60201 · 708-491-1277

Norman Wolmark · Ravitch Professor of Surgery, University of Pittsburgh School of Medicine · Surgeon-in-Chief, Montefiore University Hospital · 3459 Fifth Avenue, Pittsburgh, PA 15213 · 412-648-6751

William C. Wood · Joseph B. Whitehead Professor & Chairman, Department of Surgery, Emory University School of Medicine · Emory University Affiliated Hospitals · 1364 Clifton Road, NE, Atlanta, GA 30322 · 404-727-5800

COLON & RECTAL CANCER
(See also Colon & Rectal Surgery, Colon & Rectal Cancer)

Herand Abcarian · Professor and Chairman, Department of Surgery, The University of Illinois College of Medicine at Chicago · The University of Illinois Hospital · 840 South Wood Street, Chicago, IL 60612 · 312-782-4828

Robert W. Beart, Jr. · Professor of Surgery, Mayo Medical School · Chairman of General Surgery, Mayo Clinic Scottsdale · 13400 East Shea Boulevard, Scottsdale, AZ 85259 · 602-391-8000

Kirby I. Bland · Professor and Associate Chairman, Department of Surgery, University of Florida College of Medicine · Shands Hospital at the University of Florida · 1600 Southwest Archer Road, Room 6186, P.O. Box 100286, Gainesville, FL 32610 · 904-395-0630

Alfred Martin Cohen · Assistant Professor of Surgery, Cornell University Medical College · Memorial Sloan-Kettering Cancer Center · 1275 York Avenue, New York, NY 10021 · 212-639-2000

Edward M. Copeland III · The Edward R. Woodward Professor and Chairman, Department of Surgery, University of Florida College of Medicine · Chief of Surgery, Shands Hospital at the University of Florida · 1600 Southwest Archer Road, Room 6172, P.O. Box 100286, Gainesville, FL 32610-0286 · 904-395-0630

Jerome J. Decosse · Professor of Surgery, Cornell University Medical College · Vice-Chairman, Department of Surgery, The New York Hospital-Cornell Medical Center · 525 East 68th Street, Room F1917, New York, NY 10021 · 212-746-5414

Victor W. Fazio · Chairman, Department of Colorectal Surgery, The Cleveland Clinic Foundation · One Clinic Center, 9500 Euclid Avenue, Desk A-111, Cleveland, OH 44195 · 216-444-6672

Stanley M. Goldberg · Clinical Professor of Surgery, University of Minnesota School of Medicine · Director, Division of Colon & Rectal Surgery, University of Minnesota Hospital & Clinics · 420 Delaware Street, SE, Box 450 UMHC, Minneapolis, MN 55455 · 612-339-4534

Ira J. Kodner · Associate Professor of Surgery, Washington University School of Medicine · Director, Division of Colon & Rectal Surgery, The Jewish Hospital of St. Louis · 216 South Kingshighway Boulevard, St. Louis, MO 63110 · 314-454-7177

Glenn Steele, Jr. · The William V. McDermott Professor of Surgery, Harvard Medical School · Chairman, Department of Surgery, New England Deaconess Hospital · 110 Francis Street, Suite 3A, Boston, MA 02215 · 617-732-9780

GASTROENTEROLOGIC CANCER
(See also Gastroenterology, Gastroenterologic Cancer; Radiation Oncology, Gastroenterologic Cancer)

Murray Frederick Brennan · (Pancreatic Cancer, Adrenal Parathyroid, Islet Carcinoma) · Chairman, Department of Surgery, Memorial Sloan-Kettering Cancer Center · 1275 York Avenue, New York, NY 10021 · 212-639-6586

John L. Cameron · (Pancreatic Cancer, Biliary Cancer) · Professor and Chairman, Department of Surgery, Johns Hopkins University School of Medicine · Chief of Surgery, The Johns Hopkins Hospital · 720 Rutland Avenue, Ross Building 759, Baltimore, MD 21205 · 410-955-5166

John M. Daly · (Liver Cancer, Biliary Oncology, Pancreatic Cancer) · The Jonathan E. Rhoads Professor of Surgery, University of Pennsylvania School of Medicine · Chief, Division of Surgical Oncology, Hospital of the University of Pennsylvania · 3400 Spruce Street, Fourth Floor Silverstein, Philadelphia, PA 19104 · 215-662-7866

Joseph Fortner · (Pancreatic Cancer, Liver Cancer) · Memorial Sloan-Kettering Cancer Center · 1275 York Avenue, New York, NY 10021 · 212-639-7466

Robert E. Hermann · Chairman, Department of General Surgery, The Cleveland Clinic Foundation · One Clinic Center, 9500 Euclid Avenue, Desk A-110, Cleveland, OH 44195 · 216-444-6663

Shunzaburo Iwatsuki · (Liver Cancer) · Professor of Surgery, University of Pittsburgh School of Medicine · Presbyterian University Hospital · Falk Clinic 5C., 3601 Fifth Avenue, Pittsburgh, PA 15213 · 412-648-3200

David M. Nagorney · (Liver Cancer) · Associate Professor of Surgery, Mayo Medical School · Mayo Clinic; Rochester Methodist Hospital; St. Mary's Hospital 200 First Street, SW, Rochester, MN 55905 · 507-284-2644

Mark S. Roh · (Liver Cancer) · Assistant Professor, The University of Texas Medical School at Houston · Chief, Liver Tumor Surgery, The University of Texas MD Anderson Cancer Center · Department of General Surgery, 1515 Holcombe Boulevard, Box 106, Houston, TX 77030 · 713-792-7961

Wiley W. Souba · Associate Professor of Surgery, University of Florida College of Medicine · Staff Surgeon, Gainesville Veterans Affairs Medical Center; Shands Hospital at the University of Florida · 1600 Southwest Archer Road, Room 6116, P.O. Box 100286, Gainesville, FL 32610 · 904-395-0494

Glenn Steele, Jr. · The William V. McDermott Professor of Surgery, Harvard Medical School · Chairman, Department of Surgery, New England Deaconess Hospital · 110 Francis Street, Suite 3A, Boston, MA 02215 · 617-732-9780

IMMUNOTHERAPY, BIOLOGICAL RESPONSE MODIFIERS ONCOLOGY
(See also Medical Oncology & Hematology, Immunotherapy, Biological Response Modifiers Oncology)

Donald L. Morton · (Monoclonal Antibodies, Vaccine Therapy) · Professor of Surgery, Emeritus, University of California at Los Angeles School of Medicine · Medical Director and Surgeon-in-Chief, John Wayne Cancer Institute, St. John's Hospital & Health Center · 1328 Twenty-Second Street, Santa Monica, CA 90404 310-829-8363

MELANOMA

Charles M. Balch · (Surgical Education & Research) · Professor of Immunology and Surgery, The University of Texas MD Anderson Cancer Center · Professor and Head, Division of Surgery, and Chairman, Department of General Surgery, The University of Texas MD Anderson Cancer Center · 1515 Holcombe Boulevard, Division of Surgery—112, Houston, TX 77030 · 713-792-6446

Daniel G. Coit · Assistant Professor of Surgery, Cornell University Medical College · Assistant Attending Surgeon, Memorial Sloan-Kettering Cancer Center · 1275 York Avenue, New York, NY 10021 · 212-639-8411

Donald L. Morton · (Monoclonal Antibodies, Vaccine Therapy) · Professor of Surgery, Emeritus, University of California at Los Angeles School of Medicine · Medical Director and Surgeon-in-Chief, John Wayne Cancer Institute, St. John's Hospital & Health Center · 1328 Twenty-Second Street, Santa Monica, CA 90404 310-829-8363

THORACIC SURGERY

ADULT CARDIOTHORACIC SURGERY

Cary W. Akins · Associate Clinical Professor of Surgery, Harvard Medical School Instructor in Surgery, Massachusetts General Hospital · 32 Fruit Street, Boston, MA 02114 · 617-726-8218

L. George Alexander, Jr. · Rex Hospital; Wake Medical Center; Raleigh Community Hospital · Rex Hospital Medical Office Building, 2800 Blue Ridge Boulevard, Raleigh, NC 27607 · 913-782-7900

Margaret D. Allen · (Heart Transplantation) · Assistant Professor of Surgery, and Director of Cardiac Transplantation, University of Washington School of Medicine 1959 Northeast Pacific Street, Seattle, WA 98195 · 206-543-5517

Robert W. Anderson · Professor of Surgery & Biomedical Engineering, Northwestern University Medical School · Chief, Cardiothoracic Surgery, Northwestern Memorial Hospital; Evanston Hospital · 2650 Ridge Avenue, Evanston, IL 60201 708-570-2561, 312-908-3121

John C. Baldwin · (Heart & Lung Transplantation) · Professor and Chief, Cardiothoracic Surgery, Yale University School of Medicine · Cardiothoracic Surgeon-in-Chief, Yale-New Haven Hospital · 333 Cedar Street, 121 FMB, New Haven, CT 06510 · 203-785-2704

R. Morton Bolman III · (Heart Transplantation, Lung Transplantation, Heart & Lung Transplantation) · Professor and Chief, Division of Cardiovascular and Thoracic Surgery, Department of Surgery, University of Minnesota School of Medicine · University of Minnesota Hospital & Clinics · 425 East River Road, Box 207 UMHC, Minneapolis, MN 55455 · 612-625-3902

Mortimer J. Buckley · Professor of Surgery, Harvard Medical School · Massachusetts General Hospital · 32 Fruit Street, Boston, MA 02114 · 617-726-3726

W. Randolph Chitwood, Jr. · (Mitral Valve Repair Surgery, Homograft Aortic Valve Surgery, Complex Coronary Revascularization, Arrhythmia Surgery) · Professor and Vice-Chairman, Department of Surgery, and Chief, Division of Cardiothoracic Surgery, East Carolina University School of Medicine · University Medical Center of Eastern North Carolina · 200 Stantonsburg Road, Greenville, NC 27858-4354 · 919-551-4822

Lawrence H. Cohn · Professor of Surgery, Harvard Medical School · Chief, Division of Cardiac Surgery, Brigham & Women's Hospital · 75 Francis Street, Boston, MA 02115 · 617-732-7678

Denton A. Cooley · Clinical Professor of Surgery, The University of Texas Medical School at Houston · Surgeon -in-Chief, Texas Heart Institute; Chief, Cardiovascular Surgery, St. Luke's Hospital; Texas Childrens Hospital · Texas Heart Institute, 1101 Bates Avenue, Suite P-514, P. O. Box 20345, Houston, TX 77225-0345 · 713-791-4900

Jack G. Copeland · (Heart Transplantation) · The Michael Drummond Distinguished Professor of Cardiovascular and Thoracic Surgery, The University of Arizona College of Medicine · Chief, Section of Cardiovascular & Thoracic Surgery, and Director, Cardiac Transplantation & Artificial Heart Program, and Co-Director, University Heart Center, The University of Arizona Health Sciences Center · 1501 North Campbell Avenue, Tucson, AZ 85724 · 602-626-6339

Delos (Toby) M. Cosgrove III · The Cleveland Clinic Foundation · One Clinic Center, 9500 Euclid Avenue, Cleveland, OH 44195-5066 · 216-444-6733

James L. Cox · (Electrophysiology) · Professor and Chief, Division of Cardiac and Thoracic Surgery, Washington University School of Medicine · Barnes Hospital · Queeny Tower, Suite 3108, St. Louis, MO 63110 · 314-362-6185

Pat O. Daily · Director of Cardiovascular Surgery, Sharp Memorial Hospital · 8010 Frost Street, Suite 501, San Diego, CA 92123 · 619-292-9902

Gordon K. Danielson · Roberts Professor of Surgery, and Chairman, Division of Thoracic and Cardiovascular Surgery, Mayo Medical School · St. Mary's Hospital Rochester, MN 55905 · 507-255-7062

O. H. Frazier · (Heart Transplantation) · Professor of Surgery, The University of Texas Medical School at Houston · Chief, Transplant Service, and Co-Director, Cullen Cardiovascular Research Laboratories, Texas Heart Institute · 1101 Bates Street, Suite P306, Houston, TX 77030 · 713-791-3000

William Gay · (Heart Transplantation) · Professor and Chairman, Department of Surgery, University of Utah School of Medicine · University of Utah Health Sciences Center · 50 North Medical Drive, Salt Lake City, UT 84132 · 801-581-7304

Bartley P. Griffith · (Heart Transplantation, Lung Transplantation, Heart & Lung Transplantation) · Professor of Surgery, University of Pittsburgh School of Medicine · Chief, Division of Cardiothoracic Surgery, Presbyterian University Hospital · 1084 Scaife Hall, Pittsburgh, PA 15261 · 412-648-9890

Gerard M. Guiraudon · (Electrophysiologic Surgery) · Professor of Surgery, University Hospital · 339 Windermere Road, London, Ontario N6A 5A5 · 519-663-3621

J. Donald Hill · Assistant Surgeon & Lecturer in Surgery, University of California at San Francisco School of Medicine · Director, Department of Cardiovascular Surgery, California Pacific Medical Center · 2100 Webster Street, Suite 512, San Francisco, CA 94115 · 415-563-4321

Ronald C. Hill · Associate Professor of Surgery, West Virginia University School of Medicine · Ruby Memorial Hospital · 4060 Health Sciences Center North, Morgantown, WV 26506 · 304-293-2541

Richard Alan Hopkins · Associate Professor of Surgery, Georgetown University School of Medicine · Georgetown University Medical Center · Four Pasquerilla Health Care Center, 3800 Reservoir Road, NW, Washington, DC 20007 · 202-687-1265

O. Wayne Isom · Professor of Surgery, Cornell University Medical College · Chairman, Cardiothoracic Division, and Surgeon-in-Chief, The New York Hospital-Cornell Medical Center · 525 East 68th Street, Room 2103, New York, NY 10021 · 212-746-5151

Ellis L. Jones · (Valve, Coronary and Electrophysiology Surgery) · Professor of Cardiothoracic Surgery, Emory University School of Medicine · Emory University Affiliated Hospitals · 1365 Clifton Road, NE, Atlanta, GA 30322 · 404-248-3484

Kent W. Jones · Clinical Professor of Surgery, University of Utah School of Medicine · Attending Surgeon, Division of Cardiovascular & Thoracic Surgery, Latter Day Saints Hospital · 324 Tenth Avenue, Suite 160, Salt Lake City, UT 84103 · 801-322-0563

Robert H. Jones · (Nuclear Cardiology) · Mary & Deryl Hart Professor of Surgery, Duke University School of Medicine · Duke University Medical Center P.O. Box 2986, Durham, NC 27710 · 919-684-6077

Jerome Harold Kay · Clinical Professor of Surgery, University of Southern California School of Medicine · Attending Physician, The Hospital of the Good Samaritan · 123 South Alvarado Street, Los Angeles, CA 90057 · 213-413-5220

James K. Kirklin · (Heart Transplantation) · Professor of Surgery, The University of Alabama School of Medicine · The University of Alabama Hospital · Birmingham, AL 35294 · 205-934-3368

Nicholas T. Kouchoukos · Professor, Department of Surgery, Washington University School of Medicine · Surgeon-in-Chief, The Jewish Hospital of St. Louis; Barnes Hospital; St. Louis Children's Hospital · 216 South Kingshighway Boulevard, St. Louis, MO 63110 · 314-454-7175

Hillel Laks · Professor and Chief of Cardiothoracic Surgery, University of California at Los Angeles School of Medicine · Chief of Cardiothoracic Surgery, and Director of Heart and Lung Transplantation, University of California at Los Angeles Hospital/Clinic · UCLA Medical Center, Room 62-182A, Division TS, Los Angeles, CA 90024-1741 · 310-206-8232

Floyd D. Loop · Chairman, Board of Governors, The Cleveland Clinic Foundation · One Clinic Center, 9500 Euclid Avenue, Cleveland, OH 44195-5108 · 216-444-2300

Bruce W. Lytle · Staff Surgeon, The Cleveland Clinic Foundation · One Clinic Center, 9500 Euclid Avenue, Cleveland, OH 44195-5066 · 216-444-6962

Jon F. Moran · Professor and Chairman, Department of Cardiothoracic Surgery, University of Kansas School of Medicine · University of Kansas Medical Center · 3901 Rainbow Boulevard, Department of Cardiothoracic Surgery, Room 1232 Bell, Kansas City, KS 66160-7373 · 913-588-2840

Gordon F. Murray · Professor and Chairman, Department of Surgery, West Virginia University School of Medicine · West Virginia University Health Sciences Center · Health Sciences Center North, Morgantown, WV 26506 · 304-293-4869

Hassan Najafi · Professor of Surgery, Rush Medical College · Chairman, Department of Cardiovascular-Thoracic Surgery, Rush-Presbyterian-St. Luke's Medical Center · Jelke Building, 1653 West Congress Parkway, Room 714, Chicago, IL 60612 · 312-942-6373

David A. Ott · Clinical Professor of Surgery, The University of Texas Medical School at Houston · Associate Surgeon, Texas Heart Institute; St. Luke's Episcopal Hospital; Texas Children's Hospital · Texas Heart Institute, 1101 Bates Avenue, Suite P-514, Houston, TX 77030 · 713-791-4917

Philip E. Oyer · (Heart Transplantation) · Professor of Cardiothoracic Surgery, Stanford University School of Medicine · Stanford University Hospital · Department of Cardiac Surgery, CVRB Upper Level North, Stanford Medical Center, Stanford, CA 94305 · 415-723-5771

J. Scott Rankin · Professor of Surgery and Chief, Division of Cardiothoracic Surgery, University of California at San Francisco School of Medicine · University of California at San Francisco Medical Center · 505 Parnassus Avenue, Room M-593, Box 0118, San Francisco, CA 94143-0118 · 415-476-2606

Bruce A. Reitz · (Heart Transplantation, Heart & Lung Transplantation) · Professor of Surgery, Johns Hopkins University School of Medicine · Cardiac Surgeon-in-Charge, The Johns Hopkins Medical Institutions; Sinai Hospital of Baltimore · Blalock Building, 600 North Wolfe Street, Room 618, Baltimore, MD 21205 · 410-955-2800

Eric A. Rose · (Heart Transplantation) · Associate Professor of Surgery, College of Physicians & Surgeons of Columbia University · Columbia-Presbyterian Medical Center · 622 West 168th Street, New York, NY 10032 · 212-305-6380

Hartzell V. Schaff · (Coronary Bypass Surgery, Cardiac Surgery) · Associate Professor of Surgery, Mayo Medical School · Consultant, Thoracic & Cardiovascular Surgery, Mayo Clinic; Saint Marys Hospital; Rochester Methodist Hospital · Cardiovascular Surgery, 5 Joseph, 1216 Second Street, SW, Rochester, MN 55902 · 507-255-7068

Peter M. Scholz · Associate Professor of Surgery, Robert Wood Johnson Medical School-University of Medicine & Dentistry of New Jersey · Robert Wood Johnson University Hospital · One Robert Wood Johnson Place, CN-19, New Brunswick, NJ 08903-0019 · 908-937-7642

Norman E. Shumway · (Heart Transplantation) · Professor and Chairman, Department of Cardiothoracic Surgery, Stanford University School of Medicine · Stanford University Hospital · Falk Cardiovascular Research Center, Stanford, CA 94305-5247 · 415-723-5771

Frank Cole Spencer · Professor and Chairman, Department of Surgery, New York University School of Medicine · New York University Medical Center · 550 First Avenue, New York, NY 10016 · 212-263-6382

Vaughn A. Starnes · (Heart & Lung Transplantation) · Associate Professor of Cardiothoracic Surgery, Stanford University School of Medicine · Chief of the Cardiothoracic Surgical Service, Lucile Salter Packard Children's Hospital at Stanford · 300 Pasteur Drive, Stanford, CA 94305 · 415-723-5771

Edward E. Stinson · (Heart Transplantation) · The Thelma & Henry Doelger Professor of Cardiovascular Surgery, Department of Cardiothoracic Surgery, Stanford University School of Medicine · Stanford University Hospital · Falk Cardiovascular Research Center, 300 Pasteur Drive, Stanford, CA 94305-5247 · 415-723-5771

Robert B. Wallace · Professor and Chairman, Department of Surgery, Georgetown University School of Medicine · Chief, Division of Cardiovascular Thoracic Surgery, Georgetown University Medical Center · Pasquerilla Health Care Center, Fourth Floor, 3800 Reservoir Road, NW, Washington, DC 20007 · 202-687-8586

Andrew S. Wechsler · Stuart McGuire Professor and Chairman, Department of Surgery and Professor of Physiology, Virginia Commonwealth University, Medical College of Virginia · MCV Station, Box 645, Richmond, VA 23298 · 804-786-9670

Walter George Wolfe · Professor of Surgery, Duke University School of Medicine Duke University Medical Center · Department of Surgery, Box 3507, Durham, NC 27710 · 919-684-4117

GENERAL THORACIC SURGERY

John R. Benfield · Professor and Chief of Division of Cardiothoracic Surgery, and Vice-Chairman, Department of Surgery, University of California at Davis School of Medicine · University of California at Davis Medical Center · 4301 X Street, Suite 2250, Sacramento, CA 95817 · 916-734-3862

Joel D. Cooper · (Lung Transplantation) · Professor of Surgery, Washington University School of Medicine · Barnes Hospital · Suite 3108, Queeny Tower, Barnes Hospital Plaza, St. Louis, MO 63110 · 314-362-6021

Jean Deslauriers · Associate Professor of Surgery, Laval University · Chief, Thoracic Surgery Division, and Head, Thoracic Surgery, Hôpital Laval, Le Centre de Pneumologie de Laval · 2725 Chemin Sainte-Foy, Sainte-Foy, Quebec, Quebec G1V 4G5 · 418-656-4747

L. Penfield Faber · Associate Dean of Surgical Sciences & Services, and Professor of Surgery, Rush Medical College · Rush-Presbyterian-St. Luke's Medical Center 1725 West Harrison Street, Suite 218, Chicago, IL 60612 · 312-738-3732

Robert L. Ginsberg · (Esophageal Cancer, Lung Cancer) · Chief, Thoracic Surgery, Memorial Sloan-Kettering Cancer Center · 1275 York Avenue, New York, NY 10021 · 212-639-2806

Hermes C. Grillo · (Tracheal Surgery, Esophageal Surgery) · Professor of Surgery, Harvard Medical School · Chief, General Thoracic Surgery, Massachusetts General Hospital · Fruit Street, Boston, MA 02114 · 617-726-2811

E. Carmack Holmes · Professor of Surgery, Department of Surgery, Oncology, University of California at Los Angeles School of Medicine · University of California at Los Angeles Medical Center · UCLA Factor Building, Ninth Floor, Los Angeles, CA 90024 · 213-206-1028

James B. D. Mark · (Lung Cancer) · Professor of Cardiothoracic Surgery, Stanford University School of Medicine · Head, Division of Thoracic Surgery, Stanford University Hospital · Falk Cardiovascular Research Building, 300 Pasteur Drive, Stanford, CA 94305 · 415-723-6649

Douglas J. Mathisen · (Tracheal Surgery, Esophageal Surgery) · Associate Professor of Surgery, Harvard Medical School · Associate Visiting Surgeon, Massachusetts General Hospital · Warren 1109, Department of Thoracic Surgery, Boston, MA 02114 · 617-726-6826

Martin F. McKneally · Professor and Chairman, Division of Thoracic Surgery, University of Toronto School of Medicine · Head, Division of Thoracic Surgery, The Toronto Hospital · 200 Elizabeth Street, Eaton Building North, Room 10-226, Toronto, Ontario M5G 2C4 · 416-340-5033

Joseph Miller · (Esophageal Surgery) · Professor of Surgery—Cardiothoracic, Emory University School of Medicine · Chief of Thoracic Surgery, Crawford W. Long Hospital; Emory University Affiliated Hospitals · 1365 Clifton Road, N.E., Atlanta, GA 30322 · 404-248-3486

Mark B. Orringer · (Esophageal Surgery) · Professor of Surgery, The University of Michigan Medical School · The University of Michigan Medical Center · 1500 East Medical Center Drive, 2120 Taubman Center, Box 0344, Ann Arbor, MI 48109 · 313-936-4975

Peter C. Pairolero · (Esophageal Surgery) · Professor, Department of Surgery, Mayo Medical School · Head, Section of General Thoracic Surgery, Department of Surgery, Mayo Clinic · 200 First Street, SW, Rochester, MN 55905 · 507-284-2808

G. Alexander Patterson · (Lung Transplantation) · Professor of Surgery, Washington University School of Medicine · Attending Physician, Barnes Hospital · One Barnes Hospital Plaza, Suite 3108 Queeny Tower, St. Louis, MO 63110 · 314-362-6025

F. Griffith Pearson · (Tracheal Tumors, Esophageal Surgery) · University of Toronto School of Medicine · The Toronto General Hospital · 200 Elizabeth Street, Eaton Building North 10-233, Toronto, Ontario M5G 2C4 · 416-340-3432

Jack A. Roth · Professor and Chairman, Department of Thoracic Surgery, The University of Texas System Cancer Center · The University of Texas MD Anderson Cancer Center · Department of Thoracic Surgery, 1515 Holcombe Boulevard, Box 109, Houston, TX 77030 · 713-792-6932

Valerie W. Rusch · Associate Professor of Surgery, Cornell University Medical College · Associate Attending Surgeon, Memorial Sloan-Kettering Cancer Center 1275 York Avenue, New York, NY 10021 · 212-639-5873

David B. Skinner · (Esophageal Cancer) · Professor of Surgery , Cornell University Medical College · The New York Hospital-Cornell Medical Center · 525 East 68th Street, New York, NY 10021 · 212-746-4000

Victor F. Trastek · (Esophageal Cancer) · Associate Professor of Surgery, Mayo Medical School · Constultant, Section of General Thoracic Surgery, Mayo Clinic 200 First Street, SW, Rochester, MN 55905 · 507-284-2942

Harold C. Urschel, Jr. · (Thoracic Outlet Disorders) · Professor of Cardiovascular and Thoracic Surgery, The University of Texas Southwestern Medical Center at Dallas · 3600 Gaston Avenue, Suite 1201, Dallas, TX 75246 · 214-824-2503

PEDIATRIC CARDIAC SURGERY

James A. Alexander · Professor of Thoracic Surgery, University of Florida College of Medicine · Shands Hospital at the University of Florida · J Hillis Miller Health Center, P.O. Box 286, Gainesville, FL 32610 · 904-395-0630

Leonard L. Bailey · (Heart Transplantation) · Professor of Surgery, Loma Linda University School of Medicine · Head, Divison of Cardiothoracic Surgery, and Director of Cardiothoracic Residency Program, Loma Linda University Medical Center · 11234 Anderson Street, Room 2560, Loma Linda, CA 92354 · 714-824-4200

Edward L. Bove · Professor of Surgery, The University of Michigan Medical School · The University of Michigan Medical Center · 2120 Taubman Box 0344, 1500 East Medical Center Drive, Ann Arbor, MI 48109 · 313-936-4980

John William Brown · Professor of Surgery, Indiana University School of Medicine · Chief, Section of Cardiothoracic Surgery, James Whitcomb Riley Hospital for Children; Indiana University Medical Center · 545 Barnhill Drive, IUMC/EM212, Indianapolis, IN 46202 · 317-274-7150

Aldo R. Castaneda · William E. Ladd Professor of Child Surgery, Harvard Medical School · Children's Hospital · Department of Cardiac Surgery, 300 Longwood Avenue, Boston, MA 02115 · 617-735-7932

Gordon K. Danielson · Roberts Professor of Surgery, and Chairman, Division of Thoracic and Cardiovascular Surgery, Mayo Medical School · St. Mary's Hospital Rochester, MN 55905 · 507-255-7062

Richard Alan Hopkins · Associate Professor of Surgery, Georgetown University School of Medicine · Georgetown University Medical Center · Four Pasquerilla Health Care Center, 3800 Reservoir Road, NW, Washington, DC 20007 · 202-687-1265

Richard A. Jonas · Associate Professor of Surgery, Harvard Medical School · Senior Associate in Cardiac Surgery, Children's Hospital · Hunnewell Building, 300 Longwood Avenue, Room 319, Boston, MA 02115 · 617-735-7930

Hillel Laks · Professor and Chief of Cardiothoracic Surgery, University of California at Los Angeles School of Medicine · Chief of Cardiothoracic Surgery, and Director of Heart and Lung Transplantation, University of California at Los Angeles Hospital/Clinic · UCLA Medical Center, Room 62-182A, Division TS, Los Angeles, CA 90024-1741 · 310-206-8232

Constantine Mavroudis · Professor of Surgery, Northwestern University Medical School · Division Head and A.C. Buehler Professor of Cardiovascular-Thoracic Surgery, The Children's Memorial Hospital · 2300 Children's Plaza, Box 22, Chicago, IL 60614 · 312-880-4378

John E. Mayer, Jr. · Associate Professor of Surgery, Harvard Medical School · Senior Associate, Cardiac Surgery, Children's Hospital · 300 Longwood Avenue, Boston, MA 02115 · 617-735-8258

William I. Norwood · Professor of Surgery, University of Pennsylvania School of Medicine · Chief, Cardiothoracic Surgery, The Children's Hospital of Philadelphia · 34th Street and Civic Center Boulevard, Philadelphia, PA 19104 · 215-590-1000

Albert D. Pacifico · Professor and Director of Cardiothoracic Surgery, The University of Alabama School of Medicine · The University of Alabama Hospital · 1900 University Boulevard, Suite 760THT, Birmingham, AL 35294 · 205-934-2344

Francisco J. Puga · Professor of Surgery, Mayo Medical School · Head, Section of Cardiovascular Surgery, St. Mary's Hospital · 200 First Street, SW, Rochester, MN 55905 · 507-284-2644

Jan M. Quaegebeur · Chief, Pediatric Cardiothoracic Surgery, and Associate Professor of Surgery, College of Physicians & Surgeons of Columbia University · Attending Surgeon, Columbia-Presbyterian Medical Center · 177 Fort Washington Avenue, Seventh Floor, Room 435, New York, NY 10032 · 212-305-5975

Robert M. Sade · Professor of Surgery, Medical University of South Carolina · Medical University of South Carolina Hospital · 171 Ashley Avenue, Room 409, Department of Surgery, Charleston, SC 29425 · 803-792-3361

Thomas L. Spray · Associate Professor of Surgery, Washington University School of Medicine · Director, Pediatric Cardiac Surgery, Children's Hospital; Barnes Hospital · 5W24 St. Louis Children's Hospital, St. Louis, MO 63110 · 314-362-6311, 454-6165

Vaughn A. Starnes · (Heart & Lung Transplantation) · Associate Professor of Cardiothoracic Surgery, Stanford University School of Medicine · Chief of the Cardiothoracic Surgical Service, Lucile Salter Packard Children's Hospital at Stanford · 300 Pasteur Drive, Stanford, CA 94305 · 415-723-5771

George A. Trusler · Professor of Surgery, University of Toronto School of Medicine · The Hospital for Sick Children · 555 University Avenue, Suite 1525, Toronto, Ontario M5G 1X8 · 416-598-6420

Bill G. Williams · (Congenital Cardiac Surgery) · Professor of Surgery, University of Toronto School of Medicine · Chief, Cardiovascular Surgery, The Hospital for Sick Children · 555 University Avenue, Suite 1525, Toronto, Ontario M5G 1X8 · 416-597-0715

PEDIATRIC NON-CARDIAC THORACIC SURGERY

J. Alex Haller, Jr. · (Lung, Trachea, Esophagus) · Professor of Pediatric Surgery, and Professor of Emergency Medicine, Johns Hopkins University School of Medicine · Pediatric Surgeon-in-Charge of Pediatric Surgery, and Robert Garrett Professor of Pediatric Surgery, The Johns Hopkins Medical Institutions · 600 North Wolfe Street, CMSC 7-113, Baltimore, MD 21205 · 410-955-6256

H. Biemann Othersen, Jr. · (Lung, Trachea, Esophagus) · Professor of Surgery & Pediatrics, Medical University of South Carolina · Medical University of South Carolina Hospital · 171 Ashley Avenue, Charleston, SC 29425 · 803-792-3851

THORACIC ONCOLOGICAL SURGERY

John R. Benfield · Professor and Chief of Division of Cardiothoracic Surgery, and Vice-Chairman, Department of Surgery, University of California at Davis School of Medicine · University of California at Davis Medical Center · 4301 X Street, Suite 2250, Sacramento, CA 95817 · 916-734-3862

L. Penfield Faber · Associate Dean of Surgical Sciences & Services, and Professor of Surgery, Rush Medical College · Rush-Presbyterian-St. Luke's Medical Center 1725 West Harrison Street, Suite 218, Chicago, IL 60612 · 312-738-3732

Robert L. Ginsberg · (Esophageal Cancer, Lung Cancer) · Chief, Thoracic Surgery, Memorial Sloan-Kettering Cancer Center · 1275 York Avenue, New York, NY 10021 · 212-639-2806

Hermes C. Grillo · (Tracheal Surgery, Esophageal Surgery) · Professor of Surgery, Harvard Medical School · Chief, General Thoracic Surgery, Massachusetts General Hospital · Fruit Street, Boston, MA 02114 · 617-726-2811

E. Carmack Holmes · Professor of Surgery, Department of Surgery, Oncology, University of California at Los Angeles School of Medicine · University of California at Los Angeles Medical Center · UCLA Factor Building, Ninth Floor, Los Angeles, CA 90024 · 213-206-1028

James B. D. Mark · (Lung Cancer) · Professor of Cardiothoracic Surgery, Stanford University School of Medicine · Head, Division of Thoracic Surgery, Stanford University Hospital · Falk Cardiovascular Research Building, 300 Pasteur Drive, Stanford, CA 94305 · 415-723-6649

Douglas J. Mathisen · (Tracheal Surgery, Esophageal Surgery) · Associate Professor of Surgery, Harvard Medical School · Associate Visiting Surgeon, Massachusetts General Hospital · Warren 1109, Department of Thoracic Surgery, Boston, MA 02114 · 617-726-6826

Martin F. McKneally · Professor and Chairman, Division of Thoracic Surgery, University of Toronto School of Medicine · Head, Division of Thoracic Surgery, The Toronto Hospital · 200 Elizabeth Street, Eaton Building North, Room 10-226, Toronto, Ontario M5G 2C4 · 416-340-5033

Joseph Miller · (Esophageal Surgery) · Professor of Surgery—Cardiothoracic, Emory University School of Medicine · Chief of Thoracic Surgery, Crawford W. Long Hospital; Emory University Affiliated Hospitals · 1365 Clifton Road, N.E., Atlanta, GA 30322 · 404-248-3486

Mark B. Orringer · (Esophageal Surgery) · Professor of Surgery, The University of Michigan Medical School · The University of Michigan Medical Center · 1500 East Medical Center Drive, 2120 Taubman Center, Box 0344, Ann Arbor, MI 48109 · 313-936-4975

Peter C. Pairolero · (Esophageal Cancer) · Professor, Department of Surgery, Mayo Medical School · Head, Section of General Thoracic Surgery, Department of Surgery, Mayo Clinic · 200 First Street, SW, Rochester, MN 55905 · 507-284-2808

Harvey I. Pass · Senior Investigator, Surgery Branch, and Head, Thoracic Oncology Section, National Cancer Institute, National Institutes of Health · 9000 Rockville Pike, Building 10, Room 2B07, Bethesda, MD 20892 · 301-496-2128

F. Griffith Pearson · (Tracheal Tumors, Esophageal Surgery) · University of Toronto School of Medicine · The Toronto General Hospital · 200 Elizabeth Street, Eaton Building North 10-233, Toronto, Ontario M5G 2C4 · 416-340-3432

Jack A. Roth · Professor and Chairman, Department of Thoracic Surgery, The University of Texas System Cancer Center · The University of Texas MD Anderson Cancer Center · Department of Thoracic Surgery, 1515 Holcombe Boulevard, Box 109, Houston, TX 77030 · 713-792-6932

David B. Skinner · (Esophageal Cancer) · Professor of Surgery, Cornell University Medical College · The New York Hospital-Cornell Medical Center · 525 East 68th Street, New York, NY 10021 · 212-746-4000

Victor F. Trastek · (Esophageal Surgery) · Associate Professor of Surgery, Mayo Medical School · Constultant, Section of General Thoracic Surgery, Mayo Clinic 200 First Street, SW, Rochester, MN 55905 · 507-284-2942

TRANSPLANTATION
(See also Cardiovascular Disease, Heart Transplantation; General Surgery, Transplantation; Infectious Disease, Transplantation Infections)

Margaret D. Allen · (Heart Transplantation) · Assistant Professor of Surgery, and Director of Cardiac Transplantation, University of Washington School of Medicine 1959 Northeast Pacific Street, Seattle, WA 98195 · 206-543-5517

Leonard L. Bailey · (Heart Transplantation) · Professor of Surgery, Loma Linda University School of Medicine · Head, Divison of Cardiothoracic Surgery, and Director of Cardiothoracic Residency Program, Loma Linda University Medical Center · 11234 Anderson Street, Room 2560, Loma Linda, CA 92354 · 714-824-4200

John C. Baldwin · (Heart & Lung Transplantation) · Professor and Chief, Cardiothoracic Surgery, Yale University School of Medicine · Cardiothoracic Surgeon-in-Chief, Yale-New Haven Hospital · 333 Cedar Street, 121 FMB, New Haven, CT 06510 · 203-785-2704

R. Morton Bolman III · (Heart Transplantation, Lung Transplantation, Heart & Lung Transplantation) · Professor and Chief, Division of Cardiovascular and Thoracic Surgery, Department of Surgery, University of Minnesota School of Medicine · University of Minnesota Hospital & Clinics · 425 East River Road, Box 207 UMHC, Minneapolis, MN 55455 · 612-625-3902

Joel D. Cooper · (Lung Transplantation) · Professor of Surgery, Washington University School of Medicine · Barnes Hospital · Suite 3108, Queeny Tower, Barnes Hospital Plaza, St. Louis, MO 63110 · 314-362-6021

Jack G. Copeland · (Heart Transplantation) · The Michael Drummond Distinguished Professor of Cardiovascular and Thoracic Surgery, The University of Arizona College of Medicine · Chief, Section of Cardiovascular & Thoracic Surgery, and Director, Cardiac Transplantation & Artificial Heart Program, and Co-Director, University Heart Center, The University of Arizona Health Sciences Center · 1501 North Campbell Avenue, Tucson, AZ 85724 · 602-626-6339

O. H. Frazier · (Heart Transplantation) · Professor of Surgery, The University of Texas Medical School at Houston · Chief, Transplant Service, and Co-Director, Cullen Cardiovascular Research Laboratories, Texas Heart Institute · 1101 Bates Street, Suite P306, Houston, TX 77030 · 713-791-3000

William Gay · (Heart Transplantation) · Professor and Chairman, Department of Surgery, University of Utah School of Medicine · University of Utah Health Sciences Center · 50 North Medical Drive, Salt Lake City, UT 84132 · 801-581-7304

Bartley P. Griffith · (Heart Transplantation, Lung Transplantation, Heart & Lung Transplantation) · Professor of Surgery, University of Pittsburgh School of Medicine · Chief, Division of Cardiothoracic Surgery, Presbyterian University Hospital · 1084 Scaife Hall, Pittsburgh, PA 15261 · 412-648-9890

James K. Kirklin · (Heart Transplantation) · Professor of Surgery, The University of Alabama School of Medicine · The University of Alabama Hospital · Birmingham, AL 35294 · 205-934-3368

Philip E. Oyer · (Heart Transplantation) · Professor of Cardiothoracic Surgery, Stanford University School of Medicine · Stanford University Hospital · Department of Cardiac Surgery, CVRB Upper Level North, Stanford Medical Center, Stanford, CA 94305 · 415-723-5771

G. Alexander Patterson · (Lung Transplantation) · Professor of Surgery, Washington University School of Medicine · Attending Physician, Barnes Hospital · One Barnes Hospital Plaza, Suite 3108 Queeny Tower, St. Louis, MO 63110 · 314-362-6025

Bruce A. Reitz · (Heart Transplantation, Heart & Lung Transplantation) · Professor of Surgery, Johns Hopkins University School of Medicine · Cardiac Surgeon-in-Charge, The Johns Hopkins Medical Institutions; Sinai Hospital of Baltimore · Blalock Building, 600 North Wolfe Street, Room 618, Baltimore, MD 21205 · 410-955-2800

Eric A. Rose · (Heart Transplantation) · Associate Professor of Surgery, College of Physicians & Surgeons of Columbia University · Columbia-Presbyterian Medical Center · 622 West 168th Street, New York, NY 10032 · 212-305-6380

Norman E. Shumway · (Heart Transplantation) · Professor and Chairman, Department of Cardiothoracic Surgery, Stanford University School of Medicine · Stanford University Hospital · Falk Cardiovascular Research Center, Stanford, CA 94305-5247 · 415-723-5771

Vaughn A. Starnes · (Heart & Lung Transplantation) · Associate Professor of Cardiothoracic Surgery, Stanford University School of Medicine · Chief of the Cardiothoracic Surgical Service, Lucile Salter Packard Children's Hospital at Stanford · 300 Pasteur Drive, Stanford, CA 94305 · 415-723-5771

Edward E. Stinson · (Heart Transplantation) · The Thelma & Henry Doelger Professor of Cardiovascular Surgery, Department of Cardiothoracic Surgery, Stanford University School of Medicine · Stanford University Hospital · Falk Cardiovascular Research Center, 300 Pasteur Drive, Stanford, CA 94305-5247 · 415-723-5771

J. Kent Trinkle · (Lung Transplantation) · Professor and Head, Department of Cardiothoracic Surgery, The University of Texas Health Science Center at San Antonio · 7703 Floyd Curl Drive, San Antonio, TX 78284 · 512-567-5617

Paul F. Waters · (Lung Transplantation) · Clinical Assistant Professor of Surgery, University of California at Los Angeles School of Medicine · Director, Lung Transplant Program, Cedars-Sinai Medical Center · 8700 Beverly Boulevard, Suite 6215, Los Angeles, CA 90048-1869 · 213-855-3851

UROLOGY

ENDOUROLOGY

Richard K. Babayan · (Stone Disease, Ureteroscopy) · Professor of Urology, Boston University School of Medicine · The University Hospital · 720 Harrison Avenue, Suite 606, Boston, MA 02118 · 617-638-8485

Gopal H. Badlani · (Stone Disease, Ureteroscopy) · Associate Professor of Urology, Albert Einstein College of Medicine · Chief, Division of Neurourology & Prosthetics, Long Island Jewish Medical Center · 270-05 Seventy-Sixth Avenue, New Hyde Park, NY 11042 · 718-470-7225

Demetrius H. Bagley · (Stone Disease, Ureteroscopy) · Professor of Urology and Associate Professor of Radiology, Jefferson Medical College of Thomas Jefferson University · 1025 Walnut, Room 1112, Philadelphia, PA 19107 · 215-955-6961

Culley C. Carson III · (Stone Disease, Ureteroscopy) · Professor of Urology, Duke University School of Medicine · Duke University Medical Center · P.O. Box 3274, Durham NC 27710 · 919-684-2127

Ralph V. Clayman · (Stone Disease, Ureteroscopy, Percutaneous Stone Removal) Professor of Urologic Surgery and Radiology, Washington University School of Medicine · Barnes Hospital · 4960 Audubon Avenue, St. Louis, MO 63110 · 314-362-8208

George W. Drach · (Stone Disease) · Professor of Surgery, Section of Urology, The University of Arizona College of Medicine · The University of Arizona Health Sciences Center · 1501 North Campbell Avenue, Tucson, AZ 85724 · 602-626-6236

Stephen P. Dretler · (Stone Disease, Ureteroscopy) · Associate Professor of Urology, Harvard Medical School · Director of the Lithotriptor Unit, Massachusetts General Hospital · 15 Parkman Street, Boston, MA 02114 · 617-726-3512

Gerhard J. Fuchs · (Stone Disease, Ureteroscopy) · Associate Professor of Surgery/Urology, University of California at Los Angeles School of Medicine · Director of the UCLA Stone Center, University of California at Los Angeles Center for the Health Sciences · 10833 LeConte Avenue, Room CHS-BU 183, Los Angeles, CA 90024 · 310-825-1172

Donald P. Griffith · (Stone Disease, Ureteroscopy) · Professor of Urology, Baylor College of Medicine · The Methodist Hospital · 6560 Fannin Street, Suite 1002, Houston, TX 77030 · 713-798-4001

Jeffry L. Huffman · (Stone Disease, Ureteroscopy) · Associate Professor of Urology, University of Southern California School of Medicine · University of Southern California University Hospital · 1441 Eastlake Avenue, Los Angeles, CA 90033 · 213-222-2345

John C. Hulbert · (Ureteroscopy, Percutaneous Renal Surgery, Laparoscopic Urologic Surgery) · Associate Professor of Urology and Director of Endocrinology & ESWL, University of Minnesota School of Medicine · University of Minnesota Hospital & Clinics · 420 Delaware Street SE, Box 394, Minneapolis, MN 55455 612-625-3209

Alan D. Jenkins · (Stone Disease, Ureteroscopy) · Associate Professor of Urology, University of Virginia School of Medicine · University of Virginia Health Sciences Center · Hospital Drive, Box 422, Charlottesville, VA 22908 · 804-924-2224

Robert I. Kahn · (Stone Disease, Ureteroscopy) · Attending Urologist, California Pacific Medical Center · 2100 Webster Street, Suite 309, San Francisco, CA 94115 415-668-4336

James E. Lingeman · (Stone Disease, Ureteroscopy) · Director of Research, Methodist Hospital, Institute for Kidney Stone Disease · 1801 North Senate Boulevard, Suite 655, Indianapolis, IN 46202 · 317-924-1361

Glenn M. Preminger · (Stone Disease, Ureteroscopy) · Associate Professor of Urology, Radiology & Internal Medicine, The University of Texas Southwestern Medical Center at Dallas · Department of Urology, 5323 Harry Hines Boulevard, J8 112, Dallas, TX 75235-9031 · 214-688-4766

Joseph W. Segura · (Stone Disease, Ureteroscopy, Percutaneous Stone Removal) Carl Rosen Professor of Urology, Mayo Medical School · Mayo Clinic · 200 First Street, SW, Rochester, MN 55905 · 507-284-2297

Arthur D. Smith · (Stone Disease, Percutaneous Stone Removal, Ureteroscopy) Professor of Urology, Albert Einstein College of Medicine · Long Island Jewish Medical Center · New Hyde Park, NY 11042 · 718-470-7220

Raju Thomas · (Stone Disease, Ureteroscopy, Laparoscopy) · Director of Urology Program, and Associate Professor of Urology,and Chief, Section of Endourology and ESWL, Tulane University School of Medicine · Tulane University Medical Center · 1430 Tulane Avenue, New Orleans, LA 70112-2699 · 504-588-5271

Howard N. Winfield · (Stone Disease, Ureteroscopy, Percutaneous, Laparoscopic Surgery) · Assistant Professor of Urology, The University of Iowa College of Medicine · The University of Iowa Hospitals & Clinics · 200 Hawkins Drive, Room 3241 Roy Carver Pavilion, Iowa City, IA 52242 · 319-356-1895

IMPOTENCE
(See also General Surgery, General Vascular Surgery [Impotence])

David M. Barrett · Professor of Urology, and Chairman, Department of Urology, Mayo Medical School · Mayo Clinic · 200 First Street, SW, Rochester, MN 55905 507-284-2248

George S. Benson · (Implants) · Professor of Surgery (Urology), The University of Texas Medical School at Houston · Chief of Urology, Lyndon B. Johnson General Hospital; Attending Staff, Hermann Hospital · 6431 Fannin, Suite 6018, Houston, TX 77030 · 713-792-5640

Culley C. Carson III · Professor of Urology, Duke University School of Medicine Duke University Medical Center · P.O. Box 3274, Durham NC 27710 · 919-684-2127

Irving J. Fishman · (Implants) · Associate Professor of Urology, Baylor College of Medicine · St. Luke's Episcopal Hospital; The Methodist Hospital · 6624 Fannin Street, Suite 1280, Houston, TX 77030 · 713-798-5150

William P. Fitch III · (Penile Revascularization) · Clinical Associate Professor, The University of Texas Health Science Center at San Antonio · Humana San Antonio Hospital · 8042 Wurzbach, Suite 380, San Antonio, TX 78229 · 512-616-0410

Irwin Goldstein · (Microvascular Arterial Bypass Surgery for Impotence) · Professor of Urology, Boston University School of Medicine · Co-Director, New England Male Reproductive Center; The University Hospital · 720 Harrison Avenue, Suite 606, Boston, MA 02118 · 617-638-8485

Robert Krane · Professor & Chairman, Department of Urology, Boston University School of Medicine · Chief of Urology, The University Hospital · 720 Harrison Avenue, Suite 606, Boston, MA 02118 · 617-638-8485

Ronald W. Lewis · Professor of Urology, Mayo Medical School · Consultant in Urology, Mayo Clinic · 200 First Street, SW, Rochester, MN 55905 · 507-284-2511

Tom F. Lue · Associate Professor of Urology, University of California at San Francisco School of Medicine · Attending Physician, University of California at San Francisco Medical Center · 400 Parnassus Avenue, Room 610, San Francisco, CA 94143 · 415-476-0565

Arnold Melman · Professor and Chairman, Department of Urology, Albert Einstein College of Medicine · Montefiore Medical Center · 111 East 210th Street, Department of Urology, Bronx, NY 10467 · 212-920-5402

Drogo K. Montague · Head, Section of Prosthetic Surgery, Department of Urology, The Cleveland Clinic Foundation · One Clinic Center, 9500 Euclid Avenue, Cleveland, OH 44195-5041 · 216-444-5590

Alvaro Morales · Professor & Chairman of Urology, Queens University · Urologist-in-Chief, Kingston General Hospital; Urologist-in-Chief, Hotel Dieu Hospital · Victory Four, Kingston General Hospital, Kingston Ontario K7L 2V7 · 613-546-3710

John J. Mulcahy · (Implants) · Professor of Urology, Indiana University School of Medicine · Chief of Urology, Wishard Memorial Hospital; Indiana University Medical Center · 1001 West 10th Street, OPE320B, Indianapolis, IN 46202 · 317-630-6229

Jacob Rajfer · Professor of Surgery/Urology, University of California, Los Angeles School of Medicine · Chief, Division of Urology, Harbor-UCLA Medical Center; UCLA Hospital; St. Mary's Medical Center · 10833 LeConte Avenue, Los Angeles, CA 90024-1738 · 213-206-8164

NEURO-UROLOGY & VOIDING DYSFUNCTION
(See also Geriatric Medicine, Urinary Incontinence)

Rodney A. Appell · Professor and Vice-Chairman, Department of Urology, Louisiana State University School of Medicine · Director, Urodynamics Unit, Louisiana State University Medical Center; Meadowcrest Hospital; West Jefferson Medical Center · 1542 Tulane Avenue, New Orleans, LA 70112-2822 · 504-394-7000

Said A. Awad · Professor and Head, Department of Urology, Dalhousie University · Victoria General Hospital · 1278 Tower Road, Centennial Wing, Room 5014, Halifax, Nova Scotia B3H 2Y9 · 902-428-2469

David M. Barrett · Professor of Urology, and Chairman, Department of Urology, Mayo Medical School · Mayo Clinic · 200 First Street, SW, Rochester, MN 55905 507-284-2248

George S. Benson · Professor of Surgery (Urology), The University of Texas Medical School at Houston · Chief of Urology, Lyndon B. Johnson General Hospital; Attending Staff, Hermann Hospital · 6431Fannin, Suite 6018, Houston, TX 77030 · 713-792-5640

Jerry G. Blaivas · Professor of Urology, and Director of Neurourology, College of Physicians & Surgeons of Columbia University · Columbia-Presbyterian Medical Center · 622 West 168th Street, PH1043, New York, NY 10032 · 212-305-8946

Ruben F. Gittes · (Female Stress Incontinence) · Chairman, Department of Surgery, Green Hospital of Scripps Clinic; Sharp Memorial Hospital · 10666 North Torrey Pines Road, La Jolla, CA 92037 · 619-554-9881

Sender Herschorn · University of Toronto School of Medicine · Chief of Urology, Sunnybrook Health Science Center · 2075 Bayview Avenue, Suite A139, Toronto, Ontario M4N 3M5 · 416-480-4733

Gary E. Leach · Associate Clinical Professor of Urology, University of California at Los Angeles School of Medicine · Chief of Urology, Kaiser Permanente Medical Center · 4900 Sunset Boulevard, Second Floor, Department of Urology, Los Angeles, CA 90027 · 213-667-3981

J. Keith Light · Professor and Chairman, Department of Urology, State University of New York at Syracuse · Attending Staff, University Hospital · 750 East Adams Street, Syracuse, NY 13210 · 315-464-4473

Jorge L. Lockhart · (Reconstructive Urology) · Professor of Surgery and Director, Division of Urology, University South Florida College of Medicine · Tampa General Hospital, H. Lee Moffitt Cancer Center; Harbourside Medical Tower · 12902 Magnolia Drive, Tampa, FL 33612-0179 · 813-972-8479

Edward J. McGuire · (Incontinence) · Professor of Urology, The University of Michigan Medical School · Head, Section of Urology, Department of Surgery, The University of Michigan Medical Center · 2916 Taubman Center, 1500 East Medical Center Drive, Box 0330, Ann Arbor, MI 48109-0330 · 313-936-5775

Shlomo Raz · (Female Incontinence and Pelvic Floor Prolapse) · Associate Professor of Surgery & Urology, University of California at Los Angeles School of Medicine · 10833 LeConte Avenue, Room BU134F, Los Angeles, CA 90024 · 310-825-0496

David R. Staskin · Assistant Professor of Surgery (Urology), Harvard Medical School · Director of Urodynamics & Incontinence Center, Beth Israel Hospital · 330 Brookline Avenue, Libby 105, Boston, MA 02215 · 617-735-5619

Emil A. Tanagho · Professor and Chairman, Department of Urology, University of California at San Francisco School of Medicine · Moffitt-Long Hospital · Department of Urology, Box 0738, San Francisco, CA 94143-0738 · 415-476-8800

George D. Webster · Associate Professor of Neurology, Duke University School of Medicine · Head, Reconstructive Urology & Neurourology, Duke University Medical Center · P.O. Box 3146, Durham, NC 27710 · 919-684-2516

Alan J. Wein · Professor and Chairman, Division of Urology, University of Pennsylvania School of Medicine · Chief of Urology, Hospital of the University of Pennsylvania · 3400 Spruce Street, Five Silverstein, Philadelphia, PA 19104 · 215-662-2891

Jeffrey R. Woodside · Professor of Urology, The University of Texas Health Science Center at Houston · Vice-President, Hermann Hospital · 6431 Fannin Street, 6.018 MSB, Houston, TX 77030 · 713-793-5444

PEDIATRIC UROLOGY

Terry D. Allen · Professor of Urology, The University of Texas Southwestern Medical Center at Dallas · Children's Medical Center · 5323 Harry Hines Boulevard, Dallas, TX 75235 · 214-688-2740

Stuart B. Bauer · (Neurogenic Bladder Disease) · Professor of Surgery, Harvard Medical School · Senior Associate in Surgery, Children's Hospital · 300 Longwood Avenue, Hunnewell 930, Boston, MA 02115 · 617-735-7796

A. Barry Belman · (Hypospadias Repair) · Professor of Urology and Pediatrics, The George Washington University School of Medicine · Chairman, Department of Pediatric Urology, Children's National Medical Center · 111 Michigan Avenue NW, Washington, DC 20010 · 202-745-5042

John W. Duckett · (Hypospadias) · Professor of Urology, University of Pennsylvania School of Medicine · Director, Division of Urology, The Children's Hospital of Philadelphia · Division of Urology, 34th and Civic Center Boulevard, Philadelphia, PA 19104 · 215-590-2754

Richard M. Ehrlich · Professor of Surgery & Urology, University of California at Los Angeles School of Medicine · University of California at Los Angeles Medical Center · 100 University of California, Los Angeles Medical Plaza, Los Angeles, CA 90024 · 310-825-6865

Casimir F. Firlit · Professor of Urology, Northwestern University Medical School The Children's Memorial Hospital · 2300 Children's Plaza, Chicago, IL 60614 · 312-880-4428

John P. Gearhart · Associate Professor of Pediatric Urology, Johns Hopkins University School of Medicine · Director, Pediatric Urology Division, The Johns Hopkins Medical Institutions · 600 North Wolfe Street, Marburg 149, Baltimore, MD 21205 · 410-955-8710

Edmond T. Gonzales · Professor of Urology, Baylor College of Medicine · Chief, Pediatric Urology Service, and Head, Department of Surgery, Texas Children's Hospital · 6621 Fannin Street, Suite 270, Houston, TX 77030 · 713-770-3160

Ricardo Gonzalez · Professor, Urologic Surgery, University of Minnesota School of Medicine · Director, Pediatric Urology, University of Minnesota Hospital & Clinics · Mayo Building, 420 Delaware Street SE, Box 45, Minneapolis, MN 55455 · 612-625-9117

W. Hardy Hendren · Robert E. Gross Professor of Surgery, Harvard Medical School · Chief of Surgery, Children's Hospital · 300 Longwood Avenue, Boston, MA 02115 · 617-735-8001

Terry W. Hensle · Professor of Urology, College of Physicians & Surgeons of Columbia University · Director, Department of Pediatric Urology, Columbia-Presbyterian Medical Center, Babies Hospital · 3959 Broadway, Room 219 North, New York, NY 10032 · 212-305-8510

Robert D. Jeffs · Professor of Pediatric Urology, Johns Hopkins University School of Medicine · The Johns Hopkins Medical Institutions · Brady Urological Institute, The Marburg Building, 600 North Wolfe Street, Room 146, Baltimore, MD 21205 · 410-955-8710

George Kaplan · Clinical Professor of Surgery and Pediatrics, University of California at San Diego School of Medicine · Chief of Pediatric Urology, Children's Hospital & Health Center · 7930 Frost Street, Suite 407, San Diego, CA 92123 · 619-279-8527

Robert Kay · Head, Section of Pediatric Urology, Department of Urology, The Cleveland Clinic Foundation · One Clinic Center, 9500 Euclid Avenue, Cleveland, OH 44195-5041 · 216-444-5593

Panayotis P. Kelalis · Anson L. Clark Professor of Pediatric Urology, and Chair, Urology, Mayo Clinic Jacksonville · Davis Building, 4500 San Pablo Road, Jacksonville, FL 32224 · 904-223-2000

Lowell King · Head, Section of Pediatric Urology, Duke University School of Medicine · Duke University Medical Center · Box 3831, DUMC, Durham, NC 27710 · 919-684-6994

Stephen A. Koff · Professor, Department of Surgery, Ohio State University College of Medicine · Chief, Section of Pediatric Urology, Columbus Children's Hospital · 700 Children's Drive, Room D301, Columbus, OH 43205 · 614-461-6884

Barry A. Kogan · Associate Professor and Chief of Pediatric Urology, University of California, San Francisco School of Medicine · University of California, San Francisco Medical Center · 400 Parnassus Avenue, Room 610, San Francisco, CA 94143 · 415-476-8800

Stanley J. Kogan · (Pediatric Andrology, Intersex and Reconstructive Surgery) · Professor of Urology, New York Medical College; Associate Professor of Pediatrics, Albert Einstein College of Medicine · Co-Director, Pediatric Urology, Westchester County Medical Center; Attending Pediatric Urologist, Montefiore Medical Center and Affiliated Hospitals · Macy Pavillion—1053, Valhalla, NY 10595 · 914-285-8628

Selwyn B. Levitt · Clinical Professor of Urology, New York Medical College; Visiting Clinical Professor of Pediatrics, Albert Einstein College of Medicine · Co-Director, Division of Pediatric Urology, Westchester County Medical Center; Albert Einstein College Hospital; Montefiore Hospital; Nyack Hospital · Macy Pavillion, Valhalla, NY 10595 · 914-285-8628

Michael E. Mitchell · Professor of Pediatric Urology, University of Washington School of Medicine · Chief of Pediatric Urology, Children's Hospital & Medical Center · P.O. Box C5371, 4800 Sand Point Way NE, F-503, Seattle, WA 98105 · 206-527-3950

Alan D. Perlmutter · Professor of Urology, Wayne State University School of Medicine · Chief, Department of Pediatric Urology, Children's Hospital of Michigan · 3901 Beaubien Boulevard, Detroit, MI 48201 · 313-745-5588

Alan B. Retik · Reconstructive Procedures on the Urinary Tract) · Professor of Surgery, Harvard Medical School · Chief Urologist, Division of Urology, Children's Hospital · 300 Longwood Avenue, Hunnewell 390, Boston, MA 02115 · 617-735-7796

Harry Guilford (Gil) Rushton, Jr. · Assistant Professor of Urology, The George Washington University School of Medicine · Vice Chairman, Department of Pediatric Urology, Children's National Medical Center · 111 Michigan Avenue NW, Washington DC 20010 · 202-745-5042

Linda M. D. Shortliffe · Associate Professor of Urology, Stanford University School of Medicine · Chief of Pediatric Urology, Stanford University Hospital; Lucile Salter Packard Children's Hospital at Stanford · Department of Urology, S-287, Stanford University Medical Center, Stanford, CA 94305 · 415-725-5530

Howard McC. Snyder III · Associate Professor of Urology, University of Pennsylvania School of Medicine · Associate Director of Pediatric Urology, The Children's Hospital of Philadelphia · The Wood Building, 34th and Civic Center Boulevard, Third Floor, Philadelphia, PA 19104 · 215-590-2767

R. Dixon Walker · Professor of Surgery, University of Florida College of Medicine Shands Hospital at the University of Florida · 1600 Southwest Archer Road, Room 2406, P.O. Box 100247, Gainesville, FL 32610 · 904-392-2501

John R. Woodard · Clinical Professor of Surgery (Urology) and Director of Pediatric Urology, Emory University School of Medicine · Chief of Pediatric Urology, Henrietta Egleston Hospital for Children · 1901 Century Boulevard, NE, Suite 14, Atlanta, GA 30345 · 404-320-9179

RENAL HYPERTENSION

E. Darracott Vaughan, Jr. · (Adrenal Hypertension) · James J. Colt Professor of Urology, Cornell University Medical College · Attending-in-Chief, The New York Hospital-Cornell Medical Center · 525 East 68th Street, Box 94, New York, NY 10021 · 212-746-5480

TRANSPLANTATION
(See also Adult Nephrology, Kidney Transplantation; General Surgery, Transplantation; Infectious Disease, Transplantation Infections)

John M. Barry · (Kidney Transplantation) · Chairman, Division of Urology, University of Oregon · The Oregon Health Sciences University · 3181 Southwest Sam Jackson Park Road, Portland, OR 97201-3098 · 503-494-8470

Oscar Salvatierra, Jr. · (Kidney Transplantation) · Executive Director, Pacific Transplant Institute; Director, Pediatric Renal Transplantation, California Pacific Medical Center · 2340 Clay Street, San Francisco, CA 94115 · 415-923-3450

UROLOGIC ONCOLOGY

Alex F. Althausen · Associate Clinical Professor of Surgery, Harvard Medical School · Massachusetts General Hospital · One Hawthorne Place, Boston, MA 02114 · 617-726-3559

David M. Barrett · (Genito-Urinary Cancer) · Professor of Urology, and Chairman, Department of Urology, Mayo Medical School · Mayo Clinic · 200 First Street, SW, Rochester, MN 55905 · 507-284-2248

Stanley A. Brosman · (Intravesical Immunotherapy) · Clinical Professor of Surgery/Urology, University of California at Los Angeles School of Medicine · St. John's Hospital & Health Center; Santa Monica Hospital Medical Center · 1304 Fifteenth Street, Suite 200, Santa Monica, CA 90404 · 213-451-8751

William J. Catalona · (Prostate Cancer) · Professor of Urology, Washington University School of Medicine · Chief, Division of Urology, Barnes Hospital · 4960 Audubon Avenue, Second Floor, Wohl Hospital, St. Louis, MO 63110 · 314-362-8206

David E. Crawford · Professor and Chairman, Division of Urology, Department of Surgery, University of Colorado School of Medicine · University of Colorado Health Sciences Center · 4200 East Ninth Avenue, Box C-319, Denver, CO 80262 303-270-5937

Jean B. deKernion · Professor of Surgery/Urology, University of California at Los Angeles School of Medicine · Chief, Division of Urology, and Head, Urologic Oncology, University of California at Los Angeles Center for the Health Sciences 10833 LeConte Avenue, Room 66-133 CHS, Los Angeles, CA 90024 · 213-206-6453

Ralph W. deVere White · Chairman and Professor of Urology, University of California at Davis School of Medicine · University of California at Davis Medical Center · 4301 X Street, Suite 2210, Sacramento, CA 95817 · 916-734-5154

John P. Donohue · Distinguished Professor and Chairman, Department of Urology, Indiana University School of Medicine · Indiana University Medical Center 926 West Michigan Street, UH1725, Indianapolis, IN 46202-5250 · 317-274-7338

William R. Fair · Professor of Surgery & Urology, Cornell University Medical College · Chief, Urologic Surgery Service, Memorial Sloan-Kettering Cancer Center · 1275 York Avenue, C1061, New York, NY 10021 · 212-639-8139

Robert Charles Flanigan · Professor and Chairman of Urology, Loyola Stritch School of Medicine · Loyola University Medical Center · 2160 South First Avenue, Maywood, IL 60153 · 708-216-9000

H. Barton Grossman · Professor of Urology, The University of Michigan Medical School · Director, Urologic Oncology Program, The University of Michigan Cancer Center · 1500 East Medical Center Drive, Box 0330, Ann Arbor, MI 48109-0330 · 313-936-5755

Harry W. Herr · Associate Professor of Surgery, Cornell University Medical College · Associate Attending Surgeon of Urology and Pediatric Urology, Memorial Sloan-Kettering Cancer Center; The New York Hospital-Cornell Medical Center 1275 York Avenue, C1067, New York, NY 10021 · 212-639-8264

Donald L. Lamm · (Intravesical Immunotherapy) · Chairman, Department of Urology, West Virginia University School of Medicine · Ruby Memorial Hospital Health Sciences Center, Fifth Floor, Morgantown, WV 26506 · 304-293-2706

Paul Henry Lange · Professor and Chairman, Department of Urology, University of Washington School of Medicine · University of Washington Medical Center · 1959 Northeast Pacific Street, RL-10, Seattle, WA 98195 · 206-543-3918

John A. Libertino · (Kidney Reconstruction) · Assistant Clinical Professor of Surgery, Harvard Medical School · Chairman, Division of Surgery, Lahey Clinic Medical Center · 41 Mall Road, Burlington, MA 01805 · 617-273-8420

Michael M. Lieber · Professor of Urology, Mayo Medical School · Consultant in Urology, Mayo Clinic · 200 First Street, SW, Rochester, MN 55905 · 507-284-4427

Gary Lieskovsky · Associate Professor of Surgery/Urology, University of Southern California School of Medicine · The Kenneth Norris Comprehensive Cancer Center · 2025 Zonal Avenue, Suite GH5900, Los Angeles, CA 90033 · 213-224-5005

W. Marston Linehan · (Kidney Tumors) · Assistant Professor of Urology, Uniformed Services University of Health Sciences · Head, Urologic Oncology Section, Clinical Center, National Institutes of Health · 9000 Rockville Pike, Building 10, Room 2B47, Rockville, MD 20892 · 301-496-6353

Fray F. Marshall · Professor of Urology, Johns Hopkins University School of Medicine · Director, Division of Adult Urology, The Johns Hopkins Medical Institutions · 600 North Wolfe Street, Marburg 148, Baltimore, MD 21205 · 410-955-6100

James Montie · Professor of Urologic Oncology, Wayne State University School of Medicine · Harper Hospital · Harper Professional Building, 4160 John R, Suite 1017, Detroit, MI 48201 · 313-745-7381

Alvaro Morales · (Intravesical Immunotherapy) · Professor & Chairman of Urology, Queens University · Urologist-in-Chief, Kingston General Hospital; Urologist-in-Chief, Hotel Dieu Hospital · Victory Four, Kingston General Hospital, Kingston Ontario K7L 2V7 · 613-546-3710

Andrew C. Novick · Chairman, Department of Urology, and Chairman, Organ Transplant Center, The Cleveland Clinic Foundation · One Clinic Center, 9500 Euclid Avenue, Cleveland, OH 44195-5041 · 216-444-5584

Carl A. Olsson · The John K. Lattimer Professor of Urology, and Chairman, Department of Urology, College of Physicians & Surgeons of Columbia University Director, Squier Urological Clinic, The Presbyterian Hospital in the City of New York · 630 West 168th Street, New York, NY 10032 · 212-932-4139

David F. Paulson · Professor of Urologic Surgery, Duke University School of Medicine · Chief of Urologic Surgery, Duke University Medical Center · P.O. Box 2977, Durham, NC 27710 · 919-684-5057

J. Edson Pontes · Professor and Chairman, Department of Urology, Wayne State University School of Medicine · Chairman, Department of Urology, Harper Hospital · 4160 John R Street, Suite 1017, Detroit, MI 48201 · 313-745-7381

Jerome P. Richie · The Elliott C. Cutler Professor of Urological Surgery and Chairman, Harvard Program in Urology (Longwood Area), Harvard Medical School · Chief, Division of Urological Surgery, Brigham & Women's Hospital · 75 Francis Street, Boston, MA 02115 · 617-732-6325

Peter T. Scardino · Professor and Chairman, Department of Urology, Baylor College of Medicine · Baylor University Medical Center · Scurlock Tower, 6560 Fannin Street, Suite 1004, Houston, TX 77030 · 713-798-6153

Paul F. Schellhammer · Professor and Chairman, Department of Urology, Eastern Virginia Medical School · Sentara Hospitals; DePaul Medical Center; The Children's Hospital of the King's Daughters · 400 West Brambleton Avenue, Suite 100, Norfolk, VA 23510 · 804-628-2545

Donald G. Skinner · (Reconstructive Urology) · Professor and Chairman, Department of Urology, University of Southern California School of Medicine · The Los Angeles County University of Southern California Medical Center; USC Kenneth Norris, Jr. Cancer Hospital; USC University Hospital · 2025 Zonal Avenue, Suite GH-5900, Los Angeles, CA 90033 · 213-224-5005

Joseph A. Smith, Jr. · Professor and Chairman, Department of Urology, Vanderbilt University School of Medicine · Vanderbilt University Medical Center · D4314 Medical Center North, Nashville, TN 37232-2765 · 615-322-2142

Mark S. Soloway · (Intravesical Chemotherapy) · Professor of Urology, The University of Tennessee at Memphis, College of Medicine · 956 Court Avenue, Memphis, TN 38163 · 901-528-5868

Thomas Stamey · (Incontinence) · Professor and Chairman, Department of Urology, Stanford University School of Medicine · Stanford University Hospital · 300 Pasteur Drive, Palo Alto, CA 94305 · 415-725-5542

E. Darracott Vaughan, Jr. · James J. Colt Professor of Urology, Cornell University Medical College · Attending-in-Chief, The New York Hospital-Cornell Medical Center · 525 East 68th Street, Box 94, New York, NY 10021 · 212-746-5480

Andrew C. von Eschenbach · Professor of Urology, and Adjunct Professor of Cell Biology, The University of Texas MD Anderson Cancer Center, The University of Texas Health Science Center at Houston; The University of Texas Graduate School of Biomedical Sciences · Chairman, Department of Urology, The University of Texas MD Anderson Cancer Center · 1515 Holcombe Boulevard, Box 110, Houston, TX 77030 · 713-792-3250

Patrick C. Walsh · Professor of Urology, Johns Hopkins University School of Medicine · The Johns Hopkins Medical Institutions; Brady Urology Institute · 600 North Wolfe Street, Baltimore, MD 21205 · 410-955-6100

Alan J. Wein · Professor and Chairman, Division of Urology, University of Pennsylvania School of Medicine · Chief of Urology, Hospital of the University of Pennsylvania · 3400 Spruce Street, Five Silverstein, Philadelphia, PA 19104 · 215-662-2891

Richard D. Williams · Professor and Chairman, Department of Urology, The University of Iowa College of Medicine · The University of Iowa Hospitals & Clinics · Room 3240 RCP, Iowa City, IA 52242 · 319-356-2934

Horst Zincke · Professor of Urology, Mayo Medical School · Mayo Clinic · 200 First Street, SW, Rochester, MN 55905 · 507-284-8588

UROLOGICAL INFECTIONS
(See also Infectious Disease, Urinary Tract Infections)

Edwin M. Meares, Jr. · Professor of Urology, Tufts University School of Medicine New England Medical Center · 171 Harrison Avenue, Boston, MA 02111 · 617-956-5923

Anthony J. Schaeffer · Professor and Chairman, Department of Urology, Northwestern University Medical School · Northwestern Memorial Hospital · Tarry 11-715, 303 East Chicago Avenue, Chicago, IL 60611 · 312-908-8145

INDEX

A

Aaberg, Thomas Marshall · Ophthalmology, Medical Retinal Diseases; Ophthalmology, Vitreo-Retinal Surgery

Abbassi, Val · Pediatrics, Pediatric Endocrinology

Abcarian, Herand · Colon & Rectal Surgery, Colon & Rectal Cancer; Surgical Oncology, Colon & Rectal Cancer

Abel, Elizabeth A. · Dermatology, Clinical Dermatology; Dermatology, Photobiology; Dermatology, Psoriasis

Abel, Martin · Anesthesiology, Adult Cardiovascular

Abeloff, Martin D. · Medical Oncology & Hematology, Breast Cancer

Abend, Sander M. · Psychiatry, Psychoanalysis

Aberman, Arnold · Pulmonary & Critical Care Medicine, General Pulmonary & Critical Care Medicine

Abernethy, Darrell · Clinical Pharmacology

Ablon, Steven L. · Psychiatry, Psychoanalysis

Abram, Stephen E. · Anesthesiology, Pain

Abrams, Gary W. · Ophthalmology, Vitreo-Retinal Surgery

Abrams, Samuel · Psychiatry, Psychoanalysis

Abrass, Itamar B. · Geriatric Medicine, General Geriatric Medicine

Aceto, Thomas · Pediatrics, Pediatric Endocrinology

Achauer, Bruce M. · Plastic Surgery, Laser Surgery & Birthmarks; Plastic Surgery, Reconstructive Surgery

Achord, James L. · Gastroenterology, General Gastroenterology

Achuff, Stephen C. · Cardiovascular Disease, General Cardiovascular Disease

Ackerman, A. Bernard · Dermatology, Dermatopathology; Pathology, Dermatopathology

Adams, Harold P. · Neurology, Adult, Strokes

Adams, Robert M. · Dermatology, Contact Dermatitis

Adashi, Eli Y. · Obstetrics & Gynecology, Reproductive Endocrinology

Adatto, Carl P. · Psychiatry, Psychoanalysis

Adelman, Raymond D. · Pediatrics, Pediatric Nephrology

Adkinson, N. Franklin · Allergy & Immunology, Adult Allergy & Immunology

Ahmann, David L. · Medical Oncology & Hematology, Breast Cancer

Ahmann, Frederick · Medical Oncology & Hematology, Prostate Cancer

Aiello, Lloyd M. · Ophthalmology, Medical Retinal Diseases

Aiman, E. James · Obstetrics & Gynecology, Reproductive Endocrinology

Ajani, Jaffer A. · Medical Oncology, Gastrointestinal Oncology

Akhtar, Masood · Cardiovascular Disease, Electrophysiology

Akins, Cary W. · Thoracic Surgery, Adult Cardiothoracic Surgery

Akiskal, Hagop S. · Psychiatry, Affective Disorders

Al-Mefty, Ossama · Neurological Surgery, Tumor Surgery

Al-Sarraf, Muhyi · Medical Oncology & Hematology, Head & Neck Cancer

Alavi, Abass · Nuclear Medicine, Brain; Nuclear Medicine, General Nuclear Medicine

Alazraki, Naomi P. · Nuclear Medicine, General Nuclear Medicine

Albers, James W. · Neurology, Adult, Electromyography

Albert, Martin · Neurology, Adult, Behavioral Neurology

Albert, Richard K. · Pulmonary & Critical Care Medicine, General Pulmonary & Critical Care Medicine

Alberts, David · Medical Oncology & Hematology, Gynecologic Cancer

Albom, Michael J. · Dermatology, Skin Cancer Surgery & Reconstruction

Alderson, Philip O. · Nuclear Medicine, General Nuclear Medicine; Nuclear Medicine, Pulmonary

Alexander, James A. · Thoracic Surgery, Pediatric Cardiac Surgery

Alexander, L. George · Thoracic Surgery, Adult Cardiothoracic Surgery

Alexander, Randell C. · Pediatrics, Abused Children

Alexander, Steven Roy · Pediatrics, Pediatric Nephrology

Alexanian, Raymond · Medical Oncology & Hematology, Myeloma

Alford, Bobby R. · Otolaryngology, Otology/Neurotology

Allen, Jeffrey C. · Neurology, Child, Neuro-oncology

Allen, Margaret D. · Thoracic Surgery, Adult Cardiothoracic Surgery; Thoracic Surgery, Transplantation

Allen, Terry D. · Urology, Pediatric Urology

Allison, George H. · Psychiatry, Psychoanalysis

Allman, Richard M. · Geriatric Medicine, General Geriatric Medicine

Allo, Maria D. · General Surgery, Endocrine Surgery

Almquist, Edward E. · Hand Surgery, Peripheral Nerve Surgery

Alpert, Bernard S. · Plastic Surgery, Aesthetic Surgery; Plastic Surgery, Breast Surgery; Plastic Surgery, Microsurgery; Plastic Surgery, Reconstructive Surgery

Althausen, Alex F. · Urology, Urologic Oncology

Altman, R. Peter · General Surgery, Pediatric Surgery

Altman, Roy D. · Rheumatology, Osteoarthritis; Rheumatology, Paget's Disease; Rheumatology, Scleroderma

Altshuler, Kenneth Z. · Psychiatry, General Psychiatry; Psychiatry, Psychoanalysis

Alvarado, Jorge A. · Ophthalmology, Glaucoma

Amadio, Peter C. · Hand Surgery, General Hand Surgery

Ambrose, John · Cardiovascular Disease, Cardiac Catheterization

Amend, William J. C. · Nephrology, Kidney Transplantation

Amonette, Rex A. · Dermatology, Skin Cancer Surgery & Reconstruction

Amstey, Marvin S. · Obstetrics & Gynecology, Infectious Disease

Amstutz, Harlan C. · Orthopaedic Surgery, Hip Surgery

Anderman, Fredrick · Neurology, Adult, Epilepsy; Neurology, Child, Epilepsy

Anders, Thomas F. · Psychiatry, Child Psychiatry

Andersen, Arnold E. · Psychiatry, Eating Disorders

Anderson, Dana K. · General Surgery, Endocrine Surgery

Anderson, Douglas R. · Ophthalmology, Glaucoma

Anderson, Garland D. · Obstetrics & Gynecology, Maternal & Fetal Medicine

Anderson, John Albert · Allergy & Immunology, Pediatric Allergy & Immunology

Anderson, Kathryn Duncan · General Surgery, Pediatric Surgery

Anderson, Larry G. · Rheumatology, General Rheumatology

Anderson, Richard L. · Ophthalmology, Oculoplastic & Orbital Surgery

Anderson, Robert W. · Thoracic Surgery, Adult Cardiothoracic Surgery

Anderson, Tom · Medical Oncology & Hematology, Breast Cancer; Medical Oncology & Hematology, Lymphomas

Andiman, Warren A. · Pediatrics, Pediatric Infectious Disease

Andreasen, Nancy C. · Psychiatry, Schizophrenia

Andreoli, Sharon P. · Pediatrics, Pediatric Nephrology

Andrews, James R. · Orthopaedic Surgery, Sports Medicine

Andriole, Vincent T. · Infectious Disease, General Infectious Disease

Anhalt, Grant J. · Dermatology, Cutaneous Immunology

Antel, Jack P. · Neurology, Adult, Infectious & Demyelinating Diseases

Anthony, Elwyn James · Psychiatry, Child Psychiatry; Psychiatry, Psychoanalysis

Antman, Karen · Medical Oncology & Hematology, Bone Marrow Transplantation; Medical Oncology & Hematology, Breast Cancer

Apfelberg, David B. · Plastic Surgery, Laser Surgery & Birthmarks

Appel, Gerald B. · Nephrology, Glomerular Diseases

Appelbaum, Frederick R. · Medical Oncology & Hematology, Bone Marrow Transplantation

Appelbaum, Paul S. · Psychiatry, Forensic Psychiatry

Appell, Rodney A. · Urology, Neuro-Urology & Voiding Dysfunction

Applegate, William B. · Geriatric Medicine, General Geriatric Medicine

Apuzzo, Michael L. J. · Neurological Surgery, Stereotactic Radiosurgery

Arant, Billy S. · Pediatrics, Pediatric Nephrology

Arbus, Gerald Stanley · Pediatrics, Pediatric Nephrology

Archer, David P. · Anesthesiology, Neuroanesthesia

Archer, Gordon L. · Infectious Disease, General Infectious Disease

Ariyan, Stephan · Plastic Surgery, Head & Neck Surgery

Arlin, Zalmen Amos · Medical Oncology, Leukemia

Arlow, Jacob A. · Psychiatry, Psychoanalysis

Armitage, James O. · Medical Oncology & Hematology, Bone Marrow Transplantation; Medical Oncology & Hematology, Lymphomas

Armstrong, Donald · Infectious Disease, AIDS; Infectious Disease, Cancer & Infections; Cardiovascular Disease, Echocardiography

Arnason, Barry G. W. · Neurology, Adult, Degenerative Diseases; Neurology, Adult, Infectious & Demyelinating Diseases

Arndt, Kenneth A. · Dermatology, Clinical Dermatology; Dermatology, Laser Surgery

Arnold, James E. · Otolaryngology, Pediatric Otolaryngology

Arnold, Phillip G. · Plastic Surgery, Reconstructive Surgery

Aronson, Gerald J. · Psychiatry, Psychoanalysis

Arseneau, James Charles · Medical Oncology & Hematology, Gynecologic Cancer

Aruffo, Roy N. · Psychiatry, Psychoanalysis

Arvin, Ann M. · Pediatrics, Pediatric Infectious Disease

Asbury, Arthur K. · Neurology, Adult, General Adult Neurology; Neurology, Adult, Neuromuscular Disease

Asch, Ricardo H. · Obstetrics & Gynecology, Reproductive Endocrinology

Ascher, Nancy L. · General Surgery, Transplantation

Ashburn, William L. · Nuclear Medicine, General Nuclear Medicine

Aston, Sherrell Jerome · Plastic Surgery, Facial Aesthetic Surgery

Astrachan, Boris M. · Psychiatry, General Psychiatry

Atkins, Harold L. · Nuclear Medicine, General Nuclear Medicine

Atkinson, Arthur J. · Clinical Pharmacology

Attie, Joseph N. · General Surgery, Endocrine Surgery

Auerbach, Robert · Dermatology, Psoriasis

Aufses, Arthur H. · General Surgery, Gastroenterologic Surgery

Augsburger, James · Ophthalmology, Ocular Oncology

August, Gilbert Paul · Pediatrics, Pediatric Endocrinology

Austin, John · Radiology, Chest

Averette, Hervy E. · Obstetrics & Gynecology, Gynecologic Cancer

Awad, Said A. · Urology, Neuro-Urology & Voiding Dysfunction

Axel, Leon · Radiology, Cardiovascular Disease; Radiology, Magnetic Resonance
Imaging

Axelrod, Lloyd · Endocrinology & Metabolism, Diabetes

B

Babayan, Richard K. · Urology, Endourology

Bada, Henrietta Salvilla · Pediatrics, Neonatal-Perinatal Medicine

Baden, Howard P. · Dermatology, Psoriasis

Badlani, Gopal H. · Urology, Endourology

Bagley, Demetrius H. · Urology, Endourology

Bagshaw, Malcolm A. · Radiation Oncology, Genito-Urinary Cancer

Bailey, Byron J. · Otolaryngology, Head & Neck Surgery; Otolaryngology, Laryngology

Bailey, Harold Randolph · Colon & Rectal Surgery, General Colon & Rectal Surgery

Bailey, Leonard L. · Thoracic Surgery, Pediatric Cardiac Surgery; Thoracic Surgery, Transplantation

Bailin, Philip L. · Dermatology, Clinical Dermatology; Dermatology, Laser Surgery; Dermatology, Skin Cancer Surgery & Reconstruction

Baim, Donald S. · Cardiovascular Disease, Cardiac Catheterization

Baker, Carol Jane · Pediatrics, Pediatric Infectious Disease

Baker, Daniel C. · Plastic Surgery, Facial Aesthetic Surgery

Baker, F. M. · Psychiatry, Geriatric Psychiatry

Baker, Lester · Pediatrics, Pediatric Endocrinology

Baker, Thomas J. · Plastic Surgery, Facial Aesthetic Surgery

Baker, William Henry · General Surgery, General Vascular Surgery

Balch, Charles M. · Surgical Oncology, Melanoma

Baldassare, Andrew R. · Rheumatology, General Rheumatology

Baldessarini, Ross J. · Psychiatry, Psychopharmacology

Baldwin, David S. · Nephrology, Glomerular Diseases

Baldwin, John C. · Thoracic Surgery, Adult Cardiothoracic Surgery; Thoracic Surgery, Transplantation

Balfe, J. Williamson · Pediatrics, Pediatric Nephrology

Balfour, Henry H. · Pediatrics, Pediatric Infectious Disease

Balkany, Thomas J. · Otolaryngology, Otology/Neurotology

Ball, Gene V. · Rheumatology, General Rheumatology

Ballenger, James C. · Psychiatry, Affective Disorders; Psychiatry, Psychopharmacology

Baluarte, H. Jorge · Pediatrics, Pediatric Nephrology

Bancalari, Eduardo · Pediatrics, Neonatal-Perinatal Medicine

Bandyk, Dennis F. · General Surgery, General Vascular Surgery

Banks, Peter M. · Pathology, Hematopathology

Barash, Paul G. · Anesthesiology, Adult Cardiovascular

Barbieri, Robert L. · Obstetrics & Gynecology, Reproductive Endocrinology

Barbul, Adrian · General Surgery, Wound Healing

Bardana, Emil J. · Allergy & Immunology, Adult Allergy & Immunology

Baringer, Richard J. · Neurology, Adult, Infectious & Demyelinating Diseases

Barker, Clyde F. · General Surgery, Transplantation

Barkin, Jamie S. · Gastroenterology, Endoscopy; Gastroenterology, Pancreatic Disease

Barlogie, Bart · Medical Oncology & Hematology, Myeloma

Barnes, Leon · Pathology, ENT Pathology

Barnes, Robert W. · General Surgery, General Vascular Surgery

Barnett, Henry J. · Neurology, Adult, Strokes

Barr, Joseph S. · Orthopaedic Surgery, Spine Surgery

Barrett, David M. · Urology, Impotence; Urology, Neuro-Urology & Voiding Dysfunction; Urology, Urologic Oncology

Barry, John M. · Urology, Transplantation

Barry, Patricia P. · Geriatric Medicine, General Geriatric Medicine

Bartels, Loren J. · Otolaryngology, Otology/Neurotology

Bartlett, John G. · Infectious Disease, AIDS; Infectious Disease, Anaerobic Infections

Barton, Fritz E. · Plastic Surgery, Reconstructive Surgery

Bass, John Burrell · Pulmonary & Critical Care Medicine, Lung Infections

Bast, Robert C. · Medical Oncology & Hematology, Immunotherapy, Biological Response Modifiers Oncology

Bateman, J. Bronwyn · Ophthalmology, Ophthalmic Genetics

Batsakis, John G. · Pathology, ENT Pathology; Pathology, Surgical Pathology

Bauer, Charles R. · Pediatrics, Neonatal-Perinatal Medicine

Bauer, Eugene A. · Dermatology, Cutaneous Immunology

Bauer, John H. · Nephrology, Hypertension

Bauer, Stuart B. · Urology, Pediatric Urology

Baum, Jules L. · Ophthalmology, Corneal Diseases & Transplantation

Baxter, Donald E. · Orthopaedic Surgery, Foot & Ankle Surgery; Orthopaedic Sugery, Sports Medicine

Bayer, Arnold S. · Infectious Disease, General Infectious Disease

Bayless, Theodore M. · Gastroenterology, Inflammatory Bowel Disease

Baylis, Henry I. · Ophthalmology, Oculoplastic & Orbital Surgery

Bayne, Loui Garrett · Hand Surgery, Reconstructive Surgery

Bays, Jan · Pediatrics, Abused Children

Bear, David M. · Psychiatry, Violence

Beart, Robert W. · Surgical Oncology, Colon & Rectal Cancer

Beatty, Patrick G. · Medical Oncology & Hematology, Bone Marrow Transplantation

Beaudet, Arthur Louis · Pediatrics, Metabolic Diseases

Bechert, Charles H. · Ophthalmology, Anterior Segment (Cataract Surgery)

Beck, Roy W. · Ophthalmology, Neuro-Ophthalmology

Becker, David V. · Nuclear Medicine, Thyroid

Becker, Donald P. · Neurological Surgery, Trauma

Becker, Dorothy J. · Pediatrics, Pediatric Endocrinology

Becker, Ferdinand Francis · Otolaryngology, Facial Plastic Surgery

Becker, James · General Surgery, Gastroenterologic Surgery

Becker, Laurence E. · Pathology, Neuropathology

Bedwinek, John M. · Radiation Oncology, Breast Cancer

Beegle, Philip H. · Plastic Surgery, Breast Surgery; Plastic Surgery, Microsurgery

Behrens, Fred · Orthopaedic Surgery, Trauma

Behrens, Myles M. · Ophthalmology, Neuro-Ophthalmology

Beierwaltes, William H. · Nuclear Medicine, General Nuclear Medicine

Belenky, Walter M. · Otolaryngology, Pediatric Otolaryngology

Belfer, Myron L. · Psychiatry, Child Psychiatry

Bell, William · Neurology, Child, Central Nervous System Infections

Beller, George A. · Cardiovascular Disease, General Cardiovascular Disease; Cardiovascular Disease, Nuclear Cardiology

Bellows, A. Robert · Ophthalmology, Glaucoma

Belman, A. Barry · Urology, Pediatric Urology

Belsito, Donald Vincent · Dermatology, Contact Dermatitis

Belzer, Folkert O. · General Surgery, Transplantation

Benecke, James E. · Otolaryngology, Otology/Neurotology

Benedek, Elissa P. · Psychiatry, Child Abuse; Psychiatry, Child Psychiatry; Psychiatry, Forensic Psychiatry; Psychiatry, Sexual Abuse

Benedetti, Thomas J. · Obstetrics & Gynecology, Maternal & Fetal Medicine

Benfield, John R. · Thoracic Surgery, General Thoracic Surgery; Thoracic Surgery, Thoracic Oncological Surgery

Benjamin, Vallo · Neurological Surgery, Spinal Surgery

Bennett, John Eugene · Infectious Disease, Fungal Infections

Bennett, John M. · Medical Oncology & Hematology, Breast Cancer; Medical Oncology & Hematology, Leukemia; Medical Oncology & Hematology, Lymphomas

Bennett, Richard G. · Dermatology, Skin Cancer Surgery & Reconstruction

Bennett, Robert M. · Rheumatology, Fibromyalgia

Bennett, William · Nephrology, Dialysis; Nephrology, Kidney Disease

Benowitz, Neal L. · Clinical Pharmacology

Benson, D. Frank · Neurology, Adult, Behavioral Neurology

Benson, D. Woodrow · Pediatrics, Pediatric Cardiology

Benson, George S. · Urology, Impotence; Urology, Neuro-Urology & Voiding Dysfunction

Benson, William E. · Ophthalmology, Vitreo-Retinal Surgery

Benumof, Jonathan L. · Anesthesiology, Cardiothoracic Anesthesiology

Berard, Costan W. · Pathology, Hematopathology

Berek, Jonathan S. · Obstetrics & Gynecology, Gynecologic Cancer

Berenstein, Alex · Radiology, Neuroradiology

Berg, Bruce O. · Neurology, Child, General Child Neurology

Berg, Leonard · Neurology, Adult, Degenerative Diseases

Bergen, John J. · General Surgery, General Vascular Surgery

Bergenstal, Richard · Endocrinology & Metabolism, Diabetes

Berger, Joseph R. · Neurology, Adult, Infectious & Demyelinating Diseases

Bergfeld, John A. · Orthopaedic Surgery, Sports Medicine

Bergfeld, Wilma F. · Dermatology, Hair

Bergstresser, Paul R. · Dermatology, Cutaneous Immunologyl Dermatology, Photobiology

Berguer, Ramon · General Surgery, General Vascular Surgery

Berkeley, Ralph G. · Ophthalmology, Anterior Segment (Cataract Surgery)

Berkowitz, Carol D. · Pediatrics, Abused Children

Berkowitz, Henry D. · General Surgery, General Vascular Surgery

Berkowitz, Richard · Obstetrics & Gynecology, Maternal & Fetal Medicine

Berman, Bernard A. · Allergy & Immunology, Pediatric Allergy & Immunology

Berman, Daniel S. · Cardiovascular Disease, Nuclear Cardiology; Nuclear Medicine, Nuclear Cardiology

Berman, Michael L. · Obstetrics & Gynecology, Gynecologic Cancer

Bernhard, Gerson Charles · Rheumatology, General Rheumatology

Bernhard, Victor · General Surgery, General Vascular Surgery

Bernstein, Eugene F. · General Surgery, General Vascular Surgery

Bernstein, I. Leonard · Allergy & Immunology, Adult Allergy & Immunology

Bertino, Joseph · Medical Oncology & Hematology, Clinical Pharmacology

Bertolino, Arthur P. · Dermatology, Hair

Besdine, Richard W. · Geriatric Medicine, General Geriatric Medicine

Beynen, Froukje M. K. · Anesthesiology, Pediatric Cardiovascular

Bickers, David Rinsey · Dermatology, Clinical Dermatology; Dermatology, Photobiology; Dermatology, Psoriasis

Biederman, Joseph · Psychiatry, Child Psychiatry; Psychiatry, Psychopharmacology

Bienenfeld, David G. · Psychiatry, Geriatric Psychiatry

Bier, Dennis M. · Pediatrics, Pediatric Endocrinology

Bierman, C. Warren · Allergy & Immunology, Pediatric Allergy & Immunology

Bierman, Fredrick Z. · Pediatrics, Pediatric Cardiology

Bigliani, Louis Urban · Orthopaedic Surgery, Reconstructive Surgery

Biller, Hugh F. · Otolaryngology, Head & Neck Surgery; Otolaryngology, Laryngology

Biller, José · Neurology, Adult, Strokes

Billig, Nathan · Psychiatry, Geriatric Psychiatry

Binder, Perry S. · Ophthalmology, Corneal Diseases & Transplantation

Bird, Hector Ramon · Psychiatry, Child Psychiatry

Bird, Thomas D. · Neurology, Adult, Neurogenetics

Birnbaum, Gary · Neurology, Adult, Infectious & Demyelinating Diseases

Birnbaum, Neal S. · Rheumatology, General Rheumatology; Rheumatology, Rheumatoid Arthritis

Bissell, LeClair · Addiction Medicine, General Addiction Medicine

Bitran, Jacob D. · Medical Oncology & Hematology, Bone Marrow Transplantation; Medical Oncology & Hematology, Breast Cancer

Biundo, Joseph J. · Rheumatology, Rehabilitation

Bjornsson, Thorir D. · Clinical Pharmacology

Black, Paul William · Plastic Surgery, Reconstructive Surgery

Black, Peter M. · Neurological Surgery, General Neurological Surgery

Blackwell, Richard Edgar · Obstetrics & Gynecology, Reproductive Endocrinology

Blaese, Robert Michael · Allergy & Immunology, Pediatric Allergy & Immunology

Blaine, Jack David · Psychiatry, Addiction Medicine

Blaisdell, William F. · General Surgery, General Vascular Surgery

Blaivas, Jerry G. · Urology, Neuro-Urology & Voiding Dysfunction

Bland, Kirby I. · Surgical Oncology, Breast Cancer; Surgical Oncology, Colon & Rectal Cancer

Blankenship, George W. · Ophthalmology, Medical Retinal Diseases; Ophthalmology, Vitreo-Retinal Surgery

Blaschke, Terrence F. · Clinical Pharmacology

Blaufox, M. Donald · Nuclear Medicine, Kidney

Blazer, Dan G. · Psychiatry, Geriatric Psychiatry

Bleyer, W. Archie · Pediatrics, Pediatric Hematology-Oncology

Blitzer, Andrew · Otolaryngology, Laryngology

Blizzard, Robert M. · Pediatrics, Pediatric Endocrinology

Bloch, George Edward · General Surgery, Gastroenterologic Surgery

Block, A. Jay · Pulmonary & Critical Care Medicine, Pulmonary Disease

Block, Peter C. · Cardiovascular Disease, Cardiac Catheterization

Block, Sidney R. · Rheumatology, General Rheumatology

Bloom, Joseph D. · Psychiatry, Forensic Psychiatry

Bloomer, Joseph R. · Gastroenterology, Hepatology

Bloomfield, Clara D. · Medical Oncology, Leukemia; Medical Oncology, Lymphomas

Bluestein, Marlene · Geriatric Medicine, General Geriatric Medicine

Bluestone, Charles D. · Otolaryngology, Pediatric Otolaryngology

Bluestone, Rodney · Rheumatology, General Rheumatology

Blum, Harold Philip · Psychiatry, Psychoanalysis

Blume, Karl G. · Medical Oncology & Hematology, Bone Marrow Transplantation

Blume, Sheila Bierman · Psychiatry, Addiction Medicine

Blumenkranz, Mark S. · Ophthalmology, Medical Retinal Diseases; Ophthalmology, Vitreo-Retinal Surgery

Blumenthal, Malcolm N. · Allergy & Immunology, Adult Allergy & Immunology

Boat, Thomas F. · Pediatrics, Pediatric Pulmonology

Bodey, Gerald P. · Infectious Disease, Cancer & Infections

Boehm, Frank H. · Obstetrics & Gynecology, Maternal & Fetal Medicine

Boesky, Dale · Psychiatry, Psychoanalysis

Bohlman, Henry Hubert · Orthopaedic Surgery, Spine Surgery

Bollinger, R. Randal · General Surgery, Transplantation

Bolman, R. Morton · Thoracic Surgery, Adult Cardiothoracic Surgery; Thoracic Surgery, Transplantation

Bolton, W. Kline · Nephrology, Glomerular Diseases

Bone, Lawrence Brunton · Orthopaedic Surgery, Trauma

Bone, Roger C. · Pulmonary & Critical Care Medicine, General Pulmonary & Critical Care Medicine

Bonow, Robert Ogden · Cardiovascular Disease, Cardiac Positron Emission Tomography (PET); Cardiovascular Disease, Nuclear Cardiology

Bonte, Frederick J. · Nuclear Medicine, Brain

Bora, Frank William · Hand Surgery, Peripheral Nerve Surgery; Orthopaedic Surgery, Peripheral Nerve Surgery

Bordelon, R. Luke · Orthopaedic Surgery, Foot & Ankle Surgery

Borden, Ernest C. · Medical Oncology & Hematology, Immunotherapy, Biological Response Modifiers Oncology

Borden, Lester S. · Orthopaedic Surgery, Reconstructive Surgery

Borkowsky, William · Pediatrics, Pediatric Infectious Disease

Boronow, Richard C. · Obstetrics & Gynecology, Gynecologic Cancer

Borson, Soo · Psychiatry, Geriatric Psychiatry

Boruchoff, S. Arthur · Ophthalmology, Corneal Diseases & Transplantation

Bosl, George Joseph · Medical Oncology & Hematology, Genito-Urinary Cancer

Bosse, Michael J. · Orthopaedic Surgery, Trauma

Bostwick, John · Plastic Surgery, Breast Surgery

Boswell, John Iverson · Psychiatry, Psychoanalysis

Botvinick, Elias H. · Cardiovascular Disease, Nuclear Cardiology; Nuclear Medicine, Nuclear Cardiology

Boucher, Charles A. · Cardiovascular Disease, Nuclear Cardiology

Bourne, William M. · Ophthalmology, Corneal Diseases & Transplantation

Bove, Edward L. · Thoracic Surgery, Pediatric Cardiac Surgery

Bowers, Malcolm B. · Psychiatry, Schizophrenia/Psychopharmacology

Bowes, Watson A. · Obstetrics & Gynecology, Maternal & Fetal Medicine

Bowie, William R. · Infectious Disease, Sexually Transmitted Disease

Boyajian, Michael John · Plastic Surgery, Pediatric Plastic Surgery

Boyce, H. Worth · Gastroenterology, Endoscopy; Gastroenterology, Esophageal Disease

Boyce, John G. · Obstetrics & Gynecology, Gynecologic Cancer

Boyd, Aubrey E. · Endocrinology & Metabolism, Diabetes

Boyer, James L. · Gastroenterology, Hepatology

Bozymski, Eugene M. · Gastroenterology, General Gastroenterology

Braasch, John W. · General Surgery, Gastroenterologic Surgery

Brackmann, Derald E. · Otolaryngology, Otology/Neurotology

Braddom, Randall Lee · Physical Medicine & Rehabilitation, Electromyography

Bradford, David S. · Orthopaedic Surgery, Pediatric Orthopaedic Surgery; Orthopaedic Surgery, Spine

Bradley, Edward L. · General Surgery, Endocrine Surgery

Bradley, Walter G. · Neurology, Adult, Neuromuscular Disease

Brady, Luther W. · Radiation Oncology, Breast Cancer

Braly, Patricia S. · Obstetrics & Gynecology, Gynecologic Cancer

Brandstater, Murray E. · Physical Medicine & Rehabilitation, Electromyography

Brandt, Kenneth D. · Rheumatology, General Rheumatology; Rheumatology, Osteoarthritis

Brandt, Lawrence J. · Gastroenterology, Inflammatory Bowel Disease

Brasel, Jo Anne · Pediatrics, Pediatric Endocrinology

Brater, D. Craig · Clinical Pharmacology

Braun, Bennett G. · Psychiatry, Dissociative Disorders; Psychiatry, Post-Traumatic Stress Disorders

Braun, Martin · Dermatology, Skin Cancer Surgery & Reconstruction

Braun, Norma M. T. Wang · Pulmonary & Critical Care Medicine, Pulmonary Disease

Braun, Richard M. · Hand Surgery, Peripheral Nerve Surgery; Orthopaedic Surgery, Peripheral Nerve Surgery

Braunwald, Eugene · Cardiovascular Disease, Heart Failure

Braverman, Irwin M. · Dermatology, Clinical Dermatology

Braverman, Lewis E. · Endocrinology & Metabolism, Thyroid

Bray, George A. · Eating Disorders

Braylan, Raul C. · Pathology, Hematopathology

Breier, Alan Francis · Psychiatry, Schizophrenia/Psychopharmacology

Bremner, William J. · Endocrinology & Metabolism, Reproductive Endocrinology

Brennan, Murray Frederick · General Surgery, Endocrine Surgery; Surgical Oncology, Gastroenterologic Cancer

Brenner, Charles · Psychiatry, Psychoanalysis

Brent, Burton D. · Plastic Surgery, Reconstructive Surgery

Brent, David A. · Psychiatry, Child Psychiatry; Psychiatry, Suicidology

Bresnick, George H. · Ophthalmology, Medical Retinal Diseases

Brewer, L. Eileen Doyle · Pediatrics, Pediatric Nephrology

Brewster, David C. · General Surgery, General Vascular Surgery

Briggaman, Robert Alan · Dermatology, Cutaneous Immunology

Briggs, Dick D. · Pulmonary & Critical Care Medicine, General Pulmonary & Critical Care Medicine

Briney, Walter G. · Rheumatology, General Rheumatology

Brinker, Jeffrey A. · Cardiovascular Disease, Cardiac Catheterization

Brint, Stephen F. · Ophthalmology, Anterior Segment (Cataract Surgery)

Britton, B. Hill · Otolaryngology, Otology/Neurotology

Brodsky, Linda S. · Otolaryngology, Pediatric Otolaryngology

Bromley, Jess W. · Addiction Medicine, General Addiction Medicine

Brooke, Michael H. · Neurology, Adult, Neuromuscular Disease

Brookler, Kenneth H. · Otolaryngology, Otology/Neurotology

Brooks, Benjamin R. · Neurology, Adult, Infectious & Demyelinating Diseases

Brooks, John G. · Pediatrics, Pediatric Pulmonology

Brosman, Stanley A. · Urology, Urologic Oncology

Brott, Thomas G. · Neurology, Adult, Strokes

Brown, Burnell R. · Anesthesiology, Hepatic Disease

Brown, David L. · Anesthesiology, Complications of Anesthesia; Anesthesiology, Orthopaedic Procedures

Brown, Elizabeth Ruth · Addiction Medicine, Addicted Pregnant Women; Pediatrics, Neonatal-Perinatal Medicine

Brown, John William · Thoracic Surgery, Pediatric Cardiac Surgery

Brown, Manuel L. · Nuclear Medicine, General Nuclear Medicine

Brown, Orval E. · Otolaryngology, Pediatric Otolaryngology

Brown, Reay H. · Ophthalmology, Glaucoma

Brown, Robert H. · Neurology, Adult, Degenerative Diseases; Neurology, Adult, Neuromuscular Disease

Browne, Thomas Reed · Neurology, Adult, Epilepsy

Browner, Bruce D. · Orthopaedic Surgery, Trauma

Brubaker, Richard · Ophthalmology, Glaucoma

Bruce, Derek A. · Neurological Surgery, Pediatric Neurological Surgery

Brucker, Alexander J. · Ophthalmology, Medical Retinal Diseases; Ophthalmology, Vitreo-Retinal Surgery

Brumback, Robert · Orthopaedic Surgery, Trauma

Brummel-Smith, Kenneth V. · Geriatric Medicine, General Geriatric Medicine

Brunell, Philip A. · Pediatrics, Pediatric Infectious Disease

Brunham, Robert C. · Infectious Disease, Sexually Transmitted Disease

Brunning, Richard D, · Pathology, Hematopathology

Brusilow, Saul W. · Pediatrics, Metabolic Diseases

Brust, John C. M. · Neurology, Adult, General Adult Neurology

Bryan, Nick R. · Radiology, Neuroradiology

Bryson, Yvonne J. · Pediatrics, Pediatric Infectious Disease

Buchanan, George R. · Pediatrics, Pediatric Hematology-Oncology

Bucholz, Robert W. · Orthopaedic Surgery, Trauma

Buckley, Edward G. · Ophthalmology, Pediatric Ophthalmology

Buckley, Jerome M. · Allergy & Immunology, Pediatric Allergy & Immunology

Buckley, Mortimer J. · Thoracic Surgery, Adult Cardiothoracic Surgery

Buckley, Rebecca · Allergy & Immunology, Pediatric Allergy & Immunology

Buist, Neil R. M. · Pediatrics, Metabolic Diseases

Bukowski, Ronald M. · Medical Oncology & Hematology, Genito-Urinary Cancer

Bullard, Dexter Means · Psychiatry, Child Psychiatry

Buncke, Harry J. · Hand Surgery, Microsurgery; Plastic Surgery, Reconstructive Surgery

Bunn, Paul A. · Medical Oncology & Hematology, Lung Cancer; Medical Oncology & Hematology, Lymphomas

Burde, Ronald M. · Neurology, Adult, Neuro-Ophthalmology; Ophthalmology, Neuro-Ophthalmology

Burger, Peter C. · Pathology, Neuropathology

Burgess, Andrew R. · Orthopaedic Surgery, Trauma

Burget, Gary C. · Plastic Surgery, Reconstructive Surgery

Burke, John P. · Infectious Disease, Hospital-Acquired Infections

Burke, M. Shannon · Obstetrics & Gynecology, Maternal & Fetal Medicine

Burki, Nausherwan K. · Pulmonary & Critical Care Medicine, General Pulmonary & Critical Care Medicine

Burr, Ian M. · Pediatrics, Pediatric Endocrinology

Burton, Claude S. · Dermatology, Wound Healing

Burton, John Russell · Geriatric Medicine, Urinary Incontinence

Burton, Richard Irving · Hand Surgery, Reconstructive Surgery

Bush, Robert K. · Allergy & Immunology, Adult Allergy & Immunology

Busse, William W. · Allergy & Immunology, Adult Allergy & Immunology

Buster, John E. · Obstetrics & Gynecology, Reproductive Endocrinology

Busuttil, Ronald W. · General Surgery, Transplantation

Butler, Ian J. · Neurology, Child, General Child Neurology; Neurology, Child, Movement Disorder

Butler, James Johnson · Pathology, Hematopathology

Butler, Robert N. · Psychiatry, Geriatric Psychiatry

Buxton, Alfred E. · Cardiovascular Disease, Electrophysiology

Bystryn, Jean-Claude · Dermatology, Cutaneous Immunology

C

Cabanillas, Fernando · Medical Oncology & Hematology, Lymphomas

Cabaniss, Micki L. · Obstetrics & Gynecology, Maternal & Fetal Medicine

Cady, Blake · General Surgery, Endocrine Surgery

Cahalan, Michael K. · Anesthesiology, Adult Cardiovascular

Caine, Eric Douglas · Psychiatry, Behavioral Disorders; Psychiatry, Geriatric Psychiatry; Psychiatry, Neuropsychiatry

Cairncross, J. Gregory · Medical Oncology & Hematology, Neuro-oncology; Neurology, Adult, Neuro-oncology

Calcaterra, Thomas C. · Otolaryngology, Head & Neck Surgery; Otolaryngology, Laryngology

Call, Justin David · Psychiatry, Child Psychiatry; Psychiatry, Psychoanalysis

Callahan, Mark J. · Cardiovascular Disease, General Cardiovascular Disease

Callahan, Michael A. · Ophthalmology, Oculoplastic & Orbital Surgery

Callen, Jeffrey P. · Dermatology, Clinical Dermatology

Calne, Donald B. · Neurology, Adult, Movement Disorders

Calverley, John R. · Neurology, Adult, General Adult Neurology

Cambor, C. Glenn · Psychiatry, Psychoanalysis

Cameron, John L. · General Surgery, Gastroenterologic Surgery; Surgical Oncology, Gastroenterologic Cancer

Campbell, J. Keith · Neurology, Adult, Headache

Campbell, James N. · Neurological Surgery, Peripheral Nerve Surgery

Campbell, Magda · Psychiatry, Autism; Psychiatry, Child Psychiatry; Psychiatry, Schizophrenia; Psychiatry, Violence

Campbell, Preston W. · Pediatrics, Pediatric Pulmonology

Canellos, George P. · Medical Oncology & Hematology, Breast Cancer; Medical Oncology & Hematology, Hematological Malignancies; Medical Oncology & Hematology, Lymphomas

Cantrell, Robert W. · Otolaryngology, Head & Neck Surgery

Cantwell, Dennis P. · Psychiatry, Child Psychiatry

Capizzi, Robert L. · Medical Oncology & Hematology, Leukemia

Caplan, Daniel B. · Pediatrics, Pediatric Gastroenterology

Caplan, Louis R. · Neurology, Adult, Strokes

Caplan, Robert A. · Anesthesiology, Complications of Anesthesia

Caranasos, George J. · Geriatric Medicine, General Geriatric Medicine

Carey, Larry C. · General Surgery, Gastroenterologic Surgery

Caritis, Steve N. · Obstetrics & Gynecology, Maternal & Fetal Medicine

Carlow, Thomas J. · Neurology, Adult, Neuro-Ophthalmology; Ophthalmology, Neuro-Ophthalmology

Carlsen, Lloyd N. · Plastic Surgery, Body Contouring; Plastic Surgery, Breast Surgery; Plastic Surgery, Facial Aesthetic Surgery

Carlson, Dru E. · Obstetrics & Gynecology, Maternal & Fetal Medicine

Carlson, Gabrielle A. · Psychiatry, Child Psychiatry

Caronna, John J. · Neurology, General Adult Neurology

Carpenter, Charles B. · Nephrology, Kidney Transplantation

Carpenter, John Topham · Medical Oncology & Hematology, Breast Cancer

Carpenter, William T. · Psychiatry, Schizophrenia

Carr, Bruce R. · Obstetrics & Gynecology, Reproductive Endocrinology

Carraway, James Howard · Plastic Surgery, Facial Aesthetic Surgery

Carroll, Bernard J. · Psychiatry, Affective Disorders; Psychiatry, Psychopharmacology

Carroll, Richard P. · Ophthalmology, Oculoplastic & Orbital Surgery

Carson, Culley C. · Urology, Endourology; Urology, Impotence

Carson, Sandra A. · Obstetrics & Gynecology, Reproductive Endocrinology

Carter, Jonathan L. · Neurology, Adult, Infectious & Demyelinating Diseases

Cascino, Terrence · Medical Oncology & Hematology, Neuro-oncology; Neurology, Adult, Neuro-oncology

Caserio, Rebecca Jo Ann · Dermatology, Hair

Caspari, Rich · Orthopaedic Surgery, Sports Medicine

Casper, James J. · Pediatrics, Pediatric Hematology-Oncology

Casper, Regina Klaere · Psychiatry, Eating Disorders

Cassady, George · Pediatrics, Neonatal-Perinatal Medicine

Cassady, J. Robert · Radiation Oncology, Pediatric Radiation Oncology

Cassel, Christine K. · Geriatric Medicine, General Geriatric Medicine

Cassisi, Nicholas John · Otolaryngology, Head & Neck Surgery

Castaneda, Aldo R. · Thoracic Surgery, Pediatric Cardiac Surgery

Castell, Donald O. · Gastroenterology, Esophageal Disease

Castelnuovo-Tedesco, Pietro · Psychiatry, Psychoanalysis

Castro, Joseph · Radiation Oncology, Particle Beam Radiation

Catalona, William J. · Urology, Urologic Oncology

Catanzaro, Antonino · Pulmonary & Critical Care Medicine, Pulmonary Disease

Cate, Thomas R. · Infectious Disease, Respiratory Infections

Cavalieri, Ralph R. · Endocrinology & Metabolism, Thyroid

Cavanaugh, James L. · Psychiatry, Forensic Psychiatry

Cavenar, Jesse O. · Psychiatry, Psychopharmacology

Cederbaum, Stephen · Pediatrics, Metabolic Diseases

Cefalo, Robert C. · Obstetrics & Gynecology, Maternal & Fetal Medicine

Ceilley, Roger I. · Dermatology, Skin Cancer Surgery & Reconstruction

Cetrulo, Curtis L. · Obstetrics & Gynecology, Maternal & Fetal Medicine

Chabner, Bruce A. · Medical Oncology & Hematology, Clinical Pharmacology

Chadwick, David L. · Pediatrics, Abused Children

Chaitman, Bernard R. · Cardiovascular Disease, Clinical Exercise Testing

Champlin, Richard · Medical Oncology, Bone Marrow Transplantation; Medical Oncology, Leukemia

Chandler, John · Ophthalmology, Corneal Diseases & Transplantation

Chandler, William F. · Neurological Surgery, Tumor Surgery

Chang, R. Jeffrey · Obstetrics & Gynecology, Reproductive Endocrinology

Chang, Stanley · Ophthalmology, Vitreo-Retinal Surgery

Chapman, Michael W. · Orthopaedic Surgery, Reconstructive Surgery; Orthopaedic Surgery, Trauma

Chappel, John Nelson · Psychiatry, Addiction Medicine

Char, Devron H. · Ophthalmology, Ocular Oncology

Charles, Steven Thomas · Ophthalmology, Vitreo-Retinal Surgery

Charney, Dennis S. · Psychiatry, Affective Disorders; Psychiatry, General Psychiatry; Psychiatry, Psychopharmacology

Chase, H. Peter · Pediatrics, Pediatric Endocrinology

Chasnoff, Ira J. · Addiction Medicine, Addicted Pregnant Women; Pediatrics, Neonatal-Perinatal Medicine

Chatterjee, Kanu · Cardiovascular Disease, General Cardiovascular Disease; Cardiovascular Disease, Heart Failure

Cheney, Frederick W. · Anesthesiology, Complications of Anesthesia

Chernausek, Steven D. · Pediatrics, Pediatric Endocrinology

Chervenak, Frank A. · Obstetrics & Gynecology, Maternal & Fetal Medicine

Chestnut, David H. · Anesthesiology, Obstetric Anesthesia

Cheung, Laurence Y. · General Surgery, Gastroenterologic Surgery

Chevalier, Robert L. · Pediatrics, Pediatric Nephrology

Chez, Ronald A. · Obstetrics & Gynecology, Maternal & Fetal Medicine

Chin, Y. T. · Pediatrics, Metabolic Diseases

Chitwood, W. Randolph · Thoracic Surgery, Adult Cardiothoracic Surgery

Chobanian, Sarkis John · Gastroenterology, General Gastroenterology

Choi, Noah C. · Radiation Oncology, Lung Cancer

Christie, Dennis L. · Pediatrics, Pediatric Gastroenterology

Chrousos, George Panagiotis · Endocrinology & Metabolism, Neuroendocrinology; Pediatrics, Pediatric Endocrinology

Chubick, Andrew · Rheumatology, General Rheumatology

Church, Joseph A. · Allergy & Immunology, Pediatric Allergy & Immunology

Chused, Judith Fingert · Psychiatry, Psychoanalysis

Chutorian, Abraham M. · Neurology, Child, General Child Neurology

Ciccone, J. Richard · Psychiatry, Forensic Psychiatry

Ciraulo, Domenic A. · Psychiatry, Addiction Medicine

Ciric, Ivan S. · Neurological Surgery, General Neurological Surgery

Clancy, William · Orthopaedic Surgery, Sports Medicine

Clarfield, A. Mark · Geriatric Medicine, General Geriatric Medicine

Clark, Edward B. · Pediatrics, Pediatric Cardiology

Clark, Orlo H. · General Surgery, Endocrine Surgery

Clark, R. M. · Radiation Oncology, Breast Cancer

Clark, Steven L. · Obstetrics & Gynecology, Maternal & Fetal Medicine

Clarke, William L. · Pediatrics, Pediatric Endocrinology

Clarke-Pearson, Daniel L. · Obstetrics & Gynecology, Gynecologic Cancer

Clarkson, John G. · Ophthalmology, Medical Retinal Diseases; Vitreo-Retinal Surgery

Clayman, Henry M. · Ophthalmology, Anterior Segment (Cataract Surgery)

Clayman, Ralph V. · Urology, Endourology

Clayton, Paula J. · Psychiatry, Affective Disorders; Psychiatry, Psychopharmacology

Clearfield, Harris Reynold · Gastroenterology, General Gastroenterology; Gastroenterology, Inflammatory Bowel Disease; Gastroenterology, Peptic Disorders

Clements, Phillip J. · Rheumatology, Scleroderma

Clendenning, William E. · Dermatology, Psoriasis

Clewell, William H. · Obstetrics & Gynecology, Maternal & Fetal Medicine

Cobbs, C. Glenn · Infectious Disease, General Infectious Disease

Coburn, Jack W. · Nephrology, Kidney Disease

Coccia, Peter F. · Pediatrics, Pediatric Hematology-Oncology

Coffman, Jay D. · Cardiovascular Disease, Vaso-Spastic Diseases

Cofield, Robert H. · Orthopaedic Surgery, Reconstructive Surgery

Coggins, Cecil H. · Nephrology, General Nephrology

Cohen, Alfred Martin · Surgical Oncology, Colon & Rectal Cancer

Cohen, Benjamin E. · Plastic Surgery, Breast Surgery

Cohen, Bernard Alan · Dermatology, Pediatric Dermatology; Pediatrics, Pediatric Dermatology

Cohen, Carmel · Obstetrics & Gynecology, Gynecologic Cancer

Cohen, Donald J. · Psychiatry, Autism; Psychiatry, Child Psychiatry

Cohen, Gene D. · Psychiatry, Geriatric Psychiatry

Cohen, Harvey J. · Pediatrics, Pediatric Hematology-Oncology

Cohen, Harvey Jay · Geriatric Medicine, General Geriatric Medicine

Cohen, I. Kelman · Plastic Surgery, Breast Surgery; Plastic Surgery, Wound Healing

Cohen, Lawrence S. · Cardiovascular Disease, General Cardiovascular Disease

Cohen, Michael E. · Neurology, Child, Neuro-oncology

Cohen, Noel L. · Otolaryngology, Otology/Neurotology

Cohen, Sheila Evelyn · Anesthesiology, Obstetric Anesthesia

Cohen, Sidney · Gastroenterology, Gastrointestinal Motility

Cohen, Zane · Colon & Rectal Surgery, General Colon & Rectal Surgery

Cohn, Jay N. · Cardiovascular Disease, Heart Failure

Cohn, Lawrence H. · Thoracic Surgery, Adult Cardiothoracic Surgery

Coit, Daniel G. · Surgical Oncology, Melanoma

Coker, Newton J. · Otolaryngology, Otology/Neurotology

Colarusso, Calvin A. · Psychiatry, Child Psychiatry; Psychiatry, Psychoanalysis

Cole, Barbara R. · Pediatrics, Pediatric Nephrology

Cole, Jonathan O. · Psychiatry, General Psychiatry; Psychiatry, Psychopharmacology

Coleman, C. Norman · Radiation Oncology, General Radiation Oncology

Coleman, D. Jackson · Ophthalmology, Vitreo-Retinal Surgery

Coleman, John J. · Plastic Surgery, Head & Neck Surgery; Plastic Surgery, Reconstructive Surgery

Coleman, Morton · Medical Oncology & Hematology, Hematological Malignancies; Medical Oncology & Hematology, Lymphomas

Coleman, Ralph Edward · Nuclear Medicine, Brain; Nuclear Medicine, General Nuclear Medicine

Colenda, Christopher C. · Psychiatry, Geriatric Psychiatry

Coll, Patrick P. · Geriatric Medicine, General Geriatric Medicine

Colle, Eleanor · Pediatrics, Pediatric Endocrinology

Collier, B. David · Nuclear Medicine, Bone

Collins, Allan J. · Nephrology, Dialysis

Collins, Robert C. · Neurology, Adult, General Adult Neurology

Collins, Robert D. · Pathology, Hematopathology

Coltman, Charles A. · Medical Oncology & Hematology, Lymphomas

Colwell, Clifford W. · Orthopaedic Surgery, Reconstructive Surgery

Comis, Robert L. · Medical Oncology, Lung Cancer

Condemi, John J. · Allergy & Immunology, Adult Allergy & Immunology

Conley, Susan B. · Pediatrics, Pediatric Nephrology

Conn, Doyt LaDean · Rheumatology, General Rheumatology

Connell, Bruce F. · Plastic Surgery, Facial Aesthetic Surgery

Connolly, Edward S · Neurological Surgery, Spinal Surgery

Connolly, James L. · Pathology, Breast Pathology

Connor, Edward M. · Pediatrics, Pediatric Infectious Disease

Connors, Joseph M. · Medical Oncology & Hematology, Lymphomas

Conte, Felix A. · Pediatrics, Pediatric Endocrinology

Conti, C. Richard · Cardiovascular Disease, General Cardiovascular Disease

Conway, James J. · Nuclear Medicine, Pediatric

Cook, D. Ryan · Anesthesiology, Pediatric Anesthesiology

Cooley, Denton A. · Thoracic Surgery, Adult Cardiothoracic Surgery

Cooney, Leo M. · Geriatric Medicine, General Geriatric Medicine

Cooney, William Patrick · Hand Surgery, General Hand Surgery

Coonrad, Ralph W. · Hand Surgery, Elbow Surgery; Orthopaedic Surgery, Reconstructive Surgery

Coons, Philip M. · Psychiatry, Dissociative Disorders

Cooper, Alan Bruce · Psychiatry, Psychoanalysis

Cooper, Arnold M. · Psychiatry, Psychoanalysis

Cooper, Joel D. · Thoracic Surgery, General Thoracic Surgery; Thoracic Surgery, Transplantation

Cooper, Kevin D. · Dermatology, Atopic Dermatitis; Dermatology, Eczema

Cooper, Max D. · Allergy & Immunology, Adult Allergy & Immunology; Allergy & Immunology, Pediatric Allergy & Immunology

Cooper, Paul Richard · Neurological Surgery, Spinal Surgery

Copeland, Edward M. · Surgical Oncology, Breast Cancer; Surgical Oncology, Colon & Rectal Cancer

Copeland, Jack G. · Thoracic Surgery, Adult Cardiothoracic Surgery; Thoracic Surgery, Transplantation

Copeland, Larry J. · Obstetrics & Gynecology, Gynecologic Cancer

Coran, Arnold G. · General Surgery, Pediatric Surgery

Corbett, James J. · Neurology, Adult, Neuro-Ophthalmology

Corey, Lawrence · Infectious Disease, Herpes Virus Infections; Infectious Disease, Sexually Transmitted Disease

Corry, Robert J. · General Surgery, Transplantation

Cortese, Denis A. · Pulmonary & Critical Care Medicine, Bronchoesophegology

Cosgrove, Delos (Toby) M. · Thoracic Surgery, Adult Cardiothoracic Surgery

Cossman, Jeffrey · Pathology, Hematopathology

Cotton, David B. · Obstetrics & Gynecology, Maternal & Fetal Medicine

Cotton, Deborah J. · Infectious Disease, AIDS

Cotton, Peter · Gastroenterology, Endoscopy

Cotton, Robert B. · Pediatrics, Neonatal-Perinatal Medicine

Cotton, Robin T. · Otolaryngology, Pediatric Otolaryngology

Cottrel, James E. · Anesthesiology, Neuroanesthesia

Coughlin, Michael · Orthopaedic Surgery, Foot & Ankle Surgery

Courtiss, Eugene H. · Plastic Surgery, Aesthetic Surgery; Plastic Surgery, Body Contouring

Couser, William G. · Nephrology, Glomerular Diseases

Cousins, Larry M. · Obstetrics & Gynecology, Maternal & Fetal Medicine

Coustan, Don · Obstetrics & Gynecology, Maternal & Fetal Medicine

Coutts, Richard D. · Orthopaedic Surgery, Reconstructive Surgery

Cowley, Michael Joseph · Cardiovascular Disease, Cardiac Catheterization

Cox, James D. · Radiation Oncology, Lung Cancer

Cox, James L. · Thoracic Surgery, Adult Cardiothoracic Surgery

Crabbe, Henry F. · Psychiatry, Mental Retardation /Mental Health: Dual Diagnosis

Cracchiolo, Andrea · Orthopaedic Surgery, Foot & Ankle Surgery; Orthopaedic Surgery, Rheumatoid Arthritis

Craig, William A. · Infectious Disease, Antibiotic Pharmacology

Crandall, Alan S. · Ophthalmology, Anterior Segment (Cataract Surgery)

Craven, Donald Edward · Infectious Disease, AIDS; Infectious Disease, Hospital-Acquired Infections

Crawford, David E. · Urology, Urologic Oncology

Crawford, John D. · Pediatrics, Pediatric Endocrinology

Crawford, Michael H. · Cardiovascular Disease, Echocardiography

Creager, Mark A. · Cardiovascular Disease, Vaso-Spastic Diseases

Creasman, William T. · Obstetrics & Gynecology, Gynecologic Cancer

Creasy, Robert K. · Obstetrics & Gynecology, Maternal & Fetal Medicine

Crenshaw, Marion Carlyle · Obstetrics & Gynecology, Maternal & Fetal Medicine

Creticos, Peter S. · Allergy & Immunology, Adult Allergy & Immunology

Criley, John Michael · Cardiovascular Disease, Cardiac Catheterization

Crist, William Miles · Pediatrics, Pediatric Hematology-Oncology

Crofford, Oscar B. · Endocrinology & Metabolism, Diabetes

Croft, Joseph David · Rheumatology, General Rheumatology; Rheumatology, Rheumatoid Arthritis

Crone, Robert K. · Anesthesiology, Pediatric Anesthesiology; Pediatrics, Pediatric Critical Care

Crosby, Gregory · Anesthesiology, Neuroanesthesia

Crowell, Robert M. · Neurological Surgery, Vascular Neurological Surgery

Crowley, Thomas J. · Psychiatry, Addiction Medicine

Crowley, William F. · Endocrinology & Metabolism, Reproductive Endocrinology

Cruikshank, Dwight P. · Obstetrics & Gynecology, Maternal & Fetal Medicine

Crumley, Roger L. · Otolaryngology, Facial Plastic Surgery, Otolaryngology, Laryngology; Otolaryngology, Skull-Base Surgery

Crumpacker, Clyde S. · Infectious Disease, Herpes Virus Infections

Cryer, Philip E. · Endocrinology & Metabolism, Diabetes

Crysdale, William S. · Otolaryngology, Pediatric Otolaryngology

Cucchiara, Roy F. · Anesthesiology, Neuroanesthesia

Cuckler, John M. · Orthopaedic Surgery, Hip Surgery

Culbertson, William · Ophthalmology, Uveitis

Cummings, Bernard J. · Radiation Oncology, Gastroenterologic Cancer

Cummings, Charles W. · Otolaryngology, Head & Neck Surgery; Otolaryngology, Laryngology

Cummings, Jeffrey Lee · Neurology, Adult, Neuropsychiatry

Cunningham-Rundles, Charlotte · Allergy & Immunology, Adult Allergy & Immunology

Curd, John G. · Rheumatology, General Rheumatology

Curry, Stephen L. · Obstetrics & Gynecology, Gynecologic Cancer

Curtis, Homer C. · Psychiatry, Psychoanalysis

Cuyler, James P. · Otolaryngology, Pediatric Otolaryngology

D

D'Alton, Mary E. · Obstetrics & Gynecology, Genetics; Obstetrics & Gynecology, Maternal & Fetal Medicine

D'Amico, Donald J. · Ophthalmology, Vitreo-Retinal Surgery

D'Ercole, A. Joseph · Pediatrics, Pediatric Endocrinology

Dacey, Ralph G. · Neurological Surgery, General Neurological Surgery

Dahl, Mark V. · Dermatology, Clinical Dermatology

Dahms, William · Pediatrics, Pediatric Endocrinology

Dailey, Thomas · Colon & Rectal Surgery, General Colon & Rectal Surgery

Daily, Pat O. · Thoracic Surgery, Adult Cardiothoracic Surgery

Dalrymple, Glenn V. · Nuclear Medicine, General Nuclear Medicine

Dalton, William Steven · Medical Oncology & Hematology, General Medical Oncology & Hematology

Daly, John M. · Surgical Oncology, Gastroenterologic Cancer

Damasio, Antonio · Neurology, Adult, Behavioral Neurology, Neurology, Adult, Degenerative Diseases

Daneman, Denis · Pediatrics, Pediatric Endocrinology

Daniel, Dale · Orthopaedic Surgery, Sports Medicine

Daniel, Rollin K. · Plastic Surgery, Facial Aesthetic Surgery

Daniels, Gilbert H. · Endocrinology & Metabolism, Thyroid

Danielson, Gordon K. · Thoracic Surgery, Adult Cardiothoracic Surgery; Thoracic Surgery, Pediatric Cardiac Surgery

Danto, Bruce Leonard · Psychiatry, Suicidology; Psychiatry, Violence

Dantzker, David R. · Pulmonary & Critical Care Medicine, General Pulmonary & Critical Care Medicine

Dardik, Herbert · General Surgery, General Vascular Surgery

Daroff, Robert B. · Neurology, Adult, Neuro-Ophthalmology

Datta, Sanjay · Anesthesiology, Obstetric Anesthesia

Dattel, Bonnie J. · Obstetrics & Gynecology, Maternal & Fetal Medicine

Daube, Jasper R. · Neurology, Adult, Electromyography

Daum, Fredric · Pediatrics, Pediatric Gastroenterology

David, Raphael R. · Pediatrics, Pediatric Endocrinology

Davidson, Jonathan R. T. · Psychiatry, General Psychiatry; Psychiatry, Psychopharmacology

Davidson, Mayer B. · Endocrinology & Metabolism, Diabetes

Davidson, Nancy E. · Medical Oncology & Hematology, Bone Marrow Transplantation; Medical Oncology & Hematology, Breast Cancer

Davis, Carl L. · Psychiatry, Psychoanalysis

Davis, John M. · Psychiatry, Schizophrenia/Psychopharmacology

Davis, John S. · Rheumatology, General Rheumatology

Davis, Larry E. · Neurology, Adult, Infectious & Demyelinating Diseases

Davis, Richard L. · Pathology, Neuropathology

Davis, William J. · Allergy & Immunology, Pediatric Allergy & Immunology

Dawson, David Michael · Neurology, Adult, Neuromuscular Disease

Day, Arthur L. · Neurological Surgery, Vascular Neurological Surgery

De Cherney, Alan H. · Obstetrics & Gynecology, Reproductive Endocrinology

De La Cruz, Antonio · Otolaryngology, Otology/Neurotology

De Lisa, Joel Alan · Physical Medicine & Rehabilitation, Electromyography

De Maria, Anthony Nicholas · Cardiovascular Disease, General Cardiovascular Disease

De Vivo, Darryl C. · Neurology, Child, Metabolic Diseases

Dean, J. Michael · Pediatrics, Pediatric Critical Care

Dean, Richard H. · General Surgery, General Vascular Surgery

Debas, Haile T. · General Surgery, Gastroenterologic Surgery

Decosse, Jerome J. · Surgical Oncology, Colon & Rectal Cancer

Dedo, Herbert H. · Otolaryngology, Laryngology

DeGroot, Leslie J. · Endocrinology & Metabolism, Thyroid

DeHaven, Kenneth E. · Orthopaedic Surgery, Sports Medicine

deKernion, Jean B. · Urology, Urologic Oncology

DeLeo, Vincent A. · Dermatology, Clinical Dermatology; Dermatology, Contact Dermatitis; Dermatology, Photobiology

Dellon, A. Lee · Hand Surgery, Peripheral Nerve Surgery; Plastic Surgery, Peripheral Nerve Surgery

DeMeester, Tom R. · General Surgery, Gastroenterologic Surgery

Denckla, Martha Bridge · Neurology, Adult, Behavioral Neurology

DePalma, Ralph G. · General Surgery, General Vascular Surgery

DePaulo, J. Raymond · Psychiatry, Affective Disorders

DePetrillo, Amodio Dennis · Obstetrics & Gynecology, Gynecologic Cancer

Depp, O. Richard · Obstetrics & Gynecology, Maternal & Fetal Medicine

DePuey, Ernest Gordon · Nuclear Medicine, Nuclear Cardiology

DeSanctis, Roman W. · Cardiovascular Disease, General Cardiovascular Disease

Deslauriers, Jean · Thoracic Surgery, General Thoracic Surgery

Desnick, Robert J. · Pediatrics, Metabolic Diseases

deVere White, Ralph W. · Urology, Urologic Oncology

DeVillez, Richard L. · Dermatology, Hair

Devoe, Lawrence D. · Obstetrics & Gynecology, Maternal & Fetal Medicine

Dewald, Paul A. · Psychiatry, Psychoanalysis

Diaz, Luis A. · Dermatology, Cutaneous Immunology

Diaz-Buxo, Jose A. · Nephrology, Dialysis

Dick, Harold Michael · Hand Surgery, Pediatric Orthopaedic Surgery; Orthopaedic Surgery, Pediatric Orthopaedic Surgery

Dick, Macdonald · Pediatrics, Pediatric Cardiology

Dickins, John Roddey Edwards · Otolaryngology, Otology/Neurotology

Diethelm, Arnold G. · General Surgery, Transplantation

Dietz, Park E. · Psychiatry, Forensic Psychiatry; Psychiatry, Violence

DiGeorge, Angelo M. · Pediatrics, Pediatric Endocrinology

Dillman, Robert Owen · Medical Oncology & Hematology, Hematological Malignancies; Medical Oncology & Hematology, Immunotherapy, Biological Response Modifiers Oncology

DiMarco, John P. · Cardiovascular Disease, General Cardiovascular Disease

DiSaia, Philip J. · Obstetrics & Gynecology, Gynecologic Cancer

Dismukes, William Ernest · Infectious Disease, Fungal Infections

Dixon, Richard E. · Infectious Disease, Hospital-Acquired Infections

Dobie, Robert A. · Otolaryngology, Otology/Neurotology

Dobkin, Bruce · Neurology, Adult, Strokes

Dobson, Richard L. · Dermatology, Clinical Dermatology

Dodick, Jack M · Ophthalmology, Anterior Segment (Cataract Surgery)

Dodson, W. Edwin · Neurology, Child, Epilepsy

Doershuk, Carl Frederick · Pediatrics, Pediatric Pulmonology

Donadio, James V. · Nephrology, Glomerular Diseases

Donahoe, Patricia · General Surgery, Pediatric Surgery

Donald, Paul J. · Otolaryngology, Head & Neck Surgery; Otolaryngology, Skull-Base Surgery

Donaldson, John · Otolaryngology, Pediatric Otolaryngology

Donaldson, Sarah S. · Radiation Oncology, Pediatric Radiation Oncology

Donegan, William L. · Surgical Oncology, Breast Cancer

Donehower, Ross C. · Medical Oncology & Hematology, Clinical Pharmacology

Donohue, John P. · Urology, Urologic Oncology

Dooley, Sharon Lee · Obstetrics & Gynecology, Maternal & Fetal Medicine

Dorfman, Ronald F. · Pathology, Hematopathology

Dorkin, Henry Lawrence · Pediatrics, Pediatric Pulmonology

Doroshow, James H. · Medical Oncology & Hematology, Clinical Pharmacology

Dorr, Lawrence D. · Orthopaedic Surgery, Reconstructive Surgery

Dorros, Gerald · Cardiovascular Disease, Cardiac Catheterization

Dortzbach, Richard K. · Ophthalmology, Oculoplastic & Orbital Surgery

Douglas, Gordon · Ophthalmology, Glaucoma

Douglas, John M. · Infectious Disease, Herpes Virus Infections; Infectious Disease, Sexually Transmitted Disease

Douglas, John S. · Cardiovascular Disease, Cardiac Catheterization

Dover, George J. · Pediatrics, Pediatric Hematology-Oncology

Dover, Jeffrey S. · Dermatology, Laser Surgery

Dowling, Scott · Psychiatry, Psychoanalysis

Downes, John J. · Anesthesiology, Pediatric Anesthesiology; Pediatrics, Pediatric Critical Care

Downs, Allan R. · General Surgery, General Vascular Surgery

Dozois, Roger R. · Colon & Rectal Surgery, General Colon & Rectal Surgery

Drach, George W. · Urology, Endourology

Drachman, David A. · Neurology, Adult, Degenerative Diseases

Drake, Charles G. · Neurological Surgery, Vascular Neurological Surgery

Drance, Stephen M. · Ophthalmology, Glaucoma

Drash, Allan L. · Pediatrics, Pediatric Endocrinology

Drazen, Jeffrey · Pulmonary & Critical Care Medicine, Asthma

Dreifus, Leonard S. · Cardiovascular Disease, General Cardiovascular Disease

Dreifuss, Fritz E. · Neurology, Adult, Epilepsy; Neurology, Child, Epilepsy

Dretler, Stephen P. · Urology, Endourology

Drez, David · Orthopaedic Surgery, Sports Medicine

Driscoll, David J. · Pediatrics, Pediatric Cardiology

Dritschilo, Anatoly · Radiation Oncology, General Radiation Oncology

Drossman, Douglas A. · Gastroenterology, Functional Gastrointestinal Disorders

Drummond, Denis S. · Orthopaedic Surgery, Pediatric Orthopaedic Surgery; Orthopaedic Surgery, Spine Surgery

Drummond, John C. · Anesthesiology, Neuroanesthesia

Druzin, Maurice L. · Obstetrics & Gynecology, Maternal & Fetal Medicine

Dubin, William R. · Psychiatry, Violence

Dubovsky, Eva V. · Nuclear Medicine, Kidney

Dubovsky, Steven L. · Psychiatry, Affective Disorders

Duck, Stephen C. · Pediatrics, Pediatric Endocrinology

Duckett, John W. · Urology, Pediatric Urology

Duff, W. Patrick · Obstetrics & Gynecology, Infectious Disease; Obstetrics & Gynecology, Maternal & Fetal Medicine

Duffner, Patricia Kressel · Neurology, Child, Neuro-oncology

Duffy, Thomas P. · Medical Oncology & Hematology, General Medical Oncology & Hematology

Dulaney, David D. · Ophthalmology, Anterior Segment (Cataract Surgery)

Dumitru, Daniel · Physical Medicine & Rehabilitation, Electromyography

Dunn, Harold K. · Orthopaedic Surgery, Hip Surgery; Orthopaedic Surgery, Knee Surgery

Dunner, David L. · Psychiatry, Affective Disorders; Psychiatry, Psychopharmacology

Dunnigan, Ann · Pediatrics, Pediatric Cardiology

DuPont, Herbert L. · Infectious Disease, Diarrhea

Dupont, Robert Louis · Psychiatry, Addiction Medicine

Durack, David T. · Infectious Disease, Endocarditis

Durrie, Daniel S. · Ophthalmology, Corneal Diseases & Transplantation

Duthie, Edmund H. · Geriatric Medicine, General Geriatric Medicine

Dutton, Jonathan J. · Ophthalmology, Oculoplastic & Orbital Surgery

Dworetzky, Murray · Allergy & Immunology, Adult Allergy & Immunology

Dworkin, Howard J. · Nuclear Medicine, General Nuclear Medicine

Dyck, Peter J. · Neurology, Adult, Degenerative Diseases; Neurology, Adult, Neuromuscular Disease

Dyken, Mark L. · Neurology, Adult, Strokes

Dysken, Maurice William · Psychiatry, Geriatric Psychiatry

E

Eagan, Robert T. · Medical Oncology, Lung Cancer

Eaglstein, William H. · Dermatology, Wound Healing

Earle, John D. · Radiation Oncology, General Radiation Oncology

Eary, Janet F. · Nuclear Medicine, Oncology

Easterling, Thomas R. · Obstetrics & Gynecology, Maternal & Fetal Medicine

Easton, J. Donald · Neurology, Adult, Strokes

Eastwood, M. Robin · Psychiatry, Geriatric Psychiatry

Eaton, Richard G. · Hand Surgery, Reconstructive Surgery

Ebers, George Cornell · Neurology, Adult, Infectious & Demyelinating Diseases

Echt, Debra S. · Cardiovascular Disease, Electrophysiology

Eckardt, Jeffrey J. · Orthopaedic Surgery, Tumor Surgery

Eckhauser, Frederic E. · General Surgery, Gastroenterologic Surgery

Eddy, Allison A. · Pediatrics, Pediatric Nephrology

Eddy, Roger · Psychiatry, Psychoanalysis

Edelson, Richard L. · Dermatology, Cutaneous Lymphomas

Edmeads, John Gordon · Neurology, Adult, Headache

Edwards, John E. · Infectious Disease, Fungal Infections

Edwards, Libby I. E. · Dermatology, Genital Dermatological Disease

Edwards, Michael S. B. · Neurological Surgery, Pediatric Neurological Surgery

Eftekhar, Nas S. · Orthopaedic Surgery, Reconstructive Surgery

Egan, James · Psychiatry, Child Psychiatry

Eggleston, Peyton · Allergy & Immunology, Pediatric Allergy & Immunology

Ehrenfeld, William K. · General Surgery, General Vascular Surgery

Ehrlich, Richard M. · Urology, Pediatric Urology

Eichelman, Burr S. · Psychiatry, Psychopharmacology; Psychiatry, Violence

Eichhorn, John H. · Anesthesiology, Complications of Anesthesia

Eigen, Howard · Pediatrics, Pediatric Pulmonology

Einhorn, Lawrence · Medical Oncology & Hematology, Genito-Urinary Cancer; Medical Oncology & Hematology, Lung Cancer

Eisdorfer, Carl · Psychiatry, Geriatric Psychiatry

Eisen, Andrew · Neurology, Adult, Electromyography; Neurology, Adult, Neuromuscular Disease

Eisenach, James C. · Anesthesiology, Obstetric Anesthesia

Eisenberger, Mario · Medical Oncology & Hematology, Prostate Cancer

Elias, Sherman · Obstetrics & Gynecology, Genetics

Ellestad, Myrvin H. · Cardiovascular Disease, Clinical Exercise Testing

Elliott, Glen R. · Psychiatry, Child Psychiatry

Elliott, Lester Franklyn · Plastic Surgery, Breast Surgery; Plastic Surgery, Microsurgery

Ellis, Demetrius · Pediatrics, Pediatric Nephrology

Ellis, Elliot F. · Allergy & Immunology, Pediatric Allergy & Immunology

Ellis, Forrest D. · Ophthalmology, Pediatric Ophthalmology

Ellis, Stephen G. · Cardiovascular Disease, Cardiac Catheterization

Ellison, E. Christopher · General Surgery, Gastroenterologic Surgery

Ellison, George W. · Neurology, Adult, Infectious & Demyelinating Diseases

Ellsworth, Robert M. · Ophthalmology, Ocular Oncology

Elsas, Louis J. · Pediatrics, Metabolic Diseases

Emans, S. Jean · Obstetrics & Gynecology, Pediatric & Adolescent Gynecology; Pediatrics, Pediatric & Adolescent Gynecology

Emond, Jean C. · General Surgery, Transplantation

Engel, Andrew G. · Neurology, Adult, Neuromuscular Disease

Engel, Jerome · Neurology, Adult, Epilepsy

Engh, Charles · Orthopaedic Surgery, Hip Surgery

Engrav, Loren H. · Plastic Surgery, Reconstructive Surgery

Epstein, Andrew E. · Cardiovascular Disease, Electrophysiology

Epstein, Burton S. · Anesthesiology, Ambulatory Anesthesia

Epstein, David L. · Ophthalmology, Glaucoma

Epstein, Fred Jacob · Neurological Surgery, Pediatric Neurological Surgery

Epstein, John Howard · Dermatology, Clinical Dermatology; Dermatology, Photobiology

Epstein, Leon G. · Neurology, Child, AIDS; Neurology, Child, Neurovirology

Eriksson, Elof · Plastic Surgery, Reconstructive Surgery; Plastic Surgery, Wound Healing

Ernest, Joseph McDonald · Obstetrics & Gynecology, Maternal & Fetal Medicine

Ernst, Calvin · General Surgery, General Vascular Surgery

Ervin, Frank R. · Psychiatry, Violence

Ervin, Thomas J. · Medical Oncology & Hematology, Head & Neck Cancer

Eschenbach, David · Obstetrics & Gynecology, Infectious Disease

Esquivel, Carlos O. · General Surgery, Transplantation

Esselstyn, Caldwell B. · General Surgery, Endocrine Surgery

Esterly, Nancy B. · Dermatology, Clinical Dermatology

Ettenger, Robert · Pediatrics, Pediatric Nephrology

Ettinger, David S. · Medical Oncology & Hematology, Clinical Pharmacology; Medical Oncology & Hematology, Lung Cancer

Etzwiler, Donnell D. · Pediatrics, Pediatric Endocrinology

Evans, Richard · Allergy & Immunology, Pediatric Allergy & Immunology

Everett, Mark Allen · Dermatology, Clinical Dermatology

Ewald, Frederick C. · Orthopaedic Surgery, Reconstructive Surgery

Exelby, Philip R. · General Surgery, Pediatric Surgery

F

Faber, L. Penfield · Thoracic Surgery, General Thoracic Surgery; Thoracic Surgery, Thoracic Oncological Surgery

Fabri, Peter Jeffrey · General Surgery, Gastroenterologic Surgery

Fahn, Stanley · Neurology, Adult, Movement Disorders

Fair, William R. · Urology, Urologic Oncology

Fairley, H. Barrie · Anesthesiology, Cardiothoracic Anesthesiology

Falanga, Vincent · Dermatology, Wound Healing

Falk, Ronald J. · Nephrology, Glomerular Diseases

Fanaroff, Avroy Arnold · Pediatrics, Neonatal-Perinatal Medicine

Farmer, Richard G. · Gastroenterology, Inflammatory Bowel Disease

Faro, Sebastian · Obstetrics & Gynecology, Infectious Disease

Farris, Bradley K. · Neurology, Neuro-Ophthalmology; Ophthalmology, Neuro-Ophthalmology

Farrow, George M. · Pathology, Surgical Pathology

Fauci, Anthony Stephen · Infectious Disease, AIDS; Infectious Disease, Vasculitis

Fawcett, Jan · Psychiatry, Affective Disorders; Psychiatry, Psychopharmacology; Psychiatry, Suicidology

Faxon, David Parker · Cardiovascular Disease, Cardiac Catheterization

Fazio, Victor W. · Colon & Rectal Surgery, Colon & Rectal Cancer; Colon & Rectal Surgery, General Colon & Rectal Surgery; Surgical Oncology, Colon & Rectal Cancer

Feagin, John A. · Orthopaedic Surgery, Sports Medicine

Fechner, Robert E. · Pathology, Bone Pathology; Pathology, ENT Pathology

Federman, Jay L. · Ophthalmology, Vitreo-Retinal Surgery

Fee, Willard E. · Otolaryngology, Head & Neck Surgery

Feeley, Thomas William · Anesthesiology, Critical Care Medicine

Feigenbaum, Harvey · Cardiovascular Disease, Echocardiography

Feighner, John P. · Psychiatry, Affective Disorders

Feigin, Ralph D. · Pediatrics, Pediatric Infectious Disease

Fekety, Robert · Infectious Disease, Diarrhea; Infectious Disease, General Infectious Disease

Feldman, Bruce Allen · Otolaryngology, Otology

Feldman, Joel J. · Plastic Surgery, Reconstructive Surgery

Feldman, Kenneth W. · Pediatrics, Abused Children

Fenoglio-Preiser, Cecilia M. · Pathology, Surgical Pathology

Ferrante, F. Michael · Anesthesiology, Pain

Ferry, George D. · Pediatrics, Pediatric Gastroenterology

Fiatarone, Maria A. · Geriatric Medicine, General Geriatric Medicine

Fiedler, Virginia C. · Dermatology, Hair

Fields, Alan I. · Pediatrics, Pediatric Critical Care

Fields, Suzanne L. · Geriatric Medicine, General Geriatric Medicine

Filler, Robert M. · General Surgery, Pediatric Surgery

Filston, Howard Church · General Surgery, Pediatric Surgery

Fine, I. Howard · Ophthalmology, Anterior Segment (Cataract Surgery)

Fine, Jo-David · Dermatology, Cutaneous Immunology

Fine, Robert M. · Dermatology, Clinical Dermatology

Fine, Stuart L. · Ophthalmology, Medical Retinal Diseases

Finegold, Sydney M. · Infectious Disease, Anaerobic Infections

Fink, Jordan N. · Allergy & Immunology, Adult Allergy & Immunology

Finkel, Martin A. · Pediatrics, Abused Children

Finkel, Sanford I. · Psychiatry, Geriatric Psychiatry

Finkelstein, Fredric O. · Nephrology, Dialysis

Finlay, Jonathan L. · Pediatrics, Pediatric Hematology-Oncology

Finnegan, Loretta P. · Addiction Medicine, Addicted Pregnant Women; Pediatrics, Neonatal-Perinatal Medicine

Finster, Mieczyslaw · Anesthesiology, Obstetric Anesthesia

Fireman, Philip · Allergy & Immunology, Pediatric Allergy & Immunology

Firlit, Casimir F. · Urology, Pediatric Urology

First, M. Roy · Nephrology, Kidney Transplantation

Fischer, Josef E. · General Surgery, Gastroenterologic Surgery

Fischer, Newell · Psychiatry, Psychoanalysis

Fischer, Thomas Joseph · Allergy & Immunology, Pediatric Allergy & Immunology

Fischl, Margaret A. · Medical Oncology & Hematology, AIDS

Fish, James E. · Pulmonary & Critical Care Medicine, General Pulmonary & Critical Care Medicine

Fisher, C. Miller · Neurology, Adult, Strokes

Fisher, Jack · Plastic Surgery, Breast Surgery

Fisher, John D. · Cardiovascular Disease, Electrophysiology

Fisher, Richard · Medical Oncology & Hematology, Hematological Malignancies; Medical Oncology & Hematology, Lymphomas

Fisher, Robert S. · Gastroenterology, Functional Gastrointestinal Disorders; Gastroenterology, Gastrointestinal Motility; Gastroenterology, Peptic Disorders

Fisher, Yale L. · Ophthalmology, Ultrasound

Fishman, Irving J. · Urology, Impotence

Fishman, Robert A. · Neurology, Adult, Infectious & Demyelinating Diseases

Fitch, William P. · Urology, Impotence

FitzGerald, Garret A. · Clinical Pharmacology

Fitzgerald, Robert H. · Orthopaedic Surgery, Hip Surgery

Fitzpatrick, Peter · Radiation Oncology, Skin Cancer

Fixler, David E. · Pediatrics, Pediatric Cardiology

Flamm, Eugene S. · Neurological Surgery, Vascular Neurological Surgery

Flanagan, Joseph C. · Ophthalmology, Oculoplastic & Orbital Surgery

Flanigan, Robert Charles · Urology, Urologic Oncology

Fleischer, David E. · Gastroenterology, Endoscopy

Flynn, Harry Weisiger · Ophthalmology, Vitreo-Retinal Surgery

Flynn, John T. · Ophthalmology, Pediatric Ophthalmology

Fogel, Barry S. · Psychiatry, Geriatric Psychiatry; Psychiatry, Neuropsychiatry

Fogoros, Richard N. · Cardiovascular Disease, Electrophysiology

Foley, Cornelius James · Geriatric Medicine, General Geriatric Medicine

Foley, Kathleen M. · Medical Oncology & Hematology, Neuro-oncology; Neurology, Adult, Neuro-oncology

Foley, Thomas P. · Pediatrics, Pediatric Endocrinology

Folks, David G. · Psychiatry, Geriatric Psychiatry

Folstein, Marshal F. · Psychiatry, Geriatric Psychiatry

Folstein, Susan E. · Psychiatry, Autism; Psychiatry, Behavioral Disorders; Psychiatry, Neuropsychiatry

Forastiere, Arlene A. · Medical Oncology & Hematology, Head & Neck Cancer

Forbes, Max · Ophthalmology, Glaucoma

Ford, Charles N. · Otolaryngology, Laryngology

Fordtran, John S. · Gastroenterology, Inflammatory Bowel Disease; Gastroenterology, Peptic Disorders

Foreman, John W. · Pediatrics, Pediatric Nephrology

Forman, Stephen J. · Medical Oncology, Bone Marrow Transplantation; Medical Oncology, Leukemia

Forrester, James S. · Cardiovascular Disease, Cardiac Catheterization

Fortner, Joseph · Surgical Oncology, Gastroenterologic Cancer

Foster, C. Stephen · Ophthalmology, Uveitis

Foster, Jeffrey Robert · Psychiatry, Geriatric Psychiatry

Foucar, M. Kathryn · Pathology, Hematopathology

Foulks, Gary I. · Ophthalmology, Corneal Diseases & Transplantation

Fowble, Barbara · Radiation Oncology, Breast Cancer

Fowler, John A. · Psychiatry, Psychoanalysis

Fowler, Wesley C. · Obstetrics & Gynecology, Gynecologic Cancer

Frances, Richard J. · Psychiatry, Addiction Medicine

Frank, Alvin R. · Psychiatry, Psychoanalysis

Franklin, Rudolph M. · Ophthalmology, Uveitis

Frasier, S. Douglas · Pediatrics, Pediatric Endocrinology

Frazier, O. H. · Thoracic Surgery, Adult Cardiothoracic Surgery; Thoracic Surgery, Transplantation

Frazier, Shervert H. · Psychiatry, General Psychiatry

Fredrickson, John M. · Otolaryngology, Head & Neck Surgery

Freed, Michael David · Pediatrics, Pediatric Cardiology

Freedberg, Irwin M. · Dermatology, Clinical Dermatology; Dermatology, Eczema; Dermatology, Psoriasis

Freedman, David A. · Psychiatry, Psychoanalysis

Freedman, Michael L. · Geriatric Medicine, General Geriatric Medicine

Freeman, Arnold I. · Pediatrics, Pediatric Hematology-Oncology

Freeman, Carolyn R. · Radiation Oncology, Pediatric Radiation Oncology

Freeman, Hal MacKenzie · Ophthalmology, Vitreo-Retinal Surgery

Freeman, John M. · Neurology, Child, Epilepsy; Neurology, Child, General Child Neurology

Freeman, Leonard M. · Nuclear Medicine, General Nuclear Medicine

Freeman, Roger K. · Obstetrics & Gynecology, Maternal & Fetal Medicine

Frei, Emil · Medical Oncology & Hematology, General Medical Oncology & Hematology

Freireich, Emil J · Medical Oncology, Leukemia

Fretwell, Marsha D. · Geriatric Medicine, General Geriatric Medicine

Frick, Oscar L. · Allergy & Immunology, Pediatric Allergy & Immunology; Pediatrics, Pediatric Allergy & Immunology

Frieden, Ilona · Dermatology, Pediatric Dermatology; Pediatrics, Pediatric Dermatology

Friedland, Gerald H. · Infectious Disease, AIDS

Friedland, Jack A. · Plastic Surgery, Facial Aesthetic Surgery

Friedman, Allan H. · Neurological Surgery, Peripheral Nerve Surgery

Friedman, Eli A. · Nephrology, Dialysis; Nephrology, Kidney Disease

Friedman, Ellen M. · Otolaryngology, Pediatric Otolaryngology

Friedman, Henry J. · Psychiatry, Psychoanalysis

Friedman, Henry S. · Pediatrics, Pediatric Hematology-Oncology

Friedman, Marc Jay · Orthopaedic Surgery, Sports Medicine

Friedman, William A. · Neurological Surgery, Stereotactic Radiosurgery

Friedman, William F. · Pediatrics, Pediatric Cardiology

Friesinger, Gottlieb C. · Cardiovascular Disease, General Cardiovascular Disease

Frigoletto, Fredric D. · Obstetrics & Gynecology, Maternal & Fetal Medicine

Frizzera, Glauco · Pathology, Hematopathology

Froelicher, Victor F. · Cardiovascular Disease, Clinical Exercise Testing

Frohman, Lawrence A. · Endocrinology & Metabolism, Neuroendocrinology

Frosch, William A. · Psychiatry, Addiction Medicine; Psychiatry, Psychoanalysis

Frost, J. James · Nuclear Medicine, Brain

Frueh, Bartley R. · Ophthalmology, Oculoplastic & Orbital Surgery

Frye, Robert · Cardiovascular Disease, General Cardiovascular Disease

Fryer, Christopher · Radiation Oncology, Pediatric Radiation Oncology

Fu, Karen King-Wah · Radiation Oncology, Brachytherapy; Radiation Oncology, Head & Neck Cancer

Fuchs, Gerhard J. · Urology, Endourology

Fuhrman, Bradley P. · Pediatrics, Pediatric Critical Care

Fuks, Zvi Y. · Radiation Oncology, Genito-Urinary Cancer

Fulkerson, William J. · Pulmonary & Critical Care Medicine, General Pulmonary & Critical Care Medicine

Fung, John · General Surgery, Transplantation

Furakawa, Clifton T. · Allergy & Immunology, Pediatric Allergy & Immunology

Furlan, Anthony J. · Neurology, Adult, Strokes

Fuster, Valentine · Cardiovascular Disease, General Cardiovascular Disease

G

Gabbe, Steven G. · Obstetrics & Gynecology, Maternal & Fetal Medicine

Gahl, William · Pediatrics, Metabolic Diseases

Gaitz, Charles Milton · Psychiatry, Geriatric Psychiatry

Galaburda, Albert M. · Neurology, Adult, Behavioral Neurology

Galante, Jorge O. · Orthopaedic Surgery, Reconstructive Surgery

Galanter, Marc · Psychiatry, Addiction Medicine

Galatzer-Levy, Robert Milton · Psychiatry, Psychoanalysis

Galetta, Steven L. · Neurology, Adult, Neuro-Ophthalmology

Galicich, Joseph H. · Neurological Surgery, Tumor Surgery

Gallagher, John J. · Cardiovascular Disease, Electrophysiology

Gallagher, T. James · Anesthesiology, Critical Care Medicine

Gallant, Donald M. · Psychiatry, Addiction Medicine

Gammon, W. Ray · Dermatology, Cutaneous Immunology

Gamsu, Gordon · Radiology, Chest

Ganaway, George K. · Psychiatry, Dissociative Disorders

Gant, Norman F. · Obstetrics & Gynecology, Maternal & Fetal Medicine

Gantz, Bruce J. · Otolaryngology, Otology/Neurotology

García, Celso-Ramón · Obstetrics & Gynecology, Reproductive Endocrinology; Obstetrics & Gynecology, Reproductive Surgery

Garcia, Jairo E. · Obstetrics & Gynecology, Reproductive Endocrinology

Garden, Jerome M. · Dermatology, Laser Surgery

Gardner, Gale · Otolaryngology, Otology/Neurotology

Gardner, M. Robert · Psychiatry, Psychoanalysis

Garfinkel, Paul Earl · Psychiatry, Eating Disorders

Garibaldi, Richard A. · Infectious Disease, Hospital-Acquired Infections

Garite, Thomas J. · Obstetrics & Gynecology, Maternal & Fetal Medicine

Garnick, Marc B. · Medical Oncology & Hematology, Genito-Urinary Cancer

Garrett, John Calvin · Orthopaedic Surgery, Sports Medicine

Garrett, William E. · Orthopaedic Surgery, Sports Medicine

Garson, Arthur · Pediatrics, Pediatric Cardiology

Gaskill, Herbert Stockton · Psychiatry, Psychoanalysis

Gass, J. Donald M. · Ophthalmology, Medical Retinal Diseases

Gathright, J. Byron · Colon & Rectal Surgery, General Colon & Rectal Surgery

Gatter, Robert A. · Rheumatology, General Rheumatology

Gawin, Frank H. · Addiction Medicine, Medical Treatment for Drug Abusers

Gay, William · Thoracic Surgery, Adult Cardiothoracic Surgery; Thoracic Surgery, Transplantation

Gaz, Randall David · General Surgery, Endocrine Surgery

Gearhart, John P. · Urology, Pediatric Urology

Gedo, John E. · Psychiatry, Psychoanalysis

Geenen, Joseph E. · Gastroenterology, Endoscopy; Gastroenterology, Pancreatic Disease

Geha, Raif S. · Allergy & Immunology, Pediatric Allergy & Immunology

Gelb, Adrian · Anesthesiology, Neuroanesthesia

Gelband, Henry · Pediatrics, Pediatric Cardiology

Gelberman, Richard H. · Hand Surgery, Peripheral Nerve Surgery; Orthopaedic Surgery, Peripheral Nerve Surgery

Gelenberg, Alan J. · Psychiatry, Affective Disorders

Gelfand, Erwin W. · Allergy & Immunology, Pediatric Allergy & Immunology

Geller, Anne · Addiction Medicine, General Addiction Medicine

Gelman, Simon · Anesthesiology, Hepatic Disease

Geltman, Edward M. · Cardiovascular Disease, Cardiac Positron Emission Tomography (PET)

Gentry, Layne O. · Infectious Disease, Bone Infections

Genuth, Saul · Endocrinology & Metabolism, Diabetes

George, Ronald B. · Pulmonary & Critical Care Medicine, General Pulmonary & Critical Care Medicine

Georgitis, John W. · Allergy & Immunology, Pediatric Allergy & Immunology

Gerber, Naomi Lynn · Rheumatology, Rehabilitation

Gerding, Dale Nicholas · Infectious Disease, General Infectious Disease

Gerety, Meghan B. · Geriatric Medicine, General Geriatric Medicine

Germain, Bernard F. · Rheumatology, General Rheumatology

Gerner, Robert H. · Psychiatry, Affective Disorders

Geronemus, Roy G. · Dermatology, Laser Surgery; Dermatology, Skin Cancer Surgery & Reconstruction

Gershell, William Jay · Psychiatry, General Psychiatry

Gershenson, David M. · Obstetrics & Gynecology, Gynecologic Cancer

Gershon, Anne A. · Pediatrics, Pediatric Infectious Disease

Gershon, Elliot Sheldon · Psychiatry, Affective Disorders

Gersony, Welton M. · Pediatrics, Pediatric Cardiology

Gertner, Joseph M. · Pediatrics, Pediatric Endocrinology

Gessner, Ira H. · Pediatrics, Pediatric Cardiology

Giannotta, Steven L. · Neurological Surgery, Vascular Neurological Surgery

Gibbons, Raymond J. · Cardiovascular Disease, Nuclear Cardiology

Gibbs, Frederic A. · Radiation Oncology, Hypothermia

Gibbs, Ronald S. · Obstetrics & Gynecology, Infectious Disease

Gifford, Ray W. · Nephrology, Hypertension

Gilchrest, Barbara A. · Dermatology, Aging Skin

Gilday, David L. · Nuclear Medicine, Pediatric

Gilden, Donald H. · Neurology, Adult, Infectious & Demyelinating Diseases

Gilles, Floyd H. · Pathology, Neuropathology

Gillespie, Robert · Orthopaedic Surgery, Pediatric Orthopaedic Surgery

Gillette, Paul C. · Pediatrics, Pediatric Cardiology

Gilliland, Robert M. · Psychiatry, Psychoanalysis

Gilman, Sid · Neurology, Adult, Degenerative Diseases; Neurology, Adult, Movement Disorders

Gilsdorf, Janet R. · Pediatrics, Pediatric Infectious Disease

Gilstrap, Larry C. · Obstetrics & Gynecology, Maternal & Fetal Medicine

Gimbel, Howard V. · Ophthalmology, Anterior Segment (Cataract Surgery)

Ginsberg, Robert L. · Thoracic Surgery, General Thoracic Surgery; Thoracic Surgery, Thoracic Oncological Surgery

Ginsberg-Fellner, Fredda · Pediatrics, Pediatric Endocrinology

Ginsburg, William W. · Rheumatology, General Rheumatology

Giordano, Joseph Martin · General Surgery, General Vascular Surgery

Gitlow, Stanley · Addiction Medicine, General Addiction Medicine

Gitnick, Gary · Gastroenterology, Hepatology

Gitter, Kurt A. · Ophthalmology, Medical Retinal Diseases

Gittes, Ruben F. · Urology, Neuro-Urology & Voiding Dysfunction

Gittinger, John W. · Ophthalmology, Neuro-Ophthalmology

Giuliano, Armando E. · General Surgery, Endocrine Surgery; Surgical Oncology, Breast Cancer

Gladstein, Arthur H. · Dermatology, Skin Cancer Surgery & Reconstruction; Radiation Oncology, Skin Cancer Surgery & Reconstruction

Glaser, Bert M. · Ophthalmology, Vitreo-Retinal Surgery

Glaser, Joel S. · Neurology, Adult, Neuro-Ophthalmology; Ophthalmology, Neuro-Ophthalmology

Glasscock, Michael E. · Otolaryngology, Otology/Neurotology

Glassman, Alexander H. · Psychiatry, Affective Disorders; Psychiatry, Psychopharmacology

Glassock, Richard J. · Nephrology, Glomerular Diseases

Glassroth, Jeffrey · Pulmonary & Critical Care Medicine, AIDS; Pulmonary & Critical Care Medicine, Lung Infections

Glatstein, Eli · Radiation Oncology, Lung Cancer

Glazer, Gary M. · Radiology, Chest

Glazer, William M. · Psychiatry, Schizophrenia/Psychopharmacology

Glenn, Jules · Psychiatry, Psychoanalysis

Glew, Richard H. · Infectious Disease, General Infectious Disease

Glick, John H. · Medical Oncology, Breast Cancer; Medical Oncology, Lymphomas

Glode, L. Michael · Medical Oncology & Hematology, Genito-Urinary Cancer; Medical Oncology & Hematology, Prostate Cancer; Medical Oncology & Hematology, Solid Tumors

Glorieux, Francis H. · Pediatrics, Pediatric Endocrinology

Gloviczki, Peter · General Surgery, General Vascular Surgery

Gluckman, Jack Louis · Otolaryngology, Head & Neck Surgery

Go, Raymundo Tiu · Nuclear Medicine, Nuclear Cardiology

Gode, Richard O. · Psychiatry, Child Psychiatry

Godine, John E. · Endocrinology & Metabolism, Diabetes

Godwin, J. David · Radiology, Chest

Goepfert, Helmuth · Otolaryngology, Head & Neck Surgery

Goetz, Christopher G. · Neurology, Adult, Movement Disorders

Goetzl, Edward J. · Allergy & Immunology, Adult Allergy & Immunology

Goffinet, Don R. · Radiation Oncology, Brachytherapy; Radiation Oncology, Head & Neck Cancer

Goin, Donald W. · Otolaryngology, Otology/Neurotology

Golbus, Mitchell S. · Obstetrics & Gynecology, Genetics

Gold, Mark S. · Addiction Medicine, General Addiction Medicine

Gold, Philip M. · Pulmonary & Critical Care Medicine, General Pulmonary & Critical Care Medicine

Goldberg, Arnold I. · Psychiatry, Psychoanalysis

Goldberg, Stanley M. · Surgical Oncology, Colon & Rectal Cancer

Goldberg, Victor M. · Orthopaedic Surgery, Reconstructive Surgery

Goldberger, Marianne R. · Psychiatry, Psychoanalysis

Golden, David Bryant K. · Allergy & Immunology, Adult Allergy & Immunology

Golden, Gerald S. · Neurology, Child, Child Development

Goldenberg, Don Lee · Rheumatology, Fibromyalgia; Rheumatology, Infectious Arthritis

Goldfarb, Alvin F. · Obstetrics & Gynecology, Pediatric & Adolescent Gynecology

Goldsmith, Lowell A. · Dermatology, Clinical Dermatology; Dermatology, Hair

Goldsmith, Stanley J. · Nuclear Medicine, General Nuclear Medicine

Goldstein, David E. · Pediatrics, Pediatric Endocrinology

Goldstein, Ellie J. C. · Infectious Disease, Anaerobic Infections

Goldstein, Franz · Gastroenterology, General Gastroenterology

Goldstein, Irwin · Urology, Impotence

Goldstein, Marion Zucker · Psychiatry, Geriatric Psychiatry

Goldstein, Mary Kane · Geriatric Medicine, General Geriatric Medicine

Goldstein, Richard A. · Cardiovascular Disease, Cardiac Positron Emission Tomography (PET)

Goldstone, Jerry · General Surgery, General Vascular Surgery

Goldwyn, Robert M. · Plastic Surgery, Reconstructive Surgery

Golomb, Harvey M. · Medical Oncology, Leukemia

Golper, Thomas Alan · Nephrology, Dialysis

Goltz, Robert W. · Dermatology, Clinical Dermatology

Gomes, J. Anthony · Cardiovascular Disease, Electrophysiology

Gonik, Bernard · Obstetrics & Gynecology, Maternal & Fetal Medicine

Gonnering, Russell S. · Ophthalmology, Oculoplastic & Orbital Surgery

Gonwa, Thomas A. · Nephrology, Kidney Transplantation

Gonzales, Edmond T. · Urology, Pediatric Urology

Gonzalez, Ricardo · Urology, Pediatric Urology

Good, Robert A. · Allergy & Immunology, Adult Allergy & Immunology; Allergy & Immunology, Pediatric Allergy & Immunology

Goodkin, Donald E. · Neurology, Adult, Infectious & Demyelinating Diseases

Goodman, Lawrence R. · Radiology, Chest

Goodman, Robert L. · Radiation Oncology, Breast Cancer; Radiation Oncology, Lymphomas

Goodman, Stanley · Psychiatry, Psychoanalysis

Goodman, Stephen I. · Pediatrics, Metabolic Diseases

Goodson, William H. · Surgical Oncology, Breast Cancer

Goodwin, Frederick K. · Psychiatry, Affective Disorders

Goodwin, James A. · Neurology, Adult, Neuro-Ophthalmology

Goodwin, Jean Patricia · Psychiatry, Sexual Abuse

Goodwin, W. Jarrard · Otolaryngology, Head & Neck Surgery

Gorbach, Sherwood L. · Infectious Disease, Anaerobic Infections; Infectious Disease, Diarrhea

Gordon, Howard L. · Plastic Surgery, Facial Aesthetic Surgery

Gordon, Philip H. · Colon & Rectal Surgery, General Colon & Rectal Surgery

Gorman, Colum A. · Endocrinology & Metabolism, Thyroid

Gorman, Jack M. · Psychiatry, Affective Disorders; Psychiatry, Psychopharmacology

Gospodarowicz, Mary K. · Radiation Oncology, Genito-Urinary Cancer; Radiation Oncology, Lymphomas

Gotch, Frank A. · Nephrology, Dialysis

Gottlieb, Gary L. · Psychiatry, Geriatric Psychiatry

Gottlieb, Michael S. · Infectious Disease, AIDS

Gould, John Samuel · Orthopaedic Surgery, Foot & Ankle Surgery

Goulet, James A. · Orthopaedic Surgery, Trauma

Gradinger, Gilbert P. · Plastic Surgery, Facial Aesthetic Surgery

Graft, David F. · Allergy & Immunology, Pediatric Allergy & Immunology

Gragoudas, Evangelos S. · Ophthalmology, Ocular Oncology

Graham, Malcolm D. · Otolaryngology, Otology/Neurotology

Graham, Thomas P. · Pediatrics, Pediatric Cardiology

Gralla, Richard J. · Medical Oncology & Hematology, Lung Cancer

Grand, Richard J. · Pediatrics, Pediatric Gastroenterology

Grant, Clive S. · General Surgery, Endocrine Surgery

Grant, J. Andrew · Allergy & Immunology, Adult Allergy & Immunology

Gray, Paul · Psychiatry, Psychoanalysis

Gray, Steven D. · Otolaryngology, Pediatric Otolaryngology

Grazer, Frederick M. · Plastic Surgery, Aesthetic Surgery; Plastic Surgery, Body Contouring

Greco, F. Anthony · Medical Oncology & Hematology, Genito-Urinary Cancer; Medical Oncology & Hematology, Lung Cancer

Greeley, William J. · Anesthesiology, Pediatric Cardiovascular

Green, Arthur H. · Psychiatry, Child Abuse; Psychiatry, Child Psychiatry; Psychiatry, Psychoanalysis; Psychiatry, Sexual Abuse

Green, Christopher G. · Pediatrics, Pediatric Pulmonology

Green, David P. · Hand Surgery, General Hand Surgery

Green, Mark R. · Medical Oncology & Hematology, Lung Cancer

Green, Neil E. · Orthopaedic Surgery, Pediatric Orthopaedic Surgery

Green, Richard M. · General Surgery, General Vascular Surgery

Green, Thomas P. · Pediatrics, Pediatric Critical Care

Greenberg, Barry H. · Cardiovascular Disease, Heart Failure

Greenberg, Harry S. · Neurology, Adult, Neuro-oncology

Greenberg, Jack O. · Neurology, Adult, Magnetic Resonance Imaging

Greenberg, Richard M. · Psychiatry, Psychoanalysis

Greenberger, Paul Allen · Allergy & Immunology, Adult Allergy & Immunology

Greene, Bruce M. · Infectious Disease, Tropical Diseases

Greene, James Allen · Psychiatry, Geriatric Psychiatry

Greenfield, Lazar J. · General Surgery, General Vascular Surgery

Greenhill, Laurence L. · Psychiatry, Child Psychiatry; Psychiatry, Psychopharmacology

Greenson, Daniel Peter · Psychiatry, Psychoanalysis

Greenspan, Francis S. · Endocrinology & Metabolism, Thyroid

Greenspan, Susan L. · Geriatric Medicine, General Geriatric Medicine

Greenway, Hubert T. · Dermatology, Skin Cancer Surgery & Reconstruction

Gregory, George · Anesthesiology, Pediatric Anesthesiology; Pediatrics, Pediatric Critical Care

Gregory, Richard O. · Plastic Surgery, Laser Surgery & Birthmarks

Greifer, Ira · Pediatrics, Pediatric Nephrology

Grekin, Roy C. · Dermatology, Skin Cancer Surgery & Reconstruction

Grieco, Michael Henry · Allergy & Immunology, Adult Allergy & Immunology

Griffin, Jerry C. · Cardiovascular Disease, Pacemakers

Griffin, John W. · Neurology, Adult, Neuromuscular Disease

Griffin, Paul P. · Orthopaedic Surgery, Pediatric Orthopaedic Surgery

Griffin, Thomas W. · Radiation Oncology, General Radiation Oncology

Griffith, Bartley P. · Thoracic Surgery, Adult Cardiothoracic Surgery; Thoracic Surgery, Transplantation

Griffith, Donald P. · Urology, Endourology

Griggs, Robert C. · Neurology, Adult, Neuromuscular Disease

Grillo, Hermes C. · Thoracic Surgery, General Thoracic Surgery; Thoracic Surgery, Thoracic Oncological Surgery

Grinstein, Alexander · Psychiatry, Psychoanalysis

Grogan, Thomas M. · Pathology, Hematopathology

Groopman, Jerome E. · Medical Oncology & Hematology, AIDS

Grosfeld, Jay L. · General Surgery, Pediatric Surgery

Gross, Charles W. · Otolaryngology, Pediatric Otolaryngology; Otolaryngology, Sinus & Nasal Surgery

Grossberg, George T. · Psychiatry, Geriatric Psychiatry

Grossman, H. Barton · Urology, Urologic Oncology

Grossman, Robert G. · Neurological Surgery, Epilepsy Surgery

Grossman, Robert I. · Radiology, Neuroradiology

Grossman, William · Cardiovascular Disease, Cardiac Catheterization; Cardiovascular Disease, General Cardiovascular Disease

Grotta, James · Neurology, Adult, Strokes

Grotting, James C. · Plastic Surgery , Breast Surgery; Plastic Surgery , Microsurgery

Grove, Arthur S. · Ophthalmology, Oculoplastic & Orbital Surgery

Growdon, John H. · Neurology, Adult, Degenerative Diseases

Grumbach, Melvin M. · Pediatrics, Pediatric Endocrinology

Grundfast, Kenneth Martin · Otolaryngology, Pediatric Otolaryngology

Gruss, Joseph S. · Plastic Surgery, Maxillofacial Surgery

Guiraudon, Gerard M. · Thoracic Surgery, Adult Cardiothoracic Surgery

Gullane, Patrick Joseph · Otolaryngology, Head & Neck Surgery; Otolaryngology, Skull-Base

Gulya, A. Julianna · Otolaryngology, Otology/Neurotology

Gunderson, John G. · Psychiatry, Schizophrenia

Gunderson, Leonard L. · Radiation Oncology, Gastroenterologic Cancer

Gunter, Jack Pershing · Plastic Surgery, Facial Aesthetic Surgery

Gurian, Bennett S. · Psychiatry, Geriatric Psychiatry

Gutgesell, Howard P. · Pediatrics, Pediatric Cardiology

Gutin, Philip H. · Neurological Surgery, Stereotactic Radiosurgery; Neurological Surgery, Tumor Surgery

Gutmann, Ludwig · Neurology, Adult, Electromyography; Neurology, Adult, Neuromuscular Disease

Gutsche, Brett B. · Anesthesiology, Obstetric Anesthesia

Gutterman, Jordan U. · Medical Oncology & Hematology, Immunotherapy, Biological Response Modifiers Oncology

Guttmann, Ronald D. · Nephrology, Kidney Transplantation

Guyton, David L. · Ophthalmology, Optics & Refraction; Ophthalmology, Pediatric Ophthalmology

Guze, Samuel B. · Psychiatry, Psychopharmacology

Gwirtsman, Harry Edward · Psychiatry, Eating Disorders

H

Hachinski, Vladimir C. · Neurology, Adult, Strokes

Hahn, Bevra Hannahs · Rheumatology, Lupus

Hait, William N. · Medical Oncology & Hematology, General Medical Oncology & Hematology

Hakim, Raymond M. · Nephrology, Dialysis

Halbach, Van V. · Radiology, Neuroradiology

Halberg, Francine E. · Radiation Oncology, Breast Cancer

Hales, Robert E. · Psychiatry, Neuropsychiatry

Hall, Caroline Breese · Pediatrics, Pediatric Infectious Disease

Hall, John E. · Orthopaedic Surgery, Pediatric Orthopaedic Surgery; Orthopaedic Surgery, Spine Surgery

Hall, Russell P. · Dermatology, Cutaneous Immunology

Halleck, Seymour L. · Psychiatry, Forensic Psychiatry

Haller, Daniel G. · Medical Oncology, Gastrointestinal Oncology

Haller, J. Alex · Thoracic Surgery, Pediatric Non-Cardiac Thoracic Surgery

Hallett, Mark · Neurology, Adult, Electromyography

Halmi, Katherine A. · Psychiatry, Eating Disorders

Halpern, Abraham L. · Psychiatry, Forensic Psychiatry

Halushka, Perry V. · Clinical Pharmacology

Ham, Richard T. · Geriatric Medicine, General Geriatric Medicine

Hamilton, William G. · Orthopaedic Surgery, Foot & Ankle Surgery; Orthopaedic Surgery, Sports Medicine

Hamlin, Charles · Hand Surgery, Paralytic Disorders

Hammond, Charles B. · Obstetrics & Gynecology, Reproductive Endocrinology

Hammond, Mary G. · Obstetrics & Gynecology, Reproductive Endocrinology

Hamra, Sam T. · Plastic Surgery , Facial Aesthetic Surgery

Hanauer, Stephen B. · Gastroenterology, Inflammatory Bowel Disease

Hand, W. Lee · Infectious Disease, General Infectious Disease

Handsfield, H. Hunter · Infectious Disease, Sexually Transmitted Disease

Handwerger, Stuart · Pediatrics, Pediatric Endocrinology

Haney, Arthur F. · Obstetrics & Gynecology, Reproductive Endocrinology

Hanifin, Jon M. · Dermatology, Atopic Dermatitis; Dermatology, Eczema

Hankins, Gary D. V. · Obstetrics & Gynecology, Maternal & Fetal Medicine

Hanks, Gerald Eugene · Radiation Oncology, Genito-Urinary Cancer

Hannallah, Raafat S. · Anesthesiology, Pediatric Anesthesiology

Hansen, Dolly D. · Anesthesiology, Pediatric Cardiovascular

Hansen, Ronald C. · Dermatology, Pediatric Dermatology; Pediatrics, Pediatric Dermatology

Hansen, Sigvard T. · Orthopaedic Surgery, Foot & Ankle Surgery; Orthopaedic Surgery, Trauma

Hanson, David G. · Otolaryngology, Laryngology

Hardy, Jules · Neurological Surgery, Tumor Surgery

Hardy, Mark A. · General Surgery, Transplantation

Hargreave, Frederick E. · Pulmonary & Critical Care Medicine, Asthma

Harmon, William E. · Pediatrics, Pediatric Nephrology

Harrell, James H. · Pulmonary & Critical Care Medicine, Bronchoesophegology

Harrington, J. Timothy · Rheumatology, General Rheumatology

Harris, Gerald J. · Ophthalmology, Oculoplastic & Orbital Surgery

Harris, Jay R. · Radiation Oncology, Breast Cancer

Harris, Nancy · Pathology, Hematopathology

Harris, William H. · Orthopaedic Surgery, Hip Surgery

Harrison, Gunyon · Pediatrics, Pediatric Pulmonology

Harrison, Louis Benjamin · Radiation Oncology, Brachytherapy

Harrison, Michael R. · General Surgery, Pediatric Surgery

Hart, Robert G. · Neurology, Adult, Strokes

Harthorne, J. Warren · Cardiovascular Disease, Pacemakers

Hartmann, William H. · Pathology, Breast Pathology

Hartrampf, Carl R. · Plastic Surgery, Breast Surgery

Hartzler, Geoffrey O. · Cardiovascular Disease, Cardiac Catheterization

Harwood, Ivan R. · Pediatrics, Pediatric Pulmonology

Haskell, Charles M. · Medical Oncology, Breast Cancer

Hatch, Kenneth D. · Obstetrics & Gynecology, Gynecologic Cancer

Hauser, Stephen L. · Neurology, Adult, Infectious & Demyelinating Diseases

Hauth, John C. · Obstetrics & Gynecology, Maternal & Fetal Medicine

Hawkins, Donald B. · Otolaryngology, Pediatric Otolaryngology

Hawkins, Randall · Nuclear Medicine, Brain; Nuclear Medicine, Oncology

Hawkins, Richard J. · Orthopaedic Surgery, Reconstructive Surgery

Hay, Donald Peter · Psychiatry, Geriatric Psychiatry

Hay, Ian D. · Endocrinology & Metabolism, Thyroid

Haymond, Morey W. · Pediatrics, Pediatric Endocrinology

Haynie, Thomas Powell · Nuclear Medicine, Oncology

Hayward, James N. · Neurology, Adult, General Adult Neurology

Hazzard, William R. · Geriatric Medicine, General Geriatric Medicine

Headington, John T. · Dermatology, Hair; Pathology, Dermatopathology

Heagarty, Margaret C. · Pediatrics, Pediatric Infectious Disease

Healey, Louis A. · Rheumatology, General Rheumatology; Rheumatology, Rheumatoid Arthritis

Healy, Gerald B. · Otolaryngology, Pediatric Otolaryngology

Hebert, Adelaide A. · Dermatology, Pediatric Dermatology

Hebert, Diane · Pediatrics, Pediatric Nephrology

Heckenlively, John R. · Ophthalmology, Ophthalmic Genetics

Heckler, Frederick R. · Plastic Surgery, Reconstructive Surgery

Hedges, Thomas R. · Neurology, Adult, Neuro-Ophthalmology; Ophthalmology, Neuro-Ophthalmology

Hedley, Anthony K. · Orthopaedic Surgery, Reconstructive Surgery

Hedley-Whyte, E. Tessa · Pathology, Neuropathology

Heger, Astrid H. · Pediatrics, Abused Children

Heijn, Cornelis · Psychiatry, Psychoanalysis

Heilbrun, Peter · Neurological Surgery, Stereotactic Radiosurgery

Heilman, Kenneth M. · Neurology, Adult, Behavioral Neurology

Heimarck, Gregory J. · Psychiatry, Child Psychiatry

Heitzman, E. Robert · Radiology, Chest

Helfer, Ray E. · Pediatrics, Abused Children

Helfet, David L. · Orthopaedic Surgery, Trauma

Hellenbrand, William E. · Pediatrics, Pediatric Cardiology

Helveston, Eugene M. · Ophthalmology, Pediatric Ophthalmology

Hench, Kahler P. · Rheumatology, General Rheumatology

Henderson, I. Craig · Medical Oncology & Hematology, Breast Cancer

Hendin, Herbert M. · Psychiatry, Suicidology

Hendren, W. Hardy · General Surgery, Pediatric Surgery; Urology, Pediatric Urology

Henkin, Robert E. · Nuclear Medicine, General Nuclear Medicine

Hensinger, Robert N. · Orthopaedic Surgery, Pediatric Orthopaedic Surgery

Hensle, Terry W. · Urology, Pediatric Urology

Hentz, Vincent R. · Hand Surgery, Paralytic Disorders; Hand Surgery, Reconstructive Surgery

Hepler, Robert S. · Ophthalmology, Neuro-Ophthalmology

Herbst, Arthur L. · Obstetrics & Gynecology, Gynecologic Cancer

Herfkens, Robert J. · Radiology, Cardiovascular Disease; Radiology, Magnetic Resonance Imaging

Herman, Stephen Paul · Psychiatry, Child Psychiatry

Hermann, Robert E. · General Surgery, Gastroenterologic Surgery; urgical Oncology, Gastroenterologic Cancer

Herndon, Robert · Neurology, Adult, Infectious & Demyelinating Diseases

Heros, Roberto C. · Neurological Surgery, Vascular Neurological Surgery

Herr, Harry W. · Urology, Urologic Oncology

Herschorn, Sender · Urology, Neuro-Urology & Voiding Dysfunction

Herscovitch, Peter · Nuclear Medicine, Brain

Hershman, Jerome M. · Endocrinology & Metabolism, Thyroid

Hertzer, Norman R. · General Surgery, General Vascular Surgery

Herz, Marvin Ira · Psychiatry, Schizophrenia

Herzig, Geoffrey P. · Medical Oncology, Bone Marrow Transplantation; Medical Oncology, Leukemia; Medical Oncology, Lymphomas

Herzog, David B. · Psychiatry, Child Psychiatry; Psychiatry, Eating Disorders

Hester, T. Roderick · Plastic Surgery, Aesthetic Surgery; Plastic Surgery, Breast Surgery

Hetherington, John N. · Ophthalmology, Glaucoma

Heuer, Dale K. · Ophthalmology, Glaucoma

Heyman, Melvin B. · Pediatrics, Pediatric Gastroenterology

Heyman, Sydney · Nuclear Medicine, Pediatric

Hickey, Paul R. · Anesthesiology, Pediatric Cardiovascular

Hicks, Jeanne E. · Physical Medicine & Rehabilitation, Rheumatology; Rheumatology, Rehabilitation

Hieshima, Grant B. · Radiology, Neuroradiology

Higginbotham, Eve J. · Ophthalmology, Glaucoma

Higgins, Charles B. · Radiology, Cardiovascular Disease; Radiology, Magnetic Resonance Imaging

Hilal, Sadek K. · Radiology, Neuroradiology

Hilaris, Basil S. · Radiation Oncology, Brachytherapy

Hill, Harry R. · Allergy & Immunology, Pediatric Allergy & Immunology

Hill, J. Donald · Thoracic Surgery, Adult Cardiothoracic Surgery

Hill, Ronald C. · Thoracic Surgery, Adult Cardiothoracic Surgery

Hillis, L. David · Cardiovascular Disease, Cardiac Catheterization

Hilman, Bettina C. · Allergy & Immunology, Pediatric Allergy & Immunology; Pediatrics, Pediatric Pulmonology

Hintz, Raymond · Pediatrics, Pediatric Endocrinology

Hirsch, Martin S. · Infectious Disease, AIDS; Infectious Disease, Virology

Hirschfeld, Robert M. A. · Psychiatry, Affective Disorders; Psychiatry, General Psychiatry

Hitchcock, John · Psychiatry, Psychoanalysis

Ho, Monto · Infectious Disease, Transplantation Infections

Hoagland, H. Clark · Medical Oncology & Hematology, General Medical Oncology & Hematology

Hobbins, John C. · Obstetrics & Gynecology, Maternal & Fetal Medicine

Hobson, Robert W. · General Surgery, General Vascular Surgery

Hoch, Samuel · Psychiatry, Psychoanalysis

Hochberg, Fred H. · Neurology, Adult, Neuro-oncology

Hoff, Julian T. · Neurological Surgery, Tumor Surgery

Hoffer, Paul B. · Nuclear Medicine, General Nuclear Medicine

Hoffman, Harold J. · Neurological Surgery, Pediatric Neurological Surgery

Hoffman, Julien I. E. · Pediatrics, Pediatric Cardiology

Hogan, Walter J. · Gastroenterology, Endoscopy; Gastroenterology, General Gastroenterology

Holbrook, Peter R. · Pediatrics, Pediatric Critical Care

Holinger, Lauren D. · Otolaryngology, Pediatric Otolaryngology

Holladay, Jack T. · Ophthalmology, Optics & Refraction

Holland, Gary N. · Ophthalmology, Uveitis

Holland, James F. · Medical Oncology & Hematology, Solid Tumors

Holliday, Michael J. · Otolaryngology, Otology/Neurotology; Otolaryngology, Skull-Base Surgery

Hollier, Larry H. · General Surgery, General Vascular Surgery

Holloway, William J. · Infectious Disease, General Infectious Disease

Holman, B. Leonard · Nuclear Medicine, Brain; Nuclear Medicine, General Nuclear Medicine

Holmes, David R. · Cardiovascular Disease, Cardiac Catheterization

Holmes, E. Carmack · Thoracic Surgery, General Thoracic Surgery; Thoracic Surgery, Thoracic Oncological Surgery

Holmes, Gregory L. · Neurology, Child, Epilepsy

Holmes, King K. · Infectious Disease, AIDS; Infectious Disease, Sexually Transmitted Disease

Holsclaw, Douglas S. · Pediatrics, Pediatric Pulmonology

Homesley, Howard D. · Obstetrics & Gynecology, Gynecologic Cancer

Hong, Richard · Allergy & Immunology, Pediatric Allergy & Immunology

Hong, Waun Ki · Medical Oncology & Hematology, Head & Neck Cancer

Honig, Paul Joseph · Dermatology, Pediatric Dermatology; Pediatrics, Pediatric Dermatology

Hook, Edward W. · Infectious Disease, Sexually Transmitted Disease

Hopewell, Philip · Pulmonary & Critical Care Medicine, AIDS; Pulmonary & Critical Care Medicine, Lung Infections

Hopkins, L. Nelson · Neurological Surgery, Vascular Neurological Surgery

Hopkins, Richard Alan · Thoracic Surgery, Adult Cardiothoracic Surgery; Thoracic Surgery, Pediatric Cardiac Surgery

Hoppe, Richard T. · Radiation Oncology, Lymphomas

Hordinsky, Maria K. · Dermatology, Hair

Hornbein, Thomas F. · Anesthesiology, Cardiothoracic Anesthesiology

Hornblass, Albert · Ophthalmology, Oculoplastic & Orbital Surgery

Horning, Sandra J. · Medical Oncology & Hematology, Lymphomas

Hornstein, Nancy Louise · Psychiatry, Dissociative Disorders

Horowitz, Marc E. · Pediatrics, Pediatric Hematology-Oncology

Hortobagyi, Gabriel N. · Medical Oncology, Breast Cancer

Horwitz, Melton Jay · Otolaryngology, Otology/Neurotology

Hoskins, H. Dunbar · Ophthalmology, Glaucoma

Hoskins, William J. · Obstetrics & Gynecology, Gynecologic Cancer

Hotaling, Andrew Jay · Otolaryngology, Pediatric Otolaryngology

Houghton, Alan N. · Medical Oncology & Hematology, Immunotherapy, Biological Response Modifiers Oncology

Houpt, Jeffrey L. · Psychiatry, Psychopharmacology

House, James H. · Hand Surgery, Paralytic Disorders; Hand Surgery, Reconstructive Surgery

House, John W. · Otolaryngology, Otology/Neurotology

House, William F. · Otolaryngology, Otology/Neurotology

Howell, David S. · Rheumatology, Osteoarthritis

Howell, Stephen B. · Medical Oncology, Clinical Pharmacology

Howes, Anthony E. · Radiation Oncology, General Radiation Oncology

Howie, John S. · Psychiatry, Psychoanalysis

Hoyt, Creig S. · Ophthalmology, Pediatric Ophthalmology

Hoyt, John William · Anesthesiology, Critical Care Medicine

Hoyt, William · Neurology, Adult, Neuro-Ophthalmology

Huddleston, John F. · Obstetrics & Gynecology, Maternal & Fetal Medicine

Hudson, Alan R. · Neurological Surgery, Peripheral Nerve Surgery

Hudson, James I. · Psychiatry, Eating Disorders

Hudson, Leonard D. · Pulmonary & Critical Care Medicine, Asthma; Pulmonary & Critical Care Medicine, Pulmonary Disease

Huff, J. Clark · Dermatology, Cutaneous Immunology; Dermatology, Herpes Virus Infections

Huff, Robert W. · Obstetrics & Gynecology, Maternal & Fetal Medicine

Huffman, Jeffry L. · Urology, Endourology

Hughes, Gordon Blackistone · Otolaryngology, Otology/Neurotology

Hughes, James L. · Orthopaedic Surgery, Trauma

Hughes, Walter · Pediatrics, Pediatric Infectious Disease

Hulbert, John C. · Urology, Endourology

Hume, Michael · General Surgery, General Vascular Surgery

Humphreys, Robin P. · Neurological Surgery, Pediatric Neurological Surgery

Hunder, Gene G. · Rheumatology, Vasculitis

Hung, Weillington · Pediatrics, Pediatric Endocrinology

Hungerford, David S. · Orthopaedic Surgery, Reconstructive Surgery

Hunkeler, John D. · Ophthalmology, Anterior Segment (Cataract Surgery)

Hunt, Richard H. · Gastroenterology, Endoscopy; Gastroenterology, Peptic Disorders

Hunt, Sharon A. · Cardiovascular Disease, Heart Transplantation

Hunt, Thomas K. · General Surgery, Wound Healing

Hunter, James M. · Hand Surgery, Reconstructive Surgery

Hurley, James R. · Endocrinology & Metabolism, Thyroid; Nuclear Medicine, Thyroid

Hurst, David Michael · Psychiatry, Psychoanalysis

Hurwitz, Jeffrey J. · Ophthalmology, Oculoplastic & Orbital Surgery

Hurwitz, Sidney · Dermatology, Pediatric Dermatology; Pediatrics, Pediatric Dermatology

Hussey, David H. · Radiation Oncology, General Radiation Oncology

Hutchinson, B. Thomas · Ophthalmology, Glaucoma

Hutson, Peggy B. · Psychiatry, Psychoanalysis

Huttenlocher, Peter R. · Neurology, Child, Child Development; Neurology, Child, General Child Neurology

Hutter, Adolph M. · Cardiovascular Disease, General Cardiovascular Disease

Hyers, Thomas Morgan · Pulmonary & Critical Care Medicine, General Pulmonary & Critical Care Medicine

Hyman, Allen I. · Anesthesiology, General Anesthesiology

I

Iams, Jay D. · Obstetrics & Gynecology, Maternal & Fetal Medicine

Ihde, Daniel C. · Medical Oncology & Hematology, Lung Cancer

Iliff, Nicholas T. · Ophthalmology, Oculoplastic & Orbital Surgery

Ing, Malcolm R. · Ophthalmology, Pediatric Ophthalmology

Ingelfinger, Julie R. · Pediatrics, Pediatric Nephrology

Ingle, James N. · Medical Oncology, Breast Cancer

Inglis, Allan E. · Orthopaedic Surgery, Reconstructive Surgery

Ingram, Roland H. · Pulmonary & Critical Care Medicine, Asthma

Insall, John Nevil · Orthopaedic Surgery, Knee Surgery

Irvin, George L. · General Surgery, Endocrine Surgery

Irvine, Patrick W. · Geriatric Medicine, General Geriatric Medicine

Iseman, Michael D. · Pulmonary & Critical Care Medicine, Lung Infections

Isenberg, Jon I. · Gastroenterology, Peptic Disorders

Iskandrian, Ami S. · Cardiovascular Disease, Nuclear Cardiology

Isom, O. Wayne · Thoracic Surgery, Adult Cardiothoracic Surgery

Iwatsuki, Shunzaburo · Surgical Oncology, Gastroenterologic Cancer

J

Jabaley, Michael E. · Hand Surgery, Peripheral Nerve Surgery; Plastic Surgery, Peripheral Nerve Surgery

Jabs, Douglas A. · Ophthalmology, Uveitis

Jackler, Robert K. · Otolaryngology, Otology/Neurotology

Jackman, Warren M. · Cardiovascular Disease, Electrophysiology

Jackson, C. Gary · Otolaryngology, Otology/Neurotology

Jackson, Carol A. · Otolaryngology, Otology/Neurotology

Jackson, Douglas W. · Orthopaedic Surgery, Sports Medicine

Jackson, Ian T. · Plastic Surgery, Craniofacial Surgery; Plastic Surgery, Head & Neck Surgery

Jacobs, Alvin H. · Dermatology, Pediatric Dermatology; Pediatrics, Pediatric Dermatology

Jacobs, Charlotte · Medical Oncology & Hematology, Head & Neck Cancer

Jacobs, Richard F. · Pediatrics, Pediatric Infectious Disease

Jacobs, Samuel A. · Medical Oncology, General Medical Oncology

Jacobson, Harry R. · Nephrology, General Nephrology

Jacobson, Jacob G. · Psychiatry, Psychoanalysis

Jaffe, Bernard M. · General Surgery, Gastroenterologic Surgery

Jaffe, Elaine S. · Pathology, Hematopathology

Jaffe, Jerome Herbert · Psychiatry, Addiction Medicine

Jaffe, Robert B. · Obstetrics & Gynecology, Reproductive Endocrinology

Jagelman, David G. · Colon & Rectal Surgery, General Colon & Rectal Surgery

Jahnigen, Dennis W. · Geriatric Medicine, General Geriatric Medicine

Jahrsdoerfer, Robert A. · Otolaryngology, Otology/Neurotology

Jampol, Lee M. · Ophthalmology, Medical Retinal Diseases

Jampolsky, Arthur · Ophthalmology, Pediatric Ophthalmology

Jane, John A. · Neurological Surgery, Tumor Surgery

Jankovic, Joseph · Neurology, Adult, Movement Disorders

Jankowski, Joseph J. · Psychiatry, Child Psychiatry

Jannetta, Peter J. · Neurological Surgery, Cranial Nerve Surgery; Neurological Surgery, Tumor Surgery

Jansen, G. Thomas · Dermatology, Clinical Dermatology

Jarvik, Lissy F. · Psychiatry, Geriatric Psychiatry

Jasinski, Donald R. · Addiction Medicine, Medical Treatment of Drug Abusers

Jefferson, Larry S. · Pediatrics, Pediatric Critical Care

Jeffs, Robert D. · Urology, Pediatric Urology

Jegasothy, Brian V. · Dermatology, Clinical Dermatology

Jelks, Glenn W. · Ophthalmology, Oculoplastic & Orbital Surgery; Plastic Surgery, Oculoplastic & Orbital Surgery

Jellinek, Michael · Psychiatry, Child Psychiatry

Jenkenson, Steven · Pulmonary & Critical Care Medicine, General Pulmonary & Critical Care Medicine

Jenkins, Alan D. · Urology, Endourology

Jenkins, Herman A. · Otolaryngology, Otology/Neurotology

Jenkins, Roger L. · General Surgery, Transplantation

Jenny, Carole · Pediatrics, Abused Children

Jensen, Dennis · Gastroenterology, Endoscopy; Gastroenterology, Gastrointestinal Bleeding

Jeste, Dilip V. · Psychiatry, Geriatric Psychiatry

Jimenez, Sergio A. · Rheumatology, Scleroderma

Jobe, Frank W. · Orthopaedic Surgery, Sports Medicine

Jobes, David R. · Anesthesiology, Pediatric Cardiovascular

Johnson, Calvin M. · Otolaryngology, Facial Plastic Surgery

Johnson, Charles Felzen · Pediatrics, Abused Children

Johnson, David · Medical Oncology & Hematology, Lung Cancer; Medical Oncology & Hematology, Prostate Cancer

Johnson, Ernest W. · Physical Medicine & Rehabilitation, Electromyography

Johnson, George · General Surgery, General Vascular Surgery

Johnson, Glen Dwight · Otolaryngology, Otology/Neurotology

Johnson, Jerry C. · Geriatric Medicine, General Geriatric Medicine

Johnson, John Settle · Rheumatology, General Rheumatology

Johnson, John W. C. · Obstetrics & Gynecology, Maternal & Fetal Medicine

Johnson, Jonas T. · Otolaryngology, Head & Neck Surgery

Johnson, K. Wayne · General Surgery, General Vascular Surgery

Johnson, Kenneth A. · Orthopaedic Surgery, Foot & Ankle Surgery

Johnson, Kenneth D. · Orthopaedic Surgery, Trauma

Johnson, Kenneth P. · Neurology, Adult, Infectious & Demyelinating Diseases

Johnson, Lanny Leo · Orthopaedic Surgery, Sports Medicine

Johnson, Lynne L. · Cardiovascular Disease, General Cardiovascular Disease; Cardiovascular Disease, Nuclear Cardiology

Johnson, Richard T. · Neurology, Adult, Infectious & Demyelinating Diseases

Johnson, Robert J. · Orthopaedic Surgery, Sports Medicine

Johnson, Stephen H. · Ophthalmology, Anterior Segment (Cataract Surgery)

Johnson, Warren D. · Infectious Disease, Tropical Diseases

Johnston, James O. · Orthopaedic Surgery, Tumor Surgery

Johnstone, Murray · Ophthalmology, Glaucoma

Jonas, Richard A. · Thoracic Surgery, Pediatric Cardiac Surgery

Jones, Barry · Psychiatry, Schizophrenia

Jones, Dan B. · Ophthalmology, Corneal Diseases & Transplantation

Jones, Ellis L. · Thoracic Surgery, Adult Cardiothoracic Surgery

Jones, Georgeanna Seegar · Obstetrics & Gynecology, Reproductive Endocrinology

Jones, Howard W. · Obstetrics & Gynecology, Reproductive Endocrinology

Jones, Kent W. · Thoracic Surgery, Adult Cardiothoracic Surgery

Jones, Neil F. · Hand Surgery, General Hand Surgery

Jones, R. Scott · General Surgery, Gastroenterologic Surgery

Jones, Robert H. · Thoracic Surgery, Adult Cardiothoracic Surgery

Jones, Stephen E. · Medical Oncology & Hematology, Lymphomas

Jordon, Robert E. · Dermatology, Cutaneous Immunology

Jorizzo, Joseph L. · Dermatology, Clinical Dermatology

Josephson, Mark E. · Cardiovascular Disease, Electrophysiology

Judd, Lewis L. · Psychiatry, Affective Disorders

Judson, Franklyn N. · Infectious Disease, Sexually Transmitted Disease

Jupiter, Jesse B. · Hand Surgery, Reconstructive Surgery

Jurisson, Mary · Physical Medicine & Rehabilitation, Rheumatology; Rheumatology, Rehabilitation

K

Kadin, Marshall Edward · Pathology, Hematopathology

Kafka, John S. · Psychiatry, Psychoanalysis

Kahan, Barry Donald · General Surgery, Transplantation

Kahler, Stephen G. · Pediatrics, Metabolic Diseases

Kahn, Robert I. · Urology, Endourology

Kaiser, Allen B. · Infectious Disease, Hospital-Acquired Infections

Kalayoglu, Munci · General Surgery, Transplantation

Kaliner, Michael Aron · Allergy & Immunology, Adult Allergy & Immunology

Kalinich, Lila Joyce · Psychiatry, Psychoanalysis

Kallar, Surinder K. · Anesthesiology, Ambulatory Anesthesia

Kamer, Frank M. · Otolaryngology, Facial Plastic Surgery

Kamerer, Donald B. · Otolaryngology, Otology/Neurotology

Kane, John Michael · Psychiatry, Schizophrenia/Psychopharmacology

Kang, Yoogoo · Anesthesiology, Hepatic Disease

Kanner, Richard E. · Pulmonary & Critical Care Medicine, Asthma; Pulmonary & Critical Care Medicine, Pulmonary Disease

Kantarjian, Hagop · Medical Oncology, Leukemia

Kantoff, Philip W. · Medical Oncology & Hematology, Genito-Urinary Cancer

Kaplan, Alex H. · Psychiatry, Psychoanalysis

Kaplan, Allen Phillip · Allergy & Immunology, Adult Allergy & Immunology

Kaplan, Bernard S. · Pediatrics, Pediatric Nephrology

Kaplan, Edwin L. · General Surgery, Endocrine Surgery

Kaplan, George · Urology, Pediatric Urology

Kaplan, Henry J. · Ophthalmology, Uveitis

Kaplan, Herbert · Rheumatology, Rheumatoid Arthritis

Kaplan, Marshall M. · Gastroenterology, Hepatology

Kaplan, Selna L. · Pediatrics, Pediatric Endocrinology

Kaplan, William D. · Nuclear Medicine, Oncology

Kappy, Michael Steven · Pediatrics, Pediatric Endocrinology

Karam, John H. · Endocrinology & Metabolism, Diabetes

Karchmer, Adolf W. · Infectious Disease, Endocarditis

Karpati, George · Neurology, Adult, Neuromuscular Disease

Kartush, Jack M. · Otolaryngology, Otology/Neurotology

Kase, Carlos S. · Neurology, Adult, Strokes

Kashima, Haskins K. · Otolaryngology, Laryngology

Kass, Michael A. · Ophthalmology, Glaucoma

Katon, Ronald Melvin · Gastroenterology, Endoscopy

Katowitz, James A. · Ophthalmology, Oculoplastic & Orbital Surgery

Katz, Ira R. · Psychiatry, Geriatric Psychiatry

Katz, Jack L. · Psychiatry, Eating Disorders

Katz, Robert · Rheumatology, General Rheumatology

Katz, Roger M. · Allergy & Immunology, Pediatric Allergy & Immunology

Katz, Samuel L. · Pediatrics, Pediatric Infectious Disease

Katz, Stephen I. · Dermatology, Clinical Dermatology; Dermatology, Cutaneous Immunology

Katz, Warren A. · Rheumatology, General Rheumatology

Katzen, Leeds (Jack) · Ophthalmology, Anterior Segment (Cataract Surgery)

Katzman, Robert · Neurology, Adult, Degenerative Diseases

Kauffman, Gordon Lee · General Surgery, Gastroenterologic Surgery

Kaufman, Edward R. · Psychiatry, Addiction Medicine

Kaufman, Francine R. · Pediatrics, Pediatric Endocrinology

Kaufman, Herbert E. · Ophthalmology, Corneal Diseases & Transplantation

Kaufman, Raymond H. · Obstetrics & Gynecology, Genital Dermatological Disease

Kawamoto, Henry K. · Plastic Surgery, Craniofacial Surgery; Plastic Surgery, Maxillofacial Surgery

Kay, Jerome Harold · Thoracic Surgery, Adult Cardiothoracic Surgery

Kay, Robert · Urology, Pediatric Urology

Kaye, Bernard L. · Plastic Surgery, Facial Aesthetic Surgery

Kaye, Donald · Infectious Disease, General Infectious Disease; Infectious Disease, Urinary Tract Infections

Keane, James R. · Neurology, Adult, Neuro-Ophthalmology; Ophthalmology, Neuro-Ophthalmology

Keates, Richard H. · Ophthalmology, Corneal Diseases & Transplantation

Keating, James P. · Pediatrics, Pediatric Gastroenterology

Keating, Michael J. · Medical Oncology, Leukemia

Keats, Arthur S. · Anesthesiology, Complications of Anesthesia

Keeffe, Emmet B. · Gastroenterology, Hepatology

Keenan, Joseph M. · Geriatric Medicine, General Geriatric Medicine

Keenan, Richard L. · Anesthesiology, Complications of Anesthesia

Keith, Charles R. · Psychiatry, Child Psychiatry; Psychiatry, Violence

Keith, Samuel J. · Psychiatry, Schizophrenia

Kelalis, Panayotis P. · Urology, Pediatric Urology

Kelch, Robert P. · Pediatrics, Pediatric Endocrinology

Keller, Martin B. · Psychiatry, Affective Disorders

Kelley, John Fredric · Psychiatry, Child Psychiatry

Kelley, Mark A. · Pulmonary & Critical Care Medicine, General Pulmonary & Critical Care Medicine

Kelly, A. Paul · Dermatology, Clinical Dermatology

Kelly, David L. · Neurological Surgery, Spinal Surgery

Kelly, John · Neurology, Adult, Electromyography

Kelly, Keith A. · General Surgery, Gastroenterologic Surgery

Kelly, Patrick J. · Neurological Surgery, Stereotactic Radiosurgery; Neurological Surgery, Tumor Surgery

Kelsen, David P. · Medical Oncology, Gastrointestinal Oncology

Keltner, John L. · Ophthalmology, Neuro-Ophthalmology

Kemeny, Nancy E. · Medical Oncology, Gastrointestinal Oncology

Kemink, John L. · Otolaryngology, Otology/Neurotology

Kemp, James P. · Allergy & Immunology, Pediatric Allergy & Immunology

Kennedy, B. J. · Medical Oncology, Breast Cancer

Kennedy, David W. · Otolaryngology, Sinus & Nasal Surgery

Kennedy, Gary J. · Psychiatry, Geriatric Psychiatry

Kennedy, J. Ward · Cardiovascular Disease, General Cardiovascular Disease

Kennedy, Robert D. · Geriatric Medicine, General Geriatric Medicine

Kennerdell, John S. · Ophthalmology, Oculoplastic & Orbital Surgery

Kenney, John Andrew · Dermatology, Clinical Dermatology; Dermatology, Depigmenting Diseases

Kent, Kenneth M. · Cardiovascular Disease, Cardiac Catheterization

Kenyon, Kenneth R. · Ophthalmology, Corneal Diseases & Transplantation

Kepecs, Joseph G. · Psychiatry, Psychoanalysis

Kepes, John J. · Pathology, Neuropathology

Kerber, Richard E. · Cardiovascular Disease, Echocardiography

Kern, Eugene B. · Otolaryngology, Sinus & Nasal Surgery

Kern, Morton J. · Cardiovascular Disease, Cardiac Catheterization

Kernan, Nancy A. · Pediatrics, Pediatric Hematology-Oncology

Kernberg, Otto F. · Psychiatry, Psychoanalysis

Kernberg, Paulina · Psychiatry, Child Psychiatry; Psychiatry, Psychoanalysis

Kerr, Douglas S. · Pediatrics, Metabolic Diseases

Kersey, John H. · Pediatrics, Pediatric Hematology-Oncology

Kestenbaum, Clarice J. · Psychiatry, Child Psychiatry

Ketcham, Alfred S. · Surgical Oncology, Breast Cancer

Key, L. Lyndon · Pediatrics, Pediatric Endocrinology

Keye, William Richard · Obstetrics & Gynecology, Reproductive Endocrinology

Keyes, John W. · Nuclear Medicine, General Nuclear Medicine

Khantzian, Edward J. · Psychiatry, Addiction Medicine

Kienzle, Michael G. · Cardiovascular Disease, Electrophysiology

Killam, Allen · Obstetrics & Gynecology, Maternal & Fetal Medicine

Kim, E. Edmund · Nuclear Medicine, Oncology

Kim, Moon H. · Obstetrics & Gynecology, Reproductive Endocrinology

Kinder, Barbara · General Surgery, Endocrine Surgery

King, Lloyd E. · Dermatology, Clinical Dermatology

King, Lowell · Urology, Pediatric Urology

King, Robert A. · Psychiatry, Child Psychiatry

King, Spencer B. · Cardiovascular Disease, Cardiac Catheterization

King, Talmadge E. · Pulmonary & Critical Care Medicine, Pulmonary Disease

Kinne, David W. · General Surgery, Breast Surgery; Surgical Oncology, Breast Cancer

Kinney, Sam E. · Otolaryngology, Otology/Neurotology

Kinsella, Timothy J. · Radiation Oncology, General Radiation Oncology

Kirchner, Peter T. · Nuclear Medicine, General Nuclear Medicine

Kirkland, John Lindsey · Pediatrics, Pediatric Endocrinology

Kirklin, James K. · Thoracic Surgery, Adult Cardiothoracic Surgery; Thoracic Surgery, Transplantation

Kirschner, Barbara S. · Pediatrics, Pediatric Gastroenterology

Kirsner, Joseph Barnett · Gastroenterology, Inflammatory Bowel Disease

Kisslo, Joseph · Cardiovascular Disease, Echocardiography

Kjeldsberg, Carl R. · Pathology, Hematopathology

Kjellstrand, Carl M. · Nephrology, Kidney Disease

Klahr, Saulo · Nephrology, General Nephrology

Klatsky, Stanley A. · Plastic Surgery, Aesthetic Surgery; Plastic Surgery, Facial Aesthetic Surgery

Klein, Donald F. · Psychiatry, Affective Disorders; Psychiatry, Psychopharmacology

Klein, George J. · Cardiovascular Disease, Electrophysiology

Klein, Jerome O. · Pediatrics, Pediatric Infectious Disease

Kleinberg, David Lewis · Endocrinology & Metabolism, Neuroendocrinology

Kleinman, Charles · Pediatrics, Pediatric Cardiology

Kleinman, Joel Edward · Psychiatry, Schizophrenia/Psychopharmacology

Kleinman, William · Hand Surgery, General Hand Surgery

Kletzky, Oscar A. · Obstetrics & Gynecology, Reproductive Endocrinology

Klibanski, Anne · Endocrinology & Metabolism, Neuroendocrinology

Kligfield, Paul David · Cardiovascular Disease, Clinical Exercise Testing

Kliman, Gilbert Wallace · Psychiatry, Child Psychiatry

Klimo, Paul · Medical Oncology & Hematology, Hematological Malignancies

Kline, David G. · Neurological Surgery, Peripheral Nerve Surgery

Kline, Lanning B. · Neurology, Adult, Neuro-Ophthalmology; Ophthalmology, Neuro-Ophthalmology

Klingensmith, Georgeanna · Pediatrics, Pediatric Endocrinology

Klintmalm, Goran B. · General Surgery, Transplantation

Kluft, Richard P. · Psychiatry, Dissociative Disorders

Klykylo, William Michael · Psychiatry, Child Psychiatry

Knight, Edward H. · Psychiatry, Psychoanalysis

Knighton, David R. · General Surgery, General Vascular Surgery; General Surgery, Wound Healing

Knowles, Daniel M. · Pathology, Hematopathology

Knowles, Michael Ray · Pulmonary & Critical Care Medicine, Cystic Fibrosis

Knox, G. Eric · Obstetrics & Gynecology, Maternal & Fetal Medicine

Koch, Douglas D. · Ophthalmology, Anterior Segment (Cataract Surgery)

Koch, Paul S. · Ophthalmology, Anterior Segment (Cataract Surgery)

Kochanek, Patrick M. · Pediatrics, Pediatric Critical Care

Kochenour, Neil K. · Obstetrics & Gynecology, Maternal & Fetal Medicine

Kochis, George P. · Psychiatry, Psychoanalysis

Kodner, Ira J. · Surgical Oncology, Colon & Rectal Cancer

Koenigsberger, Merton Richard · Neurology, Child, General Child Neurology; Neurology, Child, Neonatal Neurology

Koff, Stephen A. · Urology, Pediatric Urology

Kogan, Barry A. · Urology, Pediatric Urology

Kogan, Stanley J. · Urology, Pediatric Urology

Kohaut, Edward C. · Pediatrics, Pediatric Nephrology

Kolker, Allan E. · Ophthalmology, Glaucoma

Koller, William C. · Neurology, Adult, Movement Disorders

Kolterman, Orville G. · Endocrinology & Metabolism, Diabetes

Kopf, Alfred Walter · Dermatology, Skin Cancer Surgery & Reconstruction

Korelitz, Burton I. · Gastroenterology, Inflammatory Bowel Disease

Korones, Sheldon Bernarr · Pediatrics, Neonatal-Perinatal Medicine

Kosten, Thomas R. · Psychiatry, Addiction Medicine

Kouchoukos, Nicholas T. · Thoracic Surgery, Adult Cardiothoracic Surgery

Kozarek, Richard A. · Gastroenterology, Endoscopy

Kozin, Franklin · Rheumatology, General Rheumatology

Krachmer, Jay H. · Ophthalmology, Corneal Diseases & Transplantation

Krackow, Kenneth A. · Orthopaedic Surgery, Reconstructive Surgery

Kraff, Manus C. · Ophthalmology, Anterior Segment (Cataract Surgery)

Kramer, Selma · Psychiatry, Psychoanalysis

Kramer, Steven G. · Ophthalmology, Corneal Diseases & Transplantation

Krane, Robert · Urology, Impotence

Krane, Stephen M. · Rheumatology, Osteoporosis

Krasinski, Keith Michael · Pediatrics, Pediatric Infectious Disease

Krause, Charles J. · Otolaryngology, Facial Plastic Surgery; Otolaryngology, Head & Neck Surgery; Otolaryngology, Laryngology

Kreiger, Allan E. · Ophthalmology, Vitreo-Retinal Surgery

Kremer, Joel M. · Rheumatology, General Rheumatology

Kris, Anton O. · Psychiatry, Psychoanalysis

Kris, Mark G. · Medical Oncology & Hematology, Lung Cancer

Krom, Ruud A.F. · General Surgery, Transplantation

Krueger, Gerald G. · Dermatology, Psoriasis

Krugman, Richard D. · Pediatrics, Abused Children

Krull, Edward Alexander · Dermatology, Mucous Membrane Diseases; Dermatology, Skin Cancer Surgery & Reconstruction

Krupin, Theodore · Ophthalmology, Glaucoma

Kuhl, David E. · Nuclear Medicine, Brain

Kuhlman, Kathleen A. · Obstetrics & Gynecology, Maternal & Fetal Medicine

Kun, Larry E. · Radiation Oncology, Pediatric Radiation Oncology

Kunin, Calvin M. · Infectious Disease, Hospital-Acquired Infections; Infectious Disease, Urinary Tract Infections

Kupersmith, Mark J. · Neurology, Adult, Neuro-Ophthalmology; Ophthalmology, Neuro-Ophthalmology

Kupfer, David J. · Psychiatry, Affective Disorders; Psychiatry, Psychopharmacology

Kurtzberg, Joanne · Pediatrics, Pediatric Hematology-Oncology

Kushner, Burton J. · Ophthalmology, Pediatric Ophthalmology

Kutz, Joseph E. · Hand Surgery, Peripheral Nerve Surgery

Kveton , John · Otolaryngology, Otology/Neurotology

Kyle, Richard F. · Orthopaedic Surgery, Trauma

Kyle, Robert A. · Medical Oncology & Hematology, Myeloma

L

Ladenson, Paul W. · Endocrinology & Metabolism, Thyroid

LaForce, F. Marc · Infectious Disease, Hospital-Acquired Infections

LaFranchi, Stephen Henry · Pediatrics, Pediatric Endocrinology

Lagasse, Leo D. · Obstetrics & Gynecology, Gynecologic Cancer

Lagios, Michael D. · Pathology, Breast Pathology

Laibson, Peter R. · Ophthalmology, Corneal Diseases & Transplantation

Laine, Loren A. · Gastroenterology, Endoscopy; Gastroenterology, Gastrointestinal Bleeding

Lake, Alan M. · Pediatrics, Pediatric Gastroenterology

Laks, Hillel · Thoracic Surgery, Adult Cardiothoracic Surgery; Thoracic Surgery, Pediatric Cardiac Surgery

Lam, Arthur M. · Anesthesiology, Neuroanesthesia

Lamb, H. Richard · Psychiatry, Schizophrenia

Lambros, Vasilios · Plastic Surgery , Facial Aesthetic Surgery

Lamm, Donald L. · Urology, Urologic Oncology

Lampkin, Beatrice C. · Pediatrics, Pediatric Hematology-Oncology

Landau, William M. · Neurology, Adult, General Adult Neurology

Lane, Alfred T. · Dermatology, Pediatric Dermatology; Pediatrics, Pediatric Dermatology

Lane, Joseph M. · Orthopaedic Surgery, Tumor Surgery

Lane, Stephen S. · Ophthalmology, Anterior Segment (Cataract Surgery)

Lang, Anthony E. · Neurology, Adult, Movement Disorders

Lange, Paul Henry · Urology, Urologic Oncology

Langer, Oded · Obstetrics & Gynecology, Maternal & Fetal Medicine

Langman, Craig B. · Pediatrics, Pediatric Nephrology

Langston, J. William · Neurology, Adult, Movement Disorders

Lanier, William L. · Anesthesiology, Neuroanesthesia

Lapey, Allen · Allergy & Immunology, Pediatric Allergy & Immunology; Pediatrics, Pediatric Pulmonology

Laramore, George E. · Radiation Oncology, Head & Neck Cancer

Laros, Russell K. · Obstetrics & Gynecology, Maternal & Fetal Medicine

Larsen, Gary L. · Pediatrics, Pediatric Pulmonology

Larsen, P. Reed · Endocrinology & Metabolism, Thyroid

Larson, C. Philip · Anesthesiology, Neuroanesthesia

Larson, David A. · Radiation Oncology, Brain Cancer; Radiation Oncology, Radiosurgery

Larson, David Lee · Plastic Surgery, Breast Surgery; Plastic Surgery, Head & Neck Surgery

Larson, Richard A. · Medical Oncology & Hematology, Hematological Malignancies; Medical Oncology & Hematology, Leukemia

Larson, Sanford J. · Neurological Surgery, Spinal Surgery

Larson, Steven Mark · Nuclear Medicine, Oncology

Lass, Jonathan H. · Ophthalmology, Corneal Diseases & Transplantation

Lauer, Ronald M. · Pediatrics, Pediatric Cardiology

Laurie, John Andrew · Medical Oncology, General Medical Oncology

Lavin, Patrick J. · Neurology, Adult, Neuro-Ophthalmology

Lawley, Thomas J. · Dermatology, Cutaneous Immunology

Laws, Edward R. · Neurological Surgery, Tumor Surgery

Lawson, William · Otolaryngology, Sinus & Nasal Surgery

Layden, William E. · Ophthalmology, Glaucoma

Layzer, Robert B. · Neurology, Adult, Neuromuscular Disease

Lazarus, Gerald S. · Dermatology, Psoriasis

Lazarus, J. Michael · Nephrology, Dialysis

Lazarus, Lawrence W. · Psychiatry, Geriatric Psychiatry

Le Blanc, Raymond P. · Ophthalmology, Glaucoma

Le Jentel, Thierry H. · Cardiovascular Disease, Heart Failure

Leach, Gary E. · Urology, Neuro-Urology & Voiding Dysfunction

Lean, John S. · Ophthalmology, Vitreo-Retinal Surgery

Leather, Robert P. · General Surgery, General Vascular Surgery

Leavitt, Maimon · Psychiatry, Psychoanalysis

Leckman, James F. · Psychiatry, Child Psychiatry

Ledger, William J. · Obstetrics & Gynecology, Infectious Disease

Lee, Lela A. · Dermatology, Cutaneous Immunology

Lee, Peter A. · Pediatrics, Pediatric Endocrinology

Lee, Ray A. · Obstetrics & Gynecology, Reproductive Surgery

Leffert, Robert D. · Hand Surgery, Peripheral Nerve Surgery; Orthopaedic Surgery, Shoulder Surgery

Lehman, Anthony F. · Psychiatry, Schizophrenia

Lehman, Glen A. · Gastroenterology, Endoscopy

Lehmann, Michael H. · Cardiovascular Disease, Electrophysiology

Leibel, Steven A. · Radiation Oncology, Brain Cancer

Leier, Carl V. · Cardiovascular Disease, Heart Failure

Leighton, Barbara L. · Anesthesiology, Obstetric Anesthesia

Lemanske, Robert F. · Allergy & Immunology, Pediatric Allergy & Immunology

Lemen, Richard John · Pediatrics, Pediatric Pulmonology

Lemons, James A. · Pediatrics, Neonatal-Perinatal Medicine

Lemp, Michael A. · Ophthalmology, Corneal Diseases & Transplantation

Leon, Martin B. · Cardiovascular Disease, Cardiac Catheterization

Leonard, James A. · Physical Medicine & Rehabilitation, Electromyography

Leonetti, John P. · Otolaryngology, Otology/Neurotology

Leppik, Ilo E. · Neurology, Adult, Epilepsy

Leppo, Jeffrey A. · Cardiovascular Disease, Nuclear Cardiology

LeRoy, E. Carwile · Rheumatology, Scleroderma

Lesavoy, Malcolm A. · Plastic Surgery, Reconstructive Surgery

Leshner, Robert T. · Neurology, Adult, Electromyography; Neurology, Child, General Child Neurology

Lessell, Simmons · Neurology, Adult, Neuro-Ophthalmology; Ophthalmology, Neuro-Ophthalmology

Lessner, Howard E. · Medical Oncology & Hematology, General Medical Oncology & Hematology

Leuchter, Andrew F. · Psychiatry, Geriatric Psychiatry

Leung, Donald Y. M. · Allergy & Immunology, Pediatric Allergy & Immunology

Levenson, Steven · Geriatric Medicine, General Geriatric Medicine

Leventhal, Brigid G. · Pediatrics, Pediatric Hematology-Oncology

Leventhal, Elaine Annette · Geriatric Medicine, General Geriatric Medicine

Levin, Barry · Nephrology, Kidney Transplantation

Levin, Bernard · Medical Oncology, Gastrointestinal Oncology

Levin, Daniel L. · Pediatrics, Pediatric Critical Care

Levin, Nathan W. · Nephrology, Dialysis

Levin, Victor A. · Neurology, Adult, Neuro-oncology

Levine, Alexandra M. · Medical Oncology & Hematology, AIDS; Medical Oncology & Hematology, Hematological Malignancies; Medical Oncology & Hematology, Lymphomas

Levine, Howard L. · Otolaryngology, Sinus & Nasal Surgery

Levine, Paul A. · Otolaryngology, Head & Neck Surgery

Levine, Samuel C. · Otolaryngology, Otology/Neurotology

Levitsky, Lynne Lipton · Pediatrics, Pediatric Endocrinology

Levitt, Selwyn B. · Urology, Pediatric Urology

Levitt, Seymour · Radiation Oncology, Breast Cancer; Radiation Oncology, Hodgkins Disease

Levy, Harvey L. · Pediatrics, Metabolic Diseases

Levy, Howard B. · Pediatrics, Abused Children

Levy, Moise L. · Dermatology, Pediatric Dermatology; Pediatrics, Pediatric Dermatology

Levy, Robert M. · Neurological Surgery, General Neurological Surgery

Levy, Ronald · Medical Oncology & Hematology, Immunotherapy, Biological Response Modifiers Oncology

Lewis, David C. · Addiction Medicine, General Addiction Medicine

Lewis, Dorothy Otnow · Psychiatry, Child Psychiatry; Psychiatry, Violence

Lewis, Edmund J. · Nephrology, Glomerular Diseases

Lewis, Hilel · Ophthalmology, Medical Retinal Diseases; Ophthalmology, Vitreo-Retinal Surgery

Lewis, John L. · Obstetrics & Gynecology, Gynecologic Cancer

Lewis, Melvin · Psychiatry, Child Psychiatry

Lewis, Michael M. · Orthopaedic Surgery, Tumor Surgery

Lewis, Myron · Gastroenterology, General Gastroenterology

Lewis, Richard A. · Ophthalmology, Medical Retinal Diseases; Ophthalmology, Ophthalmic Genetics

Lewis, Ronald W. · Urology, Impotence

Leyden, James J. · Dermatology, Acne; Dermatology, Aging Skin

Liberman, Robert Paul · Psychiatry, Schizophrenia

Libertino, John A. · Urology, Urologic Oncology

Libow, Leslie S. · Geriatric Medicine, General Geriatric Medicine

Libshitz, Herman I. · Radiology, Chest

Lichter, Allen S. · Radiation Oncology, Breast Cancer; Radiation Oncology, Genito-Urinary Cancer; Radiation Oncology, Lung Cancer

Lichter, Paul R. · Ophthalmology, Glaucoma

Lieber, Michael M. · Urology, Urologic Oncology

Lieberman, Phillip L. · Allergy & Immunology, Adult Allergy & Immunology

Liebowitz, Michael R. · Psychiatry, Affective Disorders; Psychiatry, Psychopharmacology

Lieff, Jonathan D. · Psychiatry, Geriatric Psychiatry

Liesegang, Thomas John · Ophthalmology, Corneal Diseases & Transplantation

Lieskovsky, Gary · Urology, Urologic Oncology

Lietman, Paul S. · Clinical Pharmacology

Light, J. Keith · Urology, Neuro-Urology & Voiding Dysfunction

Light, Richard W. · Pulmonary & Critical Care Medicine, General Pulmonary & Critical Care Medicine

Light, Terry Richard · Hand Surgery, Reconstructive Surgery

Lightfoot, Robert W. · Rheumatology, General Rheumatology; Rheumatology, Vasculitis

Lilleskov, Roy K. · Psychiatry, Psychoanalysis

Lilly, John · General Surgery, Pediatric Surgery

Linberg, John V. · Ophthalmology, Oculoplastic & Orbital Surgery

Lindberg, Robert Dery · Radiation Oncology, Head & Neck Cancer; Radiation Oncology, Sarcomas

Lindstrom, Richard L. · Ophthalmology, Corneal Diseases & Transplantation

Linehan, W. Marston · Urology, Urologic Oncology

Ling, Walter · Psychiatry, Addiction Medicine

Lingeman, James E. · Urology, Endourology

Link, Michael P. · Pediatrics, Pediatric Hematology-Oncology

Linker, Charles Albert · Medical Oncology, Leukemia

Linscheid, Ronald · Hand Surgery, Reconstructive Surgery

Lion, John R. · Psychiatry, General Psychiatry; Psychiatry, Violence

Lippe, Barbara M. · Pediatrics, Pediatric Endocrinology

Lippman, Marc E. · Medical Oncology & Hematology, Breast Cancer

Lipschitz, David A. · Geriatric Medicine, General Geriatric Medicine

Lipshutz, William H. · Gastroenterology, General Gastroenterology

Lipsitz, Lewis A. · Geriatric Medicine, General Geriatric Medicine

Liptzin, Benjamin · Psychiatry, Geriatric Psychiatry

Lisak, Robert P. · Neurology, Adult, Infectious & Demyelinating Diseases

Lisman, Richard D. · Ophthalmology, Oculoplastic & Orbital Surgery

Lister, George · Pediatrics, Pediatric Critical Care

Lister, Graham D. · Hand Surgery, Microsurgery; Hand Surgery, Reconstructive Surgery

Little, James H. · Ophthalmology, Anterior Segment (Cataract Surgery)

Little, John William · Plastic Surgery, Breast Surgery

Littman, Robert M. · Psychiatry, Suicidology

Liu, James H. · Obstetrics & Gynecology, Reproductive Endocrinology

Livingston, Robert B. · Medical Oncology & Hematology, Breast Cancer; Medical Oncology & Hematology, Lung Cancer

Lloyd-Still, John D. · Pediatrics, Pediatric Gastroenterology

Lo Gerfo, Paul · General Surgery, Endocrine Surgery

Lobo, Rogerio A. · Obstetrics & Gynecology, Reproductive Endocrinology

Lobuglio, Albert S. · Medical Oncology & Hematology, Immunotherapy, Biological Response Modifiers Oncology

Lock, James E. · Pediatrics, Pediatric Cardiology

Lockey, Richard F. · Allergy & Immunology, Adult Allergy & Immunology

Lockhart, Jorge L. · Urology, Neuro-Urology & Voiding Dysfunction

Lockwood, Ted E. · Plastic Surgery, Body Contouring

Loeffler, Jay S. · Radiation Oncology, Brain Cancer

Loehrer, Patrick J. · Medical Oncology & Hematology, Genito-Urinary Cancer

Loewenstein, Richard J. · Psychiatry, Dissociative Disorders

Lomax, James Welton · Psychiatry, Psychoanalysis

Long, Donlin · Neurological Surgery, Tumor Surgery

Long, Sarah S. · Pediatrics, Pediatric Infectious Disease

Longo, Dan L. · Medical Oncology & Hematology, Lymphomas

Lookingbill, Donald Paul · Dermatology, Acne

Loop, Floyd D. · Thoracic Surgery, Adult Cardiothoracic Surgery

Loriaux, D. Lynn · Endocrinology & Metabolism, Neuroendocrinology

Lotke, Paul A. · Orthopaedic Surgery, Reconstructive Surgery

Loughlin, Gerald M. · Pediatrics, Pediatric Pulmonology

Louis, Dean S. · Hand Surgery, Reconstructive Surgery

Low, Phillip A. · Neurology, Adult, Neuromuscular Disease

Lowe, Nicholas J. · Dermatology, Clinical Dermatology; Dermatology, Laser Surgery; Dermatology, Photobiology; Dermatology, Psoriasis

Lowensohn, Richard I. · Obstetrics & Gynecology, Maternal & Fetal Medicine

Lowenstein, Edward · Anesthesiology, Adult Cardiovascular

Lowinson, Joyce H. · Psychiatry, Addiction Medicine

Luce, Edward Andrew · Plastic Surgery, Maxillofacial Surgery

Luce, John M. · Pulmonary & Critical Care Medicine, General Pulmonary & Critical Care Medicine

Lucey, Jerold F. · Pediatrics, Neonatal-Perinatal Medicine

Luchi, Robert J. · Geriatric Medicine, General Geriatric Medicine

Lucky, Anne · Dermatology, Pediatric Dermatology; Pediatrics, Pediatric Dermatology

Ludbrook, Philip A. · Cardiovascular Disease, Cardiac Catheterization

Lüders, Hans O. · Neurology, Adult, Epilepsy

Ludwig, Jurgen · Pathology, Liver Pathology

Ludwig, Stephen · Pediatrics, Abused Children

Lue, Tom F. · Urology, Impotence

Luetje, Charles M. · Otolaryngology, Otology/Neurotology

Luft, Benjamin J. · Infectious Disease, AIDS; Infectious Disease, Lyme Disease

Lukes, Robert J. · Pathology, Hematopathology

Lumb, Philip D. · Anesthesiology, Critical Care Medicine

Lunsford, L. Dade · Neurological Surgery, Stereotactic Radiosurgery

Lusk, Rodney P. · Otolaryngology, Pediatric Otolaryngology; Otolaryngology, Sinus & Nasal Surgery

Luxford, William M. · Otolaryngology, Otology/Neurotology

Lyle, Andrew W. · Ophthalmology, Anterior Segment (Cataract Surgery)

Lyles, Kenneth W. · Geriatric Medicine, General Geriatric Medicine

Lynch, Joseph P. · Pulmonary & Critical Care Medicine, General Pulmonary & Critical Care Medicine

Lynch, Peter John · Dermatology, Clinical Dermatology; Dermatology, Genital Dermatological Disease

Lytle, Bruce W. · Thoracic Surgery, Adult Cardiothoracic Surgery

M

Macdonald, John S. · Medical Oncology, Gastrointestinal Oncology

MacEwen, G. Dean · Orthopaedic Surgery, Pediatric Orthopaedic Surgery

MacGillivray, Margaret Hilda · Pediatrics, Pediatric Endocrinology

Machemer, Robert · Ophthalmology, Vitreo-Retinal Surgery

Machleder, Herbert I. · General Surgery, General Vascular Surgery

MacIntyre, Neil · Pulmonary & Critical Care Medicine, General Pulmonary & Critical Care Medicine

Mack, Eberhard · General Surgery, Endocrine Surgery

MacKeigan, John M. · Colon & Rectal Surgery, General Colon & Rectal Surgery

MacKinnon, Roger A. · Psychiatry, Psychoanalysis

Mackinnon, Susan E. · Plastic Surgery, Peripheral Nerve Surgery

MacLean, Ian C. · Physical Medicine & Rehabilitation, Electromyography

MacLeod, John Adams · Psychiatry, Psychoanalysis

MacRae, Scott M. · Ophthalmology, Corneal Diseases & Transplantation

Maddahi, Jamshid · Cardiovascular Disease, Nuclear Cardiology; Nuclear Medicine, Nuclear Cardiology

Maddens, Michael E. · Geriatric Medicine, General Geriatric Medicine

Maddrey, Willis C. · Gastroenterology, Hepatology

Madoc-Jones, Hywel · Radiation Oncology, Gynecologic Cancer

Maguire, Leo J. · Ophthalmology, Corneal Diseases & Transplantation

Mahmoud, Adel A. F. · Infectious Disease, Tropical Diseases

Mahon, Eugene J. · Psychiatry, Child Psychiatry; Psychiatry, Psychoanalysis

Maibach, Howard I. · Dermatology, Contact Dermatitis; Dermatology, Psoriasis

Main, Denise M. · Obstetrics & Gynecology, Maternal & Fetal Medicine

Mair, Douglas D. · Pediatrics, Pediatric Cardiology

Maisels, M. Jeffrey · Pediatrics, Neonatal-Perinatal Medicine

Maize, John C. · Dermatology, Dermatopathology

Major, Francis J. · Obstetrics & Gynecology, Gynecologic Cancer

Maki, Dennis G. · Infectious Disease, Hospital-Acquired Infections

Malawer, Martin Miles · Orthopaedic Surgery, Tumor Surgery

Maletta, Gabe J. · Psychiatry, Geriatric Psychiatry

Malinak, L. Russell · Obstetrics & Gynecology, Reproductive Endocrinology; Obstetrics & Gynecology, Reproductive Surgery

Malkinson, Frederick D. · Dermatology, Clinical Dermatology

Mallory, Susan B. · Dermatology, Pediatric Dermatology; Pediatrics, Pediatric Dermatology

Mallory, Thomas H. · Orthopaedic Surgery, Reconstructive Surgery

Malmud, Leon S. · Nuclear Medicine, General Nuclear Medicine

Malone, John I. · Pediatrics, Pediatric Endocrinology

Mancall, Elliott L. · Neurology, Adult, General Adult Neurology

Mandell, Gerald L. · Infectious Disease, General Infectious Disease

Mangano, Dennis T. · Anesthesiology, Adult Cardiovascular

Mangham, Charles · Psychiatry, Child Psychiatry; Psychiatry, Psychoanalysis

Mankin, Henry J. · Orthopaedic Surgery, Tumor Surgery

Mann, Roger A. · Orthopaedic Surgery, Foot & Ankle Surgery

Mannick, John A. · General Surgery, General Vascular Surgery

Manninen, Pirjo H. · Anesthesiology, Neuroanesthesia

Manning, Frank A. · Obstetrics & Gynecology, Maternal & Fetal Medicine

Manske, Paul R. · Hand Surgery, Reconstructive Surgery

Manson, Paul N. · Plastic Surgery, Craniofacial Surgery; Plastic Surgery, Maxillofacial Surgery

March, Charles M. · Obstetrics & Gynecology, Reproductive Endocrinology; Obstetrics & Gynecology, Reproductive Surgery

Marchlinski, Francis E. · Cardiovascular Disease, Electrophysiology

Marcus, Robert B. · Radiation Oncology, Pediatric Radiation Oncology

Marder, Stephen R. · Psychiatry, Schizophrenia/Psychopharmacology

Margolese, Richard G. · Surgical Oncology, Breast Cancer

Margolin, Richard Alan · Psychiatry, Geriatric Psychiatry

Margolis, Marvin O. · Psychiatry, Psychoanalysis

Marini, John J. · Pulmonary & Critical Care Medicine, General Pulmonary & Critical Care Medicine

Marinoff, Stanley C. · Obstetrics & Gynecology, Genital Dermatological Disease

Mark, Daniel B. · Cardiovascular Disease, Clinical Exercise Testing

Mark, James B. D. · Thoracic Surgery, General Thoracic Surgery; Thoracic Surgery, Thoracic Oncological Surgery

Markman, Maurie · Medical Oncology & Hematology, Gynecologic Cancer

Marks, James Garfield · Dermatology, Contact Dermatitis

Marmer, Stephen S. · Psychiatry, Dissociative Disorders

Marmor, Leonard · Orthopaedic Surgery, Knee Surgery

Marney, Samuel R. · Allergy & Immunology, Adult Allergy & Immunology

Maroon, Joseph C. · Neurological Surgery, General Neurological Surgery

Marrs, Richard P. · Obstetrics & Gynecology, Reproductive Endocrinology

Marsh, Bernard R. · Otolaryngology, Laryngology

Marsh, Jeffrey L. · Plastic Surgery, Craniofacial Surgery; Plastic Surgery, Pediatric Plastic Surgery; Plastic Surgery, Reconstructive Surgery

Marshall, Fray F. · Urology, Urologic Oncology

Marshall, John C. · Endocrinology & Metabolism, Reproductive Endocrinology

Marshall, Lawrence F. · Neurological Surgery, Trauma

Martin, Daniel Clyde · Obstetrics & Gynecology, Reproductive Surgery

Martin, David Charles · Geriatric Medicine, General Geriatric Medicine

Martin, David H. · Infectious Disease, Sexually Transmitted Disease

Martin, Gerard Robert · Pediatrics, Pediatric Cardiology

Martin, Joseph B. · Neurology, Adult, Movement Disorders

Martin, Mary C. · Obstetrics & Gynecology, Reproductive Endocrinology

Martin, Robert G. · Ophthalmology, Anterior Segment (Cataract Surgery)

Martinez, Alvaro A. · Radiation Oncology, Brachytherapy

Martinez, Serge Anthony · Otolaryngology, Otology/Neurotology

Masket, Samuel · Ophthalmology, Anterior Segment (Cataract Surgery)

Massey, E. Wayne · Neurology, Adult, General Adult Neurology

Massey, Janice M. · Neurology, Adult, Electromyography; Neurology, Adult, Neuromuscular Disease

Mast, Jeffrey W. · Orthopaedic Surgery, Trauma

Mastroianni, Luigi · Obstetrics & Gynecology, Reproductive Endocrinology

Masur, Henry · Infectious Disease, AIDS

Mathes, Stephen J. · Plastic Surgery, Breast Surgery

Mathew, Ninan T. · Neurology, Adult, Headache

Mathias, John R. · Gastroenterology, Gastrointestinal Motility

Mathisen, Douglas J. · Thoracic Surgery, General Thoracic Surgery; Thoracic Surgery, Thoracic Oncological Surgery

Mathison, David A. · Allergy & Immunology, Adult Allergy & Immunology

Matjasko, Mary Jane · Anesthesiology, Neuroanesthesia

Matloub, Hani S. · Hand Surgery, Microsurgery

Matsen, Frederick A. · Orthopaedic Surgery, Reconstructive Surgery

Matta, Joel M. · Orthopaedic Surgery, Trauma

Matthay, Michael Anthony · Pulmonary & Critical Care Medicine, General Pulmonary & Critical Care Medicine

Matthay, Richard A. · Pulmonary & Critical Care Medicine, General Pulmonary & Critical Care Medicine

Mattison, Richard E. · Psychiatry, Child Psychiatry

Mattox, Douglas E. · Otolaryngology, Otology/Neurotology

Mattox, Kenneth L. · General Surgery, General Vascular Surgery

Mattson, Richard · Neurology, Adult, Epilepsy

Mattsson, Ake Erik · Psychiatry, Child Psychiatry

Mauch, Peter M. · Radiation Oncology, General Radiation Oncology; Radiation Oncology, Lymphomas

Mauer, S. Michael · Pediatrics, Pediatric Nephrology

Maumenee, Irene H. · Ophthalmology, Ophthalmic Genetics

Maves, Michael · Otolaryngology, Head & Neck Surgery

Mavroudis, Constantine · Thoracic Surgery, Pediatric Cardiac Surgery

Maxwell, G. Patrick · Plastic Surgery, Aesthetic Surgery; Plastic Surgery, Breast Surgery

May, James W. · Plastic Surgery, Breast Surgery; Plastic Surgery, Microsurgery

Mayer, John E. · Thoracic Surgery, Pediatric Cardiac Surgery

Mayer, Robert J. · Medical Oncology, Gastrointestinal Oncology; Medical Oncology, Leukemia

Mayeux, Richard · Neurology, Adult, Degenerative Diseases

Mayhall, C. Glen · Infectious Disease, Hospital-Acquired Infections

Maynard, C. Douglas · Nuclear Medicine, General Nuclear Medicine

Mazier, W. Patrick · Colon & Rectal Surgery, General Colon & Rectal Surgery

Mazow, Malcolm L. · Ophthalmology, Pediatric Ophthalmology

Mazziotta, John C. · Neurology, Adult, General Adult Neurology; Nuclear Medicine, Brain

McAllister, Thomas W. · Psychiatry, Neuropsychiatry

McArthur, Justin C. · Neurology, Adult, Infectious & Demyelinating Diseases

McBride, John T. · Pediatrics, Pediatric Pulmonology

McCabe, Edward R. B. · Pediatrics, Metabolic Diseases

McCain, Glenn A. · Rheumatology, Fibromyalgia

McCarthy, Joseph G. · Plastic Surgery, Craniofacial Surgery; Plastic Surgery, Maxillofacial Surgery

McCarty, Daniel J. · Rheumatology, General Rheumatology; Rheumatology, Gout

McComb, J. Gordon · Neurological Surgery, Pediatric Neurological Surgery

McCord, Clinton D. · Ophthalmology, Oculoplastic & Orbital Surgery

McCormack, William M. · Infectious Disease, Sexually Transmitted Disease

McCormick, Beryl · Radiation Oncology, Breast Cancer

McCracken, George · Pediatrics, Pediatric Infectious Disease

McCrary, John A. · Neurology, Adult, Neuro-Ophthalmology; Ophthalmology, Neuro-Ophthalmology

McCraw, John B. · Plastic Surgery, Breast Surgery; Plastic Surgery, Reconstructive Surgery

McCuen, Brooks Walton · Ophthalmology, Vitreo-Retinal Surgery

McCulley, James P. · Ophthalmology, Corneal Diseases & Transplantation

McDermott, John F. · Psychiatry, Child Psychiatry

McDonald, Charles J. · Dermatology, Clinical Dermatology

McDonald, Marguerite B. · Ophthalmology, Corneal Diseases & Transplantation

McDonough, Paul G. · Obstetrics & Gynecology, Reproductive Endocrinology

McDowell, Charles Lindsey · Hand Surgery, Paralytic Disorders

McDowell, Fletcher H. · Neurology, Adult, Neuro Rehabilitation

McEnery, Paul T. · Pediatrics, Pediatric Nephrology

McFadden, E. R. · Pulmonary & Critical Care Medicine, Asthma

McFarlane, William R. · Psychiatry, Schizophrenia

McFarlin, Dale E. · Neurology, Adult, Infectious & Demyelinating Diseases

McGill, Trevor · Otolaryngology, Pediatric Otolaryngology

McGinty, John B. · Orthopaedic Surgery, Sports Medicine

McGlashan, Thomas H. · Psychiatry, Schizophrenia

McGowan, John E. · Infectious Disease, Hospital-Acquired Infections

McGrath, Mary H. · Plastic Surgery, Breast Surgery

McGraw, Robert William · Orthopaedic Surgery, Reconstructive Surgery

McGregor, James A. · Obstetrics & Gynecology, Infectious Disease

McGuire, Edward J. · Urology, Neuro-Urology & Voiding Dysfunction

McGuire, Joseph · Dermatology, Pediatric Dermatology; Pediatrics, Pediatric Dermatology

McGuire, William P. · Medical Oncology & Hematology, Gynecologic Cancer

McGuirt, William Frederick · Otolaryngology, Head & Neck Surgery

McHenry, Paul L. · Cardiovascular Disease, Clinical Exercise Testing

McHugh, Margaret T. · Pediatrics, Abused Children

McHugh, Paul R. · Psychiatry, Behavioral Disorders; Psychiatry, Neuropsychiatry

McIntosh, Kenneth · Pediatrics, Pediatric Infectious Disease

McIntyre, David J. · Ophthalmology, Anterior Segment (Cataract Surgery)

McKay, Marilynne · Dermatology, Genital Dermatological Disease

McKenna, Robert W. · Pathology, Hematopathology

McKenzie, J. Maxwell · Endocrinology & Metabolism, Thyroid

McKinney, Peter · Plastic Surgery, Facial Aesthetic Surgery

McKneally, Martin F. · Thoracic Surgery, General Thoracic Surgery; Thoracic Surgery, Thoracic Oncological Surgery

McKusick, Kenneth A. · Nuclear Medicine, General Nuclear Medicine

McLaughlin, James T. · Psychiatry, Psychoanalysis

McLean, Robert H. · Pediatrics, Pediatric Nephrology

McLeod, Rima Linnea · Infectious Disease, Toxoplasmosis

McLone, David G. · Neurological Surgery, Pediatric Neurological Surgery

McLoud, Theresa C. · Radiology, Chest

McMahon, William Martin · Psychiatry, Child Psychiatry

McNeese, Marsha Diane · Radiation Oncology, Breast Cancer

McNulty, John Haynes · Cardiovascular Disease, Electrophysiology

McPherson, Robert W. · Anesthesiology, Neuroanesthesia

Mead, Philip B. · Obstetrics & Gynecology, Infectious Disease

Meals, Roy A. · Hand Surgery, General Hand Surgery

Meares, Edwin M. · Urology, Urological Infections

Mears, Dana Christopher · Orthopaedic Surgery, Trauma

Mecklenburg, Robert S. · Endocrinology & Metabolism, Diabetes

Medina, Jesus Edilberto · Otolaryngology, Head & Neck Surgery

Medsger, Thomas A. · Rheumatology, Scleroderma

Meek, Robert Norman · Orthopaedic Surgery, Trauma

Mehlman, Robert D. · Psychiatry, Psychoanalysis

Meier, Diane · Geriatric Medicine, General Geriatric Medicine

Meis, Paul J. · Obstetrics & Gynecology, Maternal & Fetal Medicine

Meisler, David M. · Ophthalmology, Corneal Diseases & Transplantation; Ophthalmology, Uveitis

Meldrum, David Roy · Obstetrics & Gynecology, Reproductive Endocrinology

Melish, Marian E. · Infectious Disease, Pediatric Infectious Disease

Mellins, Robert B. · Pediatrics, Pediatric Pulmonology

Melman, Arnold · Urology, Impotence

Melmed, Shlomo · Endocrinology & Metabolism, Neuroendocrinology

Meltzer, Eli Owen · Allergy & Immunology, Pediatric Allergy & Immunology

Meltzer, Herbert Yale · Psychiatry, Schizophrenia/Psychopharmacology

Melvin, John L. · Physical Medicine & Rehabilitation, Electromyography

Mendell, Jerry R. · Neurology, Adult, Neuromuscular Disease

Mendelson, Jack H. · Addiction Medicine, Medical Treatment of Drug Abusers

Mendenhall, Nancy P. · Radiation Oncology, Breast Cancer

Mendenhall, William M. · Radiation Oncology, Head & Neck Cancer

Mendez, Hermann A. · Pediatrics, Pediatric Infectious Disease

Meneilly, Graydon S. · Geriatric Medicine, General Geriatric Medicine

Menezes, Arnold H. · Neurological Surgery, Pediatric Neurological Surgery

Menkes, John H. · Neurology, Child, General Child Neurology; Neurology, Child, Inherited Biochemical Disorders

Mennuti, Michael T. · Obstetrics & Gynecology, Genetics; Obstetrics & Gynecology, Maternal & Fetal Medicine

Menolascino, Frank · Psychiatry, Mental Retardation/Mental Health: Dual Diagnosis

Menter, M. Alan · Dermatology, Psoriasis

Mentser, Mark I. · Pediatrics, Pediatric Nephrology

Meredith, Travis A. · Ophthalmology, Vitreo-Retinal Surgery

Mertz, Gregory J. · Infectious Disease, Herpes Virus Infections

Messick, Joseph M. · Anesthesiology, Neuroanesthesia

Messner, Hans A. · Medical Oncology & Hematology, Bone Marrow Transplantation

Mesulam, Marek-Marsel · Neurology, Adult, Behavioral Neurology

Metz, Henry S. · Ophthalmology, Pediatric Ophthalmology

Meyer, Jon Keith · Psychiatry, Psychoanalysis

Meyer, Roger E. · Psychiatry, Addiction Medicine

Meyer, Roger F. · Ophthalmology, Corneal Diseases & Transplantation

Meyers, Barnett Samuel · Psychiatry, Affective Disorders; Psychiatry, Geriatric Psychiatry

Meyers, Joel D. · Infectious Disease, Cancer & Infections; Infectious Disease, Transplantation Infections

Meyers, Robert Weigel · Psychiatry, Psychoanalysis

Meyers, William C. · General Surgery, Gastroenterologic Surgery

Michaels, David D. · Ophthalmology, Anterior Segment (Cataract Surgery); Ophthalmology, Optics & Refraction

Michels, Robert · Psychiatry, Psychoanalysis

Michenfelder, John D. · Anesthesiology, Neuroanesthesia

Migeon, Claude J. · Pediatrics, Pediatric Endocrinology

Mikuta, John J. · Obstetrics & Gynecology, Gynecologic Cancer

Milde, Leslie N. · Anesthesiology, Neuroanesthesia

Milder, Benjamin · Ophthalmology, Optics & Refraction

Millard, D. Ralph · Plastic Surgery , Reconstructive Surgery

Millender, Lewis H. · Hand Surgery, Reconstructive Surgery

Miller, Aaron E. · Neurology, Adult, Infectious & Demyelinating Diseases

Miller, Edward D. · Anesthesiology, Adult Cardiovascular

Miller, Fletcher A. · Cardiovascular Disease, General Cardiovascular Disease

Miller, Frank C. · Obstetrics & Gynecology, Maternal & Fetal Medicine

Miller, Joseph · Thoracic Surgery, General Thoracic Surgery; Thoracic Surgery, Thoracic Oncological Surgery

Miller, Laurence Herbert · Dermatology, Clinical Dermatology

Miller, Michael E. · Orthopaedic Surgery, Trauma

Miller, Neil R. · Neurology, Adult, Neuro-Ophthalmology; Ophthalmology, Neuro-Ophthalmology

Miller, Robert Gordon · Neurology, Adult, Electromyography; Neurology, Adult, Neuromuscular Disease; Neurology, Child, Neuromuscular Disease

Miller, Robert H. · Otolaryngology, Head & Neck Surgery; Otolaryngology, Pediatric Otolaryngology; Otolaryngology, Sinus & Nasal Surgery

Miller, Ronald D. · Anesthesiology, General Anesthesiology; Anesthesiology, Pharmacology

Miller, Sheldon I. · Psychiatry, Addiction Medicine

Miller, Thomas A. · General Surgery, Gastroenterologic Surgery

Miller, Thomas P. · Medical Oncology & Hematology, Lymphomas

Millikan, Larry E. · Dermatology, Clinical Dermatology

Million, Rodney Reiff · Radiation Oncology, Head & Neck Cancer

Millman, Robert B. · Psychiatry, Addiction Medicine

Mills, John · Infectious Disease, AIDS

Mills, Richard P. · Ophthalmology, Glaucoma

Mills, Stacey E. · Pathology, ENT Pathology

Minaker, Kenneth L. · Geriatric Medicine, General Geriatric Medicine

Minckler, Donald S. · Ophthalmology, Glaucoma

Mindell, Eugene R. · Orthopaedic Surgery, Tumor Surgery

Minkoff, Howard L. · Obstetrics & Gynecology, Infectious Disease

Minna, John Dorrance · Medical Oncology, Lung Cancer

Mintun, Mark A. · Nuclear Medicine, Brain

Mirin, Steven M. · Psychiatry, Addiction Medicine

Mirkin, Bernard L. · Clinical Pharmacology

Mirro, Joseph · Pediatrics, Pediatric Hematology-Oncology

Mischke, Robert E. · Otolaryngology, Otology/Neurotology

Mischler, Elaine H. · Pediatrics, Pediatric Pulmonology

Mishell, Daniel R. · Obstetrics & Gynecology, Reproductive Endocrinology

Mitchell, James E. · Psychiatry, Eating Disorders

Mitchell, Malcolm S. · Medical Oncology & Hematology, Immunotherapy, Biological Response Modifiers Oncology

Mitchell, Michael E. · Urology, Pediatric Urology

Miyamoto, Richard T. · Otolaryngology, Otology/Neurotology

Moak, Gary Stuart · Psychiatry, Geriatric Psychiatry

Modic, Michael T. · Radiology, Neuroradiology

Moed, Berton R. · Orthopaedic Surgery, Trauma

Moellering, Robert C. · Infectious Disease, General Infectious Disease

Moertel, Charles G. · Medical Oncology, Gastrointestinal Oncology

Mohr, J. P. · Neurology, Adult, Strokes

Molitch, Mark E. · Endocrinology & Metabolism, Neuroendocrinology

Monaco, Anthony · General Surgery, Transplantation

Monchik, Jack M. · General Surgery, Endocrine Surgery

Moncrief, Jack W. · Nephrology, Dialysis

Moncure, Ashby · General Surgery, Gastroenterologic Surgery

Montague, Drogo K. · Urology, Impotence

Montgomery, William · Otolaryngology, Laryngology; Otolaryngology, Sinus & Nasal Surgery

Montie, James · Urology, Urologic Oncology

Moody, Frank G. · General Surgery, Gastroenterologic Surgery

Mooney, Alfonso J. · Addiction Medicine, General Addiction Medicine

Moore, Gordon L. · Psychiatry, General Psychiatry

Moore, Joseph O. · Medical Oncology & Hematology, General Medical Oncology & Hematology

Moore, Michael P. · Surgical Oncology, Breast Cancer

Moore, Thomas R. · Obstetrics & Gynecology, Maternal & Fetal Medicine

Moore, Wayne V. · Pediatrics, Pediatric Endocrinology

Moore, Wesley S. · General Surgery, General Vascular Surgery

Moossa, A. R. · General Surgery, Gastroenterologic Surgery

Morady, Fred · Cardiovascular Disease, Electrophysiology

Morales, Alvaro · Urology, Impotence; Urology, Urologic Oncology

Morales, Louis · Plastic Surgery, Craniofacial Surgery; Plastic Surgery, Maxillofacial Surgery

Moran, Jon F. · Thoracic Surgery, Adult Cardiothoracic Surgery

Morawetz, Richard B. · Neurological Surgery, Vascular Neurological Surgery

Moreland, John R. · Orthopaedic Surgery, Reconstructive Surgery

Morelli, Joseph G. · Dermatology, Pediatric Dermatology; Pediatrics, Pediatric Dermatology

Morgan, Mark A. · Obstetrics & Gynecology, Maternal & Fetal Medicine

Morganroth, Melvin L. · Pulmonary & Critical Care Medicine, General Pulmonary & Critical Care Medicine

Morison, Warwick L. · Dermatology, Photobiology; Dermatology, Psoriasis

Morley, George W. · Obstetrics & Gynecology, Gynecologic Cancer

Morrey, Bernard F. · Orthopaedic Surgery, Reconstructive Surgery

Morris, Alan · Pulmonary & Critical Care Medicine, General Pulmonary & Critical Care Medicine

Morrison, John · Obstetrics & Gynecology, Maternal & Fetal Medicine

Morrissy, Raymond T. · Orthopaedic Surgery, Pediatric Orthopaedic Surgery

Morrow, C. Paul · Obstetrics & Gynecology, Gynecologic Cancer

Morrow, Monica · Surgical Oncology, Breast Cancer

Morton, Donald L. · Surgical Oncology, Immunotherapy, Biological Response Modifiers Oncology; Surgical Oncology, Melanoma

Moschella, Samuel Leonard · Dermatology, Clinical Dermatology

Moser, Kenneth · Pulmonary & Critical Care Medicine, Pulmonary Disease

Moskowitz, Roland W. · Rheumatology, Osteoarthritis

Motto, Jerome A. · Psychiatry, Suicidology

Motzer, Robert J. · Medical Oncology & Hematology, Genito-Urinary Cancer

Moxley, Richard T. · Neurology, Child, Neuromuscular Disease

Muggia, Franco M. · Medical Oncology & Hematology, Breast Cancer; Medical Oncology & Hematology, Clinical Pharmacologyl Medical Oncology & Hematology, Gynecologic Cancer; Medical Oncology & Hematology, Solid Tumors

Mulcahy, John J. · Urology, Impotence

Mulholland, Michael W. · General Surgery, Gastroenterologic Surgery

Müller, Nestor L. · Radiology, Chest

Mulliken, John B. · Plastic Surgery, Pediatric Plastic Surgery

Mullin, Walter R. · Plastic Surgery, Breast Surgery

Mullins, Charles Edward · Pediatrics, Pediatric Cardiology

Munro, Ian R. · Plastic Surgery, Craniofacial Surgery; Plastic Surgery, Maxillofacial Surgery

Munsat, Theodore L. · Neurology, Adult, Neuromuscular Disease

Muntz, Harlan R. · Otolaryngology, Pediatric Otolaryngology

Murphree, A. Linn · Ophthalmology, Ophthalmic Genetics

Murphy, Sharon Boehm · Pediatrics, Pediatric Hematology-Oncology

Murphy, Shirley · Pediatrics, Pediatric Pulmonology

Murray, Andrew B. · Pediatrics, Pediatric Allergy & Immunology

Murray, Gordon F. · Thoracic Surgery, Adult Cardiothoracic Surgery

Murray, John A. · Orthopaedic Surgery, Tumor Surgery

Murray, John F. · Pulmonary & Critical Care Medicine, Pulmonary Disease

Muss, Hyman B. · Medical Oncology & Hematology, Breast Cancer; Medical Oncology & Hematology, Gynecologic Cancer

Mustoe, Thomas Anthony · Plastic Surgery, Wound Healing

Myer, Charles M. · Otolaryngology, Pediatric Otolaryngology

Myers, Charles E. · Medical Oncology & Hematology, Clinical Pharmacology

Myers, Eugene M. · Otolaryngology, Head & Neck Surgery

Myers, Lawrence W. · Neurology, Adult, Infectious & Demyelinating Diseases

Myerson, Paul G. · Psychiatry, Psychoanalysis

Myler, Richard K. · Cardiovascular Disease, Cardiac Catheterization

N

Naccarelli, Gerald V. · Cardiovascular Disease, Electrophysiology

Naclerio, Robert M. · Otolaryngology, Pediatric Otolaryngology

Nadas, Alexander S. · Pediatrics, Pediatric Cardiology

Nadler, Lee M. · Medical Oncology & Hematology, Immunotherapy, Biological Response Modifiers Oncology; Medical Oncology & Hematology, Lymphomas

Nadol, Joseph B. · Otolaryngology, Otology/Neurotology

Nagey, David Augustus · Obstetrics & Gynecology, Maternal & Fetal Medicine

Nagorney, David M. · General Surgery, Gastroenterologic Surgery; Surgical Oncology, Gastroenterologic Cancer

Nahai, Foad · Plastic Surgery, Breast Surgery; Plastic Surgery, Reconstructive Surgery

Nahrwold, David L. · General Surgery, Gastroenterologic Surgery

Naidich, David P. · Radiology, Chest

Najafi, Hassan · Thoracic Surgery, Adult Cardiothoracic Surgery

Najarian, John S. · General Surgery, Transplantation

Nalebuff, Edward A. · Hand Surgery, Reconstructive Surgery

Narcisi, Calvern E. · Psychiatry, Psychoanalysis

Nardell, Edward A. · Pulmonary & Critical Care Medicine, Lung Infections

Natale, Ronald B. · Medical Oncology & Hematology, Lung Cancer

Nathan, David M. · Endocrinology & Metabolism, Diabetes

Nathwani, Bharat N. · Pathology, Hematopathology

Naulty, J. Stephen · Anesthesiology, Obstetric Anesthesia

Neale, Henry W. · Plastic Surgery, Reconstructive Surgery

Needell, Stanley Stuart · Psychiatry, Psychoanalysis

Neel, H. Bryan · Otolaryngology, Head & Neck Surgery; Otolaryngology, Laryngology

Neely, J. Gail · Otolaryngology, Otology/Neurotology

Neff, James R. · Orthopaedic Surgery, Tumor Surgery

Nelp, Wil B. · Nuclear Medicine, General Nuclear Medicine

Nelson, Harold S. · Allergy & Immunology, Adult Allergy & Immunology; Allergy & Immunology, Pediatric Allergy & Immunology

Nelson, J. Craig · Psychiatry, Affective Disorders; Psychiatry, Psychopharmacology

Nelson, John D. · Pediatrics, Pediatric Infectious Disease

Nemeroff, Charles B. · Psychiatry, Affective Disorders; Psychiatry, Psychopharmacology

Nemiroff, Robert A. · Psychiatry, Psychoanalysis

Neppe, Vernon M. · Psychiatry, Neuropsychiatry

Nerad, Jeffrey A. · Ophthalmology, Oculoplastic & Orbital Surgery

Nesbit, Mark E. · Pediatrics, Pediatric Hematology-Oncology

Nesburn, Anthony B. · Ophthalmology, Corneal Diseases & Transplantation

Neu, Harold C. · Infectious Disease, Antibiotic Pharmacology

Neubauer, Peter B. · Psychiatry, Psychoanalysis

Neumann, Albert C. · Ophthalmology, Anterior Segment (Cataract Surgery)

Neustadt, David H. · Rheumatology, General Rheumatology

Nevins, Thomas E. · Pediatrics, Pediatric Nephrology

New, Maria I. · Pediatrics, Pediatric Endocrinology

Newburger, Jane W. · Pediatrics, Pediatric Cardiology

Newfield, Philippa · Anesthesiology, Pediatric Anesthesiology

Newman, Kenneth M. · Psychiatry, Psychoanalysis

Newman, Nancy J. · Neurology, Adult, Neuro-Ophthalmology; Ophthalmology, Neuro-Ophthalmology

Newman, Roger B. · Obstetrics & Gynecology, Maternal & Fetal Medicine

Newsome, H. H. · General Surgery, Endocrine Surgery

Nicholas, John J. · Physical Medicine & Rehabilitation, Rheumatology; Rheumatology, Rehabilitation

Nicholas, Stephen W. · Pediatrics, Pediatric Infectious Disease

Nicklas, John · Cardiovascular Disease, Heart Failure

Nicoloff, John T. · Endocrinology & Metabolism, Thyroid

Nicolson, Susan C. · Anesthesiology, Pediatric Cardiovascular

Niebyl, Jennifer R. · Obstetrics & Gynecology, Maternal & Fetal Medicine

Niederman, Michael S. · Pulmonary & Critical Care Medicine, General Pulmonary & Critical Care Medicine

Nierenberg, David · Clinical Pharmacology

Nies, Alan S. · Clinical Pharmacology

Nishimura, Rick A. · Cardiovascular Disease, General Cardiovascular Disease

Nissenson, Allen R. · Nephrology, Dialysis

Nochimson, David J. · Obstetrics & Gynecology, Maternal & Fetal Medicine

Noe, Joel M. · Plastic Surgery, Laser Surgery & Birthmarks

Nolph, Karl D. · Nephrology, Dialysis; Nephrology, Kidney Disease

Norins, Arthur L. · Dermatology, Pediatric Dermatology

Norman, David · Radiology, Neuroradiology

Norman, Douglas J. · Nephrology, Kidney Transplantation

Norman, Philip S. · Allergy & Immunology, Adult Allergy & Immunology

Norris, David A. · Dermatology, Cutaneous Immunology; Dermatology, Depigmenting Diseases

Norris, Henry J. · Pathology, Breast Pathology; Pathology, Gynecologic Pathology

Norris, Mark C. · Anesthesiology, Obstetric Anesthesia

Norton, Jeffrey A. · General Surgery, Endocrine Surgery

Norton, Larry · Medical Oncology & Hematology, Breast Cancer

Norwood, William I. · Thoracic Surgery, Pediatric Cardiac Surgery

Noseworthy, John H. · Neurology, Adult, Infectious & Demyelinating Diseases

Novick, Andrew C. · Urology, Urologic Oncology

Noyes, Frank · Orthopaedic Surgery, Knee Surgery

Noyes, Russell · Psychiatry, Affective Disorders

Nozik, Robert A. · Ophthalmology, Uveitis

Numann, Patricia J. · General Surgery, Endocrine Surgery

Nussenblatt, Robert B. · Ophthalmology, Uveitis

Nyhan, William L. · Pediatrics, Metabolic Diseases

O

O'Brien, Charles P. · Psychiatry, Addiction Medicine

O'Brien, William F. · Obstetrics & Gynecology, Maternal & Fetal Medicine

O'Connell, John B. · Cardiovascular Disease, Heart Failure; Cardiovascular Disease, Heart Transplantation

O'Connell, Michael J. · Medical Oncology, Gastrointestinal Oncology

O'Day, Denis M. · Ophthalmology, Corneal Diseases & Transplantation

O'Donnell, Thomas F. · General Surgery, General Vascular Surgery

O'Driscoll, Shawn W. · Orthopaedic Surgery, Reconstructive Surgery

O'Dwyer, Peter James · Medical Oncology & Hematology, Clinical Pharmacology

O'Neill, James A. · General Surgery, Pediatric Surgery

O'Neill, William W. · Cardiovascular Disease, Cardiac Catheterization

O'Reilly, Richard J. · Pediatrics, Pediatric Hematology-Oncology

O'Rourke, P. Pearl · Pediatrics, Pediatric Critical Care

O'Rourke, Robert Anthony · Cardiovascular Disease, General Cardiovascular Disease

Oakes, W. Jerry · Neurological Surgery, Pediatric Neurological Surgery

Oates, John A. · Clinical Pharmacology

Oberman, Harold A. · Pathology, Breast Pathology

Obstbaum, Stephen A. · Ophthalmology, Anterior Segment (Cataract Surgery)

Ochs, Hans D. · Allergy & Immunology, Pediatric Allergy & Immunology

Odom, Lorrie Furman · Pediatrics , Pediatric Hematology-Oncology

Odom, Richard B. · Dermatology, Clinical Dermatology

Offenkrantz, William C. · Psychiatry, Psychoanalysis

Oh, William · Pediatrics, Neonatal-Perinatal Medicine

Ohman, John L. · Allergy & Immunology, Adult Allergy & Immunology

Ojemann, George A. · Neurological Surgery, Epilepsy Surgery

Ojemann, Robert G. · Neurological Surgery, Tumor Surgery

Oken, Martin M. · Medical Oncology & Hematology, Lymphomas; Medical Oncology & Hematology, Myeloma

Olanow, C. Warren · Neurology, Adult, Movement Disorders

Oldham, Robert K. · Medical Oncology & Hematology, Immunotherapy, Biological Response Modifiers Oncology

Oleske, James M. · Pediatrics, Pediatric Infectious Disease

Olivier, Andre · Neurological Surgery, Epilepsy Surgery

Olsen, Edwin J. · Geriatric Medicine, General Geriatirc Medicine; Psychiatry, Geriatric Psychiatry

Olsen, Elise A. · Dermatology, Hair

Olson, Nels R. · Otolaryngology, Laryngology

Olson, Randall J. · Ophthalmology, Corneal Diseases & Transplantation

Olsson, Carl A. · Urology, Urologic Oncology

Olsson, James Edward · Otolaryngology, Otology/Neurotology

Omer, George E. · Hand Surgery, Peripheral Nerve Surgery; Orthopaedic Surgery, Peripheral Nerve Surgery

Omura, George A. · Medical Oncology & Hematology, Gynecologic Cancer

Onofrio, Burton M. · Neurological Surgery, Spinal Surgery

Opremcak, E. Mitchel · Ophthalmology, Uveitis

Orcutt, James C. · Ophthalmology, Oculoplastic & Orbital Surgery

Orenstein, David M. · Pediatrics, Pediatric Pulmonology

Orentreich, Norman · Dermatology, Hair

Oreopoulos, Dimitrios · Nephrology, Dialysis; Nephrology, Kidney Disease

Orgel, Shelley · Psychiatry, Psychoanalysis

Orkin, Frederick K. · Anesthesiology, Complications of Anesthesia

Ornstein, Anna · Psychiatry, Psychoanalysis

Ornstein, Paul H. · Psychiatry, Psychoanalysis

Orringer, Mark B. · Thoracic Surgery, General Thoracic Surgery; Thoracic Surgery, Thoracic Oncological Surgery

Orth, David H. · Ophthalmology, Medical Retinal Diseases

Orth, David N. · Endocrinology & Metabolism, Neuroendocrinology

Osborne, C. Kent · Medical Oncology & Hematology, Breast Cancer

Osborne, Michael P. · Surgical Oncology, Breast Cancer

Osher, Robert H. · Ophthalmology, Anterior Segment (Cataract Surgery)

Ossoff, Robert H. · Otolaryngology, Laryngology

Ostheimer, Gerard W. · Anesthesiology, Obstetric Anesthesia

Ostrea, Enrique M. · Pediatrics, Neonatal-Perinatal Medicine

Othersen, H. Biemann · Thoracic Surgery, Pediatric Non-Cardiac Thoracic Surgery

Ott, David A. · Thoracic Surgery, Adult Cardiothoracic Surgery

Ottinger, Leslie W. · General Surgery, Gastroenterologic Surgery

Ouslander, Joseph G. · Geriatric Medicine, Urinary Incontinence

Ousterhout, Douglas K. · Plastic Surgery, Craniofacial Surgery

Owens, Fred D. · Otolaryngology, Otology/Neurotology

Ownby, Dennis Randall · Allergy & Immunology, Pediatric Allergy & Immunology

Owsley, John Q. · Plastic Surgery, Aesthetic Surgery; Plastic Surgery, Facial Aesthetic Surgery

Oyer, Philip E. · Thoracic Surgery, Adult Cardiothoracic Surgery; Thoracic Surgery, Transplantation

Ozols, Robert · Medical Oncology & Hematology, Gynecologic Cancer

P

Pabst, Henry F. · Allergy & Immunology, Pediatric Allergy & Immunology

Pacifico, Albert D. · Thoracic Surgery, Pediatric Cardiac Surgery

Packer, Milton · Cardiovascular Disease, Heart Failure

Packer, Roger · Neurology, Child, Neuro-oncology

Packo, Kirk H. · Ophthalmology, Vitreo-Retinal Surgery

Page, David L. · Pathology, Breast Pathology

Pahwa, Savita G. · Allergy & Immunology, Pediatric Allergy & Immunology; Pediatrics, Pediatric Allergy & Immunology

Pairolero, Peter C. · Thoracic Surgery, General Thoracic Surgery; Thoracic Surgery, Thoracic Oncological Surgery

Palestine, Alan G. · Ophthalmology, Uveitis

Paller, Amy S. · Dermatology, Pediatric Dermatology; Pediatrics, Pediatric Dermatology

Palmberg, Paul F. · Ophthalmology, Glaucoma

Palmer, Jerry P. · Endocrinology & Metabolism, Diabetes

Palmer, William M. · Pediatrics, Abused Children

Paloyan, Edward · General Surgery, Endocrine Surgery

Palumbo, P. J. · Endocrinology & Metabolism, Diabetes

Pandian, Natesa G. · Cardiovascular Disease, Echocardiography

Pang, Songya · Pediatrics, Pediatric Endocrinology

Pankey, George A. · Infectious Disease, General Infectious Disease

Pannill, Fitzhugh C. · Geriatric Medicine, General Geriatric Medicine

Papile, Lu-Ann · Pediatrics, Neonatal-Perinatal Medicine

Papish, Steven · Medical Oncology & Hematology, Breast Cancer

Pappadis, Thomas L. · Psychiatry, Psychoanalysis

Pappas, Dennis G. · Otolaryngology, Otology/Neurotology

Pappas, Theodore N. · General Surgery, Gastroenterologic Surgery

Paradise, Jan E. · Pediatrics, Abused Children

Parisi, Alfred F. · Cardiovascular Disease, Echocardiography

Parisi, Valerie M. · Obstetrics & Gynecology, Maternal & Fetal Medicine

Parisier, Simon C. · Otolaryngology, Otology

Parker, Robert G. · Radiation Oncology, General Radiation Oncology

Parkinson, David R. · Medical Oncology & Hematology, Immunotherapy, Biological Response Modifiers Oncology

Parkman, Robertson · Pediatrics, Pediatric Hematology-Oncology

Parks, Marshall M. · Ophthalmology, Pediatric Ophthalmology

Parks, Wade P. · Pediatrics, Pediatric Infectious Disease

Parmley, William W. · Cardiovascular Disease, General Cardiovascular Disease; Cardiovascular Disease, Heart Failure

Parrish, Richard K. · Ophthalmology, Glaucoma

Parsonnet, Victor · Cardiovascular Disease, Pacemakers; General Surgery, General Vascular Surgery

Parsons, David S. · Otolaryngology, Pediatric Otolaryngology

Parsons, James T. · Radiation Oncology, Genito-Urinary Cancer; Radiation Oncology, Head & Neck Cancer; Radiation Oncology, Sarcomas

Pass, Harvey I. · Thoracic Surgery, Thoracic Oncological Surgery

Passaro, Edward · General Surgery, Gastroenterologic Surgery

Pastorek, Norman Joseph · Otolaryngology, Facial Plastic Surgery

Paterson, A. H. · Medical Oncology & Hematology, Breast Cancer

Patrinely, James R. · Ophthalmology, Oculoplastic & Orbital Surgery

Patterson, G. Alexander · Thoracic Surgery, General Thoracic Surgery; Thoracic Surgery, Transplantation

Patterson, James R. · Pulmonary & Critical Care Medicine, General Pulmonary & Critical Care Medicine

Patterson, Roy · Allergy & Immunology, Adult Allergy & Immunology

Patterson, Russell H. · Neurological Surgery, General Neurological Surgery

Patton, Dennis David · Nuclear Medicine, General Nuclear Medicine

Paty, Donald W. · Neurology, Adult, Infectious & Demyelinating Diseases

Paulsen, Elsa P. · Pediatrics, Pediatric Endocrinology

Paulson, David F. · Urology, Urologic Oncology

Paulson, George W. · Neurology, Adult, General Adult Neurology

Paulus, Harold A. · Rheumatology, General Rheumatology

Peacock, Warwick J. · Neurological Surgery, Pediatric Neurological Surgery

Pearlman, Alan S. · Cardiovascular Disease, Echocardiography

Pearlman, David S. · Allergy & Immunology, Pediatric Allergy & Immunology

Pearlman, Justin D. · Cardiovascular Disease, Magnetic Resonance Imaging; Radiology, Cardiovascular Disease

Pearlman, Robert A. · Geriatric Medicine, General Geriatric Medicine

Pearson, Bruce W. · Otolaryngology, Laryngology

Pearson, F. Griffith · Thoracic Surgery, General Thoracic Surgery; Thoracic Surgery, Thoracic Oncological Surgery

Peck, George C. · Plastic Surgery, Facial Aesthetic Surgery

Pedley, Timothy A. · Neurology, Adult, Epilepsy

Peerless, Sydney J. · Neurological Surgery, Vascular Neurological Surgery

Pellegrini, Carlos · General Surgery, Gastroenterologic Surgery

Pena, Alberto · General Surgery, Pediatric Surgery

Penn, Audrey S. · Neurology, Adult, Neuromuscular Disease

Penneys, Neal S. · Dermatology, Clinical Dermatology

Penry, James Kiffin · Neurology, Adult, Epilepsy

Pensak, Myles L. · Otolaryngology, Otology/Neurotology

Pepine, Carl J. · Cardiovascular Disease, Cardiac Catheterization

Perdigao, H. Gunther · Psychiatry, Psychoanalysis

Peretz, David · Psychiatry, Psychoanalysis

Perez, Carlos A. · Radiation Oncology, Breast Cancer; Radiation Oncology, Genito-Urinary Cancer; Radiation Oncology, Gynecologic Cancer; Radiation Oncology, Lung Cancer

Perez, Louis A. · Nuclear Medicine, General Nuclear Medicine

Perkins, Rodney · Otolaryngology, Otology

Perlmutter, Alan D. · Urology, Pediatric Urology

Perot, Phanor L. · Neurological Surgery, Spinal Surgery

Perry, Harold Otto · Dermatology, Clinical Dermatology

Perry, Malcolm O. · General Surgery, General Vascular Surgery

Perry, Samuel W. · Psychiatry, General Psychiatry

Person, Ethel S. · Psychiatry, Psychoanalysis

Peshock, Ronald Michael · Cardiovascular Disease, Magnetic Resonance Imaging

Petajan, Jack H. · Neurology, Adult, Infectious & Demyelinating Diseases

Peter, Georges · Pediatrics, Pediatric Infectious Disease

Peters, Lester J. · Radiation Oncology, Head & Neck Cancer

Peters, William P. · Medical Oncology & Hematology, Bone Marrow Transplantation

Peterson, Bruce A. · Medical Oncology & Hematology, Lymphomas

Peterson, Rex A. · Plastic Surgery, Facial Aesthetic Surgery

Petrek, Jeanne A. · Surgical Oncology, Breast Cancer

Petrie, Roy H. · Obstetrics & Gynecology, Maternal & Fetal Medicine

Petrozza, Patricia H. · Anesthesiology, Neuroanesthesia

Pettigrew, Roderic I. · Nuclear Medicine, Nuclear Cardiology

Petty, Thomas L. · Pulmonary & Critical Care Medicine, Asthma; Pulmonary & Critical Care Medicine, Pulmonary Disease

Pfeffer, Cynthia Roberta · Psychiatry, Child Psychiatry; Psychiatry, Suicidology

Pfefferbaum, Betty · Psychiatry, Child Psychiatry

Phair, John P. · Infectious Disease, AIDS

Phelps, Paulding · Rheumatology, General Rheumatology

Philips, Irving · Psychiatry, Child Psychiatry

Phillips, Gordon L. · Medical Oncology & Hematology, Bone Marrow Transplantation

Phillips, Lawrence H. · Neurology, Adult, Electromyography

Phillips, Peter C. · Medical Oncology & Hematology, Neuro-oncology; Neurology, Child, Neuro-oncology

Phillips, Theodore Locke · Radiation Oncology, Brain Cancer; Radiation Oncology, Gynecologic Cancer; Radiation Oncology, Head & Neck Cancer **Pickar, David** · Psychiatry, Schizophrenia/Psychopharmacology

Pickering, Larry K. · Pediatrics, Pediatric Infectious Disease

Pickoff, Arthur S. · Pediatrics, Pediatric Cardiology

Piepgras, David G. · Neurological Surgery, Vascular Neurological Surgery

Pierce, Alan K. · Pulmonary & Critical Care Medicine, General Pulmonary & Critical Care Medicine

Pierson, David J. · Pulmonary & Critical Care Medicine, General Pulmonary & Critical Care Medicine

Pierson, William E. · Allergy & Immunology, Pediatric Allergy & Immunology

Pildes, Rosita Stephan · Pediatrics, Neonatal-Perinatal Medicine

Pillsbury, Harold C. · Otolaryngology, Head & Neck Surgery; Otolaryngology, Laryngology

Pinals, Robert S. · Rheumatology, General Rheumatology

Pincus, Jonathan L. · Neurology, Adult, Behavioral Neurology

Pincus, Stephanie Hoyer · Dermatology, Genital Dermatological Disease

Pincus, Theodore · Rheumatology, General Rheumatology

Pingleton, Susan K. · Pulmonary & Critical Care Medicine, Asthma; Pulmonary & Critical Care Medicine, Pulmonary Disease

Pinkel, Donald · Pediatrics, Pediatric Hematology-Oncology

Pinkerton, Cass A. · Cardiovascular Disease, Cardiac Catheterization

Pinkus, Geraldine S. · Pathology, Hematopathology

Pinnell, Sheldon R. · Dermatology, Psoriasis

Pinsky, William W. · Pediatrics, Pediatric Cardiology

Pistenmaa, David A. · Radiation Oncology, General Radiation Oncology

Pitkin, Roy M. · Obstetrics & Gynecology, Maternal & Fetal Medicine

Pitman, Gerald H. · Plastic Surgery, Body Contouring; Plastic Surgery, Facial Aesthetic Surgery

Pitt, Henry A. · General Surgery, Gastroenterologic Surgery

Pizzo, Philip A. · Pediatrics, Pediatric Infectious Disease

Pleasure, David E. · Neurology, Adult, Neuromuscular Disease

Plotnick, Leslie P. · Pediatrics, Pediatric Endocrinology

Plum, Fred · Neurology, Adult, General Adult Neurology; Neurology, Adult, Strokes

Podos, Steven M. · Ophthalmology, Glaucoma

Podratz, Karl C. · Obstetrics & Gynecology, Gynecologic Cancer

Pohl, Marc A. · Nephrology, Glomerular Diseases

Pohost, Gerald M. · Cardiovascular Disease, Magnetic Resonance Imaging

Poka, Attila · Orthopaedic Surgery, Trauma

Polan, Mary Lake · Obstetrics & Gynecology, Reproductive Endocrinology

Poland, Warren S. · Psychiatry, Psychoanalysis

Polansky, Kenneth · Endocrinology & Metabolism, Diabetes

Polk, Hiram C. · General Surgery, Gastroenterologic Surgery

Pollack, Irvin P. · Ophthalmology, Glaucoma

Pollack, Murray M. · Pediatrics, Pediatric Critical Care

Pollock, George H. · Psychiatry, Geriatric Psychiatry; Psychiatry, Psychoanalysis

Polmar, Stephen H. · Allergy & Immunology, Pediatric Allergy & Immunology

Pomer, Sydney Lawrence · Psychiatry, Psychoanalysis

Ponsky, Jeffrey L. · General Surgery, Gastroenterologic Surgery

Pontes, J. Edson · Urology, Urologic Oncology

Pope, Richard Mitchell · Rheumatology, General Rheumatology; Rheumatology, Rheumatic Fever

Poplack, David G. · Pediatrics, Pediatric Hematology-Oncology

Popp, Richard L. · Cardiovascular Disease, Echocardiography

Porreco, Richard P. · Obstetrics & Gynecology, Maternal & Fetal Medicine

Port, Friederich K. · Nephrology, Dialysis

Porter, Arthur T. · Radiation Oncology, Genito-Urinary Cancer

Porter, John M. · General Surgery, General Vascular Surgery

Porter, Roger J. · Neurology, Adult, Epilepsy

Portlock, Carol J. · Medical Oncology & Hematology, Lymphomas

Porto, Manuel · Obstetrics & Gynecology, Maternal & Fetal Medicine

Posner, Jerome B. · Neurology, Adult, General Adult Neurology; Neurology, Adult, Neuro-oncology

Posnick, Jeffrey C. · Plastic Surgery, Craniofacial Surgery; Plastic Surgery, Maxillofacial Surgery

Post, Kalmon D. · Neurological Surgery, Tumor Surgery

Post, Robert Morton · Psychiatry, Affective Disorders; Psychiatry, Psychopharmacology

Potsic, William P. · Otolaryngology, Pediatric Otolaryngology

Potter, Donald E. · Pediatrics, Pediatric Nephrology

Potter, Jane F. · Geriatric Medicine, General Geriatric Medicine

Powers, Pauline S. · Psychiatry, Eating Disorders

Powers, William J. · Neurology, Adult, Strokes

Prakash, Udaya B. S. · Pulmonary & Critical Care Medicine, Bronchoesophegology

Prall, Robert Cooley · Psychiatry, Psychoanalysis

Prange, Arthur J. · Psychiatry, Affective Disorders

Pransky, Seth Marc · Otolaryngology, Pediatric Otolaryngology

Pratt-Johnson, John · Ophthalmology, Pediatric Ophthalmology

Preisler, Harvey D. · Medical Oncology, Leukemia

Preminger, Glenn M. · Urology, Endourology

Prensky, Arthur L. · Neurology, Child, General Child Neurology

Present, Daniel H. · Gastroenterology, Inflammatory Bowel Disease

Price, Francis W. · Ophthalmology, Corneal Diseases & Transplantation

Price, Richard W. · Neurology, Adult, Infectious & Demyelinating Diseases

Price, Thomas R. · Neurology, Adult, Strokes

Price, Trevor R. P. · Psychiatry, Neuropsychiatry

Price, Vera H. · Dermatology, Hair

Prinz, Richard A. · General Surgery, Endocrine Surgery

Pritchard, Douglas Jack · Orthopaedic Surgery, Tumor Surgery

Pritchard, Kathleen Isabel · Medical Oncology, Breast Cancer

Prose, Neil S. · Dermatology, Pediatric Dermatology; Pediatrics, Pediatric Dermatology

Prosnitz, Leonard R. · Radiation Oncology, Breast Cancer; Radiation Oncology, Lymphomas

Prough, Donald S. · Anesthesiology, Critical Care Medicine

Provost, Thomas T. · Dermatology, Cutaneous Immunology

Prystowsky, Eric Neal · Cardiovascular Disease, Electrophysiology

Puga, Francisco J. · Thoracic Surgery, Pediatric Cardiac Surgery

Pugatch, Robert D. · Radiology, Chest

Pursch, Joseph A. · Psychiatry, Addiction Medicine

Putnam, Frank W. · Psychiatry, Dissociative Disorders

Putterman, Allen · Ophthalmology, Oculoplastic & Orbital Surgery

Q

Quaegebeur, Jan M. · Thoracic Surgery, Pediatric Cardiac Surgery

Quan, Stuart F. · Pulmonary & Critical Care Medicine, General Pulmonary & Critical Care Medicine

Queenan, John P. · Obstetrics & Gynecology, Maternal & Fetal Medicine

Quencer, Robert M. · Radiology, Neuroradiology

Quest, Donald O. · Neurological Surgery, Vascular Neurological Surgery

Quie, Paul G. · Pediatrics, Pediatric Infectious Disease

Quigley, Harry A. · Ophthalmology, Glaucoma

Quinn, Kathleen May · Psychiatry, Forensic Psychiatry

Quinn, Thomas C. · Infectious Disease, AIDS; Infectious Disease, Sexually Transmitted Diseases

Quinones, Miguel A. · Cardiovascular Disease, Echocardiography

Quirk, J. Gerald · Obstetrics & Gynecology, Maternal & Fetal Medicine

Quitkin, Frederic M. · Psychiatry, Affective Disorders; Psychiatry, Psychopharmacology

R

Raber, Martin Newman · Medical Oncology, Clinical Pharmacology

Rabins, Peter Vincent · Psychiatry, Geriatric Psychiatry

Rachelefsky, Gary S. · Allergy & Immunology, Pediatric Allergy & Immunology

Racz, Gabor B. · Anesthesiology, Pain

Rada, Richard Thomas · Psychiatry, Violence

Radcliffe, Anthony B. · Addiction Medicine, General Addiction Medicine

Raffin, Thomas · Pulmonary & Critical Care Medicine, General Pulmonary & Critical Care Medicine

Raghavan, Derek · Medical Oncology & Hematology, Genito-Urinary Cancer

Ragins, Naomi · Psychiatry, Psychoanalysis

Rai, Kanti R. · Medical Oncology, Leukemia

Raimundo, Hugo S. · Anesthesiology, Pediatric Cardiovascular

Raj, P. Prithvi · Anesthesiology, Pain

Rajfer, Jacob · Urology, Impotence

Ramsay, Colin A. · Dermatology, Clinical Dermatology; Dermatology, Photobiology

Ramsay, Norma K. C. · Pediatrics , Pediatric Hematology-Oncology

Ramsey, Bonnie W. · Pediatrics, Pediatric Pulmonology

Ranawat, Chitranjan S. · Orthopaedic Surgery, Reconstructive Surgery

Rand, James A. · Orthopaedic Surgery, Reconstructive Surgery

Rangell, Leo · Psychiatry, Psychoanalysis

Rankin, J. Scott · Thoracic Surgery, Adult Cardiothoracic Surgery

Ranson, John Hugh C. · General Surgery, Gastroenterologic Surgery

Raphaely, Russell C. · Anesthesiology, Pediatric Anesthesiology; Pediatrics, Pediatric Critical Care

Rapin, Isabelle · Neurology, Child, Child Development

Rapoport, Alan Mark · Neurology, Adult, Headache

Rapoport, Judith L. · Psychiatry, Child Psychiatry; Psychiatry, Psychopharmacology

Rappaport, Henry · Pathology, Hematopathology

Rappeport, Jonas Ralph · Psychiatry, Forensic Psychiatry

Raskin, Neil H. · Neurology, Adult, Headache

Raskin, Philip · Endocrinology & Metabolism, Diabetes

Raskind, Murray A. · Psychiatry, Geriatric Psychiatry

Ratain, Mark Jeffrey · Medical Oncology & Hematology, Clinical Pharmacology

Rauck, Richard L. · Anesthesiology, Pain

Raudzens, Peter A. · Anesthesiology, Neuroanesthesia

Raz, Shlomo · Urology, Neuro-Urology & Voiding Dysfunction

Rea, Thomas H. · Dermatology, Hansen's Disease

Ready, L. Brian · Anesthesiology, Pain

Realmuto, George M. · Psychiatry, Child Psychiatry

Reaman, Gregory H, · Pediatrics, Pediatric Hematology-Oncology

Reba, Richard C. · Nuclear Medicine, General Nuclear Medicine

Rebar, Robert William · Obstetrics & Gynecology, Reproductive Endocrinology

Reber, Howard A. · General Surgery, Gastroenterologic Surgery

Recht, Abram · Radiation Oncology, Breast Cancer

Redding, Gregory J. · Pediatrics, Pediatric Pulmonology

Reece, Robert M. · Pediatrics, Abused Children

Reed, Charles E. · Allergy & Immunology, Adult Allergy & Immunology

Reed, Kathryn L. · Obstetrics & Gynecology, Maternal & Fetal Medicine

Rees, Thomas D. · Plastic Surgery, Aesthetic Surgery; Plastic Surgery, Facial Aesthetic Surgery

Reichek, Nathaniel · Cardiovascular Disease, Echocardiography; Cardiovascular Disease, Magnetic Resonance Imaging

Reichler, Robert Jay · Psychiatry, Child Psychiatry

Reichlin, Seymour · Endocrinology & Metabolism, Neuroendocrinology

Reichman, Lee Brodersohn · Pulmonary & Critical Care Medicine, Lung Infections

Reidenberg, Marcus M. · Clinical Pharmacology

Reifler, Burton V. · Psychiatry, Geriatric Psychiatry

Reilly, James S. · Otolaryngology, Pediatric Otolaryngology

Rein, Michael F. · Infectious Disease, Sexually Transmitted Disease

Reinecke, Robert D. · Ophthalmology, Pediatric Ophthalmology

Reinisch, John F. · Plastic Surgery, Pediatric Plastic Surgery

Reisberg, Barry · Psychiatry, Geriatric Psychiatry

Reisman, Robert E. · Allergy & Immunology, Adult Allergy & Immunology

Reiter, Edward O. · Pediatrics, Pediatric Endocrinology

Reitz, Bruce A. · Thoracic Surgery, Adult Cardiothoracic Surgery; Thoracic Surgery, Transplantation

Rekate, Harold L. · Neurological Surgery, Pediatric Neurological Surgery

Remington, Jack · Infectious Disease, AIDS; Infectious Disease, Toxoplasmosis; Infectious Disease, Transplantation Infections

Renik, Owen Dennis · Psychiatry, Psychoanalysis

Renlund, Dale · Cardiovascular Disease, Heart Transplantation

Rennard, Stephen I. · Pulmonary & Critical Care Medicine, General Pulmonary & Critical Care Medicine

Renowicz, Carolyn D. · Obstetrics & Gynecology, Gynecologic Cancer

Renshaw, Domeena C. · Psychiatry, Sexual Abuse

Resnick, Neil M. · Geriatric Medicine, Urinary Incontinence

Resnick, Phillip J. · Psychiatry, Forensic Psychiatry

Resnick, Richard Boyce · Psychiatry, Addiction Medicine

Resnik, Robert · Obstetrics & Gynecology, Maternal & Fetal Medicine

Retik, Alan B. · Urology, Pediatric Urology

Retzlaff, John A. · Ophthalmology, Anterior Segment (Cataract Surgery)

Reuben, David B. · Geriatric Medicine, General Geriatric Medicine

Reus, Victor I. · Psychiatry, Affective Disorders

Reves, Joseph Gerald · Anesthesiology, Adult Cardiovascular

Reynolds, Charles F. · Psychiatry, Geriatric Psychiatry

Reynolds, Herbert Y. · Pulmonary & Critical Care Medicine, Asthma; Pulmonary & Critical Care Medicine, Pulmonary Disease

Reynolds, James C. · Gastroenterology, Gastrointestinal Motility

Reynolds, Telfer B. · Gastroenterology, Hepatology

Rhame, Frank S. · Infectious Disease, Hospital-Acquired Infections

Rhead, William J. · Pediatrics, Metabolic Diseases

Rhoton, Albert L. · Neurological Surgery, Cranial Nerve Surgery

Ricci, Lawrence R. · Pediatrics, Abused Children

Rice, Dale H. · Otolaryngology, Head & Neck Surgery; Otolaryngology, Sinus & Nasal Surgery

Rice, Thomas A. · Ophthalmology, Vitreo-Retinal Surgery

Rich, Charles Lambert · Psychiatry, Suicidology

Rich, Larry F. · Ophthalmology, Corneal Diseases & Transplantation

Richards, Kent L. · Cardiovascular Disease, Echocardiography

Richardson, Mark A. · Otolaryngology, Pediatric Otolaryngology

Richardson, Ronald Lee · Medical Oncology & Hematology, Genito-Urinary Cancer

Richerson, Hal B. · Allergy & Immunology, Adult Allergy & Immunology

Richie, Jerome P. · Urology, Urologic Oncology

Richman, Douglas D. · Infectious Disease, AIDS

Richtsmeier, William J. · Otolaryngology, Head & Neck Surgery

Riddick, Daniel H. · Obstetrics & Gynecology, Reproductive Endocrinology

Riddle, Matthew C. · Endocrinology & Metabolism, Diabetes

Ridgway, E. C. · Endocrinology & Metabolism, Neuroendocrinology; Endocrinology & Metabolism, Thyroid

Rietschel, Robert L. · Dermatology, Contact Dermatitis; Dermatology, Hair

Rifkin, Harold · Endocrinology & Metabolism, Diabetes

Rikkers, Layton F. · General Surgery, Gastroenterologic Surgery

Riles, Thomas S. · General Surgery, General Vascular Surgery

Ringel, Steven P. · Neurology, Adult, Neuro Rehabilitation; Neurology, Adult, Neuromuscular Disease

Ristow, Bruno · Plastic Surgery, Facial Aesthetic Surgery

Ritchie, J. W. Knox · Obstetrics & Gynecology, Maternal & Fetal Medicine

Ritchie, James L. · Cardiovascular Disease, Nuclear Cardiology

Ritchie, Wallace P. · General Surgery, Gastroenterologic Surgery

Ritter, Frank N. · Otolaryngology, Sinus & Nasal Surgery

Ritter, Samuel Beryl · Pediatrics, Pediatric Cardiology

Ritvo, Edward R. · Psychiatry, Autism; Psychiatry, Child Psychiatry

Ritvo, Samuel · Psychiatry, Child Psychiatry; Psychiatry, Psychoanalysis

Rivera, Gaston K. · Pediatrics, Pediatric Hematology-Oncology

Rizza, Robert A. · Endocrinology & Metabolism, Diabetes

Rizzuto, Ana-Maria · Psychiatry, Psychoanalysis

Robbins, Laurence J. · Geriatric Medicine, General Geriatric Medicine

Robert, Nichoas J. · Medical Oncology & Hematology, Breast Cancer

Robertson, Dennis M. · Ophthalmology, Medical Retinal Diseases; Ophthalmology, Vitreo-Retinal Surgery

Robertson, James T. · Neurological Surgery, Tumor Surgery; Neurological Surgery, Vascular Neurological Surgery

Robertson, R. Paul · Endocrinology & Metabolism, Diabetes

Robinson, Alan G. · Endocrinology & Metabolism, Neuroendocrinology

Robinson, Bruce Eugene · Geriatric Medicine, General Geriatric Medicine

Robinson, James · Psychiatry, Psychoanalysis

Robinson, June · Dermatology, Skin Cancer Surgery & Reconstruction

Robinson, Ralph G. · Nuclear Medicine, General Nuclear Medicine; Nuclear Medicine, Nuclear Cardiology

Robinson, Robert G. · Psychiatry, Affective Disorders; Psychiatry, Neuropsychiatry

Robson, Martin C. · Plastic Surgery, Reconstructive Surgery

Robson, Martin C. · Plastic Surgery, Wound Healing

Rocchini, Albert P. · Pediatrics, Pediatric Cardiology

Rock, John A. · Obstetrics & Gynecology, Pediatric & Adolescent Gynecology; Obstetrics & Gynecology, Reproductive Endocrinology; Obstetrics & Gynecology, Reproductive Surgery

Rockoff, Mark A. · Anesthesiology, Pediatric Anesthesiology

Rockwood, Charles A. · Orthopaedic Surgery, Reconstructive Surgery

Rodgers, Bradley Moreland · General Surgery, Pediatric Surgery

Rodman, F. Robert · Psychiatry, Psychoanalysis

Rodriguez, Moses · Neurology, Adult, Infectious & Demyelinating Diseases

Rogers, Arvey I. · Gastroenterology, Inflammatory Bowel Disease

Rogers, Mark C. · Anesthesiology, Pediatric Anesthesiology; Pediatrics, Pediatric Critical Care

Rogers, Robert M. · Pulmonary & Critical Care Medicine, Asthma; Pulmonary & Critical Care Medicine, Pulmonary Disease

Rogers, Roy S. · Dermatology, Mucous Membrane Diseases

Rogol, Alan D. · Pediatrics, Pediatric Endocrinology

Roh, Mark S. · Surgical Oncology, Gastroenterologic Cancer

Roizen, Michael F. · Anesthesiology, Adult Cardiovascular

Romero, Roberto · Obstetrics & Gynecology, Maternal & Fetal Medicine

Ronald, Allan · Infectious Disease, Sexually Transmitted Disease

Roos, David B. · General Surgery, General Vascular Surgery

Root, Allen W. · Pediatrics, Pediatric Endocrinology

Rootman, Jack · Ophthalmology, Oculoplastic & Orbital Surgery

Ropper, Allan H. · Neurology, Adult, Critical Care Medicine

Rorke, Lucy B. · Pathology, Neuropathology

Rosai, Juan · Pathology, Surgical Pathology

Rosato, Ernest F. · General Surgery, Gastroenterologic Surgery

Rose, Eric A. · Thoracic Surgery, Adult Cardiothoracic Surgery; Thoracic Surgery, Transplantation

Rosen, Fred · Allergy & Immunology, Pediatric Allergy & Immunology

Rosen, Irving B. · General Surgery, Endocrine Surgery

Rosen, Mortimer G. · Obstetrics & Gynecology, Maternal & Fetal Medicine

Rosen, Paul Peter · Pathology, Breast Pathology

Rosenbaum, Arthur L. · Ophthalmology, Pediatric Ophthalmology

Rosenbaum, Arthur Louis · Psychiatry, Psychoanalysis

Rosenbaum, Gerald F. · Psychiatry, Affective Disorders; Psychiatry, Psychopharmacology

Rosenbaum, James T. · Rheumatology, Uveitis

Rosenberg, Roger N. · Neurology, Adult, Neurogenetics

Rosenberg, Saul A. · Medical Oncology & Hematology, Hematological Malignancies; Medical Oncology & Hematology, Lymphomas

Rosenberg, Steven A. · Medical Oncology & Hematology, Immunotherapy, Biological Response Modifiers Oncology

Rosenberg, Thomas D. · Orthopaedic Surgery, Sports Medicine

Rosenblatt, Allan D. · Psychiatry, Psychoanalysis

Rosenbloom, Arlen L. · Pediatrics, Pediatric Endocrinology

Rosenfeld, Ron G. · Pediatrics, Pediatric Endocrinology

Rosenfeld, Stephen I. · Allergy & Immunology, Adult Allergy & Immunology

Rosenfield, Robert L. · Pediatrics, Pediatric Endocrinology

Rosenow, Edward C. · Pulmonary & Critical Care Medicine, General Pulmonary & Critical Care Medicine

Rosenshein, Neil B. · Obstetrics & Gynecology, Gynecologic Cancer

Rosenstein, Beryl J. · Pediatrics, Pediatric Pulmonology

Rosenthal, Amnon · Pediatrics, Pediatric Cardiology

Rosenthal, Myer H. · Anesthesiology, Critical Care Medicine

Rosenwaks, Zev · Obstetrics & Gynecology, Reproductive Endocrinology

Rosenwasser, Lanny J. · Allergy & Immunology, Adult Allergy & Immunology

Roslyn, Joel · General Surgery, Gastroenterologic Surgery

Ross, Colin A. · Psychiatry, Dissociative Disorders

Ross, Douglas S. · Endocrinology & Metabolism, Thyroid

Roth, Jack A. · Thoracic Surgery, General Thoracic Surgery; Thoracic Surgery, Thoracic Oncological Surgery

Roth, Loren H. · Psychiatry, Forensic Psychiatry; Psychiatry, Violence

Rothenberg, Michael B. · Psychiatry, Child Psychiatry

Rothenberger, David A. · Colon & Rectal Surgery, General Colon & Rectal Surgery

Rothman, Richard H. · Orthopaedic Surgery, Reconstructive Surgery

Rothstein, Arnold · Psychiatry, General Psychiatry

Rothstein, Arnold Morton · Psychiatry, Psychoanalysis

Rotman, Marvin · Radiation Oncology, Gynecologic Cancer

Roubin, Gary S. · Cardiovascular Disease, Cardiac Catheterization

Roughton, Ralph Emerson · Psychiatry, Psychoanalysis

Rounsaville, Bruce J. · Psychiatry, Addiction Medicine

Rowe, Marc I. · General Surgery, Pediatric Surgery

Rowland, Lewis P. · Neurology, Adult, Neuromuscular Disease

Rowsey, J. James · Ophthalmology, Corneal Diseases & Transplantation

Roy, Alec · Psychiatry, Suicidology

Roy, Claude C. · Pediatrics, Pediatric Gastroenterology

Roy-Byrne, Peter P. · Psychiatry, Affective Disorders

Royal, Henry D. · Nuclear Medicine, Radiation Accidents

Rozanski, Alan · Cardiovascular Disease, Nuclear Cardiology; Nuclear Medicine, Nuclear Cardiology

Ruben, Robert J. · Otolaryngology, Pediatric Otolaryngology

Rubenstein, Arthur H. · Endocrinology & Metabolism, Diabetes

Rubenstein, Laurence Z. · Geriatric Medicine, General Geriatric Medicine

Rubin, Joseph E. V. · Psychiatry, Geriatric Psychiatry

Rubin, Robert H. · Infectious Disease, Transplantation Infections

Rubinstein, Arye · Allergy & Immunology, Pediatric Allergy & Immunology

Ruckdeschel, John C. · Medical Oncology & Hematology, Lung Cancer

Ruderman, Mark · Rheumatology, General Rheumatology

Rudick, Richard A. · Neurology, Adult, Infectious & Demyelinating Diseases

Rudolph, Abraham M. · Pediatrics, Pediatric Cardiology

Ruedrich, Stephen L. · Psychiatry, Mental Retardation/Mental Health: Dual Diagnosis

Ruley, Edward Jerome · Pediatrics, Pediatric Nephrology

Rusch, Valerie W. · Thoracic Surgery, General Thoracic Surgery

Rush, A. John · Psychiatry, Affective Disorders; Psychiatry, Psychopharmacology

Rushton, Harry Guilford (Gil) · Urology, Pediatric Urology

Ruskin, Jeremy N. · Cardiovascular Disease, Electrophysiology

Russell, James A. · Pulmonary & Critical Care Medicine, General Pulmonary & Critical Care Medicine

Russell, Thomas A. · Orthopaedic Surgery, Trauma

Rutherford, Robert B. · General Surgery, General Vascular Surgery

Rutsky, Edwin A. · Nephrology, Dialysis

Ryan, James Joseph · Plastic Surgery, Breast Surgery

Ryan, Kenneth J. · Obstetrics & Gynecology, Reproductive Endocrinology

Ryan, Stephen J. · Ophthalmology, Vitreo-Retinal Surgery

Ryan, Thomas F. · Cardiovascular Disease, General Cardiovascular Disease

S

Sabin, Thomas Daniel · Neurology, Adult, General Adult Neurology

Sachar, David B. · Gastroenterology, Inflammatory Bowel Disease

Sachs, David Morton · Psychiatry, Psychoanalysis

Sadavoy, Joel · Psychiatry, Geriatric Psychiatry

Sade, Robert M. · Thoracic Surgery, Pediatric Cardiac Surgery

Sadoff, Robert Leslie · Psychiatry, Forensic Psychiatry; Psychiatry, Violence

Saenger, Paul · Pediatrics, Pediatric Endocrinology

Sagel, Stuart S. · Radiology, Chest

Sagerman, Robert H. · Radiation Oncology, General Radiation Oncology

Sahn, David J. · Pediatrics, Pediatric Cardiology

Sahn, Steven Alan · Pulmonary & Critical Care Medicine, General Pulmonary & Critical Care Medicine

Saidman, Lawrence J. · Anesthesiology, General Anesthesiology

Sakauye, Kenneth M. · Psychiatry, Geriatric Psychiatry

Salant, David J. · Nephrology, Glomerular Diseases

Salasche, Stuart J. · Dermatology, Skin Cancer Surgery & Reconstruction

Sallan, Stephen E. · Pediatrics, Pediatric Hematology-Oncology

Salmon, Sydney · Medical Oncology & Hematology, Myeloma

Salter, Robert B. · Orthopaedic Surgery, Pediatric Orthopaedic Surgery

Salusky, Isidro B. · Pediatrics, Pediatric Nephrology

Salvaggio, John E. · Allergy & Immunology, Adult Allergy & Immunology

Salvati, Eduardo A. · Orthopaedic Surgery, Hip Surgery

Salvatierra, Oscar · Urology, Transplantation

Salyer, Kenneth Everett · Plastic Surgery, Craniofacial Surgery; Plastic Surgery, Reconstructive Surgery

Salzman, Carl · Psychiatry, Psychopharmacology

Sampson, Hugh A. · Allergy & Immunology, Pediatric Allergy & Immunology

Sams, W. Mitchell · Dermatology, Cutaneous Immunology

Samuels, Martin A. · Neurology, Adult, General Adult Neurology

Sande, Merle A. · Infectious Disease, AIDS; Infectious Disease, Endocarditis

Sanders, Charles V. · Infectious Disease, General Infectious Disease

Sanders, Donald B. · Neurology, Adult, Electromyography; Neurology, Adult, Neuromuscular Disease

Sanders, Jean E. · Pediatrics, Pediatric Hematology-Oncology

Sanders, Richard J. · General Surgery, General Vascular Surgery

Sanders, Roy W. · Orthopaedic Surgery, Trauma

Sanders, Stephen P. · Pediatrics, Pediatric Cardiology

Sanderson, David R. · Pulmonary & Critical Care Medicine, Bronchoesophegology

Sandok, Burton A. · Neurology, Adult, General Adult Neurology

Sanfilippo, Joseph S. · Obstetrics & Gynecology, Pediatric & Adolescent Gynecology

Sanford, Robert Alex · Neurological Surgery, Pediatric Neurological Surgery

Santana, Victor M. · Pediatrics, Pediatric Hematology-Oncology

Santiago, Julio V. · Pediatrics, Pediatric Endocrinology

Saper, Joel R. · Neurology, Adult, Headache

Saravolatz, Louis D. · Infectious Disease, Hospital-Acquired Infections

Sarles, Richard M. · Psychiatry, Child Psychiatry

Sarna, Gregory P. · Medical Oncology & Hematology, Hematological Malignancies

Sarr, Michael G. · General Surgery, Gastroenterologic Surgery

Sasaki, Clarence T. · Otolaryngology, Laryngology

Sataloff, Robert Thayer · Otolaryngology, Laryngology

Satlin, Andrew · Psychiatry, Geriatric Psychiatry

Sauder, Daniel N. · Dermatology, Clinical Dermatology

Savin, Ronald C. · Dermatology, Hair

Savino, Peter J. · Neurology, Adult, Neuro-Ophthalmology; Ophthalmology, Neuro-Ophthalmology

Saxon, Andrew · Allergy & Immunology, Adult Allergy & Immunology

Scanlon, Patrick J. · Cardiovascular Disease, Cardiac Catheterization

Scardino, Peter T. · Urology, Urologic Oncology

Schachat, Andrew P. · Ophthalmology, Medical Retinal Diseases

Schachner, Lawrence · Dermatology, Pediatric Dermatology; Pediatrics, Pediatric Dermatology

Schachter, Judith S. · Psychiatry, Psychoanalysis

Schade, David S. · Endocrinology & Metabolism, Diabetes

Schaefer, Steven · Otolaryngology, Sinus & Nasal Surgery

Schaeffer, Anthony J. · Urology, Urological Infections

Schaff, Hartzell V. · Thoracic Surgery, Adult Cardiothoracic Surgery

Schaffner, William · Infectious Disease, Hospital-Acquired Infections

Schanzlin, David J. · Ophthalmology, Corneal Diseases & Transplantation

Schapiro, Randall T. · Neurology, Adult, Infectious & Demyelinating Diseases

Schapiro, Robert H. · Gastroenterology, Endoscopy

Scharfman, Melvin A. · Psychiatry, Psychoanalysis

Schatz, Howard · Ophthalmology, Medical Retinal Diseases

Schatz, Michael · Allergy & Immunology, Adult Allergy & Immunology

Schatz, Norman · Ophthalmology, Neuro-Ophthalmology

Schatzberg, Alan F. · Psychiatry, Affective Disorders; Psychiatry, General Psychiatry; Psychiatry, Psychopharmacology

Schatzker, Joseph · Orthopaedic Surgery, Trauma

Schaumburg, Herbert H. · Neurology, Adult, Neuromuscular Disease

Schechter, Gary L. · Otolaryngology, Head & Neck Surgery

Scheckler, William E. · Infectious Disease, Hospital-Acquired Infections

Schecter, Gisela F. · Pulmonary & Critical Care Medicine, Lung Infections

Scheiman, Melvin M. · Cardiovascular Disease, Electrophysiology

Scheinberg, Labe C. · Neurology, Adult, Infectious & Demyelinating Diseases

Scheithauer, Bernd W. · Pathology, Neuropathology

Schelbert, Heinrich R. · Nuclear Medicine, Nuclear Cardiology

Scheld, W. Michael · Infectious Disease, General Infectious Disease

Schellhammer, Paul F. · Urology, Urologic Oncology

Scher, Howard Isador · Medical Oncology & Hematology, Genito-Urinary Cancer

Schetky, Diane H. · Psychiatry, Child Abuse; Psychiatry, Child Psychiatry

Schidlow, Daniel V. · Pediatrics, Pediatric Pulmonology

Schiff, Eugene R. · Gastroenterology, Hepatology

Schiffer, Charles A. · Medical Oncology, Leukemia

Schiffer, Randolph B. · Psychiatry, Neuropsychiatry

Schild, Joyce A. · Otolaryngology, Laryngology

Schiller, Lawrence · Gastroenterology, Gastrointestinal Motility

Schiller, Nelson B. · Cardiovascular Disease, Echocardiography

Schilsky, Richard L. · Medical Oncology & Hematology, Clinical Pharmacology

Schlant, Robert C. · Cardiovascular Disease, Heart Failure

Schmidt, Cecilia L. · Obstetrics & Gynecology, Reproductive Endocrinology

Schneider, Lawrence H. · Hand Surgery, General Hand Surgery

Schneider, Max A. · Addiction Medicine, General Addiction Medicine

Schneider, Sanford · Neurology, Child, General Child Neurology

Schnitt, Stuart J. · Pathology, Breast Pathology

Schnoll, Sidney H. · Addiction Medicine, Addicted Pregnant Women

Schoetz, David J. · Colon & Rectal Surgery, General Colon & Rectal Surgery

Schold, S. Clifford · Medical Oncology & Hematology, Neuro-oncology; Neurology, Adult, Neuro-oncology

Scholz, Peter M. · Thoracic Surgery, Adult Cardiothoracic Surgery

Schooley, Robert T. · Infectious Disease, Virology

Schorr, William F. · Dermatology, Contact Dermatitis

Schowalter, John E. · Psychiatry, Child Psychiatry

Schramm, Victor L. · Otolaryngology, Head & Neck Surgery

Schreiber, James R. · Obstetrics & Gynecology, Reproductive Endocrinology

Schrier, Robert W. · Nephrology, General Nephrology

Schrock, Theodore R. · Colon & Rectal Surgery, General Colon & Rectal Surgery

Schroeder, John S. · Cardiovascular Disease, General Cardiovascular Disease

Schuckit, Marc Alan · Psychiatry, Addiction Medicine

Schuh, Sara Elizabeth · Pediatrics, Abused Children

Schuller, David E. · Otolaryngology, Facial Plastic Surgery; Otolaryngology, Head & Neck Surgery; Otolaryngology, Laryngology

Schulz, Charles S. · Psychiatry, Schizophrenia/Psychopharmacology

Schumacher, H. Ralph · Rheumatology, General Rheumatology

Schuster, Marvin M. · Gastroenterology, Gastrointestinal Motility

Schut, Luis · Neurological Surgery, Pediatric Neurological Surgery

Schwaber, Evelyne Albrecht · Psychiatry, Psychoanalysis

Schwaber, Mitchell K. · Otolaryngology, Otology/Neurotology

Schwade, James G. · Radiation Oncology, General Radiation Oncology

Schwaiger, Markus · Nuclear Medicine, Nuclear Cardiology

Schwartz, Gordon F. · Surgical Oncology, Breast Cancer

Schwartz, Howard J. · Allergy & Immunology, Adult Allergy & Immunology

Schwartz, Lawrence H. · Psychiatry, Psychoanalysis

Schwartz, Lester · Psychiatry, Psychoanalysis

Schwartz, Peter E. · Obstetrics & Gynecology, Gynecologic Cancer

Schwartz, Robert H. · Allergy & Immunology, Pediatric Allergy & Immunology; Pediatrics, Pediatric Allergy & Immunology

Schwartz, Robert S. · Geriatric Medicine, General Geriatric Medicine

Schwarz, I. Gene · Psychiatry, Psychoanalysis

Schwarz, Marvin I. · Pulmonary & Critical Care Medicine, Pulmonary Disease

Schwenn, Molly · Pediatrics, Pediatric Hematology-Oncology

Scommegna, Antonio · Obstetrics & Gynecology, Reproductive Endocrinology

Scott, Alan B. · Ophthalmology, Pediatric Ophthalmology

Scott, Gwendolyn B. · Pediatrics, Pediatric Infectious Disease

Scott, R. Michael · Neurological Surgery, Pediatric Neurological Surgery

Scott, Richard David · Orthopaedic Surgery, Reconstructive Surgery

Scott, W. Norman · Orthopaedic Surgery, Sports Medicine

Scott, William E. · Ophthalmology, Pediatric Ophthalmology

Scully, Robert E. · Pathology, Gynecologic Pathology

Sedman, Aileen B. · Pediatrics, Pediatric Nephrology

Seeds, John · Obstetrics & Gynecology, Maternal & Fetal Medicine

Segura, Joseph W. · Urology, Endourology

Seibold, James Richard · Rheumatology, Scleroderma

Seid, Allan B. · Otolaryngology, Pediatric Otolaryngology

Seiden, Anne Maxwell · Psychiatry, Addiction Medicine

Seigelman, Stanley S. · Radiology, Chest

Sekhar, Laligam N. · Neurological Surgery, Tumor Surgery

Selcow, Jay E. · Allergy & Immunology, Pediatric Allergy & Immunology; Pediatrics, Pediatric Allergy & Immunology

Selhorst, John B. · Neurology, Adult, Neuro-Ophthalmology

Sellers, Edward M. · Addiction Medicine, Medical Treatment of Drug Abusers

Selner, John C. · Allergy & Immunology, Adult Allergy & Immunology

Senay, Edward C. · Psychiatry, Addiction Medicine

Sergent, John S. · Rheumatology, General Rheumatology

Sergott, Robert C. · Ophthalmology, Neuro-Ophthalmology

Service, F. John · Endocrinology & Metabolism, Diabetes

Sessions, Roy B. · Otolaryngology, Head & Neck Surgery; Otolaryngology, Laryngology

Settlage, Calvin F. · Psychiatry, Child Psychiatry; Psychiatry, Psychoanalysis

Sever, John L. · Pediatrics, Pediatric Infectious Disease

Seward, James Bernard · Cardiovascular Disease, Echocardiography

Seyfer, Alan E. · Hand Surgery, Reconstructive Surgery; Plastic Surgery, Reconstructive Surgery

Shader, Richard I. · Psychiatry, Psychopharmacology

Shaffer, David · Psychiatry, Child Psychiatry; Psychiatry, Suicidology

Shalita, Alan R. · Dermatology, Acne

Shamoian, Charles A. · Psychiatry, Geriatric Psychiatry

Shamoon, Harry · Endocrinology & Metabolism, Diabetes

Shapiro, Barry A. · Anesthesiology, Critical Care Medicine

Shapiro, Gail Greenberg · Allergy & Immunology, Pediatric Allergy & Immunology

Shapiro, Louis B. · Psychiatry, Psychoanalysis

Shapiro, Theodore · Psychiatry, Child Psychiatry

Shapiro, William R. · Medical Oncology & Hematology, Neuro-oncology; Neurology, Adult, Neuro-oncology

Shapshay, Stanley M. · Otolaryngology, Laryngology

Sharma, Om P. · Pulmonary & Critical Care Medicine, Pulmonary Disease

Sharpe, James A. · Neurology, Adult, Neuro-Ophthalmology

Sharrock, Nigel E. · Anesthesiology, Orthopaedic Procedures

Shaw, Byers W. · General Surgery, Transplantation

Shea, M. Coyle · Otolaryngology, Otology

Shearer, William Thomas · Allergy & Immunology, Pediatric Allergy & Immunology

Shearing, Steven P. · Ophthalmology, Anterior Segment (Cataract Surgery)

Sheehan, David V. · Psychiatry, Affective Disorders; Psychiatry, Psychopharmacology

Sheehy, James L. · Otolaryngology, Otology

Sheen, Jack H. · Plastic Surgery, Facial Aesthetic Surgery

Sheets, John H. · Ophthalmology, Anterior Segment (Cataract Surgery)

Sheffer, Albert L. · Allergy & Immunology, Adult Allergy & Immunology

Sheftell, Fred D. · Psychiatry, Headache

Shelley, Walter B. · Dermatology, Clinical Dermatology

Shengold, Leonard L. · Psychiatry, Psychoanalysis

Shepherd, John R. · Ophthalmology, Anterior Segment (Cataract Surgery)

Sheppard, Dean · Pulmonary & Critical Care Medicine, Asthma

Sherman, David · Neurology, Adult, Strokes

Sherman, Fredrick Todd · Geriatric Medicine, General Geriatric Medicine

Sherrill, Kimberly A. · Psychiatry, Geriatric Psychiatry

Sherwin, Robert S. · Endocrinology & Metabolism, Diabetes

Shields, Jerry A. · Ophthalmology, Medical Retinal Diseases; Ophthalmology, Ocular Oncology

Shields, M. Bruce · Ophthalmology, Glaucoma

Shingleton, Hugh M. · Obstetrics & Gynecology, Gynecologic Cancer

Shipley, William U. · Radiation Oncology, Genito-Urinary Cancer

Shnider, Sol M. · Anesthesiology, Obstetric Anesthesia

Shopper, Moisy · Psychiatry, Psychoanalysis

Shore, John W. · Ophthalmology, Oculoplastic & Orbital Surgery

Shorr, Norman · Ophthalmology, Oculoplastic & Orbital Surgery

Shortliffe, Linda M. D. · Urology, Pediatric Urology

Shoulson, Ira · Neurology, Adult, Movement Disorders

Shucart, William · Neurological Surgery, General Neurological Surgery

Shults, William Thomas · Ophthalmology, Neuro-Ophthalmology

Shumway, Norman E. · Thoracic Surgery, Adult Cardiothoracic Surgery; Thoracic Surgery, Transplantation

Shure, Deborah · Pulmonary & Critical Care Medicine, General Pulmonary & Critical Care Medicine

Sibley, William A. · Neurology, Adult, Infectious & Demyelinating Diseases

Sicard, Gregorio A. · General Surgery, General Vascular Surgery

Siegal, Alan P. · Psychiatry, Geriatric Psychiatry

Siegel, Barry A. · Nuclear Medicine, General Nuclear Medicine

Siegel, Norman · Pediatrics, Pediatric Nephrology

Siegel, Sheldon C. · Allergy & Immunology, Pediatric Allergy & Immunology

Siggins, Lorraine D. · Psychiatry, Psychoanalysis

Silber, Austin · Psychiatry, Psychoanalysis

Silberstein, Edward B. · Nuclear Medicine, General Nuclear Medicine

Silberstein, Stephen David · Neurology, Adult, Headache

Silen, William · General Surgery, Gastroenterologic Surgery

Silver, Jonathan M. · Psychiatry, Neuropsychiatry; Psychiatry, Violence

Silverman, Arnold · Pediatrics, Pediatric Gastroenterology

Silverman, Martin A. · Psychiatry, Psychoanalysis

Silverman, Norman H. · Pediatrics, Pediatric Cardiology

Silverstein, Fred E. · Gastroenterology, Endoscopy

Silverstein, Herbert · Otolaryngology, Otology/Neurotology

Silverstein, Janet · Pediatrics, Pediatric Endocrinology

Sim, Franklin H. · Orthopaedic Surgery, Tumor Surgery

Simmons, Richard · Ophthalmology, Glaucoma

Simmons, Richard L. · General Surgery, Transplantation

Simon, Michael A. · Orthopaedic Surgery, Tumor Surgery

Simons, Frances Estelle Reed · Pediatrics, Pediatric Allergy & Immunology

Simons, Richard C. · Psychiatry, Psychoanalysis

Simpson, George M. · Psychiatry, Schizophrenia/Psychopharmacology

Simpson, Joe Leigh · Obstetrics & Gynecology, Genetics

Simpson, John B. · Cardiovascular Disease, Cardiac Catheterization

Sinaiko, Alan R. · Pediatrics, Pediatric Nephrology

Singer, Frederick R. · Endocrinology & Metabolism, Paget's Disease

Singer, Mark I. · Otolaryngology, Laryngology

Singer, Peter A. · Endocrinology & Metabolism, Thyroid

Singerman, Lawrence J. · Ophthalmology, Medical Retinal Diseases

Singleton, George Terrell · Otolaryngology, Otology

Sinskey, Robert · Ophthalmology, Anterior Segment (Cataract Surgery)

Siris, Ethel Silverman · Endocrinology & Metabolism, Paget's Disease

Sivak, Michael V. · Gastroenterology, Endoscopy

Skinner, David B. · Thoracic Surgery, General Thoracic Surgery; Thoracic Surgery, Thoracic Oncological Surgery

Skinner, Donald G. · Urology, Urologic Oncology

Skorton, David J. · Cardiovascular Disease, Echocardiography

Skyler, Jay S. · Endocrinology & Metabolism, Diabetes

Slaby, Andrew Edmund · Psychiatry, Suicidology

Sladen, Robert N. · Anesthesiology, Critical Care Medicine

Slater, James M. · Radiation Oncology, Particle Beam Radiation

Slavin, Raymond G. · Allergy & Immunology, Adult Allergy & Immunology

Slavney, Philip R. · Psychiatry, Personality Disorder

Sledge, Clement Blount · Orthopaedic Surgery, Reconstructive Surgery

Sloane, Philip D. · Geriatric Medicine, General Geriatric Medicine

Slogoff, Stephen · Anesthesiology, Adult Cardiovascular

Sly, R. Michael · Allergy & Immunology, Pediatric Allergy & Immunology

Small, Gary W. · Psychiatry, Geriatric Psychiatry

Smith, Arnold L. · Pediatrics, Pediatric Infectious Disease

Smith, Arthur D. · Urology, Endourology

Smith, David E. · Addiction Medicine, General Addiction Medicine

Smith, David John · Hand Surgery, Reconstructive Surgery; Plastic Surgery, Reconstructive Surgery

Smith, Hugh · Cardiovascular Disease, General Cardiovascular Disease

Smith, J. Lawton · Neurology, Adult, Neuro-Ophthalmology; Ophthalmology, Neuro-Ophthalmology

Smith, James P. · Pulmonary & Critical Care Medicine, General Pulmonary & Critical Care Medicine

Smith, Joseph A. · Urology, Urologic Oncology

Smith, Lee E. · Colon & Rectal Surgery, Colon & Rectal Cancer; Colon & Rectal Surgery, General Colon & Rectal Surgery

Smith, Mansfield F. W. · Otolaryngology, Otology/Neurotology

Smith, Peter G. · Otolaryngology, Otology/Neurotology; Otolaryngology, Skull-Base Surgery

Smith, Ronald E. · Ophthalmology, Corneal Diseases & Transplantation; Ophthalmology, Uveitis

Smith, Thomas J. · Surgical Oncology, Breast Cancer

Smythe, Hugh A. · Rheumatology, Fibromyalgia

Snape, William J. · Gastroenterology, Gastrointestinal Motility

Snead, O. Carter · Neurology, Child, Epilepsy

Snider, A. Rebecca · Pediatrics, Pediatric Cardiology

Snider, Gordon L. · Pulmonary & Critical Care Medicine, Asthma; Pulmonary & Critical Care Medicine, Lung Infections; Pulmonary & Critical Care Medicine, Pulmonary Disease

Snyder, Howard McC. · Urology, Pediatric Urology

Snyder, Peter Joseph · Endocrinology & Metabolism, Neuroendocrinology

Sobel, Jack D. · Infectious Disease, Sexually Transmitted Disease

Socol, Michael L. · Obstetrics & Gynecology, Maternal & Fetal Medicine

Sokol, Robert J. · Addiction Medicine, Addicted Pregnant Women; Obstetrics & Gynecology, Maternal & Fetal Medicine

Solin, Lawrence J. · Radiation Oncology, Breast Cancer

Sollinger, Hans W. · General Surgery, Transplantation

Solnit, Albert J. · Psychiatry, Child Psychiatry; Psychiatry, Psychoanalysis

Solomon, Lawrence M. · Dermatology, Pediatric Dermatology; Pediatrics, Pediatric Dermatology

Solomon, Rebecca Z. · Psychiatry, Psychoanalysis

Solomon, Seymour · Neurology, Adult, Headache

Solomon, William R. · Allergy & Immunology, Adult Allergy & Immunology

Soloway, Mark S. · Urology, Urologic Oncology

Sonnenblick, Edmond H. · Cardiovascular Disease, Heart Failure

Sonntag, Volker K. H. · Neurological Surgery, Spinal Surgery

Sontheimer, Richard D. · Dermatology, Cutaneous Immunology

Soper, David E. · Obstetrics & Gynecology, Infectious Disease

Soper, Nathaniel J. · General Surgery, Gastroenterologic Surgery

Sorensen, Ricardo U. · Pediatrics, Pediatric Allergy & Immunology

Sorkin, Michael I. · Nephrology, Dialysis

Sorrell, Michael F. · Gastroenterology, Hepatology

Soter, Nicholas Arthur · Dermatology, Clinical Dermatology; Dermatology, Photobiology

Sotos, Juan F. · Pediatrics, Pediatric Endocrinology

Souba, Wiley W. · Surgical Oncology, Gastroenterologic Cancer

Soules, Michael Roy · Obstetrics & Gynecology, Reproductive Endocrinology

Sovner, Robert · Psychiatry, Mental Retardation/Mental Health: Dual Diagnosis

Spaeth, George L. · Ophthalmology, Glaucoma

Spear, Scott L. · Plastic Surgery, Breast Surgery

Spector, Sheldon L. · Allergy & Immunology, Adult Allergy & Immunology

Spellacy, William N. · Obstetrics & Gynecology, Maternal & Fetal Medicine

Spencer, Dennis · Neurological Surgery, Epilepsy Surgery

Spencer, Frank Cole · Thoracic Surgery, Adult Cardiothoracic Surgery

Sperling, Mark A. · Pediatrics, Pediatric Endocrinology

Speroff, Leon · Obstetrics & Gynecology, Reproductive Endocrinology

Spetzler, Robert F. · Neurological Surgery, Vascular Neurological Surgery

Spiegel, David · Psychiatry, Dissociative Disorders

Spies, Stewart M. · Nuclear Medicine, General Nuclear Medicine

Spinner, Morton · Hand Surgery, Peripheral Nerve Surgery; Orthopaedic Surgery, Peripheral Nerve Surgery

Spraker, Mary K. · Dermatology, Pediatric Dermatology; Pediatrics, Pediatric Dermatology

Spray, Thomas L. · Thoracic Surgery, Pediatric Cardiac Surgery

Spriggs, David R. · Medical Oncology & Hematology, Clinical Pharmacology

Springfield, Dempsey S. · Orthopaedic Surgery, Tumor Surgery

Spruiell, Vann · Psychiatry, Psychoanalysis

Stack, Richard S. · Cardiovascular Disease, Cardiac Catheterization

Stager, David R. · Ophthalmology, Pediatric Ophthalmology

Staheli, Lynn T. · Orthopaedic Surgery, Pediatric Orthopaedic Surgery

Stamey, Thomas · Urology, Urologic Oncology

Stamm, Walter E. · Infectious Disease, Sexually Transmitted Disease

Stamper, Robert L. · Ophthalmology, Glaucoma

Stanger, Paul · Pediatrics, Pediatric Cardiology

Stanley, Charles · Pediatrics, Metabolic Diseases

Stanley, James C. · General Surgery, General Vascular Surgery

Stanley, John Roger · Dermatology, Cutaneous Immunology

Stapleton, F. Bruder · Pediatrics, Pediatric Nephrology

Stark, Walter J. · Ophthalmology, Anterior Segment (Cataract Surgery); Ophthalmology, Corneal Diseases & Transplantation

Starke, Jeffrey R. · Pediatrics, Pediatric Infectious Disease

Starling, James R. · General Surgery, Gastroenterologic Surgery

Starnes, Vaughn A. · Thoracic Surgery, Adult Cardiothoracic Surgery; Thoracic Surgery, Pediatric Cardiac Surgery; Thoracic Surgery, Transplantation

Starzl, Thomas E. · General Surgery, Transplantation

Staskin, David R. · Urology, Neuro-Urology & Voiding Dysfunction

Stauffer, Richard N. · Orthopaedic Surgery, Reconstructive Surgery

Steadman, J. Richard · Orthopaedic Surgery, Sports Medicine

Stechschulte, Daniel J. · Allergy & Immunology, Adult Allergy & Immunology

Steele, Brandt F. · Psychiatry, Psychoanalysis

Steele, Glenn · Surgical Oncology, Colon & Rectal Cancer; Surgical Oncology, Gastroenterologic Cancer

Stehman, Frederick D. · Obstetrics & Gynecology, Gynecologic Cancer

Steichen, James Baptiste · Hand Surgery, Microsurgery

Stein, Bennett M. · Neurological Surgery, Tumor Surgery; Neurological Surgery, Vascular Neurological Surgery

Stein, Elliott M. · Psychiatry, Geriatric Psychiatry

Stein, Fernando · Pediatrics, Pediatric Critical Care

Stein, Leonard I. · Psychiatry, Schizophrenia

Steiner, Ladislau · Neurological Surgery, Stereotactic Radiosurgery

Steinert, Roger · Ophthalmology, Anterior Segment (Cataract Surgery); Ophthalmology, Corneal Diseases & Transplantation

Steinglass, Peter J. · Psychiatry, Addiction Medicine

Steinman, Theodore Irving · Nephrology, General Nephrology

Stenchever, Morton A. · Obstetrics & Gynecology, Reproductive Surgery

Sterioff, Sylvester · General Surgery, Transplantation

Stern, Peter Joseph · Hand Surgery, General Hand Surgery

Stern, Robert · Dermatology, Allergic Reactions of the Skin

Stern, Robert C. · Pediatrics, Pediatric Pulmonology

Stevens, Mary Betty · Rheumatology, General Rheumatology

Stevenson, David K. · Pediatrics, Neonatal-Perinatal Medicine

Stevenson, Donald D. · Allergy & Immunology, Adult Allergy & Immunology

Steward, David J. · Anesthesiology, Pediatric Anesthesiology; Anesthesiology, Pediatric Cardiovascular

Stewart, Robert · Radiation Oncology, General Radiation Oncology

Stewart, William J. · Cardiovascular Disease, Echocardiography

Stiehm, E. Richard · Allergy & Immunology, Pediatric Allergy & Immunology

Stillman, Robert J. · Obstetrics & Gynecology, Reproductive Endocrinology

Stimmel, Barry · Addiction Medicine, General Addiction Medicine

Stinson, Edward E. · Thoracic Surgery, Adult Cardiothoracic Surgery; Thoracic Surgery, Transplantation

Stitik, Frederick P. · Radiology, Chest

Stiver, H. Grant · Infectious Disease, General Infectious Disease

Stoelting, Robert · Anesthesiology, General Anesthesiology

Stokes, Peter E. · Psychiatry, Affective Disorders

Stoller, James K. · Pulmonary & Critical Care Medicine, General Pulmonary & Critical Care Medicine

Stoller, Ronald G. · Medical Oncology, General Medical Oncology

Stolov, Walter C. · Physical Medicine & Rehabilitation, Electromyography

Stone, Alan A. · Psychiatry, Forensic Psychiatry; Psychiatry, General Psychiatry

Stone, Edwin M. · Ophthalmology, Ophthalmic Genetics

Stone, Leo · Psychiatry, Psychoanalysis

Stoney, Ronald J. · General Surgery, General Vascular Surgery

Stool, Sylvan E. · Otolaryngology, Pediatric Otolaryngology

Storch, Gregory A. · Pediatrics, Pediatric Infectious Disease

Storrs, Frances J. · Dermatology, Clinical Dermatology; Dermatology, Contact Dermatitis

Stoudemire, Alan · Psychiatry, Geriatric Psychiatry

Stover, Diane E. · Pulmonary & Critical Care Medicine, AIDS

Strafford, Maureen A. · Anesthesiology, Pediatric Cardiovascular

Strandness, D. Eugene · General Surgery, General Vascular Surgery

Straus, Stephen E. · Infectious Disease, Herpes Virus Infections

Strauss, H. William · Nuclear Medicine, Nuclear Cardiology

Strauss, John S. · Dermatology, Acne

Strauss, John S. · Psychiatry, Schizophrenia

Strauss, José · Pediatrics, Pediatric Nephrology

Strickland, James W. · Hand Surgery, Reconstructive Surgery

Striker, Theodore W. · Anesthesiology, Pediatric Anesthesiology

Strom, Terry B. · Nephrology, Kidney Transplantation

Strong, William Bryan · Pediatrics, Pediatric Cardiology

Strunk, Robert C. · Allergy & Immunology, Pediatric Allergy & Immunology

Stubbs, William King · Otolaryngology, Sinus & Nasal Surgery

Studenski, Stephanie A. · Geriatric Medicine, General Geriatric Medicine

Stulberg, Bernard N. · Orthopaedic Surgery, Reconstructive Surgery

Stulberg, David · Orthopaedic Surgery, Reconstructive Surgery

Stulting, R. Doyle · Ophthalmology, Corneal Diseases & Transplantation

Stunkard, Albert J. · Psychiatry, Eating Disorders

Styne, Dennis M. · Pediatrics, Pediatric Endocrinology

Suen, James Y. · Otolaryngology, Head & Neck Surgery

Sugar, Alan · Ophthalmology, Corneal Diseases & Transplantation

Sugar, Joel · Ophthalmology, Corneal Diseases & Transplantation

Suit, Herman D. · Radiation Oncology, General Radiation Oncology; Radiation Oncology, Particle Beam Radiation

Suki, Wadi N. · Nephrology, Dialysis; Nephrology, General Nephrology; Nephrology, Kidney Transplantation

Sullivan, Timothy J. · Allergy & Immunology, Adult Allergy & Immunology

Summer, Warren R. · Pulmonary & Critical Care Medicine, General Pulmonary & Critical Care Medicine

Sumner, Austin J. · Neurology, Adult, Electromyography

Sumner, David Spurgeon · General Surgery, General Vascular Surgery

Sundaresan, Narayan (Sunny) · Neurological Surgery, Spinal Surgery

Sundt, Thoralf M. · Neurological Surgery, Vascular Neurological Surgery

Surawicz, Christina M. · Gastroenterology, General Gastroenterology

Sussman, Karl E. · Endocrinology & Metabolism, Diabetes

Suthanthiran, Manikkam · Nephrology, Kidney Transplantation

Sutherland, David E. · General Surgery, Transplantation

Sutton, Leslie N. · Neurological Surgery, Pediatric Neurological Surgery

Sveum, Richard J. · Allergy & Immunology, Pediatric Allergy & Immunology

Swaiman, Kenneth F. · Neurology, Child, Inherited Biochemical Disorders

Swain, Sandra M. · Medical Oncology, Breast Cancer

Swanson, Neil A. · Dermatology, Skin Cancer Surgery & Reconstruction

Swartz, Morton N. · Infectious Disease, General Infectious Disease

Swartz, William M. · Plastic Surgery, Breast Surgery; Plastic Surgery, Microsurgery

Sweet, Richard L. · Obstetrics & Gynecology, Infectious Disease

Swerdloff, Ronald S. · Endocrinology & Metabolism, Reproductive Endocrinology

Swerdlow, Bernard · Psychiatry, Headache

Swezey, Robert L. · Rheumatology, Rehabilitation

Swift, Thomas R. · Neurology, Adult, Electromyography; Neurology, Adult, Neuromuscular Disease

Swiontkowski, Marc F. · Orthopaedic Surgery, Trauma

Szefler, Stanley J. · Allergy & Immunology, Pediatric Allergy & Immunology

Szymanski, Ludwik · Psychiatry, Child Psychiatry

T

Taft, Lawrence T. · Neurology, Child, Child Development

Taillefer, Raymond · Nuclear Medicine, Nuclear Cardiology

Tajik, A. Jamil · Cardiovascular Disease, Echocardiography

Talbert, Luther Marcus · Obstetrics & Gynecology, Reproductive Endocrinology

Talbott, Douglas G. · Addiction Medicine, General Addiction Medicine

Talbott, John Andrew · Psychiatry, General Psychiatry

Taleisnik, Julio · Hand Surgery, Reconstructive Surgery

Taler, George · Geriatric Medicine, General Geriatric Medicine

Talner, Norman S. · Pediatrics, Pediatric Cardiology

Talpos, Gary B. · General Surgery, Endocrine Surgery

Tamborlane, William V. · Pediatrics, Pediatric Endocrinology

Tamminga, Carol A. · Psychiatry, Schizophrenia/Psychopharmacology

Tan, Oon Tian · Dermatology, Pediatric Dermatology; Pediatrics, Pediatric Dermatology

Tanagho, Emil A. · Urology, Neuro-Urology & Voiding Dysfunction

Tanguay, Peter E. · Psychiatry, Child Psychiatry

Tanney, Bryan L. · Psychiatry, Suicidology

Tannock, Ian F. · Medical Oncology, Breast Cancer

Tarbell, Nancy J. · Radiation Oncology, Pediatric Radiation Oncology

Tardiff, Kenneth · Psychiatry, Violence

Tardy, M. Eugene · Otolaryngology, Facial Plastic Surgery

Tatum, James L. · Nuclear Medicine, Nuclear Cardiology

Taussig, Lynn M. · Pediatrics, Pediatric Pulmonology

Tavassoli, Fattaneh · Pathology, Breast Pathology

Taylor, Andrew · Nuclear Medicine, Kidney

Taylor, James S. · Dermatology, Contact Dermatitis

Taylor, Michael Alan · Psychiatry, Neuropsychiatry

Tchou, Patrick J. · Cardiovascular Disease, Electrophysiology

Tebbetts, John B. · Plastic Surgery, Breast Surgery; Plastic Surgery, Facial Aesthetic Surgery

Teimourian, Bahman · Plastic Surgery, Body Contouring

Tejani, Amir · Pediatrics, Pediatric Nephrology

Teplick, Richard · Anesthesiology, Critical Care Medicine

Tepper, Joel E. · Radiation Oncology, Gastroenterologic Cancer; Radiation Oncology, General Radiation Oncology

Terezakis, Nia · Dermatology, Hair

Terkelsen, Kenneth · Psychiatry, Schizophrenia

Terr, Abba I. · Allergy & Immunology, Adult Allergy & Immunology

Terr, Lenore C. · Psychiatry, Child Psychiatry

Tew, John M. · Neurological Surgery, Cranial Nerve Surgery

Tharp, Michael D. · Dermatology, Cutaneous Immunology

Thase, Michael E. · Psychiatry, Affective Disorders

Thedinger, Bradley S. · Otolaryngology, Otology/Neurotology

Thiele, Brian L. · General Surgery, General Vascular Surgery

Thigpen, James Tate · Medical Oncology & Hematology, Gynecologic Cancer

Thistlethwaite, J. Richard · General Surgery, Transplantation

Thoene, Jess G. · Pediatrics, Metabolic Diseases

Thomas, Colin G. · General Surgery, Endocrine Surgery

Thomas, J. Regan · Otolaryngology, Facial Plastic Surgery

Thomas, Raju · Urology, Endourology

Thomas, William H. · Orthopaedic Surgery, Rheumatoid Arthritis

Thompson, Ann E. · Pediatrics, Pediatric Critical Care

Thompson, Francesca M. · Orthopaedic Surgery, Foot & Ankle Surgery

Thompson, H. Stanley · Ophthalmology, Neuro-Ophthalmology

Thompson, James C. · General Surgery, Gastroenterologic Surgery

Thompson, Jerome W. · Otolaryngology, Pediatric Otolaryngology

Thompson, Norman W. · General Surgery, Endocrine Surgery

Thompson, Roby Calvin · Orthopaedic Surgery, Tumor Surgery

Thompson, Sumner Edward · Infectious Disease, Sexually Transmitted Disease

Thorner, Michael O. · Endocrinology & Metabolism, Neuroendocrinology

Thornhill, Thomas · Orthopaedic Surgery, Reconstructive Surgery

Thornton, George F. · Infectious Disease, General Infectious Disease

Thornton, Spencer Phillips · Ophthalmology, Anterior Segment (Cataract Surgery)

Thorp, James A. · Obstetrics & Gynecology, Maternal & Fetal Medicine

Thrall, James H. · Nuclear Medicine, General Nuclear Medicine

Thys, Daniel · Anesthesiology, Adult Cardiovascular

Tigelaar, Robert E. · Dermatology, Cutaneous Lymphomas

Tile, Marvin · Orthopaedic Surgery, Trauma

Tindall, Elizabeth A. · Rheumatology, General Rheumatology

Tindall, George T. · Neurological Surgery, Tumor Surgery

Tinetti, Mary E. · Geriatric Medicine, General Geriatric Medicine

Tinker, John · Anesthesiology, General Anesthesiology

Titchener, James Lampton · Psychiatry, Psychoanalysis

Todd, Michael M. · Anesthesiology, Neuroanesthesia

Tolo, Vernon Thorpe · Orthopaedic Surgery, Pediatric Orthopaedic Surgery

Tolpin, Paul H. · Psychiatry, Psychoanalysis

Tompkins, Ronald K. · General Surgery, Gastroenterologic Surgery

Tonino, Richard P. · Geriatric Medicine, General Geriatric Medicine

Tonnesen, Alan S. · Anesthesiology, Critical Care Medicine

Toole, James F. · Neurology, Adult, Strokes

Tooms, Robert E. · Orthopaedic Surgery, Reconstructive Surgery

Toonkel, Leonard M. · Radiation Oncology, Breast Cancer

Topol, Eric Jeffrey · Cardiovascular Disease, Cardiac Catheterization

Torg, Joseph S. · Orthopaedic Surgery, Sports Medicine

Tormey, Douglass C. · Medical Oncology & Hematology, Breast Cancer

Torti, Frank M. · Medical Oncology & Hematology, Genito-Urinary Cancer

Towne, Jonathan B. · General Surgery, General Vascular Surgery

Townley, Robert Gordon · Allergy & Immunology, Adult Allergy & Immunology

Townsend, Timothy R. · Infectious Disease, Hospital-Acquired Infections

Trafton, Peter G. · Orthopaedic Surgery, Trauma

Trastek, Victor F. · Thoracic Surgery, General Thoracic Surgery; Thoracic Surgery, Thoracic Oncological Surgery

Travis, Luther B. · Pediatrics, Pediatric Nephrology

Treiman, David M. · Neurology, Adult, Epilepsy

Treves, Salvadore · Nuclear Medicine, Pediatric

Trigg, Michael Edward · Pediatrics, Pediatric Hematology-Oncology

Trinkle, J. Kent · Thoracic Surgery, Transplantation

Trobe, Jonathan D. · Neurology, Adult, Neuro-Ophthalmology; Ophthalmology, Neuro-Ophthalmology

Trokel, Stephen Lewis · Ophthalmology, Oculoplastic & Orbital Surgery

Troost, B. Todd · Neurology, Adult, Neuro-Ophthalmology; Ophthalmology, Neuro-Ophthalmology

Trumbull, Dianne W. · Psychiatry, Child Psychiatry

Trump, Donald L. · Medical Oncology & Hematology, Clinical Pharmacology; Medical Oncology & Hematology, Genito-Urinary Cancer

Trusler, George A. · Thoracic Surgery, Pediatric Cardiac Surgery

Trzepacz, Paula T. · Psychiatry, Neuropsychiatry

Tsai, Luke Y. · Psychiatry, Child Psychiatry

Tse, David T. · Ophthalmology, Oculoplastic & Orbital Surgery

Tucker, Gary J. · Psychiatry, Behavioral Disorders; Psychiatry, Neuropsychiatry; Psychiatry, Psychopharmacology

Tucker, John A. · Otolaryngology, Pediatric Otolaryngology

Tuffanelli, Denny L. · Dermatology, Clinical Dermatology; Dermatology, Cutaneous Immunology

Tullos, Hugh S. · Orthopaedic Surgery, Hip Surgery

Tunnessen, Walter W. · Pediatrics, Pediatric Dermatology

Tupin, Joe P. · Psychiatry, Schizophrenia/Psychopharmacology; Psychiatry, Violence

Tupper, Jack W. · Hand Surgery, Peripheral Nerve Surgery; Orthopaedic Surgery, Peripheral Nerve Surgery

Turck, Marvin · Infectious Disease, General Infectious Disease

Turner, Maria L. · Dermatology, Genital Dermatological Disease

Turner, Roderick H. · Orthopaedic Surgery, Hip Surgery

Turrisi, Andrew T. · Radiation Oncology, Lung Cancer

Twiggs, Leo B. · Obstetrics & Gynecology, Gynecologic Cancer

Tyrrell, J. Blake · Endocrinology & Metabolism, Neuroendocrinology

Tyson, Robert L. · Psychiatry, Psychoanalysis

U

Uhde, Thomas Whitley · Psychiatry, Affective Disorders; Psychiatry, Psychopharmacology

Ultmann, John E. · Medical Oncology, General Medical Oncology; Medical Oncology, Lymphomas

Underwood, Louis E. · Pediatrics, Pediatric Endocrinology

Underwood, Paul · Obstetrics & Gynecology, Gynecologic Cancer

Urbaniak, James R. · Hand Surgery, Microsurgery; Hand Surgery, Peripheral Nerve Surgery; Hand Surgery, Reconstructive Surgery; Orthopaedic Surgery, Reconstructive Surgery

Uretsky, Barry F. · Cardiovascular Disease, Heart Failure

Urschel, Harold C. · Thoracic Surgery, General Thoracic Surgery

V

Valenstein, Arthur F. · Psychiatry, Psychoanalysis

Valentine, Martin Douglas · Allergy & Immunology, Pediatric Allergy & Immunology

Valle, David · Pediatrics, Metabolic Diseases

Van Beek, Allen L. · Hand Surgery, Peripheral Nerve Surgery; Plastic Surgery, Peripheral Nerve Surgery

Van Buskirk, E. Michael · Ophthalmology, Glaucoma

van den Noort, Stanley · Neurology, Adult, Infectious & Demyelinating Diseases

van der Kolk, Bessel A. · Psychiatry, Post-Traumatic Stress Disorders

Van Dooren, Hugo · Psychiatry, Geriatric Psychiatry

van Heerden, Jon · General Surgery, Endocrine Surgery

van Nagell, John R. · Obstetrics & Gynecology, Gynecologic Cancer

Van Putten, Theodore · Psychiatry, Schizophrenia/Psychopharmacology

Van Scoy, Robert · Infectious Disease, General Infectious Disease

Van Wyk, Judson J. · Pediatrics, Pediatric Endocrinology

Vance, Mary Lee · Endocrinology & Metabolism, Neuroendocrinology

VanDorsten, J. Peter · Obstetrics & Gynecology, Maternal & Fetal Medicine

VanEcho, David Andrew · Medical Oncology & Hematology, Clinical Pharmacology

Vardiman, James W. · Pathology, Hematopathology

Vasconez, Luis Oswaldo · Plastic Surgery, Reconstructive Surgery

Vaughan, E. Darracott · Urology, Renal Hypertension; Urology, Urologic Oncology

Vaughan, William P. · Medical Oncology, Bone Marrow Transplantation; Medical Oncology, Breast Cancer; Medical Oncology, Leukemia

Veidenheimer, Malcolm C. · Colon & Rectal Surgery, Colon & Rectal Cancer; Colon & Rectal Surgery, General Colon & Rectal Surgery

Veith, Frank J. · General Surgery, General Vascular Surgery

Veith, Richard C. · Psychiatry, Geriatric Psychiatry

Verani, Mario S. · Cardiovascular Disease, Nuclear Cardiology

Vetrovec, George W. · Cardiovascular Disease, Cardiac Catheterization

Vetter, Victoria L. · Pediatrics, Pediatric Cardiology

Vick, Nicholas A. · Neurology, Adult, Neuro-oncology

Vietti, Teresa J. · Pediatrics, Pediatric Hematology-Oncology

Villavicencio, J. Leonel · General Surgery, General Vascular Surgery

Vinuela, Fernando · Radiology, Neuroradiology

Vogel, Charles L. · Medical Oncology, Breast Cancer; Medical Oncology, General Medical Oncology

Vogler, W. Ralph · Medical Oncology, Leukemia

Vokes, Everett E. · Medical Oncology & Hematology, Head & Neck Cancer

Volberding, Paul A. · Medical Oncology & Hematology, AIDS

Volkan, Vamik D. · Psychiatry, Psychoanalysis

Volkmar, Fred R. · Psychiatry, Autism; Psychiatry, Child Psychiatry

Volpe, Joseph J. · Neurology, Child, Neonatal Neurology

Volpe, Peter A. · Colon & Rectal Surgery, General Colon & Rectal Surgery

Volpé, Robert · Endocrinology & Metabolism, Thyroid

Volz, Robert G. · Orthopaedic Surgery, Reconstructive Surgery

von Eschenbach, Andrew C. · Urology, Urologic Oncology

Von Hoff, Daniel D. · Medical Oncology, Clinical Pharmacology; Medical Oncology, General Medical Oncology

von Noorden, Gunter K. · Ophthalmology, Pediatric Ophthalmology

Voorhees, John J. · Dermatology, Psoriasis

W

Wackers, Frans · Cardiovascular Disease, Nuclear Cardiology

Wade, James C. · Infectious Disease, Cancer & Infections

Wagner, Henry N. · Nuclear Medicine, Brain; Nuclear Medicine, General Nuclear Medicine

Wagonfeld, Samuel · Psychiatry, Psychoanalysis

Wahl, Richard L. · Nuclear Medicine, Oncology

Waldman, Steven D. · Anesthesiology, Pain

Waldmann, Thomas A. · Allergy & Immunology, Adult Allergy & Immunology

Walker, Marion L. · Neurological Surgery, Pediatric Neurological Surgery

Walker, R. Dixon · Urology, Pediatric Urology

Walker, Roger Dale · Psychiatry, Addiction Medicine

Walker, Russell W. · Medical Oncology & Hematology, Neuro-oncology; Neurology, Child, Neuro-oncology

Wall, Michael · Neurology, Adult, Neuro-Ophthalmology; Ophthalmology, Neuro-Ophthalmology

Wall, Michael A. · Pediatrics, Pediatric Pulmonology

Wallace, Jeanne M. · Pulmonary & Critical Care Medicine, AIDS

Wallace, Robert B. · Thoracic Surgery, Adult Cardiothoracic Surgery

Wallach, Edward E. · Obstetrics & Gynecology, Reproductive Endocrinology

Wallach, Stanley · Endocrinology & Metabolism, Paget's Disease

Waller, John L. · Anesthesiology, Adult Cardiovascular

Wallerstein, Robert S. · Psychiatry, Psychoanalysis

Walsh, B. Timothy · Psychiatry, Eating Disorders

Walsh, Patrick C. · Urology, Urologic Oncology

Walsh, Thomas John · Infectious Disease, Cancer & Infections

Wang, C. C. · Radiation Oncology, Head & Neck Cancer

Wanner, Adam · Pulmonary & Critical Care Medicine, Asthma

Wara, Diane · Allergy & Immunology, Pediatric Allergy & Immunology

Wara, William M. · Radiation Oncology, Pediatric Radiation Oncology

Warady, Bradley A. · Pediatrics, Pediatric Nephrology

Ward, Paul H. · Otolaryngology, Head & Neck Surgery; Otolaryngology, Laryngology

Waring, George O. · Ophthalmology, Corneal Diseases & Transplantation

Warner, David S. · Anesthesiology, Neuroanesthesia

Warner, Mark A. · Anesthesiology, General Anesthesiology

Warnke, Roger A. · Pathology, Hematopathology

Warren, Russell F. · Orthopaedic Surgery, Sports Medicine

Warshaw, Andrew L. · General Surgery, Gastroenterologic Surgery

Warshaw, Gregg · Geriatric Medicine, General Geriatric Medicine

Wartofsky, Leonard · Endocrinology & Metabolism, Thyroid

Wasserman, Stephen I. · Allergy & Immunology, Adult Allergy & Immunology

Wassner, Steven Joel · Pediatrics, Pediatric Nephrology

Waters, Paul F. · Thoracic Surgery, Transplantation

Watkins, John B. · Pediatrics, Pediatric Gastroenterology

Watson, Charles G. · General Surgery, Endocrine Surgery

Watson, H. Kirk · Hand Surgery, Reconstructive Surgery

Waugh, Theodore R. · Orthopaedic Surgery, Foot & Ankle Surgery

Waxman, Alan D. · Nuclear Medicine, General Nuclear Medicine; Nuclear Medicine, Oncology

Way, Lawrence W. · General Surgery, Gastroenterologic Surgery

Waye, Jerome D. · Gastroenterology, Endoscopy; Gastroenterology, Gastroenterologic Cancer

Weaver, Arthur Lawrence · Rheumatology, General Rheumatology

Webb, W. Richard · Radiology, Chest

Webster, George D. · Urology, Neuro-Urology & Voiding Dysfunction

Webster, Marshall W. · General Surgery, General Vascular Surgery

Wechsler, Andrew S. · Thoracic Surgery, Adult Cardiothoracic Surgery

Wedge, John H. · Orthopaedic Surgery, Pediatric Orthopaedic Surgery

Weeks, Paul M. · Hand Surgery, Reconstructive Surgery

Weg, John G. · Pulmonary & Critical Care Medicine, General Pulmonary & Critical Care Medicine

Weichselbaum, Ralph R. · Radiation Oncology, General Radiation Oncology

Weigand, Dennis Allen · Dermatology, Clinical Dermatology

Weiland, Andrew J. · Hand Surgery, Microsurgery; Hand Surgery, Reconstructive Surgery

Wein, Alan J. · Urology, Neuro-Urology & Voiding Dysfunction; Urology, Urologic Oncology

Weinberg, Samuel · Dermatology, Pediatric Dermatology; Pediatrics, Pediatric Dermatology

Weinberger, Daniel R. · Neurology, Adult, Neuropsychiatry; Psychiatry, Neuropsychiatry; Psychiatry, Schizophrenia/Psychopharmacology

Weinberger, Miles M. · Pediatrics, Pediatric Pulmonology

Weinblatt, Michael Eliot · Rheumatology, General Rheumatology; Rheumatology, Rheumatoid Arthritis

Weiner, Donald · Cardiovascular Disease, Clinical Exercise Testing

Weiner, Myron F. · Psychiatry, Geriatric Psychiatry

Weinreb, Robert N. · Ophthalmology, Glaucoma

Weinshel, Edward M. · Psychiatry, Psychoanalysis

Weinstein, Gerald D. · Dermatology, Psoriasis

Weinstein, Howard J. · Pediatrics, Pediatric Hematology-Oncology

Weinstein, Joel M. · Ophthalmology, Neuro-Ophthalmology

Weinstein, Wilfred M. · Gastroenterology, Endoscopy

Weir, Bryce K. A. · Neurological Surgery, Vascular Neurological Surgery

Weisblatt, Steven A. · Psychiatry, Mental Retardation/Mental Health: Dual Diagnosis

Weisfeldt, Myron L. · Cardiovascular Disease, General Cardiovascular Disease

Weisman, Michael H. · Rheumatology, General Rheumatology

Weiss, Gerson · Obstetrics & Gynecology, Reproductive Endocrinology

Weiss, Martin H. · Neurological Surgery, Tumor Surgery

Weiss, Roger D. · Psychiatry, Addiction Medicine

Weiss, Samuel · Psychiatry, Psychoanalysis

Welch, K. Michael A. · Neurology, Adult, Headache; Neurology, Adult, Strokes

Weleber, Richard Gordon · Ophthalmology, Ophthalmic Genetics

Wellman, Henry N. · Nuclear Medicine, General Nuclear Medicine

Wells, Samuel A. · General Surgery, Endocrine Surgery

Wender, Paul H. · Psychiatry, Affective Disorders; Psychiatry, Child Psychiatry; Psychiatry, General Psychiatry; Psychiatry, Psychopharmacology

Wentworth, Samuel M. · Pediatrics, Pediatric Endocrinology

Wenzel, Richard P. · Infectious Disease, Hospital-Acquired Infections

Werman, David S. · Psychiatry, Psychoanalysis

Wesson, Donald · Addiction Medicine, Medical Treatment of Drug Abusers

Weston, William L. · Dermatology, Pediatric Dermatology; Pediatrics, Pediatric Dermatology

Wetchler, Bernard V. · Anesthesiology, Ambulatory Anesthesia

Wetmore, Ralph F. · Otolaryngology, Pediatric Otolaryngology

Weyman, Arthur E. · Cardiovascular Disease, Echocardiography

Weymuller, Ernest A. · Otolaryngology, Head & Neck Surgery; Otolaryngology, Sinus & Nasal Surgery

Wharam, Moody D. · Radiation Oncology, Pediatric Radiation Oncology

Wharton, J. Taylor · Obstetrics & Gynecology, Gynecologic Cancer

Wheeland, Ronald G. · Dermatology, Laser Surgery

Whisnant, Jack P. · Neurology, Adult, Strokes

Whitaker, Duane C. · Dermatology, Skin Cancer Surgery & Reconstruction

Whitaker, John N. · Neurology, Adult, Infectious & Demyelinating Diseases

Whitaker, Linton A. · Plastic Surgery, Craniofacial Surgery

White, Benjamin · Otolaryngology, Pediatric Otolaryngology

White, David P. · Pulmonary & Critical Care Medicine, Pulmonary Disease

White, Dorothy A. · Pulmonary & Critical Care Medicine, General Pulmonary & Critical Care Medicine

White, Neil H. · Pediatrics, Pediatric Endocrinology

White, Roger D. · Anesthesiology, Adult Cardiovascular

Whitehouse, Peter J. · Neurology, Adult, Degenerative Diseases

Whiting, David A. · Dermatology, Hair

Whitley, Richard J. · Pediatrics, Pediatric Infectious Disease

Whitlow, Patrick L. · Cardiovascular Disease, Cardiac Catheterization

Whittemore, Anthony D. · General Surgery, General Vascular Surgery

Whittington, Richard · Radiation Oncology, Gastroenterologic Cancer

Whitworth, Jay M. · Pediatrics, Abused Children

Whybrow, Peter C. · Psychiatry, Affective Disorders

Wiedel, Jerome D. · Orthopaedic Surgery, Hip Surgery; Orthopaedic Surgery, Knee Surgery

Wiedemann, Herbert P. · Pulmonary & Critical Care Medicine, General Pulmonary & Critical Care Medicine

Wiener, Jerry M. · Psychiatry, Child Psychiatry

Wiener, Leslie P. · Neurology, Adult, Infectious & Demyelinating Diseases

Wiernik, Peter Harris · Medical Oncology & Hematology, Leukemia

Wiet, Richard J. · Otolaryngology, Otology/Neurotology

Wilber, David James · Cardiovascular Disease, Electrophysiology

Wilbourn, Asa J. · Neurology, Adult, Electromyography

Wilde, Alan H. · Orthopaedic Surgery, Reconstructive Surgery

Wilding, George · Medical Oncology & Hematology, Genito-Urinary Cancer

Wilensky, Jacob T. · Ophthalmology, Glaucoma

Wiley, Elaine · Neurology, Child, Epilepsy

Wilfert, Catherine M. · Pediatrics, Pediatric Infectious Disease

Wilgis, E. F. Shaw · Hand Surgery, Peripheral Nerve Surgery

Wilkins, Isabelle A. · Obstetrics & Gynecology, Maternal & Fetal Medicine

Wilkins, Robert Benson · Ophthalmology, Oculoplastic & Orbital Surgery

Wilkinson, Edward J. · Pathology, Gynecologic Pathology

Willerson, James T. · Cardiovascular Disease, General Cardiovascular Disease

Willett, Christopher G. · Radiation Oncology, Gastroenterologic Cancer

Williams, Bill G. · Thoracic Surgery, Pediatric Cardiac Surgery

Williams, David O. · Cardiovascular Disease, Cardiac Catheterization

Williams, G. Melville · General Surgery, General Vascular Surgery; General Surgery, Transplantation

Williams, George A. · Ophthalmology, Vitreo-Retinal Surgery

Williams, H. Bruce · Plastic Surgery, Peripheral Nerve Surgery

Williams, John E. · Plastic Surgery, Facial Aesthetic Surgery

Williams, M. Henry · Pulmonary & Critical Care Medicine, Asthma

Williams, Mark E. · Geriatric Medicine, General Geriatric Medicine

Williams, Mary L. · Dermatology, Pediatric Dermatology; Pediatrics, Pediatric Dermatology

Williams, Richard D. · Urology, Urologic Oncology

Williams, Roberta Gay · Pediatrics, Pediatric Cardiology

Williams, Stephanie F. · Medical Oncology & Hematology, Bone Marrow Transplantation; Medical Oncology & Hematology, Breast Cancer

Williams, Stephen D. · Medical Oncology & Hematology, Genito-Urinary Cancer; Medical Oncology & Hematology, Gynecologic Cancer

Willkens, Robert F. · Rheumatology, General Rheumatology

Wilmott, Robert W. · Pediatrics, Pediatric Pulmonology

Wilske, Kenneth Ray · Rheumatology, General Rheumatology; Rheumatology, Rheumatoid Arthritis

Wilson, Charles B. · Neurological Surgery, Cranial Nerve Surgery; Neurological Surgery, Tumor Surgery; Neurological Surgery, Vascular Neurological Surgery

Wilson, J. Frank · Radiation Oncology, Brachytherapy

Wilson, Jean D. · Endocrinology & Metabolism, Reproductive Endocrinology

Wilson, John R. · Cardiovascular Disease, Heart Failure

Wilson, Richard P. · Ophthalmology, Glaucoma

Wilson, Roger S. · Anesthesiology, Critical Care Medicine

Wilson, Stuart D. · General Surgery, Endocrine Surgery

Wilson, Walter R. · Infectious Disease, Endocarditis

Winawer, Sidney J. · Gastroenterology, Gastroenterologic Cancer

Winchester, David P. · Surgical Oncology, Breast Cancer

Winchester, James F. · Nephrology, Dialysis

Windebank, Anthony J. · Neurology, Adult, Neuromuscular Disease

Winfield, Howard N. · Urology, Endourology

Winkelstein, Jerry A. · Pediatrics, Pediatric Allergy & Immunology

Winkle, Roger A. · Cardiovascular Disease, Electrophysiology

Winn, H. Richard · Neurological Surgery, Vascular Neurological Surgery

Winnie, Alon P. · Anesthesiology, Pain

Winnie, Glenna B. · Pediatrics, Pediatric Pulmonology

Winograd, Carol Hutner · Geriatric Medicine, General Geriatric Medicine

Winokur, George · Psychiatry, Affective Disorders

Winokur, Stanley · Medical Oncology, General Medical Oncology

Winquist, Robert A. · Orthopaedic Surgery, Trauma

Winterbauer, Richard · Pulmonary & Critical Care Medicine, Pulmonary Disease

Wintroub, Bruce U. · Dermatology, Allergic Reactions of the Skin

Wirtschafter, Jonathan D. · Neurology, Adult, Neuro-Ophthalmology; Ophthalmology, Neuro-Ophthalmology

Wisenberg, Gerald · Cardiovascular Disease, Magnetic Resonance Imaging

Wiss, Donald A. · Orthopaedic Surgery, Trauma

Wobig, John L. · Ophthalmology, Oculoplastic & Orbital Surgery

Wold, Lester E. · Pathology, Surgical Pathology

Wolf, Barry · Pediatrics, Metabolic Diseases

Wolf, Ernest Simon · Psychiatry, Psychoanalysis

Wolf-Klein, Gisele P. · Geriatric Medicine, General Geriatric Medicine

Wolfe, Frederick · Rheumatology, Fibromyalgia; Rheumatology, Rheumatoid Arthritis

Wolfe, S. Anthony · Plastic Surgery, Craniofacial Surgery; Plastic Surgery, Maxillofacial Surgery

Wolfe, Walter George · Thoracic Surgery, Adult Cardiothoracic Surgery

Wolff, Anna K. · Psychiatry, Psychoanalysis

Wolff, Bruce G. · Colon & Rectal Surgery, General Colon & Rectal Surgery

Wolff, Grace S. · Pediatrics, Pediatric Cardiology

Wolfsdorf, Joseph · Pediatrics, Pediatric Endocrinology

Wolinsky, Jerry S. · Neurology, Adult, Infectious & Demyelinating Diseases

Wolmark, Norman · Surgical Oncology, Breast Cancer

Wong, Harry C. · Anesthesiology, Ambulatory Anesthesia

Wood, Edwin C. · Psychiatry, Psychoanalysis

Wood, Michael B. · Hand Surgery, Microsurgery; Hand Surgery, Reconstructive Surgery

Wood, Robert E. · Pediatrics, Pediatric Pulmonology

Wood, Virchel E. · Hand Surgery, Peripheral Nerve Surgery; Hand Surgery, Reconstructive Surgery; Orthopaedic Surgery, Peripheral Nerve Surgery; Orthopaedic Surgery, Reconstructive Surgery

Wood, William C. · General Surgery, Breast Surgery; Surgical Oncology, Breast Cancer

Woodard, John R. · Urology, Pediatric Urology

Woods, James R. · Addiction Medicine, Addicted Pregnant Women; Obstetrics & Gynecology, Maternal & Fetal Medicine

Woods, John E. · Plastic Surgery, Breast Surgery; Plastic Surgery, Head & Neck Surgery

Woods, William G. · Pediatrics, Pediatric Hematology-Oncology

Woodside, Jeffrey R. · Urology, Neuro-Urology & Voiding Dysfunction

Woodson, Gayle E. · Otolaryngology, Laryngology

Woody, George E. · Psychiatry, Addiction Medicine

Wray, Betty B. · Allergy & Immunology, Adult Allergy & Immunology

Wray, Shirley H. · Neurology, Adult, Neuro-Ophthalmology

Wulc, Allan E. · Ophthalmology, Oculoplastic & Orbital Surgery

Wung, Jen-Tien · Anesthesiology, Pediatric Anesthesiology

Wyatt, Richard Jed · Psychiatry, Schizophrenia/Psychopharmacology

Wyler, Allen R. · Neurological Surgery, Epilepsy Surgery

Y

Yager, Joel · Psychiatry, Eating Disorders; Psychiatry, Psychopharmacology

Yagoda, Alan · Medical Oncology & Hematology, Genito-Urinary Cancer

Yancey, Kim B. · Dermatology, Cutaneous Immunology

Yankaskas, James R. · Pulmonary & Critical Care Medicine, Cystic Fibrosis

Yannuzzi, Lawrence A. · Ophthalmology, Medical Retinal Diseases

Yao, James See-Tao · General Surgery, General Vascular Surgery

Yarchoan, Robert · Infectious Disease, AIDS

Yates, Alayne · Psychiatry, Child Psychiatry

Yatsu, Frank M. · Neurology, Adult, Strokes

Yeager, Andrew M. · Pediatrics, Pediatric Hematology-Oncology

Yeast, John D. · Obstetrics & Gynecology, Maternal & Fetal Medicine

Yee, Robert D. · Neurology, Adult, Neuro-Ophthalmology; Ophthalmology, Neuro-Ophthalmology

Yen, Samuel S. C. · Obstetrics & Gynecology, Reproductive Endocrinology

Yesavage, Jerome A. · Psychiatry, Geriatric Psychiatry

Yogev, Ram · Pediatrics, Pediatric Infectious Disease

Yonekura, Margaret Lynn · Addiction Medicine, Addicted Pregnant Women; Obstetrics & Gynecology, Maternal & Fetal Medicine

Yood, Robert A. · Rheumatology, General Rheumatology

Young, Anne B. · Neurology, Adult, Movement Disorders

Young, Lowell S. · Infectious Disease, Transplantation Infections

Young, Robert C. · Medical Oncology & Hematology, Gynecologic Cancer; Medical Oncology & Hematology, Lymphomas

Young, Walter C. · Psychiatry, Dissociative Disorders

Young, William L. · Anesthesiology, Neuroanesthesia

Young, William P. · Obstetrics & Gynecology, Maternal & Fetal Medicine

Younge, Brian R. · Ophthalmology, Neuro-Ophthalmology

Yudofsky, Stuart C. · Psychiatry, Neuropsychiatry; Psychiatry, Psychopharmacology

Yung, W. K. Alfred · Medical Oncology & Hematology, Neuro-oncology; Neurology, Adult, Neuro-oncology

Yunginger, John W. · Allergy & Immunology, Adult Allergy & Immunology; Allergy & Immunology, Pediatric Allergy & Immunology

Z

Zacur, Howard · Obstetrics & Gynecology, Reproductive Endocrinology

Zarem, Harvey A. · Plastic Surgery, Aesthetic Surgery; Plastic Surgery, Reconstructive Surgery

Zaret, Barry L. · Cardiovascular Disease, Nuclear Cardiology

Zarins, Bertram · Orthopaedic Surgery, Sports Medicine

Zarutskie, Paul W. · Obstetrics & Gynecology, Reproductive Endocrinology

Zeiger, Robert S. · Allergy & Immunology, Pediatric Allergy & Immunology; Pediatrics, Pediatric Allergy & Immunology

Zeiss, Chester Raymound · Allergy & Immunology, Adult Allergy & Immunology

Zerhouni, Elias A. · Radiology, Cardiovascular Disease; Radiology, Magnetic Resonance Imaging

Zervas, Nicholas T. · Neurological Surgery, Tumor Surgery

Ziegler, Moritz M. · General Surgery, Pediatric Surgery

Zients, Alan Barry · Psychiatry, Psychoanalysis

Zimmerman, Bruce R. · Endocrinology & Metabolism, Diabetes

Zimmerman, Donald · Pediatrics, Pediatric Endocrinology

Zimmerman, Jerry J. · Pediatrics, Pediatric Critical Care

Zimmerman, Robert A. · Radiology, Neuroradiology

Zincke, Horst · Urology, Urologic Oncology

Zinman, Bernard · Endocrinology & Metabolism, Diabetes

Zinner, Michael J. · General Surgery, Gastroenterologic Surgery

Zitelli, John A. · Dermatology, Skin Cancer Surgery & Reconstruction; Dermatology, Wound Healing

Zonana, Howard V. · Psychiatry, Forensic Psychiatry

Zone, John · Dermatology, Cutaneous Immunology

Zuberbuhler, J. R. · Pediatrics, Pediatric Cardiology

Zweiman, Burton · Allergy & Immunology, Adult Allergy & Immunology

Zwillich, Clifford W. · Pulmonary & Critical Care Medicine, Pulmonary Disease